The Small Animal
Veterinary Nerdbook™

3rd edition

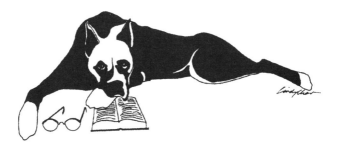

Sophia A. Yin

Cover Illustration by Cindy Chan
Text Illustrations by Mark Deamer

The Small Animal Veterinary Nerdbook™
Third Edition

Disclaimer

While a sincere effort has been made to ensure that all of the information in this book is correct, errors may be present. The author/publisher assumes no responsibility for and makes no warranty with respect to results obtained from the procedures, treatments, or drug dosages used, nor shall the author be held liable for any misstatements or errors that may have been obtained by any person or organization using this book. Should the purchaser not wish to be bound by the above, he/she may return the unused book along with a receipt of purchase within 30 days of purchase to the publisher for a full refund.

Help

Although this book has gone through numerous edits for content, grammar, and typing errors, inevitably there will be corrections and improvements that can be made. If you have any suggestions, comments, or corrections, please send them by e-mail to nerdbook@vinfoundation.org.

Order Information

To purchase the *Small Animal Veterinary Nerdbook*™ , and find information on special discount rates for bookstores and students, please visit Nerdbook.com.

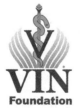

VIN Foundation
413 F Street
Davis, CA 95616
(888) 616-6506
VINFoundation.org
Nerdbook.com

Printed in the United States of America

PREFACE

Important: Read before using this book

After writing the first edition of the *Veterinary Nerdbook*™, I vowed to never write another textbook, including a new *Nerdbook*™ edition. Unfortunately, because I use the *Veterinary Nerdbook*™ myself, updating the book became a requirement.

I wrote my personal version of the first *Veterinary Nerdbook*™ in 1993 during my senior year in veterinary school. I felt that I would have gotten much more out of veterinary school if I had had such a book earlier though. In hopes that others would benefit from such a book during the **veterinary school courses, board exam preparation and clinical rotations**, I revised, expanded and published the *Veterinary Nerdbook*™ shortly thereafter.

Since writing that first edition, I have worked in private practice, then gone back into academia to study animal behavior, then taught animal behavior at the University of California, Davis, to undergraduates and then returned to private practice. Much of the time I have also spent as a pet columnist for the *San Francisco Chronicle* as well as a freelance writer for various magazines and journals including *Veterinary Forum*, *Compendium: Continuing Education for Veterinarians,* and *Bark* magazine. These experiences influenced the current *Nerdbook*™ revisions. The private practice and veterinary writing experiences have slanted the new edition to include the most clinically relevant information presented in a manner that accentuates the take-home messages.

Like the earlier editions, the third edition is organized into twenty-one sections separated by tab dividers and the information is organized into charts tables and diagrams that make the information readily accessible. This version has been extensively rewritten and updated. Additionally, the web site includes extra subchapters, diagrams, handouts, videos, and updates.

This book is intended to serve as a **guide** to **help students get through classes, clinical rotations, board exams, and early years in practice**. The information is neither all-encompassing nor does it represent the only methods of diagnosis and treatment. If you are not familiar with the ruleouts, diagnoses, or treatments discussed, or you require additional information, consult other veterinary medical references. If after reading this preface and overviewing the book you feel that it will not meet your needs, please return the unused book with a receipt to the *VIN Foundation* within 30 days of purchase for a full refund.

I believe the changes to *The Small Animal Veterinary Nerdbook*™ make this edition even more "user-friendly" and clinically useful than the first edition. The first two versions helped over 20,000 students in class and clinical rotations. I hope this updated and much improved version proves even more helpful than the first two.

Dr. Sophia Yin, DVM, MS

Nerdbook website: Nerdbook.com
Behavior website: DrSophiaYin.com
Low Stress Handling website: LowStressHandling.com

Acknowledgements

Writing a textbook is a painstaking process that requires the help of many people. I'd like to thank my editors—especially Cheryl Kolus and Dr. Kristen Franke, who edited the majority of the sections, sometimes on short notice. I especially thank my office assistant Amanda Huynh who handled the day-to-day dealings of the behavior business and publishing business, and generally kept the office running smoothly so that I had the time to revise this book. And finally, the following is a list of veterinarians who helped me by graciously reviewing sections of this book. I am deeply indebted to them for their time and effort.

Peter Pascoe BVSc
(Anesthesia)
Department of Surgical
and Radiological Science
School of Veterinary Medicine
University of California
Davis, CA 95616

Carlo Vitale DVM, DACVD
(Bacteriology, Dermatology)
San Francisco Veterinary Specialists
600 Alabama St.
San Francisco, CA 94110

Lori Siemens DVM, DACVIM
(Cardiology)
Sacramento Veterinary Surgical Services
9700 Business Park Dr. Suite 404
Sacramento, CA 95827

David Fisher DVM, DACVP
(Clinical Pathology, Cytology)
IDEXX Laboratories
Sacramento, CA

Jamie Anderson DVM, MS, DAVDC,
DACVIM (Dental)
San Francisco Veterinary Specialists
600 Alabama St.
San Francisco, CA 94110

Steve Haskins DVM, MVS, DACVA,
DACVECC (Emergency)
Department of Surgical
and Radiological Science
School of Veterinary Medicine
University of California
Davis, CA 95616

Craig Maretzki VMD, MS, DACVIM
(Endocrine, Urinary)
San Francisco Veterinary Specialists
600 Alabama St.
San Francisco, CA 94110

Alan Stewart DVM, CVA, DACVIM
(GI, Pulmonary)
San Francisco Veterinary Specialists
600 Alabama St.
San Francisco, CA 94110

Janet Foley MS, DVM, PhD
(Infectious)
Department of Medicine and
Epidemiology

School of Veterinary Medicine
University of California
Davis, CA 95616

Karen Vernau DVM
(Neurology)
Department of Surgical
and Radiological Science
School of Veterinary Medicine
University of California
Davis, CA 95616

Sally Perea DVM, MS, DACVN
(Nutrition)
Department of Molecular Biosciences
School of Veterinary Medicine
University of California
Davis, CA 95616

Carlos Rodriguez DVM, PhD, DACVIM
(Oncology)
San Francisco Veterinary Specialists
600 Alabama St.
San Francisco, CA 94110

Patrick McCallum, DVM
(Ophthalmology)
Animal Eye Specialists of San Jose
5440 Thornwood Drive Ste H
San Jose, CA 95123

Phil Watt BVSc, MACVSc, FACVS
(Orthopedics)
San Francisco Veterinary Specialists
600 Alabama St.
San Francisco, CA 94110

Autumn Davidson DVM, MS, DACVIM
(Reproduction, Infectious)
Animal Care Center
6470 Redwood Drive
Rohnert Park, CA 94928

ASPCA National Animal Poison
Control Center (Toxicology)
Sharon Gwaltney DVM, PhD, DABVT, DABT
Helen Myers DVM
Mary Schell DVM, DABT
Kristen Waratuke DVM
Tina Wismer DVM, DABT, DABVT
1717 South Philo Road
Urbana, IL 61802

Dedication

Dedicated to all veterinary students and veterinarians in need of an extracerebral source of small animal veterinary information.

TABLE of CONTENTS

CHAPTER 1: Anesthesia

COMMON DRUG CONCENTRATIONS

DRUG	CONCENTRATIONS
Acepromazine	10.0 mg/mL Or dilute to 2mg/mL or 1mg/mL with sterile water as diluent
Atipamezole	5.0 mg/mL
Atracurium	10.0 mg/mL
Atropine	0.4 mg/mL
Bupivacaine	5.0 mg/mL or 7.5 mg/mL
Buprenorphine	0.3 mg/mL
Butorphanol	10 mg/mL
Cimetidine	150 mg/mL
Diazepam	5 mg/mL
Diphenhydramine	50 mg/mL
Dopamine (40, 80, 160 mg/mL solutions. Dilute to 0.4 mg/mL)	0.4 mg/mL
Edrophonium	10 mg/mL
Etomidate	2 mg/mL
Fentanyl	50 μg/mL
Glycopyrrolate	0.2 mg/mL
Hydromorphone	4 mg/mL
Ketamine	100 mg/mL
Lidocaine	20 mg/mL
Mannitol	250 mg/mL
Medetomidine	1 mg/mL
Meperidine	50 mg/mL
Methadone	10 mg/mL
Midazolam	5 mg/mL
Morphine	15 mg/mL
Morphine (preservative free)	1 mg/mL or 25 mg/mL
Naloxone	1 mg/mL or 0.4 mg/mL
Nalbuphine	10 mg/mL
Oxymorphone	1.5 mg/mL
Propofol	10 mg/mL
Ranitidine	25 mg/mL
Telazol	100 mg/mL (50 mg/mL tiletamine + 50 mg/mL zolazepam)
Thiopental	25 mg/mL

SMALL ANIMAL ANESTHETIC DOSAGES for HEALTHY PATIENTS
(Revised from the Veterinary Medical Teaching Hospital, University of California, Davis-revised 9/05) Note: These are the dose rates for the general healthy animal. Dose rates may need to be reduced in older or debilitated animals.

Premedication Doses
Induction Doses
Maintenance
Analgesic Doses

I. **PREMEDICATION:** Administer premedications at least 15 minutes prior to IV catheterization and induction. Give morphine at least 30 minutes before such procedures. Most premedications last at least two hours. For mast cell tumor removals, antihistamines can be given at the same time as the premedications.

PREMEDICATION DOSES

Drug	Dose	Route
Acepromazine	0.01-0.06 mg/kg (max total = 3 mg)	SC, IM, dog and cat
Atipamezole (reversal agent for medetomidine)	5x the medetomidine dose	IM, dog and cat
Atropine	0.02-0.04 mg/kg	SC, IM, dog and cat
Butorphanol	0.2-0.4 mg/kg	SC, IM, dog and cat
Glycopyrrolate	0.05-0.01 mg/kg	SC, IM, dog and cat
Hydromorphone	0.05-0.1 mg/kg	SC, IM, dog and cat
Ketamine	5.0-10.0 mg/kg	SC, IM, cat
Medetomidine	5.0-10.0 µg/kg dog 10.0-15.0 µg/kg cat	IM, dog and cat
Meperidine	2.0-5.0 mg/kg	SC, IM, dog and cat
Methadone	0.2-0.5 mg/kg	SC, IM, dog and cat
Morphine	0.3-1.0 mg/kg dog 0.1-0.3 mg/kg cat	SC, IM, dog and cat
Oxymorphone	0.02-0.06 mg/kg	SC, IM, dog and cat
Telazol®	4.0-5.0 mg/kg dog 2.0-3.0 mg/kg cat	SC, IM, dog and cat
Acepromazine + Meperidine	Acepromazine 0.02-0.05 mg/kg Meperidine 4.0-5.0 mg/kg	SC, IM, dog and cat
Acepromazine + Oxymorphone	Acepromazine 0.02-0.05 mg/kg Oxymorphone 0.02-0.04 mg/kg	SC, IM, dog and cat
Acepromazine + Morphine	Acepromazine 0.02-0.05 mg/kg Morphine 0.1-0.3 mg/kg	SC, IM, dog and cat
Acepromazine + Methadone	Acepromazine 0.02-0.05 mg/kg Methadone 0.1-0.3 mg/kg	SC, IM, dog and cat
Acepromazine + Butorphanol	Acepromazine 0.02 mg/kg Butorphanol 0.1 mg/kg	SC, IM, dog and cat
Acepromazine + Ketamine	Acepromazine 0.04 mg/kg Ketamine 3.0-5.0 mg/kg	IM, cat
Telazol® + Oxymorphone	Telazol 4.0-5.0 mg/kg Oxymorphone 0.03-0.05 mg/kg	IM, dog
Telazol® + Morphine	Telazol 4.0-5.0 mg/kg Morphine 0.3-0.5 mg/kg	IM, dog
Telazol® + Butorphanol	Telazol 4.0-5.0 mg/kg Burtorphanol 0.2-0.4 mg/kg	IM, dog
Medetomidine + Butorphanol	Medetomidine 5.0-10.0 µg/kg Burtophanol 0.1 mg/kg	SC, IM, dog and cat
Medetomidine + Oxymorphone	Medetomidine 5.0-10.0 µg/kg Oxymorphone 0.03-0.05 mg/kg	SC, IM, dog and cat
Medetomidine + Methadone	Medetomidine 5.0-10.0 µg/kg Methadone 0.3-0.5 mg/kg	SC, IM, dog and cat

ANCILLARY AGENT DOSES (for Mast Cell Tumor Cases)

Drug	Dose	Route
Cimetidine	4.0 – 5.0 mg/kg	IM, SC
Diphenhydramine	0.5 – 1.0 mg/kg	IM
Ranitidine	2.0 mg/kg	IM, SC

1.2

Anesthesia (vertical, right margin)

II. INDUCTION

A. **INTRAVENOUS INDUCTION:** Rather than administering these agents in one rapid bolus which can lead to marked cardiovascular depression, titrate the induction agents to effect. Administer 1/4 dose of the first agent (e.g. etomidate, fentanyl, ketamine, thiopental) followed by 1/2 dose of diazepam or midazolam (when you are using a second agent). Then wait 30 seconds in the case of thiopental (rapid-acting barbiturate) and 60 seconds for the dissociatives and opioids. When using propofol, inject each of the 1/4 doses over 60 seconds. Faster injection leads to faster induction, but also leads to severe cardiovascular depression. Propofol has the greatest cardiovascular depressant effect of the listed injectable agents. Throughout the induction period, assess respiration rate, jaw tone, heart rate, and mucous membrane color. Intubate when the patient no longer chews when you open the mouth. Discontinue dosing if the animal becomes cyanotic or apneic. For cats, keep 0.2 mL of 2% lidocaine on hand to desensitize the laryngeal opening during intubation. If you put lidocaine on the larynx it takes 60 seconds to have an effect.

1. **Preoxygenation:** Brachycephalic animals and those that will receive opioid induction should be preoxygenated for 4 minutes at a flow of 2-4 L/minute if they will tolerate the oxygen mask. Additionally, in the case of opioid induction, the room should be quiet since animals become sensitized to sound during opioid inductions. Animals often desaturate following propofol so having the animal on oxygen during induction may minimize this.

INDUCTION (IV ADMINISTRATION, TITRATE TO EFFECT)

DRUG	DOSE	
Etomidate + Diazepam	Etomidate 1.5 mg/kg Diazepam 0.5 mg/kg	dog, cat
Etomidate + Midazolam	Etomidate 1.5 mg/kg Midazolam 0.25 mg/kg	dog, cat
Fentanyl + Diazepam	Fentanyl 10 µg/kg Diazepam 0.5 mg/kg	dog
Fentanyl + Midazolam	Fentanyl 10 µg/kg Midazolam 0.25 mg/kg	dog
Ketamine + Diazepam	Ketamine 5.0 mg/kg Diazepam 0.5 mg/kg	dog, cat
Ketamine + Midazolam	Ketamine 5.0 mg/kg Midazolam 0.25 mg/kg	dog, cat
Propofol	6.0-8.0 mg/kg	dog, cat
Propofol + Diazepam	Propofol 4.0 mg/kg Diazepam 0.2-0.3 mg/kg	dog, cat
Propofol + Midazolam	Propofol 4.0 mg/kg Midazolam 0.1-0.2 mg/kg	dog, cat
Telazol®	3.0 mg/kg	dog, cat (dilute)
Thiopental	12.5 mg/kg	dog 2.5% cat 1.25%
Thiopental + Diazepam	Thiopental 10.0 mg/kg Diazepam 0.2-0.3 mg/kg	dog, cat
Thiopental + Midazolam	Thiopental 10.0 mg/kg Midazolam 0.1-0.2 mg/kg	dog, cat

B. **GAS INDUCTION:** With gas induction, intubation must be performed more rapidly than with intravenous induction. For cats, administer 2% lidocaine onto the aretynoids and then place the mask back on. Give the lidocaine a minute to act and then remove the gas mask and intubate.

INDUCTION with GAS ANESTHETICS

DRUG	FLOW	
Halothane box	3.0-5.0% + oxygen 6.0-8.0 L/min	dog, cat
Isoflurane box	4.0-5.0% + oxygen 6.0-8.0 L/min	dog, cat
Halothane mask	0 increasing to 3% + oxygen	dog, cat
Isoflurane mask	0 increasing to 4% + oxygen	dog, cat

C. **HINTS on INTUBATION:** Be sure to use the largest diameter endotracheal tube that will comfortably fit in the animal's trachea. Larger tubes have less resistance to air. Measure the endotracheal tube against the animal so that the tip lies just in front of the thoracic inlet. Insertion past this point may place the tip past the tracheal bifurcation. Secure the endotracheal tube in place by tying roll gauze around it and then secure it around the maxilla or behind the ears. Adjust the cuff by ventilating the animal (compressing the reservoir bag while the pop-off valve is closed) to an inspiratory pressure of 15-20 cm H_2O in dogs or 10-12 cm H_2O in cats (lower if the patient has pneumothorax). Listen for airflow around the tube. Gradually inflate the cuff until you no longer hear air flowing around the tube. Also, each time the animal is ventilated, the chest should expand. Note that just inflating the cuff until the indicator is firm does not tell you anything about the cuff seal. It only tells you about pressure within the cuff. Once the cuff is sealed, check anesthetic depth and turn the vaporizer on.

1. **Other monitoring:** Now assess the cardiovascular system—mucous membrane color, capillary refill time, pulse quality, and temperature. An esophageal stethoscope and esophageal temperature probe provide convenient means for regularly assessing heart rate and temperature. A Doppler monitor or an oscillometric blood pressure monitor may be used to assess blood pressure non-invasively.

III. **MAINTENANCE:** Inhalant, Injectable, and Neuromuscular Blocking Agents

A. **INHALANT ANESTHETICS:** Be sure to review the section on anesthesia machines so that you know how to operate them correctly (Refer to www.nerdbook.com/extras). In private practice, although your technician is usually the one operating the equipment, ultimately the veterinarian is responsible for the animal's well-being. If you're unable to trouble-shoot machine malfunctions you may jeopardize the animal's safety.

INHALANT AGENTS

	LOADING DOSE		MAINTENANCE DOSE	
	Circle System	Non-rebreathing System	Circle System	Non-rebreathing System
Halothane	2.0-3.0%	1.5-2.0%	1.5-2.0%	1.0-1.75%
Isoflurane	2.5-3.0%	1.5-2.0%	2.0-2.5%	1.0-2.0%

GASES

	CIRCLE SYSTEM	NON-REBREATHING SYSTEM
Oxygen	1L/min	200 mL/kg/min (1L/min)

1. If you're having problems keeping the animal anesthetized on a fairly high vaporizer setting, check the anesthesia machine. Does the vaporizer contain anesthetic agent? Do the oxygen tanks have oxygen? Are all of the connections in place? Are there leaks in the machine set-up? These should have been checked prior to using the anesthesia machine but sometimes tubing comes loose when machines are moved from one location to another. For long procedures, oxygen tanks and vaporizers can become depleted.

B. INJECTABLE MAINTENANCE AGENTS

INJECTABLE MAINTENANCE AGENTS (IV ADMINISTRATION)

CLASSIFICATION	DRUG	DOSAGE
Opioids	Oxymorphone	0.02-0.05 mg/kg every 20 minutes
	Fentanyl	**Dogs:** Loading dose 10.0 µg/kg + 0.5-1.0 µg/kg/min infusion = 30-60 µg/kg/hr **Cats:** Loading dose 5.0 µg/kg + 0.2-0.4 µg/kg/min infusion = 12-24 µg/kg/hr
Hindered Phenol	Propofol	0.1-0.4 mg/kg/min = 6-24 mg/kg/hr
Benzodiazepines	Diazepam	0.2-0.5 mg/kg/hr
	Midazolam	0.5-1.5 µg/kg/min infusion = 30-90 µg/kg/hr

REVERSAL of OPIOID AGENTS

REVERSAL AGENT	DOSAGE
Naloxone	0.001 mg/kg increments IV for partial reversal 0.02-0.04 mg/kg IM, IV for complete reversal
Nalbuphine	0.03 mg/kg increments IV

C. NEUROMUSCULAR BLOCKING AGENTS

DRUG	DOSE
Atracurium Competitively inhibits acetylcholine at the neuromuscular junction.	0.25 mg/kg loading dose; 0.10 mg/kg redose or 0.1 mg/kg loading dose followed by 3.0-8.0 µg/kg/min infusion (180-480 µg/kg/hr)
Reversal of Atracurium's effects with Edrophonium (an anticholinesterase inhibitor)	**Edrophonium:** 0.5 mg/kg IV slowly while monitoring heart rate. Administer **atropine** 0.01-0.02 mg/kg IV before or during edrophonium injection to prevent bradycardia. If the HR ≥ 90 bpm (dog) or ≥ 120 bpm (cat), then administer atropine and edrophonium together. If HR is less than the values above, administer atropine IV and then when the HR starts to increase, inject edrophonium.

1. These agents are primarily used for ocular surgeries to ensure the eyeball remains completely still and rotated centrally during surgery. Because these drugs paralyze the animal, the animal will need to be on a ventilator.

2. **Titrating to effect:** In order to evaluate how the neuromuscular blocking agents are working, place a peripheral nerve stimulator on a hind leg. Attach the electrodes to the skin on the proximal end of the lateral side of the tibia over the peroneal nerve so that movement caused by stimulation effects only the limb and does not cause movement of the rest of the dog. Evaluate for a train of 4 twitches upon stimulation. About 5 minutes before surgical incision, infuse atracurium over 60 seconds (fast bolus may cause histamine release). Within 5 minutes the twitch response should be negative. The loading dose of atracurium should last 30 minutes. Check the twitch response every 5 minutes. When you get weak twitches infuse the maintenance dose of atracurium over 15 seconds. Redose as needed. This dose should last 10-20 minutes. Discontinue once suturing of the eye is finished. At the end of surgery, reverse the atracurium with edrophonium (and atropine) even if the patient has twitches because the twitch responses are relatively insensitive for determining the degree of residual neuromuscular blockade, and because the effects of edrophonium have a shorter duration than the effects of atracurium.

IV. **ANALGESIC AGENTS:** For painful surgeries, use a premedication with analgesic properties (usually an opioid). If the surgery lasts longer than 2 hours, an additional injection of opioid analgesic should be administered before the animal wakes up. During surgery additional analgesics can be administered if the animal shows signs of pain—heart rate, blood pressure, and respiratory rate increase in the absence of indicators of a light plane of anesthesia such as palpebral reflex, eyes rotated centrally from a downward location, and spontaneous movement. Carprofen or meloxicam are used for postoperative analgesia in conjunction with opioids and provide up to 24 hours of analgesia. Care should be taken with any patients that have received corticosteroids or who might have reduced renal perfusion.

POST-OPERATIVE ANALGESIC AGENTS
ADMINISTERED IMMEDIATELY FOLLOWING SURGERY

DRUG	DOSE	ROUTE of ADMINISTRATION
Butorphanol	0.1-0.4 mg/kg 0.1 mg/kg	SC, IM, dog and cat IV, dog and cat
Meperidine	2.0-5.0 mg/kg	SC, IM, dog and cat
Methadone	0.1-0.5 mg/kg	SC, IM, dog
Morphine	0.2-1.0 mg/kg dog 0.05-0.1 mg/kg cat	SC, IM, IV*,dog and cat
Oxymorphone	0.03-0.05 mg/kg	SC, IM, dog and cat
Carprofen	2-4 mg/kg	SC, IV, dog, cat
Meloxicam	0.1-0.2 mg/kg	SC, IV, dog; SC cat

* If morphine is given IV it should be given slowly to avoid histamine release.

POST-OPERATIVE ANALGESIC AGENTS
IN the DAYS IMMEDIATELY FOLLOWING SURGERY

DRUG	DOSE	ROUTE of ADMINISTRATION
Buprenorphine	10-20 µg/kg q 4-6 hours	SC, IM dog and cat
Butorphanol	0.1-0.2 mg/kg q 4-6 hours	SC, IM, cat
Carprofen	2.0-4.0 mg/kg q 12 hours	PO, dog and cat
Firocoxib	5.0 mg/kg SID	PO in dogs
Hydromorphone	0.05-0.2 mg/kg q 3-4 hours 0.05-0.1 mg/kg q 3-4 hours	SC, IM dog SC, IM cat
Ketoprofen	2.0 mg/kg q 8-12 hours	IM in dogs
Meloxicam	0.1-0.2 mg/kg q 12-24 hours	PO, SC, IV dog
Methadone	0.4-1.0 mg/kg q 5-6 hours	SC, IM, dog
Morphine	0.5-1.0 mg/kg q 3-4 hours 0.5 mg/kg IV diluted in 30 mL saline given slowly followed by 0.1-1.0 mg/kg/hr infusion IV (dog only) 0.1-0.3 mg/kg q 3-4 hours	SC, IM, dog SC, IM cat
Oxymorphone	0.05-0.1 mg/kg q 3-4 hours 0.05 mg/kg q 3-4 hours	SC, IM, dog SC, IM, cat

FENTANYL PATCH
Should be placed 24 hours prior to surgery

ANIMAL SIZE	SIZE FENTANYL PATCH
Cats and toy dogs (2-10kg)	25 µg/hr
Small dogs (10-20kg)	50 µg/hr
Medium dogs (20-30kg)	75 µg/hr
Large dogs (≥ 30kg)	100 µg/hr

Refer to the analgesia subchapter (p. 1.23) for information on nerve blocks and epidurals. For painful surgeries fentanyl can also be given as a constant rate infusion.

PREANESTHETIC EVALUATION and PREPARATION of the ANIMAL
Preanesthetic Evaluation
Patient Preparation

Anesthesia always carries risks, even in healthy animals presenting for routine procedures. In order to minimize risk, carefully evaluate the patient and consider the purpose of the anesthesia prior to developing an anesthetic protocol.

I. PREANESTHETIC EVALUATION of the ANIMAL
    A. HISTORY and SIGNALMENT

SIGNALMENT	In **young patients,** worry about: • Hypothermia • Decreased or increased drug metabolism: Young animals have enzyme systems that may not be well-developed. If possible, avoid thiobarbiturates in animals less than 3 months of age. Animals around 10 months of age are at the age of peak anesthetic requirement and may require higher levels of anesthetic agents. • Dehydration • **Hypoglycemia:** Use LRS + 2.5% dextrose at a flow of 10mL/kg/hr. This occurs most often in toy breeds < 10-12 weeks of age. Measure the blood glucose in the morning and during anesthesia to see whether glucose administration is necessary. If the blood glucose is low normal (< 80 mg/dL) or approaching low normal, treat with dextrose. In **older patients,** worry about: • Lower muscle mass • Organ dysfunction: especially kidney, liver, and heart • Changes within the brain: For example, the animal may have increased cerebral sensitivity to benzodiazepines and opioids; as a result, diazepam and some opioids may be more effective as a premed in older dogs than they would be in younger dogs. **Breed problems:** Avoid thiobarbiturates in Greyhounds and other sighthounds because sighthounds have a prolonged recovery time (some never recover) when on these drugs. Propofol and dissociatives can be used for these breeds.
PREVIOUS DISEASE	Evaluate for cardiac disease, seizures, renal disease, liver disease, etc. Refer to the section on anesthetics in disease situations (p.1.19).
CONCURRENT MEDICATIONS	• **Cardiac medications** may predispose the patient to hypotension and arrhythmias (e.g. vasodilators, ACE inhibitors, ß blockers). • **Diuretics:** Changes in electrolytes (e.g. hypokalemia with furosemide). The diuretics plus the anesthesia may combine to cause hypotension since these animals may already be dehydrated. • **Nephrotoxic agents:** Avoid combining methoxyflurane with other nephrotoxic agents such as gentamicin. Maintain renal perfusion. • **Carbonic anhydrase inhibitors** are used to treat glaucoma. They cause metabolic acidosis. Correct any acidosis prior to anesthesia. • **Phenylephrine** and **epinephrine** are alpha adrenergics and when used in combination with halothane, can lead to arrhythmias. Use isoflurane or sevoflurane when these drugs are used. Phenylephrine-induced hypertension can be treated with acepromazine (0.005 mg/kg IV). • **Corticosteroids:** Animals on corticosteroids are immunosuppressed and may not be able to compensate for the stress of surgery. If they've been pulled off long-term corticosteroids within one month, give a dose of corticosteroids the day of surgery.
TRAUMA	• **Pneumothorax:** Avoid nitrous oxide. It diffuses into the thorax and expands. Also avoid testing the seal on the endotracheal tube because doing so may increase thoracic pressure. If the patient has to be ventilated, use a low tidal volume and high respiratory rate. • **Pulmonary contusions** worsen under anesthesia and may result in pulmonary hemorrhage. Keep the airways expanded in order to prevent atelectasis. Avoid mechanical ventilation if possible, as it may aggravate bleeding into the lungs. • **Myocardial trauma:** Radiograph the animal first (for pulmonary trauma) and perform an ECG to look for arrhythmias.

B. **PHYSICAL EXAM**
1. **Activity level:** Calm animals require less sedation. Acepromazine can be used in young, energetic dogs. Oxymorphone is a good choice for energetic cats.
2. **Temperament:** For aggressive dogs, use a neuroleptanalgesic such as telazol or ketamine. Telazol is also good for aggressive cats. You may elect to avoid acepromazine in aggressive dogs because it takes the edge off so that the dogs look safer, but they can still attack. They often just attack more slowly.
3. **Body weight:** Fat dogs may have poor ventilation and need ventilatory support.
4. **Airway:** Observe for respiratory difficulties including those caused by brachycephalic conformation.
5. **Cardiovascular parameters:** Evaluate capillary refill time (CRT), mucous membrane (MM) color, pulses. (Refer to pp. 1.33, 3.7, and .8.5 for info on interpretation.)

C. **LABORATORY DATA**
1. **For young healthy dogs:** PCV, TP, BUN (+ glucose in very young dogs)
2. **For dogs ≥ 6 years of age:** CBC, chem panel
3. If the animal has an **arrhythmia**, perform an ECG. If it also has a murmur, consider thoracic radiographs for evaluating the heart (Refer to p.3.11 for guidelines on when to perform a preanesthetic cardiac work-up). A work-up is important because if the patient has a compensatory heart disease, drugs that decompensate the cardiovascular system may cause heart failure. Additionally, if you know the origin of the murmur, you can support the animal appropriately during surgery. For example, you would support an animal with mitral regurgitation much differently than one with aortic stenosis.

PREANESTHETIC EVALUATION – LAB FINDINGS

LAB FINDING	SIGNIFICANCE
BUN & Creatinine elevation	Indicate renal disease. Maintain blood pressure and renal perfusion. Use dopamine at 2.5-5 µg/kg/min (Refer to p.1.42)
Dehydration: Most anesthetic agents cause vasodilation. Dehydration plus vasodilation can lead to cardiovascular collapse.	Start fluids immediately upon recognition of dehydration rather than waiting until the day of surgery. If you find dehydration on the day of surgery, try to administer fluids prior to induction. **Dog:** 10-40 mL/kg IV over one hour **Cat:** 10 mL/kg IV over one hour
Anemia	If the PCV = 25-32%, consider performing a crossmatch prior to surgery. If it's < 20-25% or if the animal's lost > 30% of its circulating blood volume, perform a transfusion prior to surgery. Anemia is a concern because: • Barbiturates decrease PCV by about 6% (splenic sequestration). • Anemic animals compensate by increasing cardiac output. All anesthetic agents are cardiovascular depressants. They compromise the ability to compensate in this manner. • Fluids administered during anesthesia dilute the blood.
Hypoproteinemic: Total protein < 5g/dL Albumin < 2g/dL	These animals lose colloid osmotic pressure; thus, the animal may become hypotensive. Administer plasma or another colloid instead of crystalloids in order to combat hypotension.
Platelet or clotting factor deficiencies: (e.g. Von Willebrand's)	Give a plasma transfusion (fresh frozen or whole blood) prior to surgery. For major surgeries, perform a crossmatch since the patient may need a whole blood transfusion due to blood loss.
Potassium < 3 or > 5.5mEq/L.	Abnormal potassium levels can lead to cardiac arrhythmias. Hyperkalemia is usually more of a problem than hypokalemia. When glucose enters cells, it takes potassium with it. Thus, calcium gluconate or insulin and glucose can be used to treat hyperkalemic animals.
Hypercalcemia	Most hyperparathyroid animals are hypercalcemic which can cause renal damage. Diurese them prior to surgery with saline.
Hypocalcemia	**Hypocalcemia** can cause neuromuscular problems (e.g. muscle twitching, seizures). It can occur as a result of extremely rapid blood or plasma tranfusions because citrate, an anticoagulant in the blood, binds calcium. In cases of rapid transfusion, give $CaCl_2$ IV over 20 minutes. Avoid bolusing $CaCl_2$ as this causes **severe bradycardia.**

Anesthesia

D. CONSIDER WHY THE ANIMAL IS BEING ANESTHETIZED
   1. **Bronchoscopy:** Use the largest endotracheal tube possible for bronchoscopy. Animals with ≤ size 7 endotracheal tubes must receive injectable anesthetics or you will have to extubate them in order to perform the bronchoscopy. If the tube is > size 7, the bronchoscopy apparatus will fit within the tube.
   2. **Gastroduodenoscopy:** Avoid opioids. They cause pyloric spasms.
   3. **Ultrasound:** Opioids make dogs pant.
   4. **Myelogram:** Avoid agents that potentiate seizures (e.g. ketamine, acepromazine).
   5. **Pain:** If the surgery will be painful, use analgesics (Refer to p. 1.23 on analgesia).
   6. **Surgery involving significant blood loss:** Rhinotomies, portacaval shunts, and invasive vascular tumors among others may involve significant blood loss. Perform a crossmatch prior to anesthesia.

E. ASSESS OVERALL ANESTHETIC RISK
   1. Physical status:
      a. **Normal:** The animal has no disease or localized disease with no systemic disturbance (such as a healthy young dog with a laceration).
      b. **Mild Risk:** The patient has a slight disturbance that may or may not be related to the surgical complaint (such as a brachycephalic dog).
      c. **Moderate risk:** The patient has a moderate systemic disturbance that interferes with normal activity (such as mild renal or liver disease).
      d. **Severe risk:** The patient has an extreme systemic disturbance which seriously interferes with normal activity (such as renal or liver failure).

   2. **General risk factors** include age extremes, type and duration of surgery, skill of the surgeon, and the surgical facility. Human error is also a big risk factor. In humans, the highest percentage of anesthetic accidents occur during maintenance due to lack of vigilance.

F. DETERMINE FLUID ADMINISTRATION RATE

RATE OF FLUID ADMINISTRATION

SITUATION	ADMINISTRATION RATE
Dehydrated, hypertonic animals	20 mL/kg/hr
Normal animals	10 mL/kg/hr
Cardiovascular disease (where we're worrying about pulmonary edema)	5 mL/kg/hr
Diagnostic procedures (radiographs, CT scans)	10 mL/kg for the first hour then 5 mL/kg thereafter

G. OTHER CONSIDERATIONS
   1. **Food and water:** In general, remove food 12 hours prior to surgery and remove water 2 hours prior to surgery.
   2. Correct fluid and electrolyte imbalances prior to anesthesia.
   3. Perform a crossmatch when needed, prior to anesthesia.

ANESTHETIC AGENTS

PREMEDICATION	INDUCTION	MAINTENANCE	RECOVERY
Tranquilizers: Acepromazine Diazepam Xylazine Medetomidine Parasympatholytics: Atropine Glycopyrrolate Opioids: Oxymorphone, Morphine, Meperidine, Hydromorphone, Methadone, Butorphanol, Buprenorphine Dissociatives: Ketamine (+ diazepam) Telazol®	Barbiturates: Thiopental (± diazepam) Dissociatives: Ketamine with diazepam and Telazol® Opioids: Fentanyl± diazepam Propofol ± diazepam Etomidate ± diazepam Inhalants: Isoflurane Halothane Sevoflurane ± nitrous oxide	Gases: Isoflurane Sevoflurane Methoxyflurane Nitrous oxide Opioids: Fentanyl/diazepam Dissociatives: Ketamine/diazepam Propofol Neuromuscular blocking agents: Atracurium	Opioid reversal with Naloxone Alpha agonist reversal: Yohimbine, Atipamezole Neuromuscular blocking agent reversal: Edrophonium (+ atropine) Smoother recoveries: Acepromazine and medetomidine are sometimes used to slow (ketamine or Telazol®) recoveries down

I. **PREMEDICATIONS:** If the animal is sick, calm, stoic, or already has an IV catheter and the procedure is not very painful, you don't have to premedicate.

   A. **Purpose of premedication**
      1. To **decrease anxiety** and make the animal easier to **handle**

      2. **Decrease parasympathetic effects** such as salivation, bradycardia, and vomiting: Usually we don't have to worry about vomiting because the animal is fasted for 12 hours, and vomiting can be induced in healthy dogs and cats who've eaten within the last several hours by giving **xylazine** (0.44-1.0 mg/kg IM in cats) or morphine (in dogs).

      3. **Analgesia** helps for placing an intravenous catheter. Additionally, some of the analgesia lasts throughout the surgery and prevents the build-up of pain signals during surgery (i.e. wind-up)

      4. **To decrease the dose of other drugs (induction and maintenance) that we need:** For example, giving acepromazine as a premedication can decrease the amount of thiopental needed by 50%, and the amount of halothane needed by 30%.

      5. **Promotes a smooth recovery:** This is important in painful surgeries and in surgeries where dissociatives are the primary induction agent. Recovery from dissociatives without premedication is rough. Analgesics decrease the build-up of electrical signals during surgery so that the animal will not wake up sensitized to pain.

   B. **CLASSES of PREMEDICATIONS**

CLASSES OF PREMEDICATONS
• Parasympatholytics
• Tranquilizers
• Opioids
• Neuroleptanalgesics (e.g. an opioid + tranquilizer)
• Dissociatives
• Alpha-2 agonists

ANESTHETIC PREMEDICATIONS IN CATS and DOGS

AGENT	ACTIONS	CARDIOVASCULAR & RESPIRATORY EFFECTS	INDICATIONS	DISADVANTAGES	CONTRA-INDICATIONS
Atropine Duration: 1-1.5 hrs IV, IM, SC	**Parasympatholytic/ Vagolytic:** It blocks ACh at the muscarinic receptors of the parasympathetic nervous system (at the target organ) but does not affect the muscarinic receptors of the somatic nervous system. Decreases salivary secretions. Combats bradycardia Causes mydriasis, so don't use pupil size to assess anesthetic depth when animal has been given atropine. Glycopyrrolate, however, does not cross the blood-brain barrier.	HR: increases Respiration: bronchodilation	**Small patients** (secretions significantly decrease airway size). **When ketamine is used** (ketamine increases secretions). **Increased vagal tone or bradycardia:** e.g. eye or neck surgeries, when administering opioids, or to treat reactions to myelograms. **To combat 2° heart block** It's especially useful in situations where you need to reverse vagal tone immediately. When given IV, it starts taking effect within one minute. **In cesareans** when opioids are used on pregnant dogs/cats. Atropine also prevents bradycardia in the unborn pups/kittens.	Short duration **Crosses the blood brain barrier** and the placental barrier. Decreases cardiac esophageal sphincter tone thus increasing the likelihood of regurgitation (esophagitis). May induce arrhythmias. During inductions, 2° heartblock is more likely; after induction, PVCs are more likely. Animals on halothane are more likely to have arrhythmias. Tachycardia Dries up secretions	Pneumonia (animals need to get rid of their secretions). Also be careful in animals with tachycardia, tachyarrhythmias, hyperthyroidism, or hypertrophic cardiomyopathy.
Glycopyrrolate Duration: 3-4 hrs	**Parasympatholytic:** Decreases salivary secretions Combats bradycardia	HR: increases Respiration: bronchodilation	Similar to atropine but has a longer duration. (no mydriasis)	Similar to atropine but 1.5-2x more expensive. Slower onset when given IV (4 min)	Similar to atropine
Xylazine 0.5-1.0 mg/kg IV in cats and dogs 0.5-2.0 mg/kg IM in cats and dogs	**α₂ agonist** that decreases anxiety and sedates the animal. It also increases sympathetic and vagal tone. It induces emesis due to central emetic zone stimulation. Reversible with yohimbine It also decreases insulin and can cause hyperglycemia.	HR: decreases CO: severe decrease. Initial increase in blood pressure leads to bradycardia and decreased cardiac output—to as little as 30% of normal. Mucous membranes may be pale due to vasoconstriction. Respiration: no effect	Emetic In **healthy** animals for short procedures such as ear exams, eye exams, wound cleaning, bandage changes, or where you want to reverse the effects (with Yohimbine). Because it's a sedative, higher levels produce longer duration but not deeper anesthesia. Use blood pressure monitoring and watch for arrhythmias. Place an IV catheter beforehand.	Causes catecholamine induced arrhythmias (usually SA or AV nodal block or bradycardia). These α₂ effects outlast xylazine's α₂ effects. Thus, the animal may be fully awake and still have xylazine-induced arrhythmias. Potentiates the effects of thiopental, so decrease your thiopental induction dose by 40-90%. Decrease propofol dose by 30-90%.	Hypotensive animals. Animals with cardiac dysfunction. Not as effective in small, excitable dogs or during high catecholamine levels.

AGENT	ACTIONS	CARDIOVASCULAR & RESPIRATORY EFFECTS	INDICATIONS	DISADVANTAGES	CONTRA-INDICATIONS
Medetomidine Dose: 5-40 µg/kg IV or IM in dogs 80-100 µg/kg IV or IM in cats. For preanesthesia, use 5-10 µg/kg in dogs and 10-20 mg/kg in cats (IV or IM).	α_2 agonist: It's ten times more selective for α_2 receptors than xylazine, so it has much greater α_2 and much less α_1 effect than xylazine. Like xylazine, medetomidine decreases anxiety and sedates the animal. It also increases sympathetic and vagal tone and induces emesis. Reversal: **Atipamezole** 2-5x the medetomidine dose if given within one hour of medetomidine dose (IM). Atipamezole has 100 times more affinity for α_2 receptors than ychimbine.	HR: decreases to as low as 30 bpm in dogs. CO: severe decrease. Decreases CO to as little as 30% of normal. Respiration: no effect	Good for **healthy animals** undergoing short procedures in which you want to reverse the effects (such as ear or oral exam, laceration repair, bandage change, radiographs). Sedation develops within 1-3 minutes of IV administration and within 5-10 minutes of IM injection. 30-40 µg/kg provides sedation in lateral recumbency for 40-60 minutes without reversal. Higher doses lead to longer durations but not greater sedation. For intubation, mask dog with gaseous anesthesia first because jaw tone will probably be too tight. Can also be used in lower doses as a preanesthetic agent.	Causes marked vasoconstriction accompanied by **bradycardia**. This markedly decreases cardiac output. Can cause transient 2nd degree AV block. Use only in healthy animals. Monitor for arrhythmias and hypotension Some animals can awaken and bite suddenly. Treat animals sedated with medetomidine alone with caution.	Only use this in young healthy dogs. Do not use anticholinergics to increase heart rate as this will increase workload on the heart. Use an alpha-2 antagonist first.
Acepromazine SQ, IM, IV Onset: SQ=40min. IM= 15min.	**Tranquilizer** (phenothiazine) that works on the reticular activating system, thus it doesn't cause total CNS depression; patients will still react to stimuli. Tranquilizers have a ceiling effect. Depresses the response of the chemoreceptor trigger zone. **Sedation:** Good Good **anxiolytic** premedication (but not strong enough for thunderstorm or fireworks phobias). **Not analgesic**	HR: If the dog is energetic to start with, the heart rate will slow down as the dog calms down. In already calm dogs, the heart rate will increase. CO: no change SVR: α_1 antagonist. Dogs with sympathetic tone can experience severe hypotension with acepromazine. Respiration: no effect	Young dogs where good sedation is required. **Protects against catecholamine-induced arrhythmias:** If we premed with acepromazine, halothane won't induce arrhythmias. When ophthalmologists give 100x the dose of phenylephrine it causes increased blood pressure; 1/10th the premedication dose of acepromazine will block this change in blood pressure. To smooth recovery when ketamine or Telazol® have been used.	Not an analgesic Dogs still **respond to stimuli**, thus vicious animals may look safe but they can still be dangerous. Don't perform painful procedures on animals only sedated with acepromazine. α_1 blockade: It may cause hypotension when there's sympathetic tone (e.g. trauma, hypovolemia, cardiovascular shock). Avoid using acepromazine in animals unable to withstand further cardiovascular insult.	Trauma (avoid for 5 days following trauma) Seizure patients Myelograms Hypotensive animals Boxers (BSAVA guide) Cardiovascular disease

1.12

Drug		HR / Respiration	Use / Dose	Effects	Contraindications
Ketamine PO, SC, IM, IV IM gives the most consistent results. Peak effect: 15 minutes. Duration: 5-10 min. Can increase by giving 0.04 mg/kg acepromazine. Usually administered with diazepam.	Belongs to the only class of premedications that can bring an animal to a surgical plane of anesthesia. Low doses sedate the animal. Moderate doses can be used to restrain the animal. High doses can be used to reach a surgical plane of anesthesia. Causes increased salivation (use it with a parasympatholytic). Has a therapeutic index of about 10.	HR: increases due to increased sympathetic tone. Don't use this drug when increases in sympathetic tone are contraindicated. Respiration: Ventilation decreases a little and the pattern changes. Periodic apnea or apneustic breathing may occur.	Used in cats but not dogs as a premed. We use it when deep sedation is needed or when the animal is fractious. Ketamine can be given "intra-animal" and it has a rapid onset. Calm cats: 5 mg/kg Feisty cats: 7 mg/kg Vicious cats: 10 mg/kg. Apneusis/catalepsy can occur at doses ≥ 10mg/kg. Oral dose: 20mg/kg because there's a first pass effect.	pH is very acidic so it stings. Increases intracranial pressure Increases intraocular pressure Increases salivation Hyperthermia may occur in dogs that are recovering from ketamine.	Seizure patients Neurologic procedures where increased intracranial pressure must be avoided (e.g. CSF tap, patients with brain tumors, etc). Hypertrophic cardiomyopathy or other cardiomyopathies. Glaucoma Hyperthyroidism
Telazol® SC, IM, IV Onset: 2-3 minutes Duration: 10 min.	Tiletamine + zolazepam: a long acting dissociative plus a long acting benzodiazepine. It has the same characteristics as ketamine/diazepam but it gives much more consistent effects with better anesthesia (patients are more manageable for catheterization).	Same as with ketamine Respiration: Apneustic breathing is not usually seen.	Premed of choice for unmanageable cats as well as aggressive dogs. Cat: 2.5 mg/kg Dog: 5 mg/kg	Same as with ketamine/diazepam. Recoveries are rough. You can give acepromazine (0.01 mg/kg) to slow or smooth recovery. If the surgery was long, then it's likely that the Telazol® has worn off and the animal is waking up from the effect of the maintenance agent. Hyperthermia may occur in dogs that are recovering from Telazol®.	Same as with ketamine/diazepam
Butorphanol Duration: 1-6 hours Schedule IV drug	Opioid agonist/antagonist: μ antagonist and kappa agonist. Analgesia: fairly potent but μ agonists such as oxymorphone are more potent. Sedation: better sedation than oxymorphone especially if we use 0.3-0.4 mg/kg. Reversible with naloxone	Similar to oxymorphone (next page)	Similar to oxymorphone (next page)	Similar to oxymorphone but is less controlled.	Similar to oxymorphone Don't use it if you will be using other opioids for analgesics post-op as it is a μ-antagonist.

AGENT	ACTIONS	CARDIOVASCULAR & RESPIRATORY EFFECTS	INDICATIONS	DISADVANTAGES	CONTRAINDICATIONS
Oxymorphone SC, IM Onset: 10 minutes Duration: 3-4 hrs	Opioids act via specific receptors in the CNS and GI tract. They have some sedative effect but are primarily analgesics (against dull pain). Analgesic: Very potent μ agonist Reversible with naloxone	Minimal cardiovascular effects. Vagotonic: Opioids decrease heart rate, so use them with anticholinergics such as atropine. Ventilation decreases (both rate and tidal volume) due to decrease in medullary sensitivity to CO_2. Opioids cause panting due to resetting of thermoregulation.	Painful surgeries: Opioids help decrease build up of pain signals during surgery, thus post-op, the animal is not as painful. Cardiovascular or neurologically compromised animals: Opioids have minimal cardiovascular effects.	It causes panting and mild bradycardia. Opioids are respiratory depressants. Increased CSF pressure: Opioids decrease sensitivity to CO_2 leading to increased CO_2 and respiratory acidosis. This results in dilation of the cerebral vessels and increased CSF pressure. We can avoid this problem if we put the animal on a ventilator. Causes GI spasms followed by stasis. Controlled drug	Gastroduodenoscopy: opioids tighten the cardiac and pyloric sphincters. Hydrocephalus Pulmonary parenchymal disease: The respiratory depression may force you to put the animal on a ventilator.
Morphine Onset: 20 minutes Duration: 3-4 hrs	Opioid: μ agonist Sedation: Sedates as well as acepromazine. Reversible with naloxone	Similar to oxymorphone	Similar to oxymorphone Cat: 0.1-0.2 mg/kg. A higher dose may cause excitement. Dog: 0.5 mg/kg-1.0 mg/kg	Similar to oxymorphone Do not give it IV rapidly (histamine release).	Similar to oxymorphone Asthma or limited respiratory reserve Intradermal skin test (histamine release)
Hydromorphone Onset: 10 minutes Duration: 4-6 hrs	Opioid: μ agonist Sedation: Sedates as well as acepromazine. Reversible with naloxone	Similar to oxymorphone	Similar to oxymorphone	Similar to oxymorphone	Similar to oxymorphone
Methadone Onset: 10 minutes Duration: 4-6 hrs	Opioid: μ agonist and is also an NMDA antagonist Sedation: Sedates as well as acepromazine.	Similar to oxymorphone	Analgesia occurs within 10-20 minutes of IM or SC injection. More analgesic when administered IM. Methadone is less likely to induce vomiting than morphine and oxymorphone.	Similar to oxymorphone	Similar to oxymorphone
Meperidine: SC or IM; not IV. Onset: 10 min. Duration: 1-2hrs	Opioid: μ agonist Weak sedative/analgesic. Not good for post-op analgesia.	Similar to oxymorphone. Meperidine is the most cardiovascular depressant opioid but causes the least bradycardia.	Similar to oxymorphone but causes less respiratory depression in fetuses than morphine or methadone.	Similar to oxymorphone, but no bradycardia IV administration causes hypotension (histamine release)	Similar to oxymorphone Asthma or limited respiratory reserve Intradermal skin test (histamine release)

1.14

INDUCTION AGENTS IN CATS and DOGS

AGENT	ACTIONS	CARDIOVASCULAR & RESPIRATORY EFFECTS	INDICATIONS	DISADVANTAGES	CONTRAINDICATIONS
Thiopental 10-12.5 mg/kg for induction	Thiobarbiturate that's very lipid soluble and crosses the blood-brain barrier rapidly, leading to rapid induction. Inductions are usually smooth. Give 1/4 dose boluses and wait 30 seconds. Do not wait much longer than this or the effects may start to wear off. Excitation can occur with a relative underdose.	Vagolytic Heart rate increases in healthy animals and then levels off. HR and contractility decrease in sick animals. Decreased cardiac contractility Ventilation: barbiturate apnea. This is not the same as post-intubation apnea.	Healthy dogs. Note: puppies around 10 months of age are at their peak anesthetic requirement and may need a higher dose of thiopental in order to be anesthetized. It's often given with diazepam (0.2-0.5 mg/kg) or midazolam (0.1-0.2 mg/kg). Give 1/4 dose thiopental and flush with heparinized saline. Then give 1/2 dose diazepam and flush. Wait 30 seconds and then repeat the procedure. Use for anesthetizing animals to check for laryngeal paralysis. It decreases intracranial pressure and is an anticonvulsant.	Cardiovascular depressant Causes splenic sequestration of red blood cells (2-4% decrease in PCV). Repeated dosings of thiopental lead to slightly longer durations of action. Can cause ventricular bigeminy. Administering lidocaine (1-2 mg/kg) decreases the incidence of arrhythmias. Sighthounds have extremely prolonged recovery. Without premedication, animals go through an activation phase. If the animal tightens up, give it a little more drug. Can cause perivascular sloughing if given extravascularly (not as common with 2% thiopental as with 5% thiopental). Cats are more difficult to intubate.	Animals with cardiovascular disease Sighthounds Animals with low PCVs or that will loose a lot of blood during surgery. Animals with hepatic insufficiency, especially portocaval shunt.
Fentanyl 10 µg/kg induction or loading dose for fentanyl infusion.	Opioid: Usually doesn't provide a surgical plane of anesthesia, so we must supplement with inhalant anesthetics. Administer with 0.5 mg/kg diazepam or 0.25 mg/kg midazolam. Give 1/4 dose fentanyl, 1/2 dose diazepam, and wait 1-2 minutes.	Minimal cardiovascular effects but causes heart rate to decrease. Premedicate with a parasympatholytic to combat bradycardia. Ventilation: Respiratory depressant, so preoxygenate for 4 minutes and expect to ventilate after induction.	Only used in dogs (and in cats that are virtually dead). It causes excitement in cats. Use in older, sick patients. Avoid use in young, healthy dog. Use in dogs with cardiovascular disease.	Must preoxygenate Causes an excitement phase in young healthy dogs.	Cats Healthy dogs

INDUCTION AGENTS IN CATS and DOGS

AGENT	ACTIONS	CARDIOVASCULAR & RESPIRATORY EFFECTS	INDICATIONS	DISADVANTAGES	CONTRAINDICATIONS
Ketamine 5 mg/kg IV Duration: 10 min.	**Dissociative:** It's usually given with diazepam or midazolam. High doses can be used to reach a surgical plane of anesthesia. Causes increased salivation (use it with a parasympatholytic). Has a therapeutic index of about 10. Give 1/4 dose and then wait 1 minute. When given with diazepam or midazolam, give 1/4 ketamine then 1/2 benzodiazepine dose and wait 30 sec. Alternatively mix the ketamine/diazepam or ketamine/midazolam.	**HR:** increases due to increased sympathetic tone. Don't use this drug when the animal's cardiovascular system is already working hard (e.g. sepsis, gastric torsion, etc). **Respiration:** Ventilation decreases a little and the pattern changes. Periodic apnea or apneustic breathing.	**Routine inductions** Quick knockdowns for short Procedures. **Older patients** where thiopental can't be used.	Increases intracranial pressure. **Recoveries are rough.** You can give acepromazine (0.01 mg/kg) to slow/smooth the recovery. If the surgery was long, then it's likely that the ketamine has worn off and the animal is waking up from the effect of the maintenance agent instead.	**Seizure patients Neurologic procedures** where increased intracranial pressure must be avoided (e.g. CSF tap, patients with brain tumors, etc). **Hypertrophic cardiomyopathy** or other cardiomyopathies. **Hyperthyroidism** Renal insufficiency in cats
Telazol® 3 mg/kg IV Duration: 10 min.	**Tiletamine + zolazepam** is a long acting dissociative plus a long acting benzodiazepine. It has the same characteristics as ketamine/diazepam.	Same as with ketamine		Same as with ketamine/diazepam. Recoveries are rough. You can give acepromazine (0.01 mg/kg) to slow/smooth the recovery. If the surgery was long, then it's likely that the Telazol® has worn off and the animal is waking up from the effect of the maintenance agent.	Same as with ketamine/diazepam Renal insufficiency in cats

1.16

Propofol IV Duration: 2-5 min. Onset: fast Recovery: fast and smooth	Hindered phenol in soybean oil. It's a depressant anesthetic with rapid onset and smooth, rapid recovery. 6 mg/kg in premedicated animals; 10 mg/kg if not. Administer in 1/4 doses over 30-60 seconds and then wait 30 sec. before giving the next 1/4 dose. Often administered with diazepam (0.2-0.3 mg/kg diazepam or midazolam 0.1-0.2 mg/kg with 4 mg/kg propofol). Give 1/4 dose propofol over 60 seconds and 1/2 dose benzodiazepine and wait 30 sec.	Propofol is the most cardiovascular depressant of all of the injectable anesthetics. At low doses it's a vasodilator. It causes arteriolar dilator. It causes myocardial depression. Heart rate does not change. Giving it slowly and in 1/4 doses prevents severe cardiovascular depression. Ventilation: apnea	C-sections: It crosses the placental barrier but lasts just a short time. The puppies are usually not overly depressed when they are removed from the uterus. **Brain tumors/head trauma:** It decreases intracranial pressure. **Quick-knockdowns** (e.g. ultrasound) **Bronchoscopy** **When inhaled agents can't be used** e.g. in animals with malignant hyperthermia. Recovery is good with hepatic and renal disease.	**Cats:** Can only be used for procedures lasting under 20-30 minutes, otherwise the recoveries are prolonged (may last one day). **Expensive** The soybean oil provides a good growth medium for bacteria, thus propofol can only be kept for 6 hours once the vial has been opened.
Etomidate	Imidazole: It's a depressant anesthetic with rapid onset. Dose: 1 mg/kg Given in 1/4 boluses (30 sec between bolus). It is usually administered with diazepam (0.5 mg/kg) or midazolam (0.25 mg/kg).	Causes little cardiovascular depression Ventilation: Less respiratory depression than with barbiturates and shorter acting.	**Cats with cardiovascular disease.** We can't use opioids for induction in cats.	Potent adrenocortico-suppressive agent. Since glucocorticoids are needed for handling stress, this drug should not be used as an infusion. Excitatory: High incidence of muscle tremors on induction, thus it's often given with diazepam. High osmolality so it can cause some hemolysis. Give it with fluids. The amount of hemolysis with constant rate infusion is dangerous so don't use etomidate as a maintenance anesthetic.

INHALATIONAL ANESTHETICS

AGENT	ADVANTAGES	DISADVANTAGES	INDICATIONS	CONTRA-INDICATIONS	MAC
Halothane	Fairly rapid induction/recovery due to intermediate solubility. Quick enough for mask or box induction. Inexpensive	Sensitizes the heart to catecholamine induced arrhythmias Potent cardiovascular depressant (decreases cardiac output).		Animals with arrhythmias or who will be receiving epinephrine. Malignant hyperthermia	MAC = 200 B/G = 0.47
Isoflurane	Fast induction and recovery due to low lipid solubility. The least metabolized of the inhalant anesthetics. May be used in a halothane precision vaporizer that's been cleaned well (same partial pressure as halothane). Does not cause arrhythmias as often as halothane.	Expensive Less potent Recovery may be rough	For fast induction/recovery in surgeries > 1 hr long (e.g. in older animals or very young animals or other animals in which a quick recovery is important). When arrhythmias are a concern (or when you need to administer epinephrine).	Malignant hyperthermia	MAC = 1.4 B/G = 1.4
Sevoflurane	Fast induction and recovery due to low lipid solubility. It does not sensitize the heart to catecholamine-induced arrhythmias. Less pungent than isoflurane so mask inductions may be faster and smoother.	Very expensive Least potent of the inhalant anesthetics Recovery may be rough It reacts with soda lime to produce a compound that may be nephrotoxic. To date, no clinical studies have documented toxic concentrations of this compound.	Same as isoflurane	Kidney or liver disease Malignant hyperthermia	MAC = 2.4 B/G = 0.65

ANESTHETIC CONSIDERATIONS in SPECIFIC DISEASE SITUATIONS

	CONSIDERATIONS	ACCEPTABLE DRUGS/PROTOCOLS	DRUGS to AVOID
Cesarean Section	**Physiologic alterations:** The expanding uterus **decreases total lung capacity** so that ventilation and oxygenation during general anesthesia may be impaired, especially since the bitch will be on her back during the surgery. PCV as well as venous return may be decreased. Less anesthetic may be required. **Fetal well-being:** Fetal tissue perfusion and gas exchange are dependent upon the maternal cardiovascular system, respiratory system, and placenta. Fetal drug elimination is carried out by maternal organs. Uterine blood flow is not autoregulated, thus **maternal hypotension** can lead to fetal death. Most sympathomimetics that correct maternal hypotension decrease uterine blood flow (e.g. dopamine). Ephedrine can be used because it preserves uterine blood flow. Drugs with low molecular weight and high lipid solubility can **diffuse rapidly across the placenta**, affecting the fetuses. **First aid for newborns:** Clear the airways with towels and by swinging the neonate. Stimulate ventilation by rubbing vigorously with a towel. If the neonate fails to breathe, use **doxapram** (0.05-0.1 mL) to stimulate respiratory centers which have been depressed by barbiturate or inhalational anesthetics. It doesn't work well if the neonate is hypoxic. If opioids were used, **naloxone** (0.05-0.1 mL) can be used to reverse the effects. Neonates can be intubated and ventilated with a bulb syringe or O$_2$. If the heart stops, administer **epinephrine** (0.01-0.05 mL of 1:10,000 dilution) intravenously or **intrathoracically**. Keep neonates warm. **Post-op:** The bitch may need oxytocin to facilitate lactation and uterine involution.	Clip abdomen and perform initial scrubs prior to anesthesia. 1) **Modified inhalant:** Premedicate with an opioid and mask down with isoflurane or halothane. Use 50% N$_2$O during induction in order to speed the induction. Maintain on isoflurane or halothane and nitrous oxide. You can use a ventral midline block with 0.5-1% lidocaine at a total dose of ≤ 3-5 mg/kg. With N$_2$O, the puppies should be oxygenated for several minutes following birth. 2) IV **propofol** or IV **etomidate** works well. 3) IV **neuroleptanalgesic (dog):** Fentanyl/diazepam 4) **Epidural** with lidocaine ± morphine plus **sedation** with a neuroleptanalgesic such as oxymorphone (0.05 mg/kg) ± acepromazine (0.02 mg/kg). Use 2% lidocaine (1mL/4.5kg) epidural or (1mL/3kg) subarachnoid. 5) **Atracurium** paralysis and maintain on isoflurane or fentanyl/isoflurane. Reverse with edrophonium (pretret reversal with atropine). **Emergencies:** In emergencies, try to pre-load with fluids and pre-oxygenate. Patients with moderate to severe exhaustion don't tolerate general or regional anesthesia as well and are more likely to become hypotensive and have impaired ventilation. Sometimes a line block ± systemic analgesic sedatives are all that are required.	The following drugs result in significant neonatal depression: Barbiturates Ketamine Telazol® Xylazine You may want to avoid propofol if the bitch is already hypotensive.
Cardiac Disease	Avoid hypovolemia and hypotension: Discontinue ß blockers and ACE inhibitors the morning of surgery. Combining them with anesthetics can lead to severe hypotension. Avoid hypertension: Do not fluid overload. Avoid tachycardia: Avoid excitement during induction.	**Fentanyl/Diazepam:** Fentanyl causes only mild cardiovascular depression. **Etomidate/Diazepam** has minimal effect on heart rate, peripheral resistance, and contractility. **Ketamine/Diazepam** can be used in mitral/tricuspid regurgitation. **Acepromazine** premed can decrease catecholamine-induced arrhythmias.	Barbiturates/propofol are severe cardiovascular depressants. Avoid **atropine** unless the animal is bradycardic. Avoid **dissociatives** in cases of hypertrophic cardiomyopathy and valvular stenoses.

ANESTHETIC CONSIDERATIONS in SPECIFIC DISEASE SITUATIONS continued

	CONSIDERATIONS	ACCEPTABLE DRUGS/PROTOCOLS	DRUGS to AVOID
Diabetes	Prevent hyperglycemia, hypoglycemia, metabolic acidosis, and ketosis. Schedule the surgery for the time that the animal is at its peak insulin activity. Give 1/4–1/2 dose of insulin in the morning and then do the surgery. If you give this dose of insulin without food, most animals become hypoglycemic, so perform blood glucoses during surgery. If glucose levels drop below 120 g/dL, give dextrose or glucose by spiking the fluids (e.g. in the buretrol).		Ketamine, xylazine, and medetomidine. Xylazine and medetomidine are alpha$_2$ agonists (increase sympathetic tone) thus they are anti-insulin.
GI Disease	**GASTRIC TORSION:** Stabilize the animal. Try to decompress the stomach. Administer fluids. **Hypotension:** The enlarged stomach puts pressure on the caudal vena cava, obstructing venous return. It also puts pressure on the diaphragm, decreasing its ability to generate intrathoracic pressure, thus **lung volume is decreased.** **Cardiac arrhythmias:** PVCs can occur at any time, as can sinus or ventricular tachycardia. Treat arrhythmias > 170 bpm or arrhythmias that cause hemodynamic compensation. Treat multiform PVCs or ventricular tachycardia as they result in dramatic decreases in blood pressure. **Endotoxic shock/DIC**	Opioids produce good analgesia which results in a more stable anesthesia. Use **fentanyl/diazepam** for induction. If the animal is hypotensive on fentanyl/diazepam, use **dopamine** (5 μg/kg/min.) to increase preload, myocardial contractility (which results in increased cardiac output), and blood pressure, without decreasing peripheral perfusion. At 10–15 μg/kg/minute, you start decreasing perfusion. Have **glycopyrrolate** on hand in case of opioid-induced bradycardia. Maintain on **fentanyl/diazepam and isoflurane.** **Lidocaine** (1–4 mg/kg) for ventricular tachycardia. You may use a lidocaine constant rate infusion (CRI).	Thiopental and propofol are severe cardiac depressants.
	ENDOSCOPY (e.g. for swallowed fishhook or gastric biopsy): When the stomach is inflated, the animal may have difficulty ventilating on its own. As a result, it may get light, or it may start panting due to hypoxia. In addition, it may look like it is retching. If this occurs, deflate the stomach and evaluate the animal's stage of anesthesia. You may not need to deepen the animal; it's often easier to mechanically ventilate the animal. Endoscopy may cause vagal stimulation.	Include **atropine or glycopyrrolate** to combat vagal stimulation.	Opioids increase cardiac and pyloric sphincter tone.
	INTUSSUSCEPTION or OBSTRUCTION: **High obstruction:** More profound electrolyte imbalance (decreased HCl, Na$^+$, K$^+$). The animal is alkalotic and has decreased respiration.	Quick induction to prevent vomiting.	

Glaucoma or cataracts	The animal will be on drugs to decrease its intraocular pressure. These drugs may include mannitol, carbonic anhydrase inhibitors (cause metabolic acidosis) or lasix. The patient may be very dehydrated prior to surgery due to the medications and may be acidotic (panting). Induce mydriasis and avoid increasing intraocular pressure. The ophthalmologist may use phenylephrine to constrict vessels. This drug may induce hypertension, which can be treated with small amounts of acepromazine.	Use **Atropine** or **glycopyrrolate** premedication since the surgeon will stimulate the eye (vagostimulatory). **Meperidine** or **butorphanol** premeds are good because they don't induce vomiting (vomiting increases intraocular pressure) as do oxymorphone and morphine. **Thiopental/diazepam:** Use small doses in order to avoid hypotension. **Atracurium:** Use it to paralyze the eye so that it stays central (reverse with edrophonium and atropine).	**Ketamine** may increase intraocular pressure **Fentanyl** may cause meiosis.
Pulmonary Disease	All anesthetics are respiratory depressants. Ventilation increases as CO_2 increases, but with anesthesia, animals tolerate higher CO_2 concentrations before they increase their ventilation. Isoflurane causes more respiratory depression than halothane, and opioid induction agents in high doses cause respiratory depression. With decreased functional residual capacity (due to fluid or other abnormal contents in the thorax), the lungs become atelectic. To overcome the atelectasis, you can sigh the animal regularly, use PEEP (positive end-expiratory pressure) so the lungs don't deflate all the way, or use CPAP (continuous airway pressure). CPAP and PEEP affect O_2 but not CO_2. Use a **respirometer** (on the expiratory end of the anesthetic machine) to measure tidal volume and minute ventilation. **Blood gas:** Ventilate the animal if $pCO_2 \geq 55$ mmHg. **Pulse oximeter:** O_2 saturation should be $\geq 98\%$. **IPPV** (Intermittent Positive Pressure Ventilation): Monitor animals with pneumothorax very carefully, especially if using IPPV. Higher pCO_2s and lower tidal volumes are acceptable in these cases. With diaphragmatic hernia, you should use IPPV at lower tidal volumes since there's less intrathoracic space and a risk of re-expansion edema. **Prevent stress, especially in cats.**	Drain the thorax of air or fluid before anesthetizing. **Opioid premeds** serve as antitussives and are good for brachycephalic animals and patients with collapsing tracheas or kennel cough. **Preoxygenate** for 4 minutes (hard in brachycephalic animals), because induction is a critical period, or at least put the mask on with 100% oxygen after the initial induction. **Brachycephalic breeds:** Have gauze on a hemostat ready for clearing mucus from the throat. Use **adequate sedation** so that induction is fast. Use minimal restraint. Use **rapid-acting induction agents** in small animals such as propofol, thiopental, or etomidate. **Recovery:** Keep the animal on oxygen as long as possible. Use agents that allow rapid recovery. **Bronchoscopy:** Use injectable maintenance such as propofol. Jet ventilation can be used to ensure high enough oxygenation and adequate carbon dioxide removal.	N_2O: Avoid nitrous oxide in cases where pneumothorax may be present or where oxygenation is difficult.

ANESTHETIC CONSIDERATIONS in SPECIFIC DISEASE SITUATIONS continued

	CONSIDERATIONS	ACCEPTABLE DRUGS/PROTOCOLS	DRUGS to AVOID
Liver shunt	Prevent hypoglycemia and blood loss. The surgeon may have to shut off venous return in order to find the intrahepatic shunt. These animals have low albumin. Administer plasma if needed. Measure glucose every 15-30 minutes and give dextrose if glucose ≤ 120 g/dL. This procedure is very painful. Use analgesics (including epidural). Complications: hypoglycemia and portal hypertension.	Opioid premeds: Some animals with liver shunts have prolonged hepatic metabolism. Anticholinergics Inhalant induction is best since injectables are metabolized by the liver. The response to opioids is variable.	
Neurology	**Myelogram and disc repair:** Myelogram contrast may be seizurogenic and can increase vagal tone. Have **atropine** on hand for reactions to the contrast agent (atropine IV works very quickly whereas glycopyrrolate IV takes up to 4 min to work). Keep the head up for one hour after myelogram. Administer 0.5 mg/kg diazepam (1/4 bolus) if the animal convulses. Most contrasts are excreted via the kidneys. Make sure the animal is diuresed. Avoid increased intracranial pressure.	Thiopental and diazepam are anti-seizurogenic. Parasympatholytic premeds can help combat any bradycardia caused by the myelogram contrast.	Ketamine, acepromazine, and methohexital decrease seizure threshold. Avoid nitrous oxide if the animal is going to surgery.
Renal Disease	Anesthesia induces decreased renal blood flow, leading to decreased glomerular filtration rate, urine flow, and electrolyte excretion. Anesthetics can indirectly cause **hypotension** and changes in the endocrine system (changes in ADH, renin-angiotensin, aldosterone). Some anesthetics have a **direct nephrotoxic effect** (e.g. methoxyflurane). Don't use two nephrotoxic agents together (e.g. flunixin, an NSAID, and gentamicin, an antibiotic, are two commonly used nephrotoxic agents). **Make sure the animal is rehydrated before surgery starts** and keep it adequately hydrated during surgery. If PCV is low, you may need to crossmatch. Renal patients usually have compensated chronic anemia and depending on their PCV and the procedure, may not need to be transfused. **Hyperkalemia** is caused by the inability to excrete potassium. Monitor for hyperkalemia via ECG (bradycardia, no P wave).	**Etomidate** is the drug of choice of cats with renal failure. **Ketamine/Diazepam** maintain blood pressure but recovery may be prolonged. **Isoflurane** induction is good. **Propofol and thiopental** are okay too. **Dopamine:** 2.5-5 µg/kg/min to increase renal perfusion. Note: Cats have no dopamine receptors in the kidney, so use mannitol instead. Add dopamine if blood pressure is low. **Mannitol** (0.25-0.5 g/kg), an osmotic diuretic, can be given prior to surgery and during surgery to increase renal perfusion. We use it with kidney stones or kidney transplants. **Lasix:** a diuretic **Hyperkalemia** can be corrected by treating acidosis, giving **bicarbonate,** or administering **insulin** and **dextrose** or **calcium gluconate.**	Avoid **barbiturates** if PCV is low. In addition, the acidotic animal has more unionized barbiturate (non-protein bound); thus, these animals are more sensitive to barbiturates. Cats with renal disease have prolonged recovery when on **dissociatives.** Propofol is very hypotensive.

ANALGESIA
Preoperative Pain Management
Pain Control During Surgery
Local Anesthetic Techniques

Any animal undergoing surgery is likely to have post-operative pain because tissue damage triggers nociceptors, resulting in pain. It is best to prevent the animal from waking up in pain rather than treating for pain after it occurs. If the animal wakes up in pain, it will release norepinephrine (increased sympathetic tone) in the painful areas. Consequently, higher doses of analgesics will be needed to control the pain. In general, analgesics should be used in any surgery known to be painful in humans.

I. **PREOPERATIVE TREATMENT OF PAIN: Controlling pain prior to and during surgery:** In the absence of analgesia, build-up of neuronal pain input (termed wind-up) leads to anesthesia that is less smooth. Additionally, the animal is more sensitive to pain post-operatively than it would have been if it had received analgesics during surgery.
    A. **Reasons for preoperative analgesia**
        1. Smoother surgical plane and smoother recovery with less pain.
    B. **Preoperative management of pain**
        1. **Allay anxiety** in the animal via management and drugs: Administer anxiolytics if needed, and try to accustom the animal to the surroundings.
        2. **NSAIDS** decrease tissue inflammation. Drugs with significant COX-1 activity should not be used prior to surgery due to alterations in platelet function (increased bleeding). Drugs with predominantly COX-2 activity (e.g. carprofen, meloxicam, firocoxib, and deracoxib) do not appear to alter coagulation.
        3. **Opioid analgesics** provide sedation and good analgesia.
        4. **Alpha-2 agonists** such as xylazine and medetomidine have an analgesic effect.
        5. **Local anesthetic agents:** Bupivacaine is longer-acting than lidocaine.

II. **PAIN CONTROL DURING SURGERY:**
    A. **LOCAL TECHNIQUES** involve using local anesthetics at the surgical site. Lidocaine and bupivacaine block both sensory and motor impulses, whereas opioids bind to opioid receptors.
        1. **Epidural injections** reduce pain in the hind limbs and abdomen and are good for surgeries such as total hip replacements, cruciate ruptures, triple pelvic osteotomies, and abdominal mass removals.
        2. Specific nerve blocks
    B. **SYSTEMIC ANALGESICS** include fentanyl infusion or repeated administration of oxymorphone or other opioids. Oxymorphone can be administered every 3 hours.
    C. **POST-OPERATIVE:** Try to prevent sympathetic discharge by preventing the animal from waking up in pain.
        1. Analgesics fall into **3 categories:**
            a. **Opioids** (Morphine, methadone, oxymorphone, etc.): Opioids mimic naturally occurring peptide substances called endorphins.
                i. Morphine and fentanyl are μ agonists. Butorphanol is a competitive μ receptor antagonist but still exerts a weak analgesic effect due to its actions at the kappa receptor. Naloxone and naltrexone are antagonists and serve to reverse the effects of the μ agonists.

Opioid	Mu (μ)	Delta	Kappa
Morphine	+++		+
Fentanyl	+++		
Butorphanol	--		++
Buprenorphine	Partial agonist		--
Naloxone	---	-	--
Naltrexone	---	-	--
Opioid	**Mu (μ)**	**Delta**	**Kappa**
Agonists mediate the following	Hypothermia Analgesia Miosis (mydriasis in cats) Bradycardia Euphoria Respiratory depression GI stasis		Good sedation Weak analgesia Dysphoria

It can be difficult to distinguish pain from dysphoria. If the animal is bothered primarily when touched in a specific area (such as the surgery site), its behavior is most likely due to pain. If it reacts when touched anywhere, the behavior is more likely due to dysphoria.

b. **Non-steroidal anti-inflammatories** such as carprofen, ketoprofen and aspirin can provide analgesia.

c. **Alpha-2 antagonists** such as xylazine and medetomidine provide analgesia.

2. **Administer an analgesic before the animal wakes up.** Opioids are okay for management because they **only reduce dull pain**, so if the nonpainful animal tries to run around, it will still feel sharp pain, and thus limit its movement. Opioids are less likely to cause respiratory depression when used at analgesic doses and when used in an animal that is experiencing pain.

3. **Let the animal wake up slowly.** The goal following a painful surgery is to keep the animal sleeping/resting for 12 hours. You may need to administer a tranquilizer post-operatively to achieve this goal.

4. **FENTANYL PATCH:** (Duragesic®, Janssen Pharmaceutica, Titusville, NJ). Apply the patch to the lateral thorax or back of the dog or cat's neck 12-24 hours prior to surgery and cover it with a bandage to prevent it from falling off and being ingested. Each patch contains about 5 mg of fentanyl so ingestion may lead to intoxication— however, since much of the fentanyl is metabolized by the liver before it reaches the central circulation, risk of toxicity on ingestion is low. The patch can be left on for a total of three days. Since it's a schedule II narcotic, you may elect to remove it prior to sending the animal home.

ANIMAL SIZE	SIZE FENTANYL PATCH
Cats and toy dogs (2-10 kg)	25 µg/hr
Small dogs (10-20 kg)	50 µg/hr
Medium dogs (20-30 kg)	75 µg/hr
Large dogs (≥ 30 kg)	100 µg/hr

III. LOCAL ANESTHETIC TECHNIQUES

> **Maximum dose per animal**
> Bupivacaine = 2 mg/kg
> Lidocaine = 8 mg/kg

A. **INTRA-ARTICULAR BLOCKS**
   1. **Elbow:** Use preservative-free morphine (1.0 mg/kg diluted to 5-6 mL with sterile saline).
   2. For **other joints,** use 0.5% bupivacaine (5.0-10.0 mL ± 0.1 mg/kg preservative-free morphine). The surgeon can bathe the joint while exploring it.

B. **Paws of the cat for declawing**
   1. **Forepaw: 0.5% bupivacaine** (0.1-0.2 mL in each site). Inject into **three** sites:

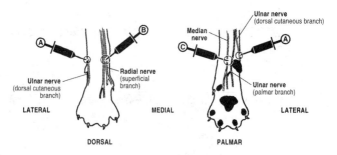

Anesthesia

    a.   **Superficial radial nerve:** Inject immediately underneath the cephalic vein as the nerve traverses the dorsal surface of the carpus.

    b.   **Dorsal cutaneous branch of the ulnar nerve:** Inject right above the pad as the nerve traverses from the plantar to dorsal surface of the paw.

    c.   **Median and ulnar nerves:** Inject on midline medial to the pad with a single injection.

C.   **FOREARM BLOCK** for procedures below the elbow. Use 0.5% bupivacaine (1 mg/kg in the medial injection site and 0.5-2.0 mL in the anterior injection site). Inject in the following locations:

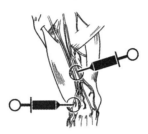

1.   **Medial, ulnar and musculocutaneous nerves:** Block with a single injection. Use a spinal needle and advance it between the triceps and biceps at a 30-45° angle to the horizontal.

2.   **Superficial radial nerves:** Identify the cephalic vein where the nerves traverse the dorsal aspect of the elbow. Insert the needle with a lateral approach and push the needle through to the other side. Inject as the needle is withdrawn.

D.   **DENTAL BLOCKS**

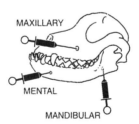

1.   **Inferior alveolar block** blocks the teeth, skin, and mucosa of the chin and lower lip. Use 0.5% bupivacaine and inject 0.5-3.0 mL (max 2 mg/kg). There are several methods for hitting this nerve.

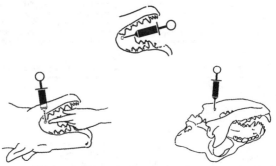

a. With the animal lying on its side or back, reach into the mouth and palpate the lingual surface of the caudal mandible until you feel the **mandibular foramen**. Then from the inside, bring the needle down beside the finger inside the mouth and inject around the nerve.

b. Alternatively, approach with the needle from the ventral aspect of the jaw by inserting through the skin, walking the needle off the ventral mandible and advancing dorsally until you reach the mandibular foramen.

2. **Mental nerve block:** This blocks the mandibular nerve to the caudal mandibular foramen. (0.5% bupivacaine: 0.3-1.0 mL; max 2 mg/kg). Use this in larger dogs. First palpate the mental foramen (ventral to PM_1 & PM_2). Insert a 26 gauge needle several mm into the foramen. Aspirate before injecting to be sure you're not injecting into a vessel.

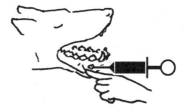

3. **Maxillary nerve block (infraorbital nerve):** This blocks the teeth and associated mucosa (also premolar and molars in cats). Inject 0.2-1.0 mL 0.5% bupivacaine (max dose = 2 mg/kg). Palpate the opening of the infraorbital canal from the inside of the mouth directly above PM_3. Insert the needle into the canal and advance caudally.

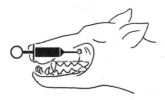

E. **Epidurals** can be used for any surgery of the caudal portion of the body including pelvic or hindlimb surgery, perianal surgery, tail amputations, and lower abdominal surgery. Epidurals should be performed on anesthetized or highly sedated animals to prevent pain during surgery. If muscle relaxation is important,

F. then the epidural should include lidocaine or bupivacaine. Bupivacaine has a longer
    duration. Both bupivacaine and lidocaine produce sympathetic block which can cause
    vasodilation and hypotension, so these animals should be on IV fluids.

Drug	Dose	Onset & Duration
Lidocaine (0.2%)	3 mg/kg	Onset: 5 minutes Duration: 60 minutes
Bupivacaine (0.5%)	2 mg/kg alone or 0.5-1.0 mg/kg when given with 0.1 mg/kg preservative-free **morphine.**	Duration: 3-4 hours
Morphine (preservative-free)	0.1 mg/kg diluted to 0.33 mL/kg in sterile saline	Duration: 24 hours
Buprenorphine	12.5 mg/kg diluted to 0.33 mL/kg with sterile saline	

Decrease by 75% if you get spinal fluid.
Maximum volume = 6 mL

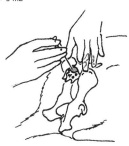

1. Inject the drug between L$_7$ and the sacral vertebrae using the wings of the
    ileum, the dorsal spinous processes of the sacral vertebrae, and the spinous
    process of L$_7$ as landmarks.
2. Insert the needle bevel forward, through a layer of skin, muscle, and ligament.
    Stop when you've gone through the ligament. If you hit bone (the dorsal
    vertebral arch), pull the needle back and then redirect either forward or
    backward.

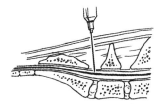

3. Next, place a glass syringe on the needle and push air into the epidural space. If
    you're in the epidural space, there should be no resistance to injection. If you
    are in muscle, you will not be able to push air in easily.
4. Inject the drug into the epidural space. Attach the syringe containing the drug
    and aspirate first. If you get blood, remove the needle and try again. If no blood
    is aspirated, inject the drug slowly (over one minute) into the epidural space. If
    you get CSF, use only 1/4 of the original amount.

MONITORING ANESTHETIC DEPTH

Animals should be monitored continuously for depth of anesthesia in order to ensure they are at an appropriate level of anesthesia for the procedure they are undergoing, and that the anesthesia is not putting them at risk for temporary or permanent physiologic damage (e.g. renal damage due to prolonged low blood pressure). Anesthetic level will need to be adjusted based on the amount of stimulation and pain associated with the segment of the procedure. For instance, the level will need to be deeper if the mesenteric root will be adjusted and lighter during the non-painful portions of the procedure.

A. **LEVEL of ANESTHESIA:** During the anesthetic process, the animal goes from an awake state (stage I) in which he responds to environmental stimuli, to the beginnings of loss of consciousness (stage II), where the CNS becomes depressed but the animal may show uncontrolled spontaneous reflex activity. Once this spontaneous motor activity ceases, the animal is in a **surgical plane** of anesthesia (Stage III)—either a light, medium, or deep plane.

> Stage 1: Awake
> Stage 2: Excitement phase (as the animal loses consciousness)
> Stage 3: Surgical level of anesthesia: Can be divided into light plane, medium
>   plane, and deep plane

B. **SIGNS of ANESTHETIC DEPTH:** A number of parameters can be used to evaluate anesthetic depth; however, some signs are more reliable than others, and multiple signs must be evaluated simultaneously to determine anesthetic depth, rather than relying on one sign alone. Note that these signs are for inhalational anesthetics and barbiturates.
    1. **Evaluate these signs first (most reliable)**
        a. **Spontaneous or purposeful movement** (excluding sporadic twitching or shivering) such as when the animal moves a leg— indicates the animal is in a light plane of anesthesia. For some surgical procedures, such a light level of anesthesia may be acceptable.
        b. **Reflex movement** such as **palpebral reflex** or leg withdrawal reflex indicates the animal is in a light plane of anesthesia. Their absence indicates a medium or deep plane of anesthesia, although some patients never show a palpebral reflex in stage III. For some surgical procedures, a light plane of anesthesia where reflex movement is seen is acceptable. Because these are reflex responses, they do not indicate pain perception. Conscious perception of pain is lost during stage II of anesthesia.
        c. **Muscle tone:** In general, the deeper the animal, the more relaxed the muscle tone. One way to evaluate muscle tone is to open the animal's mouth and estimate resistance. Some patients lose jaw tone immediately upon entering stage III of anesthesia.
        d. **Eyeball rotation:** The eyeball usually rotates ventromedially and the nictitans protrudes when the patient is in a **medium** plane of anesthesia, but it tends to go back to central position when the animal is in a light or deep plane of anesthesia.
        e. **Transient increase in heart rate, blood pressure, or respiratory rate in response to a specific surgical stimulation** such as incising the skin or pulling on the mesenteric root, indicates the animal is in a light plane of anesthesia relative to his needs at the moment. These parameters can also increase with other events such as hypoxia, hypercapnia, blood loss, etc. If these parameters increase but reflex movement, muscle tone, and eyeball rotation indicate medium or deep plane of anesthesia, this indicates the animal needs more analgesics, NOT that he is at a light plane of anesthesia.
        f. **Pupillary light response:** The pupil constricts in response to bright light when the animal is in a light or medium plane of anesthesia.

    2. **Unreliable signs: Heart rate, respiration rate, and blood pressure** should decrease with deeper anesthetic level; however they are unreliable for determining level of anesthesia. They should be measured continuously regardless, as specific actions must be taken if they are too low or too high. Additionally, change in response to specific surgical stimuli is a good indicator of anesthetic level.

1.28

> Change in heart rate, respiration rate, and blood pressure in **response to specific surgical stimuli IS** a good indicator of anesthetic level when evaluated in conjunction with change in reflexes, muscle tone, eyeball rotation, spontaneous movement, and reflexes.

    a. **Heart rate** does not reliably predict if the animal is about to experience cardiovascular collapse or wake up.

    b. **Respiration rate:** Patients often exhibit apnea during and immediately following induction until their arterial CO_2 increases above the apneic threshold, regardless of anesthetic level. Apnea also occurs with too deep levels of anesthesia. Tachypnea can occur when an animal is too light, too deep, or hypercapnic.

3. **Misleading signs:** Twitching of focal muscle groups, flaring of the nasal alae or muzzle during inspiration, and flicking of the ears (in cats) when the hairs are touched are not indicators of anesthetic level.

Monitoring Anesthetic Depth
(Inhalational anesthetics, barbiturates, and hindered phenols)

Anesthetic Level	Level Description	Spontaneous Movement	Response to Stimuli	Muscle Tone (Jaw one)	Palpebral Reflex	Pupillary Light Response (PLR)	Pupil Position	HR, RR, BP
I	Awake	+	+	+	+	+		N
II	Excitatory (start losing consciousness)	+	+	+	+	+		↑
III Surgical Level	Light	±	±	↓	+	+		N or ↑
	Medium	-	-	↓	-	±		N or ↓
	Deep	-	-	↓	-	-		↓↓

Modified from: UC Davis

Note: These signs of anesthetic depth do not pertain to ketamine or opioids. Animals in a surgical plane of anesthesia due to ketamine exhibit increased muscle tone, open eyelids, spontaneous reflexes including PLRs, and their eyeballs often remain centrally located. They may also have withdrawal reflexes even when deeply anesthetized. Opioids alone are sedatives, not anesthetic agents. A surgical level of analgesia can be reached in physiologically compromised patients, but they are not unconscious.

CARDIOVASCULAR MONITORING in THE ANESTHETIZED PATIENT
Heart Rate and Rhythm
Tissue Perfusion
Arterial Blood Pressure
Respiration

ACCEPTABLE PARAMETERS FOR THE ANESTHETIZED PATIENT

HEART RATE	BLOOD PRESSURE
Dog: 60-140 beats/minute Cat: 80-160 beats/minute	Systolic > 90 mmHg Mean > 70 mmHg

RESPIRATION
Rate: 8-10 breaths per minute Tidal Volume: 10-20 mL/kg Minute ventilation: 100-200 mL/kg per minute Inspiratory pressure in dogs: 15-20 cmH$_2$O Inspiratory pressure in cats: 10-12 cmH$_2$O Note: Measure arterial blood gases or end-tidal CO$_2$ to determine whether ventilation is adequate.

I.   **HEART RATE and RHYTHM:** The goal of the heart is to maintain the amount of blood pumped out by the left ventricle per minute (cardiac output). Cardiac output is affected by stroke volume (the amount of blood ejected with each ventricular contraction) and heart rate. Stroke volume, in turn, is determined by **cardiac contractility** (how forcefully the heart contracts), **preload** (the end-diastolic volume of the ventricle), and **afterload** (the systemic resistance against which the heart must pump blood). (Refer to the section on cardiac physiology, p. 3.2 for more information). During anesthesia, the ability to regulate these functions may be compromised.

EQUIPMENT FOR MEASURING HEART RATE and RHYTHM
Esophageal stethoscope: Allows monitoring of breath sounds in addition to HR and rhythm. **Doppler or oscillometric blood pressure monitors:** All anesthetized animals should have their blood pressure monitored. **Pulse Oximeter:** Estimates the arterial oxygenated hemoglobin as well as indicating heart rate. **EKG:** Use this in patients on anesthetic agents that potentiate catecholamine-induced arrhythmias, and in patients with diseases that cause arrhythmias (e.g. gastric dilatation-volvulus, myocardial trauma, dilated cardiomyopathy, electrolyte imbalances).

A.   **HEART RATE**
1.   **Tachycardia:** Tachycardia shortens ventricular filling time and consequently decreases preload, resulting in inadequate coronary perfusion which is followed by inadequate systemic vascular perfusion

CAUSES of TACHYCARDIA DURING ANESTHESIA
• **Light plane of anesthesia:** If the animal is not at the appropriate plane of anesthesia, it may respond to surgical stimuli. • **Pain:** Animals with pathology separate from the surgical site may become tachycardic if that area is stressed (e.g. a dog with bad hip dysplasia put in dorsal recumbency with no support for the hips). • **Hypotension/hypovolemia** leads to reflex tachycardia. • **Hypoxia** or **hypercapnea** lead to reflex tachycardia. • **Anemia** leads to hypoxia and hypercapnea. • **Fever** • **Drugs** such as ketamine, catecholamines, and parasympatholytics increase heart rate.

2. **Bradycardia** can lead to decreased cardiac output if the heart is unable to compensate by contracting forcefully enough to increase stroke volume adequately.

BRADYCARDIA

CAUSES	• **Anesthetic depth:** If the animal shows signs of a deep plane of anesthesia such as lack of jaw tone, pupils rotated downwards (or central and dilated), or loss of palpebral reflex, then start decreasing the anesthetic level and monitor for changes in heart rate. • **Premedications** such as medetomidine, xylazine, and opioids as well as **medications** such as digitalis induce bradycardia. • **Vagal tone:** Check to see if the surgeon is manipulating vagal tone by, for instance, manipulating the eyeball or esophagus. • **Hypothermia:** If the animal is or has been hypothermic for a prolonged period, heart rate will remain low until the temperature is raised. • **Hypertension** leads to reflex bradycardia. • **Terminal or end-stage hypoxia:** Check the mucous membrane color and capillary refill time as well as other parameters of oxygen content. • **Myocardial disturbance:** Check the ECG for evidence of first or second degree heart block. • **Hyperkalemia:** Check the electrolyte status
TREATMENT Dog < 60 bpm Cats < 80 bpm	Treat when the heart rate falls below about 80 beats per minute in cats and 60 beats per minute in dogs. • **Decrease anesthetic level** and monitor for increase in HR. • **Atropine:** (0.02 - 0.03 mg/kg IV). Start with **0.02 mg/kg IM.** If the heart rate is decreasing rapidly, administer atropine IV. Atropine can be used for both first and second degree AV blocks. It usually doesn't work for third degree heart block, so in cases of third degree AV block, use a sympathomimetic such as dopamine (ß$_1$ effects of increasing heart rate and contractility). • **Electrocardiogram:** Run an ECG to determine whether there's first, second, or third degree AV block. • If the animal is **hypothermic,** warm it up. • Correct any electrolyte disturbance (e.g. hyperkalemia) that might be contributing to the problem. • **Dopamine:** Give 2.5 – 20 μg/kg per minute to increase cardiac output and heart rate. • **Ephedrine** can be used instead of dopamine since it causes less vasoconstriction (Ephedrine: 0.05-0.5 mg/kg IV). It lasts for 10-15 minutes. **Blood pressure:** Check the blood pressure to see if the patient is also hypotensive. The slower the heart rate, the more time blood has to run off during diastole leading to a lower diastolic pressure. As a result, mean blood pressure decreases.

B. **ARRHYTHMIAS during ANESTHESIA:** Anesthesia occasionally induces ectopic pacemaker activity; consequently, we may see premature atrial contractions (PACs), premature ventricular contractions (PVCs), and bundle branch blocks (BBB). All can lead to decreased cardiac output due to decreased heart rate (with BBB) or decreased stroke volume.

1. **Etiology and treatment**
   a. Related to **catecholamines**
      i. Some anesthetics **lower the threshold** for catecholamine-induced arrhythmias (e.g. halothane, xylazine, medetomidine, thiopental).
      ii. Exogenous **catecholamines** can induce arrhythmias.
      iii. Some illnesses predispose the patient to arrhythmias (e.g. gastric dilatation-volvulus, traumatic myocarditis, electrolyte abnormalities, dilated cardiomyopathy). Treat the underlying cause when possible and be ready to treat for the specific arrhythmias.

   b. **Light anesthetic level:** If the animal is **light**, then surgical stimuli can lead to catecholamine release which may potentiate arrhythmias.
   c. **Hypercapnia and hypoxia** can lead to coronary damage and consequently to arrhythmias.
      i. If the animal is **too deep** it may become hypercapnic or hypoxic.
   d. **Hypovolemia** or hypotension

   e. **Electrolyte imbalance**
      i. **Hypokalemia** often leads to tall T waves (the same as hypoxia). Respiratory or metabolic alkalosis as well as glucose/insulin therapy potentiate hypokalemia. Alkalosis leads to higher potassium excretion whereas insulin and glucose draw the potassium intracellularly.
      ii. **Hyperkalemia** can cause arrhythmias (bradycardia) and is potentiated by acidosis and hypocalcemia.
      iii. **Hypercalcemia** can cause arrhythmias and is potentiated by respiratory or metabolic acidosis.

HANDLING ARRHYTHMIAS in the ANESTHETIZED PATIENT

- Check the anesthetic level and adjust by increasing the vaporizer setting if the animal is too light or decreasing the vaporizer setting if the patient is too deep.

- Check the oxygen supply and improve ventilation if the animal is hypoxic or hypercapnic. Use a ventilator if needed.

- Begin rapid fluid administration in order to improve cardiac output.

- Eliminate other obvious causes such as electrolyte disorders, acid base status, and anesthetic agents that might decrease the threshold for arrhythmias.

- Treat premature ventricular contractions if they are increasing in frequency, if they are multifocal, or when heart rate exceeds 180-200 beats per minute (dogs).
  - Lidocaine: 1-5 mg/kg IV
  - Procainamide: 1-5 mg/kg IV
  - Esmolol: 0.1-0.5 mg/kg IV
  - Propranolol: 0.05-0.3 mg/kg IV
  - Verapamil: 0.05-0.15 mg/kg IV

II. **TISSUE PERFUSION** (how well blood is delivered to the tissues) can be monitored by examining arterial pulses, capillary refill time, and color of the mucous membranes and viscera.
   A. **PULSE PRESSURE:** Pulse quality or pressure is determined by the difference between systolic and diastolic blood pressure. It is a function of stroke volume and systemic arterial resistance. **Weak pulses indicate poor tissue perfusion.**

WEAK PULSES	BOUNDING PULSES
Weak pulses occur when stroke volume is decreased as occurs when systolic pressure drops or diastolic pressure increases. • **Hypovolemia** leads to decreased preload. • **Arrhythmias** can lead to poor ventricular filling and consequently decrease preload. • **Ventricular failure:** The heart can't contract in order to eject blood from the heart. • **Pericardial disease or effusion** leads to both decreased cardiac contractility and decreased preload. • **Increased systemic vascular resistance** or subaortic stenosis	Anything that increases the systolic pressure or decreases diastolic pressure can lead to bounding pulses. **Decreased diastolic pressure** is commonly due to states where there's excessive arterial run-off such as with: • Vasodilation • Patent ductus arteriosus or other arteriovenous fistula • Aortic insufficiency **Increased systolic pressure** is commonly associated with high output states (strong contractions) such as: • Anemia • Excitement • Hyperthyroidism

B. **CAPILLARY REFILL TIME (CRT)** is determined by applying pressure with a fingertip to the oral mucosa or gums until it turns white, which indicates that blood's been forced from the tissue (blanching). Then remove the pressure and note the time needed for normal color to return. Normal capillary refill time is 1-2 seconds. Measuring CRT provides information about tissue perfusion and vasomotor tone.
   1. **Prolonged capillary refill time** is caused by **peripheral vasoconstriction**. Such vasoconstriction occurs in response to hypotension and decreased cardiac output. Etiologies of prolonged CRT include:
      a. **Hypovolemia** can occur with blood loss leading to hypotension.
      b. **Anesthesia:** Deep anesthesia can depress the vasomotor center leading to vasomotor collapse and consequently severe decrease in cardiac output.
      c. **Hypothermia** can lead to bradycardia and subsequently decreased cardiac output.
      d. **Alpha-2 agonists** decrease cardiac output causing peripheral vasoconstriction.
   2. **Shortened capillary refill time** may be caused by peripheral vasodilation or hyperperfusion. Vasodilation occurs in some forms of shock such as anaphylactic shock, reperfusion injury, etc. Vasodilation carries with it a worse prognosis. (Refer to the Emergency section on shock p. 8.5).

C. **MUCOUS MEMBRANE COLOR:** Evaluate the color of the mucous membranes.
   1. **Cyanosis** is when the arterial blood is bluish in color due to relatively high amounts of deoxygenated hemoglobin; thus, it is a measure of low oxygen content in the blood. In humans, cyanosis occurs once the patient has about 1.5g of deoxygenated hemoglobin. Anemic animals may be hypoxemic but not cyanotic if they don't have enough deoxygenated hemoglobin mass. Conversely, animals with **polycythemia vera** may look cyanotic even at normal blood oxygen levels. During anesthesia, low blood oxygen can occur due to poor delivery of oxygen to the animal or due to poor diffusion of the delivered oxygen from the lungs to the blood.
      a. **Poor oxygen delivery to the patient:** Check the machine and oxygen delivery tubing to the patient.
      b. **Poor oxygen delivery from lungs to blood** can occur with:
         i. **Primary lung disease** where there's an increased physiologic dead space due to decreased alveolar surface area.
         ii. It can also occur due to decreased vascular perfusion of the lungs (a.k.a. shunting) where the vessels may be vasoconstricted or don't reach the alveoli and thus don't receive oxygen, or when there's a right-to-left vascular shunt so that venous blood gets shunted past the lungs back to the body as with a right-to-left PDA.
   2. **Pale mucous membranes** are caused by decreased cardiac output, anemia, or peripheal vasoconstriction (as occurs with increased sympathetic tone when animals are nervous, in pain, or in shock).
   3. **Extremely red mucous membranes:** Injected mucous membranes may indicate polycythemia, hypercapnia, conditions inducing hyperdynamic states, or vasodilative shock.

III. ARTERIAL BLOOD PRESSURE is an estimate of cardiac output and tissue perfusion. It is a product of both cardiac output and vascular resistance. It's important to maintain arterial blood pressure since significant drops in pressure can lead to inadequate cerebral, renal, and coronary perfusion. With minor to moderate hypotension, the sympathetic nervous system **responds by vasoconstriction** of arterioles to maintain systemic resistance, **venous constriction** to maintain preload, and **increased cardiac contractility.**

A. ETIOLOGY and TREATMENT of HYPOTENSION

ETIOLOGY	• **Anesthetic depth:** Animal is too deep • **Anesthetic agents:** All anesthetic agents cause respiratory and cardiovascular depression but some such as thiopental and propofol cause more depression. Acepromazine may cause hypotension when there is sympathetic tone, such as in the trauma patient, by causing α_1 **blockade.** • **Hypovolemia** may result from blood loss, dehydration, anaphylaxis, sepsis, etc. • **Hypothermia**
TREATMENT Treat in dogs and cats when **diastolic** pressure is $\leq$ 80mmHg or **mean** blood pressure is $\leq$ 60mmHg	• **Decrease the anesthetics** and evaluate for anesthetic depth. Also make sure the patient is not hypothermic. • **Fluid bolus:** Administer a crystalloid fluid bolus of 20 mL/kg rapidly. • If the first two steps are ineffective, administer **dopamine** (10-15 μg/kg/minute). Dopamine is a positive inotrope (Refer to p. 1.26 for more info on dopamine). • **Dobutamine** can be administered in place of dopamine. It is a better β_1 stimulator (increases heart rate and contractility) than dopamine and has a wider margin of safety. That is, we get a wider margin of safety with a positive inotropic effect without tachycardia. It may increase cardiac output significantly without increasing blood pressure very much due to a reduction in systemic vascular resistance. • **Ephedrine** is another sympathomimetic.that can be used. • Reserve **epinephrine** for cardiac arrest or impending cardiac arrest. Start with 5 μg/kg intravenously (Refer to Emergency section p. 3.2). • **Phenylephrine** is a pure α_1 agonist that will increase blood pressure but may decrease perfusion. It is used to increase blood pressure in cases with dynamic outflow obstructions from the heart and in animals with right-to-left shunts. It helps increase pressures on the left side so that less blood is shunted right-to-left.

B. NON-INVASIVE METHODS for MEASURING ARTERIAL BLOOD PRESSURE

1. **Ultrasonic Doppler device** measures systolic blood pressure. A probe is placed over a peripheral pulse (usually over the dorsal pedal or radial artery) and an inflatable blood pressure cuff is placed on the extremity proximal to the probe. The probe contains two piezoelectric crystals—one emits ultrasonic waves and the other acts as a receiver. Moving red blood cells alter the pitch of the ultrasound. When the cuff is inflated, blood flow to the distal limb stops, consequently the ultrasonic sound stops. The cuff is then gradually deflated until you hear the pulse (first blood passing through). It's important to use a cuff with a width approximately 40% of the circumference of the leg. If it's too small, you'll need higher pressure to occlude the artery, leading to falsely elevated systolic blood pressure measurement. If the cuff is too wide, the blood pressure measurement will be falsely low.

2. **Oscillometric blood pressure monitors** automatically measure systolic, mean, and diastolic blood pressures repeatedly at a constant rate which can be adjusted. One advantage to this system is that it measures **mean blood pressure** which is a better estimate of perfusion through the capillary beds than systolic or diastolic pressures. The pulse pressure generated by systolic and diastolic pressure can be damped out by vascular resistance and compliance. When using an oscillometric device, set it to cycle every 2.5-3 minutes or less frequently. More frequent cycling, such as every minute, may lead to tissue hypoxia and ischemia. When cycling every minute, the cuff is inflated 75% of the time.

RESPIRATORY MONITORING and BLOOD GAS MEASUREMENTS
Gas Exchange and Acid Base Regulation
Blood Gas Measurements and Ventilation
Pulse Oximetry
End-tidal CO_2

I. **GAS EXCHANGE AND ACID-BASE REGULATION:** The lungs are important in gas exchange as well as acid-base regulation.

A. **GAS EXCHANGE:** Air is inhaled through the trachea and conducting airways into the lung **alveoli**. Once in the alveoli, oxygen is absorbed into the circulation and exchanged with carbon dioxide, which is blown off during exhalation.

1. The volume of air that's inhaled and exhaled with each breath is the **tidal volume**. Normal tidal volume is **10-20 mL/kg**. The total volume of air that enters the lungs per minute is the **minute ventilation**. Not all of this air participates in gas exchange. Much of it only makes it to the conducting airways (trachea and bronchi) which are not involved in gas exchange. This volume of wasted air is called **dead space**.

2. A more accurate description of the air available for gas exchange is **alveolar ventilation**, the air that reaches the alveoli. Because a fixed amount of air is used in the dead space, increased breathing depth is more effective in increasing alveolar ventilation than increased breathing rate. One implication is that an anesthetized animal with a shallow, fast respiratory character may be ventilating less than one with a slower rate but greater tidal volume. A second important point is that animals should be sighed while they are under anesthesia in order to maximize the number of alveoli available for gas exchange.

a. **Sighing an animal:** Anesthetized animals should be sighed once every 10 minutes in order to inflate the atelectic alveoli. Inflate to a pressure of 10 – 20 cmH2O (10-12 cmH2O in cats). Do not overinflate. Overinflation may damage the lungs resulting in pneumothorax. Additionally, because lung inflation hinders venous return, when you ventilate the patient, apply pressure on the bag for the duration of a normal inspiration. That is, avoid maintaining pressure on the bag for an extended period of time.

B. **Regulation of Ventilation:** Alveolar ventilation is regulated by carbon dioxide levels, pH, and oxygen, with carbon dioxide levels being the most potent regulator.

$$CO_2 + H_2O \rightleftharpoons H_2CO_3 \rightleftharpoons H^+ + HCO_3$$

Lung   Kidney takes care of this

1. **When arterial carbon dioxide levels are elevated** (e.g. with exercise), the respiratory centers are stimulated to increase alveolar respiration (hyperventilation) so that excess carbon dioxide can be blown off. If excess carbon dioxide isn't blown off, it combines with water in the blood to form carbonic acid, which breaks down to bicarbonate and hydrogen ions. The more carbon dioxide in the blood, the higher the hydrogen ion content and the lower the pH. Thus, the animal becomes acidotic (pH decreases).

2. **Conversely, when carbon dioxide is low,** the respiratory centers respond by decreasing alveolar ventilation so that less carbon dioxide is blown off. Low carbon dioxide drives the above reaction to the left. As a result, hydrogen ion concentration falls and the blood becomes more alkaline (pH increases).

C. **ACID-BASE REGULATION:** The body tries to maintain blood pH between 7.35-7.45. pH above or below these values leads to enzyme denaturation which ultimately leads to shutdown of cellular activities and consequently cell death. The respiratory and renal systems work in concert to regulate pH. That is, when over or under-ventilation leads to acid-base imbalance, the kidneys compensate by excreting or retaining compensatory amounts of H^+ and bicarbonate. Conversely, when pH is acidic or alkaline due to imbalances of H^+ and bicarbonate, the animal responds with a reflex compensatory change in respiration.

COMPENSATORY MECHANISMS of ACID-BASE IMBALANCES

PROBLEM	ETIOLOGIES	COMPENSATORY MECH.
Respiratory Acidosis: The pH of the blood is acidotic due to accumulation of carbon dioxide (hypercapnia) in the blood as a result of inadequate ventilation.	• **Insufficient neural drive for ventilation** (e.g. anesthetics, CNS disease) • **Airway obstruction** • **Pulmonary disease** • Disease **restricting lung inflation** (e.g. abdominal bloat, pleural effusion)	The kidneys compensate by excreting more H^+ in the urine and reabsorbing more HCO_3^-. This mechanism takes a few days.
Respiratory Alkalosis: The pH of the blood is alkaline due to low CO_2 levels as a result of over ventilation.	• Alveolar hyperventilation • Anxiety • Stimulation of the respiratory centers (e.g. toxic ingestion, fever, meningitis)	The kidneys compensate by retaining H^+ and by excreting HCO_3^- in the urine so that blood HCO_3^- falls. This mechanism takes a few days.
Metabolic Acidosis: The pH is low due to a gain in acid (other than H_2CO_3)or loss of bicarbonate.	• **Renal failure:** HCO_3^- is not excreted. • **Diabetes mellitus** with ketone bodies (weak acids) • **Inadequate circulation** (e.g. cardiac disease) leads to tissue hypoxia and anaerobic metabolism which produces the weak acid, lactic acid. • **Heavy exercise** produces lactic acid. • Loss of HCO_3^- from **diarrhea** (alkaline intestinal fluids)	The Respiratory system compensates in the acute situation within minutes to hours by increasing ventilation. With severe chronic metabolic acidosis (e.g. ketoacidosis), animals may develop deep, labored breathing (Kussmaul breathing). **Renal compensation:** If the original cause of acidosis is not due to renal insufficiency, the kidneys respond by increased H^+ excretion and increased resorption of HCO_3^-· This takes a few days.
Metabolic alkalosis: The pH is high due to gain in HCO_3^-or loss in H^+.	• **Iatrogenic:** Ingestion or administration of HCO_3^- • **Vomiting:** Vomit that is primarily from the stomach (e.g. pyloric obstruction or high duodenal obstruction) is acidic.	**Compensation:** Not much respiratory compensation. It would lead to decreased PO_2. **Renal:** Increased HCO_3^- excretion and increased H^+ resorption occur.

II. **BLOOD GAS MEASUREMENTS:** Is ventilation good enough?

RESPIRATION
Rate: 8-15 breaths per minute
Tidal Volume: 10-20 mL/kg
Minute ventilation: 100-200 ml/kg per minute

A respirometer can be used to evaluate tidal volume and minute ventilation. To determine whether ventilation is adequate and gases are being exchanged as expected (i.e. no perfusion abnormalities), measure the blood gases from an arterial blood sample (such as from the dorsal pedal artery). When an artery is not accessible, use the lingual vein as it gives a good approximation.

A. INTERPRETING the BLOOD-GAS MEASUREMENTS:
SIGNIFICANCE OF INDIVIDUAL PARAMETERS

PARAMETER	DESCRIPTION
pH 7.35-7.45	The pH of the blood is important because at extreme pHs, enzymes and proteins become denatured and cannot function properly. Treat the animal for acidosis if the pH < 7.2 or earlier if the pH is decreasing at a constant rate. Treat the animal for alkalosis if pH > 7.6.
$PaCO_2$ (partial pressure of arterial carbon dioxide) Dogs: normal = 37 mmHg (35-45) Cats: normal = 32 mmHg	CO_2, a soluble end product of metabolism, is made by the cells and diffuses into the blood where it is transported to the lungs and blown off. Doubling the ventilation halves the CO_2 in the blood. There are many causes of high CO_2 levels in the blood. If the animal is anesthetized, it may have an inadequate response to increased CO_2. • **Poor ventilation (hypoventilation):** Usually when cells are metabolizing faster than oxygen is being provided, the brain senses the increase in CO_2 and tells the body to ventilate more. All anesthetics decrease the brain's sensitivity to CO_2 so there must be a higher level of CO_2 in the blood in order to trigger an increase in ventilation. Opioids and barbiturates are strong respiratory depressants. • **Ventilation-perfusion mismatch** occurs when the air gets to the alveoli but can't be absorbed efficiently into the circulation. The animal is able to compensate to some extent. As the $PaCO_2$ (partial pressure of CO_2 in the arteries) increases, the chemoreceptors generally sense the change and increase ventilation so that the $PaCO_2$ decreases to close to normal. With ventilation-perfusion mismatch, the end-tidal CO_2 values are usually much lower than $PaCO_2$, because the arteries carry deoxygenated, high CO_2 blood but can't transfer the CO_2 efficiently into the alveoli to be expired
PaO_2 (partial pressure of oxygen in arteries) Normal = 5x inspired O_2	PaO_2: Arterial O_2 tells how well the lungs are picking up oxygen. The partial pressure of arterial oxygen is about 5x the inspired concentration of oxygen. Since room air is 21% oxygen, the arterial O_2 should be 105 mmHg when breathing room air. When breathing 100% oxygen (e.g. under anesthesia), the arterial O_2 theoretically should be around 500 mmHg. If the pressure of O_2 in the arteries is **less than 80 mmHg**, the animal is **hypoxemic**. An animal can have adequate PaO_2 but a low red blood cell volume leading to tissue hypoxia.
HCO_3^- Normal = 24 meq/L (21-27meq/L)	HCO_3^-: An increase in bicarbonate causes an increase in pH. Abnormal bicarbonate levels indicate a metabolic problem or uncompensated respiratory problem. For example, in cardiac arrest the animal develops increased amounts of lactic acid. The excess acid reacts with the bicarbonate resulting in a decrease in bicarbonate levels. Abnormally high bicarbonate is most commonly caused by gastric outflow obstruction and the associated vomiting of acidic vomit.
Base deficit Normal = 2meq/L	Base deficit is the amount of buffer needed to correct the pH to 7.4 when the $PaCO_2$ has been adjusted to 40 mmHg. If HCO_3 decreases from 24 to 19, then the animal has an actual base excess (ABE) of -5. The standard base excess (SBE) is the base excess standardized to a CO_2 of 40mmHg. Treat for acidosis when the standard base excess (SBE) is $\geq$ -10 meq/L or if it is expected that BE will continue to decrease (e.g. low cardiac output state).

BLOOD-GAS PARAMETER	DEFINITIONS
pH	< 7.35 = acidosis > 7.45 = alkalosis
$PaCO_2$	> 45 mmHg = **hypercapnia.** This indicates hypoventilation. < 35 mmHg = **hypocapnia.** This indicates hyperventilation.
PaO_2	< 80 mmHg = **hypoxemia**

B. **INTERPRETATION and TREATMENT of PATIENTS with ABNORMAL BLOOD-GAS MEASURMENTS**

1. **First look at the pH** and determine whether the animal is acidotic or alkalotic. Next determine whether the pH imbalance is due to the respiratory system or whether it's metabolic by evaluating arterial $PaCO_2$ and base excess.

2. **Evaluate arterial $PaCO_2$** to determine ventilatory status. An elevated arterial $PaCO_2$ indicates that the animal is **hypoventilating** and if the pH indicates acidosis, then the animal has a **respiratory acidosis.** Increase the minute ventilation and use mechanical ventilation if needed to correct the hypoventilation. Hypocapnia on the other hand indicates that the patient has been **hyperventilating** and if the pH is alkalotic, the animal has a **respiratory alkalosis.**

3. **Evaluate base excess:** If it's low and the pH is low, then the animal has **metabolic acidosis.** If it's high and the pH is high, then the animal has a **metabolic alkalosis.**

4. Next, in cases where both HCO_3 and $PaCO_2$ levels are abnormal, **determine which problem is primary and which is a compensatory mechanism.** In **compensatory states,** the $PaCO_2$ (ventilation status) and BE (metabolic status) should be abnormal but in different directions. For instance, if the pH is acidotic and it's acidotic due to metabolic reasons (BE is low), the respiratory system should respond by hyperventilating, leading to a higher than normal pCO_2 (respiratory alkalosis). Note that under anesthesia, animals can't respond well by hyperventilation because anesthesia often depresses the respiratory response. Also, note that metabolic **compensatory mechanisms bring the pH back towards normal but the compensation** is never complete. If the pH returns to normal or overshoots into the opposite range, consider a secondary disturbance.

   a. **Sample case 1:** A dog has a pH of 7.3, $PaCO_2$ of 30 mmHg, HCO_3 of 17 meq/L, and an actual base excess (ABE) of −7 meq/L. What's your interpretation?

BLOOD-GAS MEASUREMENT	INTERPRETATION
pH = 7.3	Acidosis
$PaCO_2$ = 30 mmHg	Respiratory alkalosis (hyperventilation)
HCO_3 = -17 meq/L	Metabolic acidosis
ABE = -7 meq/L	Metabolic acidosis

   The dog has a primary metabolic acidosis and the respiratory system is responding by hyperventilating, leading to respiratory alkalosis. Consequently there's minimal change in pH.

   b. **Sample case 2:** A dog given opioid induction has a pH of 7.1, $PaCO_2$ of 60 mmHg, HCO_3 of 14 meq/L, and actual base deficit of −10 meq/L.

BLOOD-GAS MEASUREMENT	INTERPRETATION
pH = 7.1	Acidotic
CO_2 = 60 mmHg	Respiratory acidosis (hypoventilation)
HCO_3 = 14 meq/L	Metabolic acidosis
ABE = -10 meq/L	Metabolic acidosis

This animal has a primary metabolic acidosis and the respiratory system is not compensating with hyperventilation because the opioid induction has caused respiratory depression. Treat by increasing the dog's ventilation and then re-measure the blood gas. If this doesn't work, then administer bicarbonate.

In general, if the base deficit is large ($\geq$ 10 meq/L), administer HCO_3. Since some of the HCO_3 is converted to CO_2, whenever bicarbonate is administered, the animal must be well ventilated.

> 0.3 (body weight in Kg) (base excess) = mEq HCO_3 to give
> 0.5 (body weight in Kg) (base excess) = mEq HCO_3 in neonates

Administer bicarbonate slowly IV. Give 1/4 to 1/2 of the dose over 30 minutes and then recheck blood gas values. Do not overshoot the mark because it will take days for the body to get rid of the excess bicarbonate.

III. **PULSE OXIMETRY** is a noninvasive method for assessing **the percent oxygenated hemoglobin** (HbO_2) in the arteries. Tests such as blood-gas measurement and end-tidal CO_2 are more reliable and sensitive measures of ventilation and PaO_2, however, pulse oximetry is non-invasive, easy to perform, and is an appropriate monitor of oxygenation during anesthesia or in critically ill patients when the limitations are kept in consideration.
   A. **INDICATIONS FOR USE**
   1. Use in patients at risk for hypoxia.
   2. Use to see if oxygen increases with oxygen supplementation.
   3. Use when continuous information on oxygenation is needed.

   B. **HOW IT WORKS**
   1. Place the oximeter probe on the patient's tongue during surgery (or on a non-pigmented pinna or paw). The probe measures light absorption of HbO_2 compared to that of deoxygenated hemoglobin. During diastole, it measures light absorption of the background venous blood and during systole it measures the light absorption in the arteries. Then it calculates the difference in absorption at both wavelengths between diastole and systole to determine the arterial hemoglobin saturation.

LIMITATIONS of the PULSE OXIMETERS
• Background pigments such as pigmented skin (and possibly icterus and methemoglobinemia) may interfere with the readings.
• Ambient light sometimes interferes.
• Pulse pressure must be strong.

   To validate the readings, check the results against blood gas measures of PaO_2.

   3. Because pulse oximetry estimates PaO_2 by measuring HbO_2, it's important to understand the oxygen-hemoglobin dissociation curve.

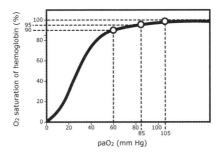

a. The oxygen-hemoglobin curve is sigmoidal— which means that at high PaO_2 values, saturation is insensitive to changes in PaO_2 whereas at lower PaO_2 levels, hemoglobin saturation is extremely sensitive to PaO_2. For instance, at PaO_2 of 80-90 mmHg, over 95% of the hemoglobin is HbO_2. That is, most is saturated with O_2. At PaO_2 of 105mmHg and above, hemoglobin is close to maximally saturated (98-100%). Notice that this means that if an animal is on 100% oxygen (which means the PaO_2 should be 500 mmHg), the Hb will be saturated and the oximeter will read 100% saturation. The patient, however, could have significant pulmonary disease such that much of the oxygen doesn't diffuse into the blood. Rather than being at 500 mmHg, the PaO_2 could be closer to 200 mmHg. At 200 mmHg, the pulse oximeter will still read at 100% saturation and thus will not detect this ventilation perfusion mismatch.

b. Note that the curve decreases more quickly at lower PaO_2 values. At 60 mmHg, the oxygen saturation is < 90%. At PaO_2 < 50 mmHg in animals with normal red blood cell counts, there's usually $\geq$ 5 g/dL of unsaturated Hb and consequently the animal is cyanotic. If the animal is polycythemic, it will become cyanotic at higher PaO_2 values, and if it's anemic, it will require lower PaO_2 levels to become cyanotic.

LIMITATIONS of the MECHANISMS
• Pulse oximetry does not provide information on acid-base status or $PaCO_2$, so we can't tell whether the animal is hypoventilated unless the animal becomes hypoxemic.
• At higher arterial PaO_2, hemoglobin is maximally saturated (100%) and consequently pulse oximetry doesn't give an estimate of arterial PaO_2. So with pulse oximetry you won't detect pulmonary disease or ventilation-perfusion mismatch until the animal becomes hypoxemic.

4. If the hemoglobin saturation falls below 90-95%, check for the following:
   a. **Mucous membrane color**
   b. **Probe placement**: If the tissues are dry or the probe has placed extended pressure on one point, the reading may be inaccurate. Reposition the probe.
   c. **Pulse quality**: If pulse quality is poor, then readings will be inaccurate. Check the blood pressure and pulse quality.
   d. **Low oxygen flow**: Check the anesthetic machine for leaks, empty O_2 tanks, and kinks in the tubing, including in the endotracheal tube.
   e. **Hypoventilation**: Evaluate tidal volume, respiratory rate, and minute ventilation.
   f. **Ventilation/perfusion mismatch**: Comparison of pulse oximetry or end-tidal CO_2 to blood gas measurements will tell if there's a ventilation perfusion-mismatch. If the inspired PO_2 is high but the arterial PaO_2 is much lower or if the end-tidal CO_2 measurement is much lower than the arterial $PaCO_2$, then there is a ventilation-perfusion mismatch. Mismatch occurs when well ventilated alveoli are poorly perfused (most common) and when perfusion is good but the alveoli are underventilated. These mismatches may be due to a variety of conditions, some of which are described in the next section.

IV. **END-TIDAL CO_2 (CAPNOGRAPHY) is a better measure of ventilation than pulse oximetry.** Capnography measures the concentration of air at the end of expiration and gives an approximation of arterial $PaCO_2$.

A. **WHY END-TIDAL MEASUREMENTS?** Expired air is a combination of dead space air (from the trachea, mouth, and nasal passages) and alveolar air. On expiration, the first air that's expired is from dead space where no gas exchange occurs, so the air is similar in composition to the air that's inspired. It isn't until the end of expiration that the air is a true representation of the air that's undergone gas exchange with the arteries—that is, alveolar air. Mid-stream expiratory air samples are a mixture of alveolar air and dead-space air. Consequently, mid-stream samples underestimate $PaCO_2$ and overestimate PaO_2 of the arteries.

1. Theoretically, with 100% diffusion of gases between the arteries and the alveoli, the end tidal CO_2 should be the same as the arterial CO_2. Generally there is a gap between the two of about 2-5 mmHg due to intrapulmonary or anatomic dead space and consequent inefficient diffusion of CO_2 from the arteries into the alveoli. Thus the end-tidal PCO_2 is lower than the arterial $PaCO_2$.

Anesthesia

2. While **end-tidal** CO_2 approximates $PaCO_2$, in some forms of ventilation-perfusion mismatch, end-tidal PCO_2 is much lower than $PaCO_2$.

B. **VENTILATION PERFUSION MISMATCH** occurs when capillary blood flows through regions where alveoli are poorly ventilated or when well-ventilated alveoli are poorly perfused by capillaries. These both lead to mismatch between expected arterial PO_2 (5 x inspired PO_2) and the actual PO_2 which often leads to hypoxemia. Ventilation perfusion mismatch is the most common cause of arterial hypoxemia in pulmonary diseases.

1. **Mismatches involving normal ventilation but low perfusion** lead to a low end-tidal PCO_2 that underestimates arterial $PaCO_2$. The gap between $ETCO_2$ and $PaCO_2$ is larger than normal.
   a. This type of mismatch is caused by increased **physiologic dead space**. The respiratory system is comprised of alveoli where gas exchange with the blood occurs and non-conducting regions such as the trachea and nasal passages where gas exchange does not occur. The non-conducting portions are referred to as **anatomic dead space**. Additionally, some portions of the **conducting zone** may conduct air but the air cannot diffuse because there is either no perfusion or there is an obstruction to diffusion (e.g. thickened membranes). The sum off all of the lung volume that does not eliminate CO_2 is called **physiologic dead space**. It includes the anatomic dead space as well as that volume of the lungs where gas exchange is impaired in spite of good ventilation. The ventilation is said to be **wasted ventilation**.
   b. The end tidal PCO_2 underestimates the amount of hypercapnia in the arteries because the CO_2 from the arteries does not diffuse into the alveoli well. Most pulmonary diseases leading to hypoxia involve physiologic dead space ventilation-perfusion mismatches.
   c. Note: Increased gap between end-tidal CO_2 and $PaCO_2$ also results from low respiratory tidal volumes which lead to incomplete alveolar emptying.

ETIOLOGY of NORMAL VENTILATION, LOW PERFUSION MISMATCH

Barriers to Diffusion
- Pulmonary edema in the interstitial spaces
- Fibrosis of the connective tissue of the lungs

Decrease in pulmonary forward blood flow/cardiac output
- Hypotension
- Bradycardia
- Pulmonary thromboembolism
- Shock
- Vasoconstriction
- **Positive pressure ventilation**: High inspiratory pressures and long inspiratory phases decrease venous return to the lungs.

---

2. Mismatches involving **low ventilation and normal perfusion: This type of mismatch**, termed **shunt**, occurs when there's air trapped in the alveoli so that the alveoli empty slowly. This allows more time for the gases between the vessels and alveoli to equilibrate. Thus, $ETCO_2$ is closer to the arterial PCO_2. That is, the gap between $ETCO_2$ and PCO_2 will be normal to decreased. The animal will be hypoxic but $ETCO_2$ will be normal. This type of mismatch is not common. It may occur with atelectasis, mucous plugs, or pulmonary secretions.

C. **Uses for $ETCO_2$ and Interpretation:** $ETCO_2$ is useful for monitoring anesthesia and monitoring response to cardiac resuscitation. $ETCO_2$ is a faster indicator of change than blood gases.
1. Sudden increase in $ETCO_2$ = not ventilating well (hypoventilation). Sudden decrease in $ETCO_2$ = no perfusion or gas exchange.
2. In respiratory arrest, CO_2 initially increases due to CO_2 accumulation.

3. Most capnographs also give a value for inspired CO_2 which gives a good indication of changes in deadspace. A stuck valve on a circle system or an exhausted soda lime canister will both give significant increases in inspired CO_2.

DOPAMINE

Dopamine works at three receptors: **dopaminergic** receptors (located in the kidneys and gut), **ß$_1$ receptors**, and indirectly on **α$_1$ receptors**. Since it works at several receptors, it has a **dose responsive effect.**

DOPAMINE'S DOSE RESPONSIVE ACTIONS

	LOW DOSE	MEDIUM DOSE	HIGH DOSE
DOSE	2-3 µg/kg/min.	5-15 µg/kg/min.	15-20 µg/kg/min.
ACTION	Works at **dopaminergic** receptors to increase renal and gut circulation by causing vasodilation.	Works at **dopaminergic** plus at the ß$_1$ **receptors** which increase cardiac contractility (positive inotrope) resulting in increased cardiac output.	Works at **dopaminergic receptors, ß$_1$ receptors,** and also at the α$_1$ **receptors** leading to vasoconstriction. When α$_1$ receptors are activated, they override the dopaminergic receptors thereby decreasing renal and gut perfusion.
WHEN to USE	Use this dose to increase renal perfusion in dogs with evidence of renal compromise (elevated BUN and creatinine). You can also use it in older animals with high-normal BUN and/or creatinine. Anesthetics usually cause mild hypotension leading to decreased renal perfusion. The goal of dopamine administration is to compensate for this effect.	Use the moderate dose in hypotensive animals where decreasing anesthetic and increasing fluid administration haven't controlled the hypotension. In these cases, we are aiming for the ß$_1$ effect (increased cardiac output). The goal is to keep **systolic blood pressure above 80 mmHg.** It's good to have dopamine on hand for cat anesthesia since their blood pressure often drops below 80 mmHg.	High doses are reserved for animals in shock or with marked vasodilation. For example, epidurals can cause hypotension due to α$_1$ blockade. High doses of dopamine stimulate release of norepinephrine which binds to α$_1$receptors and counteracts this effect. In humans, dopamine is used to treat hypotension associated with sepsis.

DETERMINING DOPAMINE INFUSION RATES: A QUICK-&-DIRTY METHOD

AMOUNT OF DOPAMINE to add to 250 mLs 0.9% NaCl	CONVERSION FACTOR to get 5µg/kg/min	CONVERSION FACTOR to get 10µg/kg/min
100 mg dopamine (2.5 mLs)	0.75 x BW(kg) = mL/hr	Multiply the 5µg/kg/min amount by 2
50 mg dopamine (1.25 mLs)	1.5 x BW(kg) = mL/hr	
25 mg dopamine (0.63 mLs)	3.0 x BW(kg) = mL/hr	

1. **Example:** If a 30kg dog has renal insufficiency and you want to infuse dopamine at a rate of 5.0µg/kg/min, mix 100 mg dopamine in 250 mls of 0.9% saline. The equation for determining mLs/hr (0.75 x 30 kg) gives a rate of 22.5 mLs/hr. So if we want to give this dog 5µg/kg/min of dopamine, we should administer the dopamine at 22.5 mL/hr.
   a. If we want to give the dog 2.5µg/kg/hr, we could give the dopamine at half this rate, which is about 11.25 mL/hr.

2. **Don't administer dopamine with an alkaline solution** because the alkaline solution will inactivate the dopamine.

THE ANESTHESIA MACHINE

I. **THE ANESTHESIA MACHINE:** Anesthesia machines can be divided into circle systems, where the path of gas flows in a circle, and non-rebreathing systems. Circle systems can quickly be converted to non-rebreathing systems by changing the attachments going to the patient. To ensure that you know how to operate your machine and check for problems, practice tracing the flow of oxygen and vaporizer throughout the system.

A. **CIRCLE SYSTEM (OUT-OF-CIRCUIT):** 99% of circle systems have the **vaporizer out of circuit (VOC)**, meaning oxygen flows directly to the vaporizer, picks up gas, and once it does so, the gas enters the circular portion of the system.
   1. In the system depicted below, the vapor goes first to the reservoir bag and then to the patient. Exhaled air goes to the CO_2 absorber which removes CO_2 and then circles around back to the reservoir bag. The flow throughout the system is unidirectional due to one-way valves.

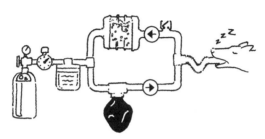

   2. In this system, change in ventilation does not affect the anesthetic concentrations delivered from the vaporizer to the patient. Due to the mixing of fresh oxygen-gas with expired air in the reservoir bag, the concentration of gas that reaches the dog is usually lower than the reading on the vaporizer; however, by increasing the oxygen flow rate, you can increase the concentration to more closely match the vaporizer setting.

Suggested flow: 30 mL/kg/min

   3. The circle system is best for dogs over 10kg because they are best able to handle the resistance created by the valves and the CO_2 absorber canister.
   4. After tracing the flow of oxygen and vapor in the machine and ensuring that all the connections are in place, check the system for leaks by closing off the pop-off valve, plugging the mouthpiece that would go to the patient, turning on the oxygen flow to fill up the reservoir bag to a pressure of 20 cm H_2O and then turning the flow down to < 500 mL/min. With no leaks, the pressure of 20 cm H_2O should be maintained.
   5. To "sigh" or "bag" the patient, fill the reservoir bag with oxygen and temporarily close the pop-off valve. Apply pressure to the bag while observing the patient's chest expand. Expand to a pressure of 10-20 cm H_2O in dogs (10-12 cm H_2O in cats). Remember to open the valve afterwards.

B. **CIRCLE SYSTEM (IN-CIRCUIT):** Probably less than 1% of anesthesia machines have **vaporizers in circuit (VIC)** but because there are some major differences in anesthesia between the two, it's important to know the differences if you have one. All vaporizers in-circuit are made with glass. If your machine does not have a glass vaporizer, it is a VOC and you can disregard this section.
   1. When the vaporizer is in circuit (**VIC**), the anesthetic gas from the vaporizer is carried by oxygen directly to the patient and then the expired air goes to the CO_2 absorber and then to the rebreathing bag. Since the system is in a circle, the exhaled gas then goes through the vaporizer along with a new influx of gas and oxygen. Because the exhaled air has some vapor in it, the net concentration of gas going to the patient may be higher than the reading on the vaporizer.

Also, because the air going through the vaporizer is warmed, it will pick up more vapor.

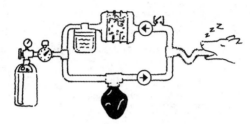

2. With VICs, increased ventilation leads to deeper anesthesia because the exhaled gases (which include unused anesthetic agent) pass through the vaporizer more often, thus becoming more saturated with anesthetic vapor. On spontaneous ventilation this allows the animal to "autoregulate" anesthetic depth to some extent. This autoregulation is removed if you begin to ventilate the patient—this may quickly overdose the patient if you don't turn the vaporizer down before beginning IPPV. Also, the lower the fresh gas flow, the higher the inspired concentration and generally it is most efficient to run these systems with very low oxygen flow rates (5 mL/kg/min).

C. **NON-REBREATHING SYSTEM:** For patients less than 10 kg, use a non-rebreathing system such as the Bain system because it requires less work on the animal's part to move the gasses in and out of the lungs.
   1. The circle system can be converted to a non-rebreathing system by using the correct attachments. In the non-rebreathing system, oxygen and vapor are delivered directly to the patient with no rebreathing of expired patient air. Instead, the inspired air flows through a separate tube which leads directly to a reservoir bag and then through the exhaust.

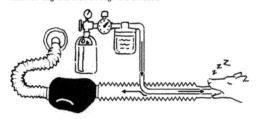

> Flow rate = 200 mL/kg per minute; Minimum flow = 1 liter.

   2. Check for leaks prior to anesthesia by closing off the exhaust valve usually on the reservoir bag, letting O_2 in and seeing if the bag can hold a pressure of 20 cm H_2O with a low flow of less than 500 mL/minute.
   3. Do a second leak check to test the integrity of the tubing from the flowmeter to the patient. On most Bain circuits this can be done by turning the flowmeter to 2-3 L/minute and then blocking the end of the smaller central tube at the patient end with a pen or similar object. The float of the flowmeter should drop as pressure increases in the animal. If it does not drop, check the connections; if everything appears to be OK, repeat the test and if the float does not drop, replace the circuit.
   4. When a patient is hooked up to the non-rebreathing system, **never** inflate the reservoir bag by pressing the oxygen valve because this O_2 goes directly to the patient.

1.44

Bacteriology

SUGGESTED READING

Morley PS, et al. 2005. Antimicrobial Drug Use in Veterinary Medicine. *Journal of Veterinary Internal Medicine* 19, pp. 617-629.

INDEX of BACTERIAL and FUNGAL DISEASES

	DOG	CAT
Abscess (The bacteria involved depend on whether the abscess is due to a dog or cat bite, cut, or foxtail).	Staphylococcus Obligate anaerobes Proteus Actinomyces/Nocardia (foxtail-associated)	Pasteurella Obligate anaerobes Enterics Actinomyces spp. (rare)
Diarrhea	Salmonella Campylobacter E. coli Clostridium	Salmonella Campylobacter Clostridium
Diskospondylitis	Staphylococcus Streptococcus Brucella canis Actinomyces	Staphylococcus Streptococcus
Endocarditis	Staphylococcus E. coli Corynebacterium Erysipelothrix	
Encephalitis/ Meningitis	Staphylococcus Pasteurella Actinomyces Nocardia Cryptococcus	Staphylococcus Pasteurella Actinomyces Nocardia Cryptococcus
Joints	Staphylococcus Streptococcus E. coli Mycoplasma Anaerobes Borrelia burgdorferi (Lyme disease—rare)	Pasteurella Mycoplasma L-form bacteria
Mastitis	E. coli Staphylococcus Streptococcus	E. coli Staphylococcus Streptococcus
Nasal Infection	Aspergillus	Cryptococcus
Osteomyelitis	Staphylococcus Streptococcus Enterics (E. coli, Enterococcus) Pasteurella Anaerobes Brucella	Staphylococcus Streptococcus Enterics Anaerobes
Otitis Externa	Pseudomonas Proteus Staphylococcus ß Streptococcus Pasteurella Malassezia pachydermatis	Pseudomonas Proteus Staphylococcus Streptococcus Pasteurella Malassezia pachydermatis
Reproductive	Brucella	
Respiratory (Upper)	B. bronchiseptica	Staphylococcus Streptococcus Pasteurella (if chronic and primary signs is conjunctivitis, then Chlamydia)

INDEX of BACTERIAL and FUNGAL DISEASES continued

	DOG	CAT
Respiratory (Lower)	E. coli Klebsiella Pasteurella Streptococcus Bordetella Staphylococcus Pseudomonas Obligate anaerobes Coccidioides immitus	Pasteurella Proteus Obligate anaerobes Moraxella Mycoplasma Cryptococcus
Septicemia	Staphylococcus E. coli Streptococcus Salmonella Proteus Pseudomonas Enterococcus Anaerobes	E.coli Klebsiella Salmonella Anaerobes
Skin Lesions	Staphylococcus Malassezia Dermatophytes (ringworm)	Staphylococcus Malassezia Dermatophytes (ringworm)
Strangles (Puppy)	Staphylococcus	
Urinary Tract	E. coli Proteus Klebsiella Enterobacter Pseudomonas Staphylococcus Streptococcus Mycoplasma Leptospira (renal)	E. coli Proteus Klebsiella Enterobacter Pseudomonas Staphylococcus Streptococcus Mycoplasma

Bacteriology

ANTIBIOTICS
General Information
General Pharmacology
When and What to Use

I. **GENERAL INFORMATION on ANTIBIOTICS:** Antibiotics are chemicals produced by microorganisms (fungi, bacteria) that suppress the growth of or destroy other microbes.

   A. **BACTERICIDAL vs. BACTERIOSTATIC ANTIBIOTICS:**
      1. **Bactericidal** antibiotics are capable of killing bacteria at clinically achievable concentrations.
      2. **Bacteriostatic** antibiotics inhibit bacterial growth but do not kill the organisms at clinically achievable concentrations. When the animal is taken off the antibiotic, the bacterial growth resumes. These antibiotics allow the animal's healthy immune system to catch up with and control the infection.

EXAMPLES OF BACTERIOSTATIC vs. BACTERICIDAL DRUGS

BACTERIOSTATIC	BACTERICIDAL
Chloramphenicol	Aminoglycosides
Lincomycin	Cephalosporins
Macrolides	Fluoroquinolones (at
Tetracycline	high doses)
	Penicillins
	Polymyxins

   B. **MBC and MIC**
      1. **Minimal bactericidal concentration (MBC)** is the lowest concentration of the antibiotic that kills 99.9% of the bacteria.
      2. **Minimal inhibitory concentration (MIC)** is the lowest concentration of the antibiotic that inhibits visible bacterial growth. To determine which antibiotic to use, culture the bacteria and measure the sensitivity (MIC) to different antibiotics. MIC is determined on bacteria in vitro. To be effective in the patient, the drug must reach MIC in the target tissues and remain at that level for some period. There are many obstacles to achieving this concentration, such as crossing the blood-brain barrier and problems with perfusion. It is important to choose an appropriate drug and dosing schedule, and to provide the appropriate route of administration to attain the proper target tissue concentrations (rather than just reading the MIC without regards to these factors). Conversely, some antimicrobials can attain a very high concentration when applied topically or as infusions (e.g. into the bladder or mammary glands). Additionally, some are actively transported into the urine (e.g. ß-lactams and cephalosporins) and consequently can achieve levels up to 200X those achieved in blood.

   B. **MECHANISM OF ACTION**

Inhibit Cell Wall Synthesis	Penicillins and cephalosporins prevent crosslinking of the peptidoglycans in the bacterial cell wall, while bacitracins inhibit transfer of building blocks to the growing cell wall. Without their cell wall, bacteria become spheroblasts and rupture. Cell wall synthesis occurs during a small interval of the bacteria's lifespan; thus, to catch the population of bacteria during this phase, the antibiotic must remain at therapeutic levels throughout treatment. • **Penicillins:** Bacteria with ß-lactamases are resistant to non-potentiated penicillins. Some penicillin products are resistant to penicillinases (oxacillin, cloxacillin) or are combined with other products to make them resistant to penicillinases (clavulanic acid). • **Cephalosporins:** Some gram-negative bacteria with ß-lactamases are resistant to cephalosporins. The penicillinase-resistant *Staphylococci* are still susceptible to this drug though. • **Bacitracins**
Affect Cell Membrane Permeability	**Polymyxin:** Polymyxin works like a detergent to disrupt the cell membrane structure, thus increasing its permeability. It is more active against **gram-negative** organisms including *Pseudomonas*. Polymyxin is nephrotoxic and neurotoxic. It is most commonly used aurally and topically (as an otic or ophthalmic). It is not absorbed orally unless the mucosa is damaged, in which case it can be fairly toxic to the animal (aminoglycosides and nystatin also have this characteristic).

MECHANISM of ACTION continued

Antimetabolite	Antimetabolites inhibit bacterial enzymes. Sulfonamides inhibit dihydrofolic acid reductase which is important for formation of nucleic acids. They are not effective at purulent sites because, here, sufficient level of nucleic acids are present for bacterial growth. The most common side effect of sulfonamides is dry eye.
Inhibit Protein Synthesis	These antibiotics **inhibit protein synthesis** by blocking transcription. • **Aminoglycosides** have primarily a gram-negative spectrum. They are not absorbed orally and are nephrotoxic. They bind with RNA to block protein synthesis but also bind with RNA in cellular debris, thus becoming less available in purulent environments. • **Spectinomycin** is structurally similar to the aminoglycosides and has a primarily gram-negative spectrum. • **Tetracyclines** are good for intracellular parasites. They have good penetration into synovial fluid and milk. • **Chloramphenicol** is widely distributed and reaches high concentrations in the liver, bile, kidney, brain, and CSF. It can cause bone marrow suppression when used at high levels or for prolonged periods. • **Macrolides** (e.g. erythromycin) have a spectrum similar to penicillin except that they work much better on gram-positive organisms. • **Lincosamides** (e.g. lincomycin, clindamycin): Clindamycin selectively concentrates in the osteum, so it's good for use in osteomyelitis. It is effective against obligate anaerobes.
Suppress Nucleic Acid Synthesis	**Fluoroquinolones** (e.g. enrofloxacin) can potentiate seizures in animals (GABA antagonists in the brain) with past seizure history (more likely when combined with NSAIDS). At doses higher than 10 mg/kg/day, enrofloxacin can cause retinal degeneration and acute vision loss in cats. Thus, the current dosing in cats is $\leq$ 5 mg/kg/day. Ciprofloxacin is dosed similarly in dogs and is safe in cats. The dose for treatment of *Pseudomonas* infections is higher (20 mg/kg/day).

Bacteriology

II. **FACTORS THAT AFFECT DRUG SUCCESS:** Systemic drugs must be absorbed into the blood stream where they travel via the circulation to the target tissue. Once at the target tissue, they may react with or compete with local factors which alter their efficacy. They are then metabolized and eliminated. Events at each stage can affect the success of the drug therapy.

   A. **DRUG ABSORPTION:** Absorption of a drug is defined as movement of the drug molecules from the administration site to the systemic circulation. The degree to which a drug is absorbed is termed its bioavailability. Thus, if 100% is absorbed, it has a bioavailability of 100% or 1.0.

   1. **Route of administration affects bioavailability and absorption rate:**
      a. Drugs administered IV have no absorption phase since they are placed directly into the circulation.
      b. Those administered IM are absorbed rapidly and almost completely. Drugs administered SC must diffuse a significant distance to reach capillaries. If they are injected into low perfusion regions such as fat, they are absorbed even more slowly and incompletely.
         i. If the animal is hypotensive (due to dehydration, shock, hypovolemia) or otherwise has poor peripheral perfusion, the drug will not be absorbed well via SC or IM routes. Examples: a diabetic patient that receives an insulin injection into a fat pad will have poor absorption and consequently poor control of glucose levels; the hypotensive animal given SC fluids will exhibit slow uptake of the fluid; comatose or immobile animals absorb drugs poorly with IM adminstration.
         ii. Drugs administered **orally** have to diffuse through the tightly arranged cellular barrier to get into the circulation. For this reason, lipophilic drugs are well absorbed in the GI tract whereas those in ionic/hydrophilic forms such as **aminoglycosides are not well absorbed.** Aminoglycosides are good for altering GI flora since they remain in the GI tract.

        iii. **Liquids** are better absorbed than pills. When changing from liquid to tablet form or vice versa, the dose may need to be modified to account for this difference in bioavailability.

        iv. **Drugs that increase sympathetic nervous tone** (e.g. epinephrine, dobutamine) as well as physiologic states of high sympathetic tone lead to vasoconstriction in the GI tract and poorer absorption of drugs.

        v. Antacids, activated charcoal, and sucralfate prevent absorption. Give other medications several hours prior to administering such drugs.

    c. **First pass metabolism by the liver**: Blood from the intestines goes directly to the liver where foreign substances can be removed and metabolized. Some drugs such as diazepam undergo extensive first-pass metabolism so that very little reaches the systemic circulation. Consequently, drugs such as diazepam (over 90% is removed with first pass elimination) aren't very effective when given orally. They can, however, be well absorbed rectally because circulation to the rectum does not go directly to the liver.

    d. **Drugs can be modified to change absorption rate.** Procaine penicillin and benzathine penicillin have side chains that delay their absorption from 24-48 hours (procaine) to up to 5 days (benzathine). Due to the prolonged absorption, they have a lower peak serum concentration. Thus, if a high serum concentration is needed, use the non-repositol version (no procaine or benzathine).

    e. **Human sustained-release drugs** often aren't absorbed well in dogs and cats due to the much shorter GI tract. Additionally, if the pills are broken, they lose their sustained release property.

B. **DRUG IS ABSORBED BUT CAN'T GET TO the TARGET SITE:**
1. **Blood-brain barrier** makes it difficult for hydrophilic drugs to get into the brain.
   a. As with the intestinal lining, the brain capillaries have endothelial cells that abut closely thus providing a barrier to hydrophilic compounds. Astrocytes and glial cells surrounding the capillaries provide a second membrane barrier through which drugs need to pass to distribute into the brain. The prostate gland and globe of the eye have similarly tight barriers that make it difficult for many drugs to penetrate.
   b. Once drugs get into the endothelial cells, **p-glycoproteins** actively transport the drugs back out, thus keeping the levels down. P-glycoprotein is found in brain, gut, and kidney cells (leading to increased excretion into the urine). Collies and other related breeds have genetically low levels of P-glycoproteins; consequently, some drugs such as ivermectin penetrate into the brain and reach much higher levels there than in other breeds. Erythromycin inhibits P-glycoprotein in normal animals as do ketoconazole and grapefruit.
2. **Protein binding:** Some drugs (e.g. NSAIDS and some antimicrobials) are highly protein- bound to albumin and globulins and only a small portion remain in the active non-bound form in the blood. In conditions where serum proteins are low, the dosages of these drugs must be reduced.
3. **Volume of distribution:** If the animal is abnormally fat, the volume of distribution will be lower and the blood concentration of drug will achieve higher concentrations. Consequently, obese dogs and cats may need a lower dose than a dog or cat of the same weight that is lean.
4. **Poor circulation:** Necrotic tissue has no circulation. Treatment of a necrotic abscess with antibiotics might yield therapeutic plasma levels, but the drug will not reach therapeutic concentrations at the site. Necrotic tissue should be debrided where appropriate and the purulent material drained. These areas may respond well to topical therapy. The topical agents will absorb systemically in such cases due to loss of skin integrity, so be careful with aminoglycosides and polymyxins.

B. **PROBLEMS at the TARGET SITE:** Even if the drug is absorbed and distributed well to the target site, up-regulation or down-regulation of receptors and competition with other drugs for receptor sites can lead to altered efficacy.
1. **Down-regulation of receptors:** Drug administration can lead to down-regulation of the receptors for that drug. For instance, dobutamine and albuterol are ß-receptor stimulants. With dobutamine, receptors decrease within hours of administration leading to a decreased response for a given amount of

dobutamine. Albuterol, on the other hand, must be taken for longer periods of time to cause down-regulation, but it's the mechanism by which asthmatics become unreceptive to rescue with these drugs.

2. **Up-regulation of receptors**: Drugs such as ß-blockers that block access of the normal substrate to the receptor can cause up-regulation (an increased number) of the receptors they block. Because of this up-regulation, when such drugs are discontinued abruptly, the heart is hypersensitive to epinephrine and norepinephrine and bouts of exercise can lead to fatal arrhythmias.

C. **METABOLISM and EXCRETION:**
1. Many drugs are metabolized to more soluble compounds (more hydrophilic) for excretion by a two-step process in the liver. The liver's cytochrome P450 system (which is also present in gut and lung cells) oxidizes the compound and then a second set of enzymes adds a hydrophilic handle. If two drugs compete for the same breakdown enzymes, both drugs will be metabolized more slowly and thus have a longer lasting effect. Additionally, both young animals under 5 weeks and aged animals have a metabolism system that is not fully functional.
   a. Drugs such as phenobarbital cause sedation initially until the cytochrome P450 system up-regulates.
2. Most drugs are excreted by the kidneys. Renal damage as well as vasoconstriction of the renal arterioles (as with hypotension) can slow GFR, leading to slower excretion.
3. **Compounds or drugs that compete for the same target receptors.**
E. **PHARMACOLOGIC PROFILE:** Once administered, the drug levels rise in the blood, hopefully above the subtherapeutic level but below the toxic threshold. The levels then drop gradually until the next dose is given. Drugs frequently have numerous dosing schedules in which a total daily dose is listed but the medication can be given SID, BID, TID, or at some other interval. When given at a higher dose less frequently, the high and low points of the serum drug levels are more extreme. For instance, if you switch from BID to SID administration of phenobarbital (same total daily dose), the animal may show signs of ataxia because the higher dose is into the toxic range. The lower dose may be subtherapeutic.

II. **ANTIBIOTICS: GUIDELINES for USE**

GUIDELINES for USE
1) Determine whether the animal has an infection (based on clinical signs, cytology, culture, bloodwork, etc.).
2) Identify the pathogen or likely pathogens and choose an antibiotic that works against them. You may need to perform a culture and sensitivity.
3) Choose a drug that reaches appropriate levels at the infection site.
4) Consider local factors such as presence of necrotic tissue and purulent material.
5) Choose a flexible dose regimen based on the pharmacokinetics of the drug and the individual needs of the patient (e.g. the animal may have liver or kidney disease etc.).
6) Keep the animal on the antibiotics for a sufficient period of time to cure infection and to prevent relapse.

A **DOES THE ANIMAL NEED ANTIBIOTICS: Is there an infectious process?** If you suspect infection, then perform cytology on an appropriate sample (e.g. mass aspirate, transtracheal wash, urinalysis, etc.) and look for intra- and extracellular bacteria. You need a lot of bacteria before you can visualize the bacteria in a sample (**1 million organisms/gram** in order to see **1 organism/oil field**). If you don't see bacteria, look for other signs of infection such as:
1. Fever
2. Leukocytosis
3. Increased fibrinogen
4. Other evidence of infection such as discospondylitis (seen on radiographs)
5. Pain or swelling
6. Purulent exudate
   If an animal has two of the above listed features, it is likely to have an infection. In addition, **any animal that is on long-term corticosteroids and has a fever or is neutropenic and has a fever should be treated with antibiotics.**

B. **IDENTIFY THE PATHOGEN OR LIKELY PATHOGENS:** Often on cytology you can identify the pathogen as a rod or cocci bacteria. Based on this morphologic finding and on the location of the infection (e.g. skin, bladder, oral cavity), you can usually make a conclusion as to the type of bacteria that may be present. Consequently, by knowing which antibiotics are effective against the likely bacteria, you can empirically choose an antibiotic for use until the culture and sensitivity results are in. Some bacteria such as *Pseudomonas, Enterococcus, Klebsiella, E. coli, Proteus,* and *Enterobacter* frequently show antibiotic resistance; therefore, culture and sensitivity should always be performed when infection involves these bacteria.

1. Make sure to interpret the MIC correctly rather than just selecting a drug solely based on the results.

INITIAL ANTIBIOTIC CHOICES

CLASSIFICATION	AGENTS to TRY	AGENTS to AVOID
Enterics and Gram-Negative Non-Enterics (e.g. Pasteurella, Actinobacillus)	• Amoxicillin/clavulanic acid (Clavamox®) • Aminoglycosides (amikacin, gentamicin) • Cephalosporins, 3rd generation (e.g. Ceftizoxime). 1st and 3rd generation cephalosporins work against Pasteurella. • Fluoroquinolones • Imipenem (restricted use) • Trimethoprim or ormethoprim sulfa (Not as useful as in the recent past with enterics) • Chloramphenicol, penicillins, and tetracycline are useful in Pasteurella infections	• Ampicillin or amoxicillin by themselves • Aminoglycosides—kanamycin or streptomycin • Cephalosporins, 1st generation: the penicillinases that enterics have also work on these (Ancef®, Keflex®). • Chloramphenicol • Tetracycline • Sulfonamides • Avoid oxacillin and cloxacillin with Pasteurella infections
Pseudomonas	• Aminoglycosides • Cephalosporins: some 3rd generations work • Enrofloxacin/ciprofloxacin • Imipenem • Ticaricillin	• Amoxicillin • Cephalosporins • Chloramphenicol • Tetracyclines • Trimethoprim sulfa
Staphylococcus	• Aminoglycosides • Amoxicillin/clavulanic acid • Cephalosporins, 1st generation (cefadroxil, cephalexin) • Chloramphenicol • Enrofloxacin (Baytril®) • Erythromycin • Lincomycin • Trimethoprim or ormethoprim	• Penicillin, ampicillin, or amoxicillin alone • Tetracycline • Note: sulfa drugs are less predictable
Streptococcus	• Penicillin • Almost any antibiotic works	
Obligate Anaerobes	• Amoxicillin/clavulanic acid = 100% • Cephalosporins (1st generation) kill 60% of anaerobes • Clindamycin • Chloramphenicol • Metronidazole = 100% • Penicillin, ampicillin, and amoxicillin kill 60%. The other 40% have penicillinases or cephalosporin-ases. • Tetracycline (70% effective)	• Aminoglycosides • Enrofloxacin
Nocardia	• Trimethoprim sulfa	
Bordetella/ Mycoplasma	• Tetracycline • Fluoroquinolones • Chloramphenicol • Clindamycin	• Enrofloxacin (inconsistent activity but good at high doses)
Actinomyces	• Penicillin	

C. **CHOOSE A DRUG THAT GETS TO THE SITE:** Drugs are carried to the infection site via the circulation. If perfusion to the infection site is poor (e.g. bone sequestrum, hypotension, necrotic tissue), of if there's a barrier to drug diffusion (e.g. cell membrane, blood-brain barrier), the drug may not reach effective levels at the site. In cases where there's a membrane barrier preventing drug diffusion, we use more lipophilic drugs such as tetracycline, chloramphenicol, macrolides, and fluoroquinolones (enrofloxacin).

DRUG PENETRATION to Specific Sites

ORGAN	DRUG
Bone	• Clindamycin • Cephalosporin (1st generation = first choice) • Clavamox • Fluoroquinolones (enrofloxacin, marbofloxacin)
Brain, CSF, Eyes	• Cephalosporins (3rd generation— cefotaxime, ceftazidime) • Chloramphenicol • Doxycycline • Imipenem (restricted use) • Macrolides (erythromycin) • Metronidazole • Trimethoprim sulfa • Note: in the presence of inflammation, ampicillin crosses the blood-brain barrier. Ampicillin is commonly used in cases of bacterial meningitis.
Intracellular	• Chloramphenicol • Doxycycline, tetracycline • Fluoroquinolones (enrofloxacin) • Azithromycin
Prostate	• Chloramphenicol • Clindamycin and lincomycin • Erythromycin base • Fluoroquinolones (enrofloxacin, marbofloxacin) • Trimethoprim sulfa, ormethoprim sulfa
Synovial Fluid	• Cephalosporins • Clavamox • Doxycycline • Fluoroquinolones (enrofloxacin, marbofloxacin)

D. **CONSIDER LOCAL FACTORS** such as the presence of **pus** and **necrotic** debris. Neither sulfa drugs nor aminoglycosides work well in this environment.

E. **CONSIDER PHARMACOKINETICS**
   1. Certain drugs such as gentamicin and potentiated ß-lactams (when used against *Staphylococcus*) just need to reach a dose 6-10X above MIC some time during the dosing interval. These drugs can be dosed less often so that they reach an appropriate level for a short period of time but then drop low enough to diffuse out of renal cells and consequently decrease the likelihood of damage to these cells
      a. In cases where you're concerned about renal function but gentamicin is the best choice, decrease the dosing interval using the following formula: new dosing interval = current interval X serum creatinine. For example, if the current interval is 24 hours and serum creatinine is 2.0 mg/dL, then the new dosing interval is every 48 hours. Check urine for casts on a daily basis as casts are a more sensitive indicator of damage than creatinine levels.
      b. Fluoroquinolones: the total area under the curve (plasma concentration of drug in the therapeutic range) is what's important.
      c. ß-lactams (penicillins and cephalosporins) should be above MIC continuously in order to inhibit cell wall synthesis in the dividing bacteria.
      d. Most bacteriostatic drugs must be above MIC at all times.

Bacteriology

INDIVIDUAL CONSIDERATIONS in ANTIBIOTIC CHOICE

PATIENT	ANTIBIOTIC CONSIDERATIONS
Puppies and Kittens	• Avoid enrofloxacin or use with extreme caution. It interferes with developing cartilage and bone formation. • Tetracycline can cause enamel hypoplasia and may affect bone development. • Decrease the antibiotic dose in puppies and kittens less than 4 weeks of age. They have juvenile liver and renal function. • Chloramphenicol can cause bone marrow suppression.
Geriatric patients	• May need decreased drug dosages due to decreased liver and renal function
Renal disease patients	• Be careful with aminoglycosides such as gentamicin. They are nephrotoxic and ototoxic. They should be administered at the less frequent dosing of SID vs. BID or TID.

G. HELP AVOID ANTIBIOTIC RESISTANCE
   1. **Use primary tier antibiotics for most infections:** These include amoxicillin, simple penicillins, tetracyclines, first generation cephalexins, and sulfonamides. Use these for most infections and while awaiting culture and sensitivity results.
   2. **Use secondary tier antibiotics** such as enrofloxacin, marbofloxacin, oxacillin, aminoglycosides, 2nd generation cephalexins, when culture and sensitivity indicate a resistance to primary drugs.

H. **TREAT LONG ENOUGH.** If the drugs are discontinued prematurely when clinical signs subside, then the remaining bacteria that are more resistant to the drug will then proliferate forming more resistance to the drug.
   1. In simple, acute infections, continue antibiotics at least 3 days after all clinical signs have subsided. Clinical signs should start subsiding within 24-48 hours.
      a. For less severe infections this amounts to 7-10 days of treatment.
      b. For severe infections (such as systemic infections) continue for 10-14 days.
      c. With fevers, once the fever breaks, continue for 4-5 days.
   2. For chronic infections, antibiotics may need to be continued for 3-4 weeks or for months.

COMMON CARDIAC MEDICATIONS

DRUG	CANINE	FELINE
Amlodipine	0.2 - 0.4 mg/kg PO BID (Start at 0.1 mg/kg PO BID)	0.625 mg (1/4 of 2.5 mg tab) to 1.25 mg per cat PO SID
Aspirin (to prevent clotting) 81 mg, 250 mg, 325 mg tablets	5 - 10 mg/kg PO q 24 -48 hr	80 mg/cat PO q 72 hr
Atenolol 25 mg, 50 mg, 100 mg	0.25 - 1.0 mg/kg PO SID-BID	1.0 mg/kg PO BID
Benazepril (Lotensin®; ACE inhibitor) 5 mg, 10 mg, 20 mg, 40 mg	0.25 - 0.5 mg/kg PO SID to BID	Same as dog
Digoxin (for supraventricular tachyarrhythmias and as a positive inotrope) Tablets: 0.125 mg, 0.25 mg Elixir: 0.05 or 0.15 mg/mL	**Loading dose** (avoid loading if possible): 2x maintenance for 24 hours. 0.011 - 0.02 mg/kg IV divided into 3-4 doses over the first 1-4 hrs. **Maintenance:** Refer to section on dilated cardiomyopathy.	
Diltiazem (Ca channel blocker) Tablets: 30, 60, 90, 120 mg Injectable: 50 mg/mL	0.5 - 1.5 mg/kg PO q 8 hrs	1.75 - 2.4 mg/kg PO TID (Cardizem CD® dose, 10 mg/kg PO SID)
Enalapril (ACE inhibitor) 2.5 , 5 , 10 , 20 mg tabs	0.5 mg/kg SID to **BID** PO	0.25 - 0.5 mg/kg SID to **BID**
Furosemide (loop diuretic) Tablets: 12.5 mg, 50 mg Elixir: 10 mg/mL or 60 mg/mL Injectable: 50 mg/mL	• 2 - 8 mg/kg IV or IM q 1-6 hr • 2 - 4 mg/kg PO q 8-48 hr • 8 mg/kg IV q 1hr if severe	• 1 - 2 mg/kg IV or IM q 1-6 hr • 0.25 - 2.0 mg/kg PO q 8-24 hr • 4 mg/kg IV q 1 hr if severe
Lovenox	N.A.	1 - 1.5 mg/kg SQ SID
Lidocaine (for arrhythmias) Injectable: 5, 10, 15, 20 mg/mL	• 2 - 4 mg/kg IV q 10 minutes (Max: 8 mg/kg over 10 min) • 25 - 75 µg/kg/min IV infusion	0.25 - 0.75 mg/kg IV slowly
Nitroglycerine	Dog & Cat: 1/8 - 1/4 inch per 7 kg cutaneously, q 4-6 h	
Pimobendan	0.5 - 2.5 mg/kg PO BID	Same as dogs
Propranolol (ß antagonist) Tablets: 10 mg, 20 mg, 40 mg Injectable: 1 mg/mL	• 0.1 - 1.0 mg/kg PO q TID • 20 - 60 µg/kg IV over 10 min	2.5 - 5.0 mg/cat PO TID
Spironolactone Tablets:25 mg, 50 mg, 100 mg	0.5 - 1.0 mg/kg PO SID	

VOLUME of 50 mg/mL FUROSEMIDE in HEART FAILURE (2 mg/kg IM or IV)					
Weight of dog or cat	5 kg	10 kg	20 kg	30 kg	40 kg
Volume of furosemide	0.2 mL	0.4 mL	0.8 mL	1.2 mL	1.6 mL

Cardiology

CARDIAC PHYSIOLOGY
Anatomy and Function of the Cardiovascular System
The Cardiac Cycle
The Heart's Short-Term Response to Acute Change
The Heart's Response to Chronic Changes

I. **ANATOMY and FUNCTION of the CARDIOVASCULAR SYSTEM**
  A. **CIRCULATION in the ADULT, FETAL, and TRANSITIONAL HEART:** The heart is
     composed of four chambers—a right and left atrium separated by an interatrial
     septum, and a right and left ventricle separated by an interventricular septum.
     Anatomically, the right and left heart are side by side, but functionally, they act as
     two pumps in series. The right side is a low pressure pump that expels blood to the
     pulmonary vasculature, and the left side is a high pressure pump that forces blood
     through the systemic circulation.
     1. **Circulation in the adult heart:** Unoxygenated blood returns to the right side
        of the heart via the cranial and caudal vena cava. It enters the right atrium and
        then travels to the right ventricle where it is pumped out into the pulmonary
        artery and into the lungs. Once in the lungs, it picks up oxygen and then travels
        via the pulmonary veins to the left atrium and then into the left ventricle. Next
        it is pumped out the aorta and into the systemic circulation. Blood also travels
        from the aorta into the coronary arteries which perfuse the heart.

     2. **Circulation in the fetal heart:**
        a. Oxygenated blood from the placenta returns to the fetus via the umbilical
           vein, which joins the **portal vein** to enter the liver. Blood either passes
           through the hepatic sinusoids or the **ductus venosus** into the caudal vena
           cava.
        b. Upon entering the right atrium, a large portion of this blood is directed
           through the **foramen ovale** into the left atrium.

        c. Most of the venous return from the cranial vena cava and the remaining
           blood flow from the caudal vena cava enters the right ventricle and is
           ejected into the main pulmonary artery. Only a small amount (10% of the
           cardiovascular output) perfuses the lungs, while the majority crosses the
           ductus arteriosus into the **descending aorta**.
           i   The reason fetal pulmonary blood flow is low (10% of the
               cardiovascular output) is that pulmonary vascular resistance is high
               due to a thick smooth muscle layer in the pulmonary arterioles. This
               layer remains constricted in the presence of a low fetal oxygen tension.
        d. The blood ejected by the left ventricle enters the ascending aorta to supply
           mainly the coronary arteries and brachiocephalic vessels.

        e. Note the following with regard to fetal circulation:
           i.   The right ventricle ejects 2/3 of the combined ventricular output.
           ii. 60% of the cardiovascular output passes from the pulmonary artery
                across the ductus arteriosus to the descending aorta.
           iii. Aortic and pulmonary artery pressures are equal, as are the right
                ventricular and left ventricular systolic pressures.
           iv. Right atrial pressure slightly exceeds left atrial pressure.

     3. The **transitional circulation:** At birth, marked changes occur in the
        cardiovascular system. These changes are primarily directed at shifting the
        origin of oxygenated blood from the placenta to the neonate's lungs.
        a. The onset of respiration and rapid rise in oxygen saturation in the lungs
           results in pulmonary arteriolar vasodilation. This vasodilation and resulting
           drop in pulmonary arteriolar vascular resistance allows blood from the right
           ventricle to flow more easily into the lungs; thus, blood flow to the lungs
           increases dramatically. Over the next few weeks of life, the muscular layer
           of the pulmonary arterioles regress and pulmonary artery resistance and
           pressure continue to fall to adult levels. Pulmonary resistance in adults is
           much lower than systemic vascular resistance.
        b. Since the right ventricle doesn't need to pump against such high pressure,
           the right ventricular walls atrophy.
        c. Constriction of the low resistance umbilical arteries increases systemic
           vascular resistance and arterial pressure so that the left heart now has to
           pump against a much higher resistance (6x higher) than the right heart.
           Increased venous return from the now perfused lungs results in increased

left atrial pressure (greater than right atrial pressure) and functional **closure of the foramen ovale**. Over time, the valve of the foramen ovale fuses with the atrial septum, preventing further shunting of blood.

d.   Finally, the increased arterial oxygen saturation (and probably other factors) causes constriction of the muscular layer of the **ductus arteriosus (functional closure)** shortly after birth, with eventual anatomic closure via thrombosis and fibrosis.

e.   Cardiac output from both ventricles equalizes as the pumps begin to function in series.

Note that during the transition period, two fetal shunts, one between the left and right atria and one between the aorta and the pulmonary artery close. If they remain open in the adult, they are called **patent foramen ovale** (which is benign) and **patent ductus arteriosus** which can have serious consequences. Another common shunt is one between the right and left ventricles called a **ventricular septal defect**.

B.   **THE VASCULAR SYSTEM**

COMPONENTS of the VASCULAR SYSTEM

- **Arteries** distribute oxygenated blood from the heart to different regions of the body. The one exception is the pulmonary artery which takes unoxygenated blood to the lungs.
- **Capillaries** are the site of gas and nutrient exchange.
- **Lymphatics** filter fluid going from the interstitial space into the circulatory system.
- **Veins** serve as a reservoir for unoxygenated blood. Blood returns to the heart via the veins. The exceptions are the pulmonary veins which bring oxygenated blood from the lungs to the left atrium.

---

1.   **The arterial side** consists of the aorta, arteries (small and large), and arterioles. The function of the arterial side is to **distribute the blood** pumped by the heart to different regions of the body. The **arterioles are the principal site of resistance to flow** within the vascular system.

a.   **Arterioles determine the distribution of blood** within the different tissues and organs of the body. They vasodilate in regions that need blood and vasoconstrict in areas that don't need as much blood. For example, in the fight/flight response, blood is shunted to the muscles and away from the gastrointestinal tract.

b.   **Arteriolar resistance determines blood pressure** and determines the pressure that the heart must generate in order to supply blood to the body. Maintaining blood pressure is vital. If the arterial blood pressure is 0 (then the difference in blood pressure between the arteriolar and venous side is 0) then blood flow is 0. Blood flows from areas of high pressure to areas of low pressure.

Blood flow = $\dfrac{\text{Aortic blood pressure - Vena Cava blood pressure}}{\text{Vessel resistance}}$

In **anaphylactic shock and septic shock** (both are cases of vasodilatory shock), there's massive vasodilation which results in a dramatic drop in systemic blood pressure. Consequently, venous return decreases, cardiac output drops precipitously, and organ perfusion is insufficient.

c.   Arteriole diameter is under neuronal control (ANS; primarily the sympathetic nerves) and local metabolic control. Local tissue metabolism (high carbon dioxide levels) cause vasodilation which allows more blood and oxygen into the areas that need it.

2.   **Capillary and lymphatic systems:**

a.   Capillaries are very small vessels with walls that are only one cell layer thick. They are the site of gas and nutrient exchange from blood to tissue and vice versa. In addition, capillaries filter fluid (plasma) going out of the vascular compartment and into the interstitial space.

b.   Conversely, the **lymphatic** system filters fluid going from the interstitial space back into the circulatory system.

Cardiology

3. **The venous side** includes the venules, small and large veins, and the cranial and caudal vena cava. The vessels contain elastic tissue and smooth muscle cells.

   a. Veins act as storage vessels or **reservoir vessels.** That is, they are responsible for **capacitance.** About 60-80% of the circulating blood volume is in the venous side of the circuit. When the veins dilate, the venous side acts as a larger reservoir. When they constrict, they act as a smaller reservoir.

   b. The venous system is under **neuronal control.**

II. THE CARDIAC CYCLE

> * **Diastole:** Relaxation phase
> * **Systole:** Contraction phase
> * **End-diastolic volume** (EDV): The volume of blood in the ventricles at the end of diastole. This is the same as **preload.**
> * **End-systolic volume** (ESV): The volume of blood in the ventricles at the end of systole.

A. THE SEQUENCE OF EVENTS

1. During **diastole,** the relaxation phase of the cycle, the AV valves (mitral on the left side, tricuspid on the right side) are open and the atria and ventricles communicate. Thus, blood pressures in the left atrium and left ventricle equalize as the ventricles fill rapidly with atrial blood. During this phase, blood flows from the venous side to fill the heart. The semilunar valves (aortic and pulmonic valves) are closed. The volume of blood in the ventricles prior to the onset of contraction is the **end-diastolic volume (EDV) or preload.**

2. When the SA node fires, it sends an electrical impulse into the atria causing the atria to depolarize and then contract. Atrial contraction takes place at the end of diastole and contributes 20% of the preload. Next, the ventricles depolarize. At the peak of the R wave, the ventricles start to contract; this marks the onset of **systole.** As soon as the ventricles start to contract (resulting in increased ventricular pressure), the mitral and tricuspid valves shut, preventing blood from flowing backwards into the atria. The **first heart sound** corresponds with the closing of the AV valves.

3. Now each ventricle is a closed chamber. As the ventricle continues to contract, blood volume remains the same but pressure increases. This is termed **isovolumetric contraction.**

4. Once the left ventricular pressure reaches or exceeds aortic diastolic pressure, the aortic valves open and blood is ejected into the aorta (**rapid ejection phase**). At the same time, the right ventricle ejects blood into the pulmonary artery. As this occurs, ventricular pressure and volume decrease. About 50-60% of the ventricular volume is ejected and about 40-50% of the systolic reserve volume remains. This remaining volume is the **end-systolic volume (ESV).**

5. As ventricular pressure falls, so does aortic pressure. When ventricular pressure falls below the pressure stored in the expanded aorta, the elastic energy of the aorta wall is released. Pressure in the aorta exceeds ventricular pressure, so the aortic valve closes. This closure and dissipation of elastic energy is responsible for the **dicrotic notch** seen on aortic pulse pressure monitors. Closure of the aortic and pulmonic valves corresponds to the **second heart sound.**

6. Now the left ventricle is once again a closed chamber. This time, the walls relax and volume remains the same but pressure decreases. This is termed **isovolumetric relaxation.**

7. While the ventricles are undergoing isovolumetric contraction, rapid ejection, and isovolumetric relaxation, the AV valves are closed. Because there are no valves between the pulmonary veins and the atria, the atria fill with blood from venous return and atrial pressures increase. Atrial pressures continue to increase while ventricular pressures decrease in isovolumetric relaxation. When atrial pressure exceeds left ventricular pressure, the AV valves open and blood from

the atria rapidly flow into the ventricles. This phase is termed the **rapid filling phase**. It marks the onset of diastole. Two additional heart sounds are sometimes heard during diastole.
a. **The third heart sound** (S3) is not normally heard. It can be heard in association with rapid ventricular filling in volume overloads.
b. **The fourth heart sound** (S4) is not normally heard. It can be heard at the beginning of atrial systole with pressure overloads and non-compliant ventricles or with 3° AV block.

III. **The HEART'S SHORT-TERM RESPONSE to CHANGE**

> • **Stroke volume** is the amount of blood ejected out of the left ventricle with **each beat**.
> • **Cardiac output** is the amount of blood pumped out of the left ventricle per minute. It is equal to **stroke volume x heart rate**.

The heart tries to maintain cardiac output. Cardiac output is affected by stroke volume and heart rate. In turn, stroke volume is determined by **cardiac contractility, preload** (end-diastolic volume), and **afterload** (the resistance that the ventricle has to pump blood out against). In other words, the heart can pump out more blood with each beat if it contracts harder, if the amount of blood filling the heart at the end of diastole increases, or if the resistance the heart is pumping blood against (systemic resistance) decreases. Increased sympathetic tone and catecholamines increase cardiac output by binding to ß receptors on the heart, which in turn **increase heart rate** and **myocardial contractility**.

A. **HEART RATE** is under neuronal, hormonal, and pressure control. In general, the heart rate increases in order to **maintain adequate blood pressure**. Maintaining adequate blood pressure is the heart's first priority. Heart rate increases with fever, exercise, excitement, hypovolemia, etc.
1. **Response to blood pressure**: When blood pressure increases, heart rate reflexively slows. Conversely, when blood pressure decreases, heart rate increases. For example, if blood pressure drops rapidly due to hemorrhage, the heart rate immediately increases to compensate. Blood pressure receptors (baroreceptors) are located in the aortic arch and carotid sinus.
2. **Increase in sympathetic tone** (as with the fight or flight response) elevates heart rate by causing the release of **norepinephrine** which binds to ß1 **receptors in the heart**. Sympathetic tone also increases heart rate by **increasing conduction through the AV node**; thus, the P-R interval becomes shorter.
a. **ß antagonists** such as propranolol, atenolol, and metoprolol decrease heart rate and can be used to slow down supraventricular tachyarrhythmias.
3. **Increase in parasympathetic tone** decreases heart rate by slowing conduction through the AV node.

B. **CARDIAC CONTRACTILITY**: The force of contraction depends on the **preload** (end-diastolic volume), **afterload** (pressure the heart has to pump against), and the **intrinsic myocardial contractility** (the ability of the cardiac muscle to generate force).
1. Calcium is the major ion involved in myocardial contractility. One method of increasing cardiac contractility is to increase the amount of calcium released from the sarcoplasmic reticulum and the rate at which it is released.
a. **Catecholamines with ß1 adrenergic activity** activate the cyclic AMP cascade which allows the sarcoplasmic reticulum to bind more calcium during diastole and then release more calcium during systole. It also increases the rate at which calcium is bound and released.

2. **Preload**: The **Frank-Starling Law** states that the greater the cardiac volume (longer muscle fiber length), the stronger the contractility. The result is that the heart can accommodate any volume that it receives. This allows the heart to compensate for beat to beat variations in volume (e.g. going from sitting to reclining = more venous return).

3. **Afterload**: The higher the resistance, the harder the heart contracts; thus, the heart can generate whatever pressure it needs in order to achieve the required stroke volume.

IV. The HEART'S CHRONIC RESPONSE to CHANGE

A. RENIN-ANGIOTENSIN-ALDOSTERONE SYSTEM (RAAS):

When cardiac output falls below normal, renin is released from the juxtaglomerular apparatus of the kidneys. Renin converts angiotensinogen, a pro-hormone made by the liver, to angiotensin I (Ang I). Ang I is then converted to Ang II by angiotensin converting enzyme (ACE) in the lungs. Ang II stimulates **aldosterone** release from the **adrenal** glands and **ADH** release from the **pituitary** gland.

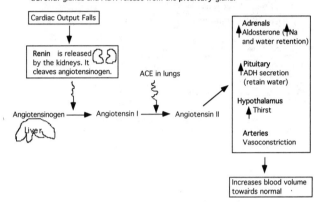

1. **Angiotensin II** is a potent vasoconstrictor that increases arteriolar resistance. It also stimulates the release of aldosterone from the adrenal glands, ADH from the pituitary gland, and stimulates the thirst centers in the hypothalamus.
2. **Aldosterone** promotes sodium and water retention, which increases total blood volume.
3. **Antidiuretic hormone** works at the distal collecting ducts of the kidneys to retain water.
   Note: Angiotensin-converting enzyme inhibitors (ACE inhibitors) can be used in volume overload patients because they act directly on the RAAS to decrease volume retention.

B. Eccentric and Concentric Hypertrophy:

Hypertrophy is an increase in cell size.

1. **Eccentric hypertrophy** is when the cardiac chamber size gets larger but the wall thickness stays the same. It occurs in response to **volume overload**. For example, in mitral regurgitation, total stroke volume remains the same but forward flow decreases and backward flow increases. As a result, systemic blood pressure initially falls. The body initially compensates by increasing systemic resistance and increasing heart rate and contractility, but for long term maintenance, the RAAS system is activated. This results in vasoconstriction and increased ADH and aldosterone. The end result is that sodium and water are retained and the total blood volume increases— resulting in an increase in preload. In order to accommodate this increased preload without increasing ventricular pressure, the ventricle must grow larger. An increase in end-diastolic ventricular pressure is detrimental because it produces increased atrial pressure and increased capillary hydrostatic pressure which results in edema or effusion. To prevent this, the ventricle grows larger by laying more sarcomeres end-to end (in series).
2. **Concentric hypertrophy** is when the cardiac chamber stays the same size but the ventricle walls get thicker and stronger (with severe hypertrophy, the internal chamber dimensions get smaller). This occurs in response to **pressure overload** (an increase in **afterload**). For instance, during systemic hypertension, the left ventricle has to pump blood against a higher resistance. In order to do this, it develops more muscle (lays down more sarcomeres in parallel) resulting in a thicker wall that can more easily pump against greater pressure.

CARDIAC PHYSICAL EXAMINATION
Inspection from a Distance
Head and Neck
Thoracic Auscultation
Abdominal Examination
Examining the Pulses

I. **PHYSICAL INSPECTION FROM A DISTANCE.** Observe the patient from a distance and note:

   A. **BREED and AGE:** Some breeds are predisposed to certain types of cardiovascular diseases. Young animals may have congenital defects while old animals are more likely to have acquired defects.

   B. **ABILITY to AMBULATE:** Many severely compromised cardiac patients are reluctant to exercise or too weak to ambulate.

   C. **ATTITUDE:** Cardiac patients that are dyspneic may stand with elbows abducted in an attempt to improve ventilation or may sit on their haunches while refusing to get up.

   D. **RESPIRATION:** Observe the rate and character. Watch the frequency, regularity, and depth as well as the effort required during inspiration and expiration. Tachypnea and coughing are frequently associated with pulmonary edema or the accumulation of pleural fluid. Coughing is a major sign of chronic heart failure in dogs but is rarely seen in cats. Cardiac disease is often associated with inspiratory dyspnea.

   E. **GENERAL BODY CONDITION:**
   1. **Cardiac cachexia:** Patients with advanced cardiovascular disease are often thin with marked loss of muscle mass (particularly noticeable along the dorsal lumbar area of large breed dogs).
   2. Patients with ascites may appear obese due to abdominal distension.

II. **HEAD and NECK**

   A. **MUCOUS MEMBRANES:** Check mucous membrane color and capillary refill time (CRT). The mucous membranes are normally moist and pink and the CRT should be between 1-2 seconds. If the animal has pigmented mucous membranes, check the ocular conjunctiva. Also compare with the posterior mucous membranes for differential cyanosis.

   1. **Mucous Membrane Color:**
      a. **Cyanosis** occurs in cases of hypoxia, which may be the result of pulmonary disease (e.g. primary pulmonary disease or severe pulmonary edema) or shunting of blood from the right side directly to the left side, consequently bypassing the lungs. This shunt results in arterial hypoxemia. Examples of right to left shunting include Tetralogy of Fallot and reverse PDA. The latter condition is characterized by differential cyanosis in which the caudal half of the body is cyanotic while the head and front legs receive blood with near normal oxygen saturation.

      b. **Pale mucous membranes** are caused by peripheral vasoconstriction which occurs as a response to any decrease in cardiac output (such as hypovolemic shock or cardiogenic shock). Mucous membranes may also appear pale in nervous animals (especially cats), animals in pain (due to increased sympathetic tone), or anemic animals.

      c. **Injected mucous membranes** may be caused by polycythemia, vasodilatory shock (e.g. septic or anaphylactic shock), or can occasionally be seen in otherwise normal patients.

   2. **Capillary refill time** is normally between 1-2 seconds.
      a. **Decreased (fast) capillary refill time** may be caused by peripheral vasodilation (vasodilatory shock) or hyperperfusion.
      b. **Increased (slowed) capillary refill time** may be caused by peripheral vasoconstriction. Vasoconstriction occurs in response to any decrease in cardiac output (e.g. hypovolemic shock, cardiogenic shock, or increased sympathetic tone).

   3. **Petechia** may be observed in patients with bleeding disorders (e.g. thrombocytopenia) and occasionally may be noted in patients with infective endocarditis.

Cardiology

B. **OCULAR FUNDUS:** Examination of the ocular fundus allows us to visually inspect and evaluate the arterioles and veins of the retina.
   1. **Retinal hemorrhages** may be present with systemic hypertension or bacterial endocarditis.
   2. **Papilledema** (swelling of the optic disc), tortuous vessels, and/or **retinal detachment** may be observed in patients with severe hypertension.
   3. **Retinal degeneration** can occur secondary to taurine deficiency in cats.

C. **JUGULAR VEINS:** Jugular distension and jugular pulses extending greater than 1/3 of the way up the neck reflect elevated venous pressure and occurs with:
   1. Right heart failure
   2. Reduced compliance of the right ventricle
   3. Pericardial disease (resulting in decreased ventricular compliance)
   4. Hypervolemia
   5. Obstruction of the cranial vena cava

III. **THORACIC AUSCULTATION:** Before ausculting the heart, listen to the lungs for increased inspiratory sounds, crackles, or wheezing. Next, palpate the chest to locate the point of maximal intensity. This represents the apex beat. The apex beat may be displaced (or reduced in intensity) by any condition that alters the position of the heart within the chest cavity (e.g. intrathoracic neoplasia, hernias, effusions, or cardiomegaly). Also note the presence and location of any palpable murmur which is termed a "thrill."

A. **GENERAL INFORMATION about AUSCULTATION:** Auscultation is a valuable part of the cardiovascular exam. It not only provides information about the heart and great vessels, but it also allows evaluation of the airways and pulmonary parenchyma. Obtain the heart rate and rhythm, check for pulse deficits, and listen for abnormal sounds.
   1. **About the stethoscope:** Use the diaphragm to hear high-pitched sounds and the bell to hear lower frequency sounds.
   2. **Location of the valves:**

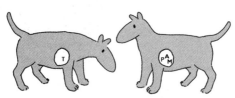

   a. **Pulmonic valve:** Left third intercostal space
   b. **Aortic valve:** Left fourth intercostal space
   c. **Mitral valve:** Left fifth intercostal space
   d. **Tricuspid valve:** Right fourth intercostal space

   Rather than locating the valves by counting rib spaces, just start listening at the point of maximal intensity (the mitral valve/apex beat) on the left side and then slowly move the stethoscope cranially and dorsally. Then listen on the right side. It's standard practice to describe the point of maximum intensity of an abnormal murmur as being at the base or apex rather than at a specific valve location (e.g. left apical systolic murmur).

   3. Cardiac sounds may be decreased due to extrathoracic fat, intrathoracic fluid, masses, or air, and pericardial fluid. Sounds may be increased in animals that are thin, hyperactive, or in high output states (e.g. hyperthyroidism, anemia, excitement).

B. THE FOUR HEART SOUNDS: Only S₁ and S₂ are normally heard in small animals.

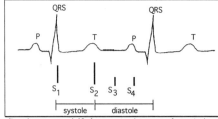

1. The first heart sound (S₁) occurs at the onset of ventricular systole and corresponds with the closure of the AV valves (mitral and tricuspid). S₁ is loudest at the palpable apex beat just prior to the rise in arterial pressure.
2. The second heart sound (S₂) occurs at the end of ventricular systole and corresponds to the closure of the semilunar valves (aortic and pulmonic). It's loudest at the base.
3. The third heart sound (S₃, the protodiastolic gallop) is a low-pitched sound associated with rapid ventricular filling. It's best heard at the left apex. S₃ is not heard in normal animals. It occurs with volume overload, thus it frequently accompanies congestive heart failure and ventricular dilatation associated with advanced mitral insufficiency or cardiomyopathy.
4. The fourth heart sound occurs at the beginning of atrial systole and is not heard in normal animals. It is due to filling of a non-compliant ventricle such as with pressure overload or hypertrophic cardiomyopathy. The fourth heart sound is low in frequency and best heard on the left side.
5. Systolic click: A high frequency extra heart sound heard between S1 and S2 in systole.
6. Split S2 is caused by asynchronous closure of the semilunar valves. It is associated with diseases that cause pulmonary or systemic hypertension as well as bundle branch blocks. It may increase on inspiration due to the drop in pulmonary pressure.

C. MURMURS arise from turbulent blood flow created when the laminar flow of blood is disrupted by 1) alterations in blood viscosity (e.g. low viscosity due to anemia), 2) vessel diameter (e.g. narrow diameter), or 3) abnormal flow patterns from insufficient valves or abnormal communications between cardiac chambers.
   1. Characteristics important in describing murmurs:
      a. Intensity:

INTENSITY OF MURMURS
Grade I: The softest audible murmur, detected only by meticulous auscultation in an optimal environment
Grade II: A faint murmur heard after a few seconds of auscultation
Grade III: A moderate intensity murmur heard immediately and easily
Grade IV: A loud murmur which does not produce a thrill
Grade V: A loud murmur which produces a thrill
Grade VI: A very loud murmur with a thrill, audible with the stethoscope just removed from the chest wall

      b. Frequency: Murmurs may be high, medium, or low in pitch, or may have mixed frequency.
      c. Shape is based on the variations in intensity during the cardiac cycle. Murmurs may be band-shaped, diamond-shaped (crescendo-decrescendo), or decrescendo.
      d. Timing: Systolic, diastolic, or continuous.
      e. Duration:
         i. Holosystolic: Throughout systole
         ii. Pansystolic: Throughout systole and including S2

Cardiology

f. **Pathologic vs. non-pathologic murmurs:** Innocent murmurs (no known anatomic abnormality) are most common in young animals. They are usually short, early systolic, low-grade murmurs heard best at the left heart base. Innocent murmurs should disappear as the juvenile animal matures. Other non-pathologic murmurs include physiologic murmurs (e.g. those caused by increased cardiac output or decreased blood viscosity in the absence of gross pathology). Like innocent murmurs, physiologic murmurs are usually low-grade, early systolic murmurs. Physiologic murmurs will be present as long as the underlying etiology is present. They do not represent cardiac disease.

2. **Systolic Murmurs:**

CHART of SYSTOLIC MURMURS

LESION	BREED PREDISPOSITIONS	TYPE OF MURMUR	POINT OF INTENSITY
Mitral Insufficiency	Acquired: Small breeds (e.g. miniature poodle) Congenital (mitral dysplasia): Large breed dogs	WM or Mw	Left Apex
Tricuspid Insufficiency	Acquired: Small breeds Congenital (tricuspid dysplasia): Labrador Retriever	WM or Mw	Right Side
Aortic (subaortic) Stenosis	Newfoundland, German shepherd, Boxer, Rottweiler, Golden Retriever	Mww	Left Base
Pulmonic Stenosis	English bulldog, Beagle, terriers	Mww	Left Base
Ventricular Septal Defect (VSD)	English bulldog, English springer spaniel	WM or Mw	Right Side
Atrial Septal Defect (ASD)	Rare	Mww	Left Side
Tetralogy of Fallot	Keeshond	Mww	Left Base

3. **Diastolic Murmurs:**

CHART of DIASTOLIC MURMURS

LESION	TYPICAL BREEDS	ETIOLOGY	POINT OF INTENSITY
Aortic Insufficiency	None	Seen most frequently in dogs with bacterial endocarditis involving the aortic valve. Also seen with subaortic stenosis and VSDs.	Left Side
Pulmonic Insufficiency	None	Rare	Left Side
Mitral Stenosis	None	Rare	Left Side
Tricuspid Stenosis	Labrador	Rare	Right Side

4. Continuous murmurs are characteristic of arteriovenous fistulas in which the pressure on the arterial side of the shunt is higher than on the venous side. This results in shunting of blood during both systole and diastole. It's heard most commonly in young animals with patent ductus arteriosus (PDA). The murmur is loudest at the left base but may radiate widely in some animals. A continuous murmur may also be heard over a peripheral arteriovenous fistula. These occasionally occur in the limbs of dogs and cats. The murmur is similar in character to that of a PDA and may be accompanied by palpable fremitus. Continuous murmurs from PDAs are heard best at the left axillary region. Sometimes they're only present in this region.

LESION	TYPICAL BREEDS	MURMUR	POINT OF INTENSITY
Patent Ductus Arteriosus	Miniature poodle, Corgi, Pomeranian, German Shepherd	Continuous murmur	Left Base

5. **To-and-fro murmurs** are a combination of a systolic and diastolic murmur (e.g. a ventricular septal defect plus aortic insufficiency)

6. **WHEN is it important to work up a murmur?** Not all murmurs are pathologic, life-threatening, or detrimental to the animal's health, and not all murmurs have to be worked up with ECG, thoracic radiographs, and cardiac ultrasound.

IT IS ESPECIALLY IMPORTANT TO WORK UP A MURMUR WHEN

- The animal has signs of cardiac disease such as ascites, harsh lung sounds, coughing, decreased exercise tolerance, pale or cyanotic mucous membranes.
- The animal has a continuous or diastolic murmur, gallop rhythm, or pulse deficits.
- The murmur has progressed since you last listened to it.
- The murmur is in a dog breed prone to dilated cardiomyopathy (DCM).
- The patient is a small breed dog with a grade III or louder murmur.
- The owner would like you to further pursue the murmur.
- Any cat with a murmur or gallop rhythm.

   a. Innocent murmurs need not be worked up. However, if you hear a short, soft, systolic murmur in a young dog, you should inform the owner that the animal has a murmur. Its thorax should be ausculted carefully at each examination and the presence or absence of the murmur noted.

   b. Murmur intensity does not always determine severity of cardiac disease; however, if the intensity of the murmur increases over time, the disease process is likely progressing. Dog breeds predisposed to DCM should receive an echocardiogram. Small breed dogs with a grade III or louder murmur should have an echocardiogram, but radiographs may be adequate for revealing cardiomegaly. In cats, murmur intensity has no correlation with severity of disease. Cats with soft murmurs can have significant heart disease (predominantly hypertrophic cardiomyopathy). Consequently, all cats with murmurs should receive an echocardiogram. Radiographs are not a sensitive diagnostic tool in feline cardiac disease.

7. **WHEN is it safe to anesthetize an animal with a murmur or with mild cardiac disease?** Cardiac disease often increases anesthetic risk, so do not fluid overload an animal with a murmur, even if the murmur is soft. If the murmur is something other than a short, grade I systolic murmur, the animal should be further evaluated with chest radiographs to determine whether there are already cardiac changes (e.g. enlarged atria) that suggest the presence of pathologic cardiac disease. If there is evidence of compensation (such as large atria), then anesthesia greatly increases the risk of decompensation and special anesthetic precautions must be taken.

IV. **ABDOMEN:** Palpate for organomegaly or ascites; use abdominal ballottement to check for fluid. Right heart failure usually results in a modified transudate due to hepatic venous congestion.

V. **CHECK PULSES:** The femoral pulse should be palpated and characterized.
   A. The strength and character of the pulse is determined by:
      1. Stroke volume and ejection rate
      2. Distensibility of the vascular bed
      3. Peripheral resistance
      4. The difference between systolic and diastolic pulse pressures

   B. **VARIATIONS in PULSE CHARACTER:**

	WEAK PULSES	BOUNDING PULSES	PULSE DEFICITS
Patho-physiology	Occur when the stroke volume is low, the pulse pressure is narrow, or there's increased peripheral resistance (vasoconstriction).	Occur when there is a large difference between systolic and diastolic blood pressures.	Occur during a premature beat when there's not enough time for the ventricles to fill before contracting.
Etiologies	• Hypovolemia (leads to vasoconstriction) • Severe subaortic stenosis • Left ventricular failure • Pericardial disease Can be weak in the pre-CHF patient.	• PDA or other arteriovenous fistulas • Aortic insufficiency • High output states (hyperthyroidism, anemia, excitement) • Vasodilatory shock (sepsis, anaphylaxis)	• Atrial fibrillation • Ventricular and atrial premature contractions

Cardiology

RADIOGRAPHIC & ECHOCARDIOGRAPHIC CHANGES

ABNORMALITY	ETIOLOGY
Enlarged Left Atrium	Mitral Insufficiency or Stenosis Patent Ductus Arteriosus (PDA) Ventricular Septal Defect (VSD) Dilated Cardiomyopathy Feline Hypertrophic, Restrictive, or Dilated Cardiomyopathy

Enlarged Left Ventricle
• Volume overload =
  eccentric hypertrophy
• Pressure overload =
  concentric hypertrophy
	Patent Ductus Arteriosus (PDA)
	Ventricular Septal Defect (VSD)
	Dilated Cardiomyopathy
	Mitral Insufficiency
	Aortic Stenosis (concentric hypertrophy)
	Systemic Hypertension (concentric hypertrophy)

Enlarged Right Atrium	Tricuspid Insufficiency or Stenosis Atrial Septal Defect (ASD) Dilated Cardiomyopathy Feline Hypertrophic, Restrictive, or Dilated Cardiomyopathy

Enlarged Right Ventricle
• Volume overload =
  eccentric hypertrophy
• Pressure overload =
  concentric hypertrophy
	Atrial Septal Defect (eccentric hypertrophy)
	Tricuspid Insufficiency (eccentric hypertrophy)
	Dilated Cardiomyopathy (eccentric hypertrophy)
	Pulmonic Stenosis (concentric hypertrophy)
	Right-to-Left PDA (concentric hypertrophy)
	Tetralogy of Fallot (concentric hypertrophy)
	Pulmonary Hypertension (concentric hypertrophy)

Enlarged Pulmonary Trunk	Anything causing pulmonary hypertension can cause an enlarged pulmonary trunk. Heartworms Pulmonic stenosis (post-stenotic dilatation)
Enlarged Aorta	Patent Ductus Arteriosus (Left-to-Right) Subaortic Stenosis (post-stenotic dilatation)

VOLUME OVERLOAD vs. PRESSURE OVERLOAD

	LEFT SIDE	RIGHT SIDE
Volume Overload	• Mitral Insufficiency • Dilated Cardiomyopathy • VSD • Aortic Insufficiency • PDA (Left-to-Right)	• Tricuspid Insufficiency • Atrial Septal Defect • Dilated Cardiomyopathy
Pressure Overload	• Aortic Stenosis • Systemic Hypertension	• Pulmonic Stenosis • Tetralogy of Fallot • PDA (Right-to-Left) • Pulmonary Hypertension

READING ELECTROCARDIOGRAMS

I. **ELECTRICAL CONDUCTION:** The electrical signal starts at the pacemaker (the sinoatrial or SA node). It travels first into the right atrium and then into the left atrium (P wave). It then travels through the AV node (P-R interval) and enters the bundle branch system which depolarizes the ventricles (QRS wave complex). Lastly, the ventricles repolarize (T wave).

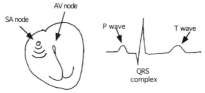

II. **STEPS in READING ECGs:**

STEPS in READING an ECG
1. Determine the **mean electrical axis:** Is the axis normal or is it deviated towards the right or left?
2. Determine the **heart rate:** Is the heart rate fast, normal, or slow?
3. Determine the **rhythm:** Is the rhythm regular or irregular? Is there a QRS for every P wave and a P wave for every QRS?
4. Determine the **wave forms, heights, and widths:** Are the P waves or QRS waves wider or taller than normal? Is the P-R interval always the same? If there are bizarre forms, are they early or late?
5. **Miscellaneous abnormalities:** Is the S-T segment depressed or elevated?

A. **Quickly determine the MEAN ELECTRICAL AXIS:** A general idea of the direction of the mean electrical axis can be easily obtained by looking at leads I and avF. For example, if both leads I and aVF show completely positive deflections, the mean electrical axis is around 0-90°. If lead I shows a completely negative deflection and avF shows a completely positive deflection, then the mean electrical axis is around 90°-180°. In a dog, this would be a right axis deviation.

MEAN ELECTRICAL AXIS	DOG	CAT
Normal Axis	40°-100°	0-160°
Right Axis Deviation	> 100°	> 160°
Left Axis Deviation	< 40°	< 0°

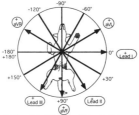

Modified from Tilley LP: *Essentials of Canine and Feline Cardiology.* 2nd Ed. Philadelphia: Lea & Febiger, 1985.

Cardiology

B. **HEART RATE:** Identify **tachycardias** and **bradycardias**. If the heart rate is irregular, a long time span should be used to determine heart rate. If it's regular, 6 seconds is a long enough time span to count.

1. **General Heart Rate:**

$$\begin{array}{ll} \text{Heart Rate} = & \underline{\text{\# beats}} \quad \text{x} \quad \underline{\text{60 seconds}} \\ \text{(beats/min)} & \text{\# seconds} \qquad \text{minute} \end{array}$$

Note that if you count the beats per 6 seconds, the formula becomes:

$$\text{Heart Rate} = \text{\# beats} \ \text{x} \ 10$$

If you only count for 3 seconds, multiply the number of beats by 20.

2. **Instantaneous Heart Rate:** Determining heart rate at any point in time is often beneficial (e.g. to determine the rate at which a ventricular focus fires in a short burst of ventricular tachycardia). To do this, measure the time between the two wave forms you are interested in (e.g. R-R interval in the case of ventricular tachycardia; P-P or R-R interval in the case of atrial tachycardia) and divide that time in seconds into 60 seconds.

$$\begin{array}{ll} \text{Instantaneous heart rate} = & \underline{\text{60 seconds/minute}} \\ \text{(beats/min)} & \text{\# seconds/beat} \end{array}$$

A quick and dirty method for determining instantaneous heart rate is to use one of the following equations (one for a paper speed of 50mm/minute and one for a paper speed of 25mm/minute):

Paper Speed	50mm/second	25mm/second
Equation for Instantaneous Heart Rate	$\dfrac{3000}{\text{\# boxes counted}}$	$\dfrac{1500}{\text{\# boxes counted}}$

C. **RHYTHM:**

1. Look at the R-R intervals and see if they are **regular** or **irregular**. If irregular, is the irregularity repeated (e.g. does it occur with respiration)? Does the heart rate increase with inspiration and decrease with expiration? This arrhythmia is called **sinus arrhythmia** and is a normal cardiac rhythm in the dog. It should disappear with exercise or with the administration of atropine. Sinus arrhythmia is not normal in the cat or horse.

2. Are there premature depolarizations?

3. Is there a P wave for every QRS complex and a QRS for every P wave?

D. **WAVEFORMS:**

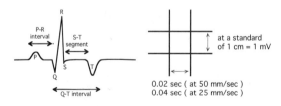

at a standard of 1 cm = 1 mV

0.02 sec (at 50 mm/sec)
0.04 sec (at 25 mm/sec)

ECG Measurements: Lead II, 50mm/sec, 1cm = 1 mV		DOG NORMALS	CAT NORMALS
P wave	Width	≤ 0.04 sec (2 boxes)	≤ 0.04 sec (2 boxes)
	Height	≤ 0.4 mV (4 boxes)	≤ 0.2 mV (2 boxes)
P-R interval	Width	0.06 - 0.13 sec (3 - 6.5 boxes)	0.05 - 0.09 sec (2.5 - 4.5 boxes)
QRS complex	Width	Small breeds ≤ 0.05 sec (2.5 boxes) Large breeds ≤ 0.06 sec (3 boxes)	0.04 sec (2 boxes)
	Height (R wave)	Small breeds ≤ 2.5 mV (25 boxes) Large breeds ≤ 3.0 mV (30 boxes)	0.9 mV (9 boxes)
S-T segment	Depression	≤ 0.2 mV (2 boxes)	No marked depression/elevation
	Elevation	≤ 0.15 mV (1.5 boxes)	No marked depression/elevation
T wave	Positive, negative, or biphasic	≤ Amplitude of the R wave	Commonly positive ≤ 0.3 mV (3 boxes)
Q-T interval	Width varies with heart rate (faster rates have shorter Q-T intervals)	0.15 - 0.25 sec (7.5 - 12.5 boxes)	0.12 - 0.18 sec (6 - 9 boxes) at normal heart rate (Range: 0.07 -0.2 sec = 3.5 - 10 boxes)

1. Wider than normal waves indicate slowed conduction while taller than normal waves indicate chamber enlargement.
   a. Tall P wave indicates right atrial enlargement.
   b. Wide P wave indicates left atrial enlargement.
   c. Notching of the P wave plus a wide P wave indicates biatrial enlargement.
   d. Wide QRS indicates slowed conduction through the ventricles. This occurs when conduction travels through the myocardium rather than through the bundle branch system (e.g. damaged bundle branch system or ectopic depolarization from within the ventricular myocardium). A small increase in QRS width may also occur with ventricular hypertrophy.
   e. Tall QRS indicates enlarged ventricles. If the deflection is positive (tall R wave), then the left ventricle is enlarged. If the deflection is negative (deep S wave), then the right ventricle is enlarged.
2. Depressed S-T segment indicates myocardial hypoxemia (an acute condition) or myocardial ischemia (a chronic condition).
3. Negatively deflected P wave indicates depolarization is starting from the lower portion of the left atrium or in the AV node.

III. DETECTING CHAMBER ENLARGEMENT:

CHAMBER ENLARGEMENT	ECG CHANGES
Right Atrial Enlargement	Tall P waves
Left Atrial Enlargement	Prolonged P waves (longer activation in the atria)
Biatrial Enlargement	Notched P waves in which the first portion is tall and the remaining portion is prolonged
Right Ventricular Enlargement	Large negative deflection (S wave) Shift of the mean electrical axis to the right
Left Ventricular Enlargement	Normal or taller than normal R waves in leads II and aVF ± prolonged QRS complexes (LBB conduction disturbance)

CARDIAC ARRHYTHMIAS

I. **CARDIAC ARRHYTHMIAS:** Arrhythmias are disturbances in the cardiac rhythm. They may occur for a number of reasons including abnormal conduction, ectopic depolarization, or the acceleration or slowing of a normal pacemaker. Electrocardiograph (ECG) recordings provide the definitive diagnosis of an arrhythmia. Diagnosis of the specific arrhythmia is crucial prior to initiating therapy.

   A. **TYPES OF ARRYTHMIAS:** Arrhythmias can be divided into those originating from the SA node, those originating from ectopic tissue (causing depolarization that is either too soon or too late), and those caused by slower or faster than normal conduction through the usual conduction pathway (e.g. Wolff-Parkinson-White Syndrome causes faster than normal conduction).

   1. **Disturbances of SA nodal activity:**
       a. Sinus arrhythmia (normal in dogs)
       b. Sinus tachycardia
       c. Sinus bradycardia
       d. Sinus arrest
       e. Atrial standstill

   2. **Conduction blocks:**
       a. **Atrioventricular (AV) blocks:**
           i.   **First degree AV block** results in prolongation of the PR interval.
           ii. **Second degree AV block (Mobitz type I or II)** results in some atrial depolarizations not reaching the ventricles.
           iii. **Third degree AV block** occurs when no atrial depolarizations reach the ventricles. This is one form of AV dissociation.

       b. **Intraventricular conduction blocks:**
           i.   Left bundle branch block (complete or partial)
           ii. Right bundle branch block (complete or partial)

   3. **Conduction bypass:**
       a. **Preexcitation Syndrome** (Formerly called Wolfe-Parkinson-White Syndrome): Faster conduction because conduction bypasses the AV node.

   4. **Ectopic depolarizations** originate from areas other than the SA node:
       a. **Escape beats or rhythms** occur when a lower pacemaker takes over the cardiac rhythm because a higher pacemaker has either failed (e.g. sinus arrest) or is blocked from stimulating a lower pacemaker (e.g. third degree AV block). Escape beats can be supraventricular, junctional, or ventricular in origin.

       b. **Premature depolarizations** (beats, contractions) occur when depolarization is initiated from an abnormal (ectopic) site **earlier than normal**. The ectopic site can be located in the atria, AV node, or bundle of His (all supraventricular), as well as in the ventricles. Premature contractions may occur singly, in pairs, as tachycardia (3 or more consecutive beats), as bigeminy (every other beat), or as trigeminy (every third beat), etc.

Schematic for Diagnosing Arrhythmias

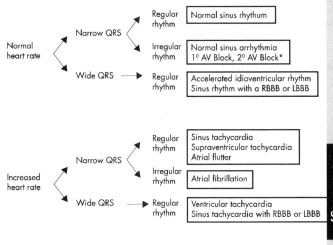

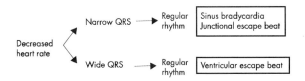

* Often the heart rate is decreased with 2° AV blocks (depends on whether it's a low-grade or hihg-grade block)

* Often the heart rate is decreased with 2° AV blocks (depends on whether it's a low-grade or high-grade block).

CARDIAC ARRHYTHMIAS - SA Node Disorders

ARRHYTHMIA	DESCRIPTION	ETIOLOGY	SIGNIFICANCE	TREATMENT
Sinus Arrhythmia	Sinus arrhythmia is a regular increase and decrease in heart rate associated with respiration. The P wave may be variably shaped because vagal tone shifts the site of depolarization outside the sinus node (wandering pacemaker). The P-QRS-T configuration is normal.	Caused by waxing and waning vagal tone in association with respiration. Vagal tone decreases on inspiration (heart rate increases) and increases on expiration (heart rate decreases).	This is a normal rhythm in the dog, but it can be classified as abnormal if it's exaggerated. An exaggerated sinus arrhythmia occurs most commonly in animals with respiratory disease in which the large swings in intrapleural pressure associated with dyspnea result in large swings in vagal tone.	Sinus arrhythmia is a normal rhythm in most dogs. Atropine and exercise should abolish this rhythm. No treatment is required.
Sinus Tachycardia	The heart rate is increased above normal for the species, but the rhythm is regular. The P-QRS-T configuration is normal.	May be caused by increased sympathetic tone, decreased parasympathetic tone, or both.	It's often seen in association with fear, excitement, pain, heart failure, shock, hyperthyroidism, and drug administration (atropine, catecholamines), thus it can be a normal physiologic response or it can indicate the presence of underlying disease.	If you suspect underlying pathology, try to determine the etiology so that you can treat it. Otherwise, no treatment is required.
Sinus Bradycardia	The heart rate is slower than normal. The P-QRS-T configuration is normal.	Can be associated with increased vagal tone, hypothermia, diseased sinus node, and administration of certain drugs.	In extremely athletic animals, sinus bradycardia can be normal, but in other animals it may be associated with increased vagal tone, drug administration (digitalis, beta adrenergic blocking agents), sinus node disease (sick sinus syndrome), hyperkalemia, or hypothermia.	Atropine can be given to determine whether vagal tone is responsible. No treatment is required unless the animal has episodes of syncope.

Sinus Arrest	A pathologic condition resulting in the cessation of sinus activity for longer than 2 R-R intervals. If it's prolonged (> 5 - 6 sec.) we may see syncope or episodes of weakness. The pause may be terminated by an **escape beat** (junctional or ventricular). The P-QRS-T configuration is normal (except for the escape beats).	Similar causes as sinus bradycardia.	Sinus arrest is a pathologic condition that may be associated with increased vagal tone, drug administration (digitalis, beta adrenergic blocking agents), sick sinus syndrome, hypothermia, or cardiac arrest.	Treat sinus arrest if it results in syncope. Atropine is the drug of choice. It will stop the sinus arrest if it's associated with increased vagal tone. If it's associated with a diseased SA node, atropine may cause partial resolution or have no effect. Animals that experience syncope from sinus arrest but do not respond to atropine may be treated with a pacemaker.
Atrial Standstill	Occurs when the atria cannot depolarize, either due to disease (a cardiomyopathy most commonly seen in English springer spaniels) or severe hyperkalemia. There are no P waves on the ECG and there is no escape rhythm.	Caused by destruction of the atria and thus the SA node. No electrical impulse occurs.	This is a pathologic condition that will progress. It may cause syncope.	Pacemaker implantation is usually not performed because progressive myocardial failure often develops.

Cardiology

CARDIAC ARRHYTHMIAS - Atrioventricular Conduction Blocks

ARRHYTHMIA	DESCRIPTION	ETIOLOGY	SIGNIFICANCE	TREATMENT
First Degree AV Block (1°)	Prolonged P-R interval	Caused by prolonged conduction through the AV node secondary to increased vagal tone, organic disease of the AV node (usually degeneration), or drug administration.	Indicates increased vagal tone, disease of the AV node, or drug administration (e.g. digitalis, beta blockers).	No treatment required
Second Degree AV Block (2°)	A more advanced AV conduction disturbance than the 1° block, characterized by complete blockage of some of the sinus depolarizations. This appears as some P waves without QRS complexes. **Mobitz type I:** The P-R interval is progressively longer until the 2° block occurs. **Mobitz type II:** The P-R interval is normal or constantly long.	Increased vagal tone, organic disease of the AV node, or drug administration.	If the AV block resolves with atropine, the block is due to elevated vagal tone. Lack of response to atropine suggests AV node pathology.	AV blocks only require therapy if the patient is showing clinical signs (syncope or weakness) or if the block is 3:1 or greater (3 P waves for every QRS). Pacemaker implantation is the treatment of choice; however, medical therapy such as terbutaline, can be tried first.
Third Degree AV Block (3°)	A form of AV dissociation. The P waves and QRS complexes are completely dissociated. Atrial rate is faster than ventricular rate and the P-R intervals are irregular. The ventricles are depolarized by either a junctional escape rhythm (40 - 60 bpm) or a ventricular escape rhythm (20-40 bpm).	Usually due to AV nodal disease.	Dogs with a ventricular escape rhythm often present for syncope, while dogs with a junctional escape rhythm often do not exhibit clinical signs.	Pacemaker implantation is the only rational therapy. IV isoproterenol may be used in emergency situations to increase ventricular rate, but this drug should be used cautiously. Complications of its use include arrhythmias and resulting hypotension.

CARDIAC ARRHYTHMIAS - Intraventricular Conduction Abnormalities

	DESCRIPTION	ETIOLOGY	SIGNIFICANCE
Right Bundle Branch Block (RBBB)	A P wave precedes every QRS and a QRS follows every P wave. The QRS is prolonged with a right axis deviation (deep S wave) in lead II. With incomplete RBBB, the QRS complex is not prolonged but right axis deviation is present along with a deep S wave. Incomplete RBBB must be differentiated from right ventricular enlargement by examining chest radiographs or ideally by echocardiography. It's easy to confuse RBBB with right ventricular hypertrophy or VPCs. RBBB usually has a regular rhythm.	RBBB is caused by interruption of conduction in the right bundle branch. It can be a benign incidental finding or can indicate disease affecting the right ventricular myocardium. The QRS complex is prolonged because conduction moves quickly through the left ventricle via the left bundle branch and then must go slowly via the myocardium to the right side. This results in deep S waves.	No treatment required, however underlying right heart disease should be ruled out.
Left Bundle Branch Block (LBBB)	ECG reveals tall, wide QRS complexes that are preceded by P waves. LBBB has a regular rhythm.	Caused by slower conduction (or interruption of conduction) through the left bundle branch.	Usually occurs in association with left ventricular disease but is occasionally seen in otherwise normal dogs. LBBB produces no hemodynamic abnormalities. It's almost always associated with left ventricular disease in cats and is most commonly found in association with hypertrophic cardiomyopathy.
Preexcitation Syndrome Formerly called Wolff-Parkinson-White Syndrome (WPW)	ECG reveals shortened P-R intervals and delta waves when in sinus rhythm.	Caused by accessory conduction fibers which produce an unusually rapid impulse that bypasses the AV node.	WPW is a tachyarrhythmia.

Cardiology

CARDIAC ARRHYTHMIAS - Supraventricular Arrhythmias

ARRHYTHMIA	DESCRIPTION	ETIOLOGY	SIGNIFICANCE	TREATMENT
Supra-ventricular Premature Contractions	Caused by ectopic foci that fire earlier than normal. Foci can be located in the atria (atrial premature contractions), the AV node, or the bundle of His (junctional premature contractions). The QRS complex is narrow. The R-R interval from the premature depolarization to the next normal depolarization is either normal or slightly prolonged. **Atrial premature contractions** have a P wave before the QRS. The P wave may be positive or negative (if the ectopic focus is in the lower region of the left atrium). The P wave may be buried in the T wave from the previous complex. **Junctional premature contractions** may not have P waves in front of the QRS or the P waves may be negative. Animals may have pulse deficits or weak pulses accompanying the premature beats.	Supraventricular premature contractions are caused by organic disease of the atria (most commonly atrial distension), disease of the AV junction, or by drug administration (e.g. digoxin, catecholamines). The R-R interval from the premature depolarization to the next normal depolarization is either normal or slightly prolonged because the ectopic depolarization is conducted retrograde to the sinus node where it discharges and resets the sinus node.	Supraventricular premature depolarizations may lead to atrial tachycardia, atrial flutter, or atrial fibrillation. Prognosis depends on the underlying disease.	Treatment is indicated when the premature contractions are frequent (occurring every sixth beat or more), or are present in runs. They are most frequently treated with calcium channel blockers, beta blockers, and/or digoxin. When supraventricular premature contractions are seen, an underlying etiology should be pursued.
Supra-ventricular Tachycardia	Supraventricular tachycardia is a series of supraventricular premature depolarizations occurring in succession. The rhythm is **regular**. The QRS complex configuration is usually normal but can be wide and bizarre if an associated bundle branch block is present, making it difficult to distinguish from ventricular tachycardia (the rate may be too fast to see P waves).	Usually associated with atrial or junctional disease. Clinical signs include weakness, or less commonly, syncope if the rate is rapid and sustained (due to decreased cardiac output).	May indicate atrial or junctional disease or can be an isolated conduction disorder. Some supraventricular tachycardias are controlled very well with drugs for many years.	Try to break the sustained runs using a chest thump, vagal maneuvers, or IV propranolol. (0.02 - 0.06 mg/kg IV given over 5-10 minutes for both dogs and cats). Long-term treatment is the same as for atrial premature depolarizations.

Atrial Flutter	The atrial rate is 400-500 bpm. Only every other (2:1) or every third (3:1) atrial depolarization gets through the AV node (functional second degree AV block). The ventricular rate can be regular or irregular. ECG shows undulating "flutter waves" instead of P waves. The QRS configurations are normal.	Atrial flutter is associated with severe atrial disease or digitalis toxicity.	Indicates severe atrial or junctional disease. It usually precedes atrial fibrillation. Animals with atrial flutter may have syncopal episodes. Atrial flutter is very rare.	Treated the same as atrial fibrillation (digitalis, β blockers, calcium channel blockers, electrical conversion).
Atrial Fibrillation	The atrial rate is 600-700 bpm. Only a small number of atrial depolarizations are conducted through the AV node to the ventricles. The rhythm is **irregular** because a variable number of depolarizations get through to the ventricles, thus the R-R intervals are variable. P waves are not visible. The baseline may be flat or undulating due to fibrillation waves. The heart sounds have variable intensities and the rate is irregular (sounds like jungle drums or tennis shoes in a dryer). Pulse deficits are present.	Occurs due to multiple sites of reentry in the atria. This usually requires a large atrial surface area (i.e. large atria because of patient size or secondary to disease).	Large breed dogs that have normal, anatomically large atria and no underlying cardiac disease can have atrial fibrillation. You may or may not elect treatment depending on the rate; many do well without treatment. Smaller animals with atrial fibrillation usually have underlying cardiac disease which results in atrial enlargement (e.g. dilated cardiomyopathy). Their underlying disease and atrial fibrillation warrants treatment, but treatment is not a true emergency unless the heart rate is so fast that it causes marked hemodynamic compromise. CHF is harder to control if the animal is in atrial fibrillation. Prognosis is good with primary atrial fibrillation and guarded when underlying cardiac disease exists.	Treatment is aimed at slowing the ventricular rate when it is rapid (> 180 bpm). Excessively rapid heart rates increase myocardial oxygen consumption and thus predispose to myocardial hypoxia and myocardial failure. In dogs with dilated cardiomyopathy, it's best to increase contractility at the same time you decrease heart rate (using digoxin). If more rapid rate control is needed, a calcium channel blocker or beta blocker is often used. When treating large dogs without underlying heart disease, the options are 1) to convert to normal sinus rhythm, 2) treat if the heart rate is rapid, or 3) not to treat if the heart rate is normal.

Cardiology

CARDIAC ARRHYTHMIAS - Ventricular Arrhythmias

ARRHYTHMIA	DESCRIPTION	ETIOLOGY	SIGNIFICANCE	TREATMENT
Ventricular Premature Contractions (VPCs)	Characterized by wide, bizarre QRS complexes that occur earlier than normal. The interval after the VPC is variable; it's usually longer than the normal R-R interval (compensatory pause). VPCs originating from the right ventricle travel the same way the mean vector normally travels; therefore, the QRS complexes are upright in leads where the normal sinus QRS complexes are normally positive. VPCs that originate from the left ventricle have negative QRS complexes in leads where the sinus QRS complexes are normally positive. A run of 3 or more VPCs is called ventricular tachycardia.	An ectopic focus in the ventricles depolarizes before sinus node depolarization is initiated or reaches the ventricles. The R-R interval following the ventricular depolarization is longer than normal because the myocardium is refractory to normal sinus depolarization. Depolarization travels retrograde to or through the AV node, canceling the sinus node depolarization before it reaches the ventricles. The next sinus depolarization comes along and depolarizes the ventricles normally.	VPCs occur in association with myocardial disease, drug administration (e.g. digitalis, anesthetic agents), hypoxia, neoplasia, electrolyte abnormalities, autonomic imbalances (e.g. gastric dilatation-volvulus), and release of myocardial depressant or irritative agents (e.g. during abdominal surgery). Occasionally they are found in normal dogs. Multiform VPCs originate from different areas in the ventricles (multifocal) and are generally considered a sign of more serious disease; consequently, they are usually treated.	VPCs should be treated when they are associated with underlying organic myocardial disease or when they occur in pairs, groups, or as tachycardia. **Ventricular tachycardia:** The faster an ectopic focus fires, the greater the chance for fibrillation. Thus, the faster the instantaneous rate, the sooner you should treat. If the rate is > 200 bpm, institute therapy as soon as possible regardless of other criteria. Rates of < 140 are relatively benign and may or may not need treatment, depending on the underlying disease. Rates between 140-200 bpm may require treatment. If so, oral antiarrhythmics are usually sufficient. Critical cases can be managed with lidocaine: 2 mg/kg IV q 10 min for up to 4 doses. If this works, put the animal on a lidocaine infusion (CRI) until it's stable enough to be released on an oral antiarrhythmic.
Ventricular Flutter and Fibrillation	Ventricular flutter is the stage between ventricular tachycardia and ventricular fibrillation. Ventricular fibrillation is more common than flutter. With flutter, the QRS complexes and T waves are no longer distinguishable from one another, and in ventricular fibrillation the undulation is smaller and grossly irregular. Both are forms of cardiac arrest.		Associated with severe heart disease or severe disease processes affecting the heart. Both produce ineffective myocardial contractions; therefore, they are forms of cardiac arrest. Prognosis is grave.	Electrical defibrillation and supportive measures (cardiopulmonary resuscitation).

CARDIAC ARRHYTHMIAS - Escape Beats

ARRHYTHMIA	DESCRIPTION	ETIOLOGY	SIGNIFICANCE	TREATMENT
Escape Beats and Rhythms • Supraventricular • Junctional • Ventricular	Escape beats that originate from the lower AV node or bundle of His (**junctional** or **supraventricular escape beats**) usually have a narrow QRS and a heart rate of 40-60 bpm. If they originate from the bundle branches or Purkinje fibers (**ventricular escape beats**), the QRS complexes are **wide** (like VPCs) and the escape rate is 20-40 bpm.	Escape beats occur because the normal pacemaking region of the heart (the SA node) has stopped (as in sinus arrest or atrial standstill) or its depolarization has been blocked from reaching the ventricles (severe second degree AV block or 3rd degree AV block). As a result, the lower pacemaking regions initiate and control depolarization of the heart.	Escape beats can be benign or indicate a pathologic condition.	Treat the underlying rhythm disturbance. Do not try to suppress the escape beats, even the ventricular ones that look like VPCs. Escape beats are a protective mechanism

Cardiology

Valvular Diseases
Mitral Regurgitation (MR)
Tricuspid Regurgitation (TR)
Aortic (Subaortic) Stenosis
Pulmonic Stenosis
Aortic Insufficiency

MITRAL REGURGITATION (MR)

ETIOLOGIES	Primary etiologies are those involving changes in the mitral valve leaflets or chordae tendineae: • **Endocardiosis** (chronic myxomatous valvular degeneration) is a common lesion seen in older dogs (especially small breeds). It is characterized of an accumulation of collagenous and myxomatous deposits in the valve leaflets resulting in thickened, nodular, stiff valve leaflets. • **Ruptured chordae tendineae** (seen in conjunction with endocardiosis): Large primary or smaller secondary and tertiary chordae tendineae break, causing a sudden worsening of regurgitation in proportion to the structural support that is lost. • **Bacterial endocarditis** is bacterial infection of the valves. • **Mitral dysplasia** is a congenital malformation of the valves. Secondary etiologies involve malpositioning of the valves: • **Left ventricular dilation** (e.g. dilated cardiomyopathy) changes the positioning of the papillary muscles and consequently pulls the valve leaflets apart, creating a gap. • **Left ventricular concentric hypertrophy** (e.g. HCM in cats)

PATHO-PHYSIOLOGY	Mitral regurgitation causes volume overload:
	   Each time the left ventricle contracts, a portion of the total stroke volume (TSV) flows in the normal forward direction (forward stroke volume, FSV) and a portion leaks backwards (reverse stroke volume, RSV) through the defect, into the low pressure left atrium. As a result, cardiac output initially decreases, thus activating the sympathetic nervous system which triggers an increase in heart rate and cardiac contractility to bring cardiac output back to normal. This sympathetic stimulation effect diminishes over several days. Meanwhile, a different system, the RAAS (Refer to p. 3.6) is activated to help the heart compensate.
	   The activated RAAS leads to an increase in water retention, which in turn results in increased preload (end-diastolic volume) for the heart to pump. Thus the total stroke volume increases. As the TSV increases, the amount that regurgitates also increases, but so does the volume of blood ejected forward. In the early stages, enough blood is ejected forward to bring cardiac output back up to normal.
	   In order for the left heart to compensate for the increase in end-diastolic blood volume without having to increase left ventricular pressure (e.g. if you fill a balloon with more air, the pressure in the balloon increases), the ventricle undergoes **eccentric hypertrophy**. In eccentric hypertrophy, sarcomeres are laid down end-to-end so that the ventricular walls get longer and the left ventricular chamber dilates (analogous to getting a bigger balloon).
	
	With chronic mitral valve disease, congestive heart failure may be the result of one of two separate entities:
	• **Congestive heart failure:** Once the heart has undergone maximal eccentric hypertrophy, the chamber stops enlarging. As preload continues to increase, pressure in the left ventricle also increases. During diastole, the left ventricle, left atrium, and pulmonary veins freely communicate (the mitral valve is open) so that the pressure is the same in all three regions. This means that left atrial pressure and pulmonary venous and capillary pressures are also elevated. The end result is pulmonary edema.
	• **Myocardial failure:** In end-stage mitral regurgitation, the cardiac muscle may begin to fail so that the heart no longer has the strength to pump fluid forward. This occurs infrequently in small dogs and when it does, it tends to be mild. Myocardial failure is more common in large breed dogs.

MITRAL REGURGITATION continued

CLINICAL SIGNS	Signs are due to congestive heart failure: • **Cough** is due to pulmonary edema or compression of the left mainstem bronchus by an enlarged left atrium. Rule out collapsing trachea and lower airway disease. • **Tachypnea and increased respiratory effort** are due to pulmonary edema leading to hypoxia. • **Exercise intolerance** and **lethargy** are due to low cardiac output. • **Syncope:** With moderate to severe disease, some animals develop baroreceptor abnormalities which result in hypotensive events and consequently episodes of fainting.
PHYSICAL EXAM	Holosystolic or pansystolic murmur due to turbulent blood flow into the left atrium. The murmur is heard best over the **left apex** but it radiates dorsally, caudally, and to the right. A **third heart sound** is sometimes present (volume overload).
RADIOGRAPHIC FINDINGS	• Early in disease, radiographs may be normal. As the disease progresses, radiographs may reveal **left atrial enlargement** which appears as loss of the caudal cardiac waist (mild disease) or left atrial bulge $\pm$ elevation or narrowing of the trachea at the carina or mainstem bronchi. These tracheal changes can cause a cough. Left atrial enlargement also appears on the DV radiographs. **Left ventricular enlargement** appears on lateral radiographs as **elevation of the trachea** or a "tall" heart. • **Pulmonary congestion** and edema appear when congestive heart failure is present. Earlier in the course of disease, the pulmonary veins may just look distended.
ECG	• Symptomatic patients often have **long P waves** (> 0.04 s) due to the **enlarged left atrium**. • The **QRS complex** may be **tall** due to left ventricular enlargement (ECG is not a sensitive indicator of ventricular enlargement but is quite specific when abnormalities are present). • **Atrial arrhythmias** become common as the left atrium enlarges (atrial fibrillation, etc). • **Ventricular arrhythmias** can occur in advanced disease. • **Increased heart rate:** Heart rate increases in patients with heart failure in order to compensate for the low stroke volume.
ECHOCARDIOGRAM	• Eccentric hypertrophy of the left ventricle + dilated left atrium • Hyperdynamic contraction of the left ventricle • Doppler echocardiography reveals mitral regurgitation
TREATMENT	Mitral insufficiency often progresses slowly and the left ventricle and atrium have time to adapt. Consequently, in cases where radiographic or echocardiogram evidence of failure exists (e.g. severely enlarged left atrium, pulmonary edema), it is controversial as to whether animals should be treated. Some studies have found early treatment with ACE inhibitors decreases disease progression whereas other studies have found no difference. The conflict in research findings may be due to the fact that heart disease has strong genetic components and genetics contribute to the onset and progression of disease. Thus far, studies have not controlled for genetics.

Cardiology

MITRAL REGURGITATION continued

TREATMENT (CONTINUED)	Cardiologists who elect to treat earlier in disease when there's significant chamber enlargement but no clinical signs of heart failure, start with ACE inhibitors, which block formation of angiotensin II (p. 3.6). Angiotensin II causes increased systemic arterial pressure by producing vasoconstriction and increasing fluid volume. ACE inhibitors block these functions.

- **ACE inhibitors:** The most commonly used ACE inhibitors include **enalapril** and **benazepril** (Lotensin®). Benazepril is usually used SID and has fewer renal effects than enalapril. Once on ACE inhibitors, bloodwork should be rechecked in one week for signs of renal disease and electrolyte imbalance (especially if the animal is also on diuretics). If the animal is on enalapril and labwork reveals renal changes, switch to benazapril. Bloodwork should be rechecked every three months with renal parameters checked during some visits and a full blood panel and CBC (with or without urinalysis) checked in the alternating three months. The CBC and chemistry panel screen for concurrent disease (e.g. liver disease) that might necessitate adjusting drug therapy or that might affect overall health. Perform a recheck **ultrasound** every 6-9 months to assess parameters such as regurgitation and chamber enlargement. As disease progresses, the next drug that can be added is spironolactone.

- **Spironolactone** (0.5 - 1.0 mg/kg PO SID), an aldosterone-blocking agent, can be used with moderate to severe disease before heart failure has developed. This drug is very safe with few side effects reported in humans. At higher doses spironolactone acts as a weak, potassium sparing diuretic.

Once the animal is showing signs of congestive heart failure, treat with diuretics such as furosemide:

- **Diuretics decrease fluid volume: Furosemide,** a loop diuretic, is one of the best cardiac drugs, especially in emergency congestive heart failure cases. Dose should be adjusted based on clinical signs.
- **ACE inhibitors** such as enalapril and benazepril also decrease fluid volume and peripheral vascular resistance but are slower acting (take effect in approximately 6 hours).

- **Pimobendan** (Vetmedin®) is an inodilator: It increases cardiac contractility, dilates blood vessels, and effectively improves the clinical signs of mitral regurgitation (Dose: 0.2 - 0.5 mg/kg PO BID).

Diuretics, ACE inhibitors, and pimobendan can be used together in patients with congestive heart failure.

- **Antitussives** can be used when collapsing trachea is a component.
- **Antiarrhythmics** are indicated to treat arrhythmias.

TRICUSPID REGURGITATION (TR)

Tricuspid regurgitation is similar to mitral regurgitation, but instead of pulmonary congestion, the TR patient develops hepatic congestion, ascites, and/or pleural effusion. Tricuspid regurgitation causes volume overload, which results in eccentric hypertrophy.

ETIOLOGIES	**Primary etiologies involve changes to the tricuspid valve leaflets or chordae tendineae:** • Endocardiosis • Ruptured chordae tendineae • Bacterial endocarditis • Tricuspid dysplasia **Secondary etiologies involve malpositioning of the valves:** • Right ventricular dilation • Right atrial dilation, especially due to pulmonary hypertension
PATHO-PHYSIOLOGY	Refer to mitral insufficiency (p. 3.26). The only difference here is that in right heart failure, hydrostatic pressure increases in the vena cava which results in abdominal or pleural effusion (a modified transudate).
CLINICAL SIGNS	**Due to congestive heart failure:** • **Distended abdomen** due to ascites • **Increased respiratory effort and tachypnea** due to pleural effusion. This is more common in cats than dogs. Animals can also be dyspneic because of severe ascites. • **Peripheral edema** (rare) **Due to low cardiac output** (end-stage disease only): • **Exercise intolerance, lethargy**
PHYSICAL EXAM	• Systolic murmur heard best over the right side. If pleural effusion is present, the heart sounds may be muffled. • Jugular distension • Jugular pulses extending more than 1/3 up the vein • Ascites
RADIOGRAPHIC FINDINGS	• Early cases may show no evidence of cardiac enlargement. As the disease progresses, **right atrial enlargement** becomes evident, followed by **right ventricular enlargement.** • In right heart failure, radiographs may reveal **hepatomegaly** and **ascites** due to hepatic congestion.
ECG	• Symptomatic patients typically have tall P waves (> 0.04 s) due to the enlarged right atrium. • The QRS complexes have deep S waves because of right ventricular enlargement. • **Atrial arrhythmias** become common as the right atrium enlarges (atrial fibrillation, etc.). • **Ventricular arrhythmias** can occur in advanced cases. • **Increased heart rate**
ECHOCARDIOGRAM	• Eccentric hypertrophy of the right ventricle • Dilated right atrium • Distension of the hepatic vessels • Normal or hyperdynamic contractions of the right ventricle • Doppler echocardiogram reveals tricuspid regurgitation
TREATMENT	In mild cases where radiographic changes aren't seen (no enlarged right atrium), treatment is unnecessary. Tricuspid insufficiency often progresses slowly and the right ventricle and atrium have time to adapt. As with mitral insufficiency, some cardiologists elect to treat once moderate atrial enlargement exists. Once the animal is showing signs of congestive heart failure, begin treating with diuretics such as furosemide. Refer to mitral regurgitation and therapy in cardiac failure for more information (p. 3.28 & 3.44).

If you see evidence of tricuspid regurgitation plus bilirubinuria or hemoglobinuria, rule out heartworm infection (caval syndrome).

Cardiology

AORTIC INSUFFICIENCY (AI)

Aortic insufficiency is a volume overload problem resulting in eccentric hypertrophy. It also involves a pressure overload component.

ETIOLOGIES	**Bacterial endocarditis:** bacterial infection of the aortic valve occurs more commonly in dogs than cats (rare). Aortic insufficiency is often seen with **subaortic stenosis** and VSDs. Dogs may also have acquired degeneration of the aortic valve.
PATHO-PHYSIOLOGY	Aortic insufficiency, like PDA, is a volume overload problem with a pressure overload component. In aortic insufficiency (AI), the left ventricle pumps blood into the aorta during systole, but during diastole a portion of this blood leaks back into the ventricle causing an increase in preload (end-diastolic volume). The heart responds to the increased preload with eccentric hypertrophy. Atrial insufficiency places a much greater workload on the heart than pure volume overloads such as mitral insufficiency (MI); while total stroke volume (TSV) is elevated in both cases, the heart must eject its entire TSV to a high pressure aorta in AI, whereas the heart pumps only a fraction of blood into the high pressure aorta in MI. A large portion gets ejected backwards into the low pressure left atrium. Because AI hearts have to do so much high-pressure work, the myocardium tires out more quickly leading to early myocardial failure when compared to MI patients with similar degrees of regurgitation.
CLINICAL SIGNS	• Signs of congestive left heart failure • Exercise intolerance and syncope • Lethargy
PHYSICAL EXAM	• **Bounding pulses:** A large blood volume is ejected into the aorta during systole, creating a normal systolic pressure. Next, blood begins leaking backwards through the aortic valve during diastole, causing systemic diastolic pressures to drop below normal. These changes result in a larger than normal difference between systolic and diastolic blood pressures. The difference between the pulse pressures produces bounding pulses. • **Diastolic decrescendo murmur** heard best over the left heart base: The severity of regurgitation correlates better with the duration of the murmur than with the intensity.
RADIOGRAPHIC FINDINGS	• No changes are seen in early regurgitation, but evidence of left ventricular enlargement may be present in chronic cases. • Pulmonary edema with congestive left heart failure
ECG	• Arrhythmias are common in patients with endocarditis. • **Tall R waves** can occur because of left ventricular enlargement. • **Increased heart rate**
ECHOCARDIOGRAM	• Left ventricular enlargement • Abnormal valve leaflets • The severity of the AI is best assessed using 2D color Doppler echocardiography
TREATMENT	• Same as for heart failure patients (p. 3.44) • Peripheral vasodilators can reduce the degree of regurgitation • **Antibiotics** long term (in cases of endocarditis)
PROGNOSIS	Guarded. In general, animals go into myocardial failure and congestive heart failure much sooner than those with mitral or tricuspid insufficiency.

AORTIC STENOSIS (SUBAORTIC STENOSIS)

TYPICAL BREEDS	• A common congenital defect in the dog; less common in cats. • Breed predispositions: Newfoundland, Boxer, German shepherd, Golden Retriever, and Rottweiler. Inherited in Newfoundlands most likely as a polygenic trait.
PATHOPHYSIOLOGY	Valvular stenosis is uncommon in dogs. In most cases of canine aortic stenosis, a subvalvular fibrous ring or band partially or completely encircles the left ventricular outflow tract. Small nodules and secondary fibrosis may occur on the aortic valve cusps. Mitral valve dysplasia is often seen concurrently with subaortic stenosis (SAS). In aortic and subaortic stenosis, the stenosis causes elevation in afterload. In order to pump blood against this increased resistance, the left ventricular walls thicken and undergo concentric hypertrophy. Thickened myocardium is able to generate higher pressures but it also has greater oxygen demands. Hypertrophied ventricular walls make coronary artery filling more difficult during diastole. Both of these oxygen factors contribute to myocardial ischemia, which in turn is associated with development of ventricular arrhythmias. **Most patients with aortic stenosis die from arrhythmias** rather than from congestive heart failure. • Often the aorta has post-stenotic dilatation due to the increased velocity of flow through the stenosis. • Mild aortic regurgitation often occurs with subaortic stenosis.
CLINICAL SIGNS	• Young dogs are usually asymptomatic but may have a history of fatigue, **exercise intolerance, or exertional syncope** caused by low cardiac output (in severe cases). • Dogs with severe aortic stenosis often die suddenly or experience syncopal episodes because of ventricular arrhythmias.
PHYSICAL EXAM FINDINGS	• A systolic ejection murmur is present at the left heart base. Loud murmurs frequently radiate well to the carotid arteries in the neck and to the right cranial thorax. If significant aortic regurgitation develops, a diastolic murmur may also be heard over the heart base. • Arterial pulses may be diminished and slow rising due to delayed ventricular ejection (in severe cases).
SCREENING FOR DISEASE	If a puppy over 12 months of age is normal on auscultation, it's probably safe to call it clear of subaortic stenosis. However, if a murmur is audible, ultrasound the dog prior to making recommendations.
ECG	• The ECG may be normal even in severe cases, or left ventricular enlargement (increased QRS amplitudes) may be evident. • ST segment deviation (at rest or post-exercise) indicates **myocardial ischemia.** • Ventricular arrhythmias are common in severe cases.
THORACIC RADIOGRAPHS	Radiographs are frequently unremarkable in young dogs and cats. Characteristic findings include: • Left ventricular enlargement • Post-stenotic dilatation of the ascending aorta
ECHOCARDIOGRAM	• Concentric left ventricular hypertrophy (thickened septal and LV wall) • Thickened aortic valve cusps • Subvalvular narrowing • Post-stenotic dilatation of the ascending aorta • Turbulent blood flow in the ascending aorta

Cardiology

AORTIC STENOSIS (Subaortic Stenosis) continued

ECHOCARDIO-GRAM	• Measure the **pressure gradient** between the left ventricle and aorta. The severity of stenosis is roughly indicated by the magnitude of the pressure gradient. There is increased risk of sudden death with **pressure gradients > 80 mmHg** (see prognosis, below). • Left ventricular end-diastolic pressure also increases with severity.
TREATMENT	• The primary goal of therapy is to control arrhythmias and to reduce myocardial oxygen demands. **Beta blockers** such as **atenolol** (1 - 2 mg/kg PO BID) and **propranolol** (1 - 2 mg/kg PO TID) help to do both. They lower myocardial oxygen demands by lowering heart rate and decreasing force of contraction. • Surgical repair requires cardiac bypass, which is technically difficult and not very successful. Balloon angioplasty is only temporarily effective.
CARDIAC CATHETERIZATION & ANGIOGRAPHY	With angioplasty, cardiac catheterization and angiography are usually performed. Contrast injection into the left ventricle reveals: • Left ventricular hypertrophy • Subaortic or aortic obstruction • Post-stenotic dilatation of the ascending aorta
PROGNOSIS	Prognosis depends on the magnitude of the pressure gradient as well as the progression of disease. • **Mild pressure gradients (30-50 mmHg):** Good prognosis. Most of these animals lead a normal life. • **Moderate pressure gradients (50-80 mmHg):** Guarded prognosis, but has the potential for a normal lifespan. • **Severe pressure gradients (> 80 mmHg):** Poor prognosis. 70% die by the age of 3 years. Death is usually sudden and due to arrhythmias. These dogs rarely live long enough to develop heart failure. Dogs with severe gradients should be treated with **beta blockers.** Pressure gradients can increase as the animal grows, but they stabilize by **one year of age.** When subaortic stenosis is diagnosed in a puppy, the puppy should be re-echoed at one year of age for final staging of the disease. Adults should be re-examined every two years or more often if they have concurrent aortic insufficiency or mitral regurgitation.

PULMONIC STENOSIS (PS)

TYPICAL BREEDS	• This is the 3rd most common congenital heart defect in dogs (behind PDA and SAS). Uncommon in cats and large animals. • Breed predisposition: English bulldog, terriers, Beagle. In Beagles, a polygenic mode of inheritance has been reported.
PATHOPHYSIOLOGY	• Valvular pathology (most common) includes thickening of cusps and fusion of cusps at the commissures. Subvalvular or supravalvular fibrous rings may occur alone or with valvular changes. • Pulmonic stenosis can occur as an isolated defect or may be combined with other defects of the conotruncal septum (e.g. Tetralogy of Fallot). • The tricuspid valve apparatus can be malformed when there is concurrent pulmonic stenosis. Pulmonic stenosis (PS) causes a pressure overload of the right ventricle which results in right ventricular concentric hypertrophy. Arrhythmias are much less common in PS than in SAS.
CLINICAL SIGNS	• Dogs are frequently asymptomatic. Severe cases may exhibit exercise intolerance and exertional syncope due to the inability to increase cardiac output. Severe arrhythmias can cause lethargy and syncope. • Signs of right heart failure (venous engorgement, hepatomegaly, ascites) may occur in severe cases if there is concurrent tricuspid regurgitation.
PHYSICAL EXAM FINDINGS	• **Systolic ejection murmur** heard best at the **left heart base** over the pulmonic area. It may be heard on the right side. • Arterial pulses are decreased in severe cases. Lung sounds are normal. Jugular pulse may be visible in severe cases with concurrent tricuspid regurgitation.
ECG	• Right ventricular hypertrophy pattern in most cases, thus the ECG may show a right axis deviation with deep S waves. • Rhythm is usually normal.
THORACIC RADIOGRAPHS	Characteristic findings include: • Right ventricular enlargement • **Post-stenotic dilatation** of the main pulmonary artery • Pulmonary vasculature is usually normal
ECHOCARDIOGRAM	• Right ventricular thickening is proportional to the severity of stenosis. • The stenotic area and post-stenotic dilatation may be visible with 2D echo. • Color doppler will show turbulence in the main pulmonary artery and **a pressure gradient across the stenosis** that is proportional to the severity of obstruction. As with SAS, 30-50 mmHg is mild, 50-80 mmHg is moderate, and > 80 mmHg indicates severe stenosis.
CARDIAC CATHETERIZATION & ANGIOGRAPHY	Right ventricular contrast injection demonstrates: • Narrowed area of stenosis or valve thickening • Post-stenotic dilatation of the main pulmonary artery • Right ventricular hypertrophy
TREATMENT	ß blockers are used to control arrhythmias and decrease force of contraction to allow for better filling. Surgery or balloon valvuloplasty is reserved for severe cases. Surgery consists of valvulotomy or patch grafting of the outflow region.
PROGNOSIS	The natural history of pulmonic stenosis is not well documented. A severe right ventricular to pulmonary artery systolic gradient (> 80 mmHg) carries a worse prognosis, but in general, this disease is not as life-threatening as subaortic stenosis. Dogs with severe gradients often do well although they can still die from arrhythmias. As with SAS, gradients are stable by one year of age. Thus, dogs should be re-echoed at one year for final staging of the gradient. Animals with combined pulmonic stenosis and tricuspid regurgitation have the worst prognosis and should be evaluated regularly for progression.

Cardiology

CONGENITAL CARDIAC SHUNTS

There are five congenital cardiac shunts. Some can be so small that they are not detected for many years. The right-to-left shunts result in cyanosis.

Patent Ductus Arteriosus—Left-to-Right
Ventricular Septal Defect
Atrial Septal Defect
Patent Ductus Arteriosus—Right-to-Left
Tetralogy of Fallot

LEFT-TO-RIGHT PATENT DUCTUS ARTERIOSUS (PDA)

As with aortic insufficiency, PDA is a volume overload.

TYPICAL BREEDS	Poodle, Collie, Pomeranian, Sheltie, German shepherd
PATHOPHYSIOLOGY	In the fetus, the ductus arteriosus allows the majority of the right ventricular output to shunt from the pulmonary artery to the aorta, away from the non-functioning lungs. Soon after birth, the ductus closes and pulmonary resistance and pressure falls to normal. Failure of ductus closure usually results in a left-to-right shunt, from the aorta to the pulmonary artery. With PDAs, blood travels from the left ventricle to the aorta. Then a portion of blood is diverted through the PDA into the low pressure pulmonary artery where it travels through the lungs and back to the left atrium. The net result is an increase in preload (end-diastolic volume). A PDA places a much greater workload on the heart than does a pure volume overload such as mitral insufficiency (MI). Although total stroke volume is elevated in both cases, with PDAs, the heart must eject its entire stroke volume into a high pressure aorta, whereas with MI, the heart only pumps a fraction of blood into the high pressure aorta. With MI, a large portion of blood gets ejected backwards into the low pressure left atrium. Because PDA hearts have to do so much pumping against normal systemic pressure, the myocardium tires out faster leading to early myocardial failure when compared to MI patients with similar degrees of diverted flow.
CLINICAL FEATURES	If clinical signs are present, they may include fatigue, dyspnea, and exercise intolerance (signs of left heart failure). Puppies with PDAs may be smaller than their littermates.
PHYSICAL EXAM FINDINGS	A **continuous murmur** is best heard at the **left heart base** over the aortic and pulmonic areas, and it often radiates widely. Listen high up under the left axilla. A palpable thrill accompanies more intense murmurs. A systolic murmur of secondary mitral insufficiency may sometimes be ausculted at the left apex. **Bounding arterial pulse:** As with aortic insufficiency, there is a rapid run-off of aortic blood. This results in a greater difference between systolic and diastolic blood pressures which creates a wider pulse pressure, resulting in a stronger-than-normal arterial pulse.
ECG	• Variable— but often there's a marked left ventricular hypertrophy pattern (increased QRS amplitude). The electrical axis is normal. • P waves may be prolonged due to left atrial enlargement. • Advanced cases may show supraventricular arrhythmias (e.g. atrial premature contractions, atrial fibrillation) or ventricular arrhythmias.
THORACIC RADIOGRAPHY	The **descending aorta** often has an **aneurysmal bulge** near the ductus on the DV view. Radiographs reveal enlargement of the: • Left atrium • Left ventricle • Aortic arch • Main pulmonary artery ± **pulmonary hypervascularity** (enlarged arteries and veins)

LEFT-TO-RIGHT PATENT DUCTUS ARTERIOSUS (PDA) continued

ECHOCARDIOGRAM	• Eccentric hypertrophy of the **left ventricle** ± dilation of the left atrium. • **Hyperdynamic** left ventricular wall motion (volume overload) early on and myocardial failure in advanced cases. • The PDA should be visible by 2D echo.
CARDIAC CATHETERIZATION & ANGIOGRAM	• Pressures are normal with small shunts. Oxygen saturation is higher in the pulmonary artery than in the right ventricle or right atrium. An aortic root or left ventricular contrast injection demonstrates the ductus arteriosus. • With larger shunts, aortic pulse pressure increases primarily due to the decrease in diastolic pressure, and left ventricular diastolic pressure rises.
TREATMENT	Medical stabilization (if there is evidence of congestive heart failure) followed by surgical ligation or coil embolization of the PDA.
PROGNOSIS	• Prognosis is excellent with surgical correction prior to the development of left heart failure. • Prognosis in animals that are not treated is guarded except in cases of small PDAs. Remember that the stresses placed on the myocardium by a PDA are the same as those placed on it by aortic insufficiency. Thus, myocardial failure is a common sequela. Mitral regurgitation also occurs secondary to ventricular dilation. • Without correction, puppies with large shunts often die before 12 weeks of age; dogs with intermediate sized shunts may live to several years of age. Dogs with small shunts can have a normal lifespan, but most left-to-right PDAs in young dogs should be surgically corrected.

Card

VENTRICULAR SEPTAL DEFECT (VSD) – Left-to-Right Shunt

VSDs are volume overloads. Their pathophysiology is similar to mitral regurgitation.

TYPICAL BREEDS	English bulldog, Siberian husky, English springer spaniel, cats
PATHO-PHYSIOLOGY	The communication typically occurs in the upper portion of the interventricular septum just below the aortic valve on the left side, and just under the anterior part of the septal leaflet of the tricuspid valve on the right. The defect is usually ringed by fibromembranous tissue. Perimembranous septal defects are most common. Pathophysiology is similar to that of mitral regurgitation (MR) in that a portion of the total stroke volume (TSV) is ejected into the aorta and a portion is ejected into a low-pressure chamber (the right ventricle/right ventricular outflow tract). The net effect is that forward stroke volume (FSV) decreases. The body initially responds by increasing heart rate and contractility. In the long run, the RAAS system is activated causing water retention and consequently an increase in total blood volume and preload. The heart handles this increase in preload by undergoing eccentric hypertrophy and the TSV increases. While a portion of the blood still flows through the VSD, the FSV increases to normal. The amount of shunted blood depends on the size of the VSD. Most VSDs are small, but small VSDs still cause loud murmurs because they create more turbulence than large VSDs. The larger the murmur defect, the more dilated the left heart will become. Two secondary problems that can occur with VSDs are aortic insufficiency— due to damage caused to the aortic cusps by the high velocity shunt— and mitral regurgitation due to stretching of the mitral valve annulus secondary to chamber dilation.
CLINICAL SIGNS	• Most patients with small defects are asymptomatic. • Large defects are rarely found. It's possible these patients may die within the first weeks of life and consequently never present to a veterinary hospital. Fatigue and dyspnea may occur with moderately-sized defects (in left-to-right shunts).
PHYSICAL EXAM FINDINGS	• The typical murmur is a mixed frequency **holosystolic murmur** loudest at the **right** side. The location is variable and it may also be heard well on the left. • Arterial pulse is usually normal but **may be bounding** with large defects in which the aortic valves are disrupted (**aortic insufficiency**). Note that aortic insufficiency with concurrent VSD results in a systolic and diastolic (to-and-fro) murmur.
ECG	Usually normal although a non-specific left ventricular enlargement pattern may be seen.
THORACIC RADIOGRAPHS	• May be unremarkable in patients with small defects. • With larger defects there is left **atrial** and left **ventricular enlargement** together with **pulmonary hyperperfusion** (increased vascular marking, both arterial and venous).
ECHOCARDIOGRAM	• Dilatation of the **left atrium** and **left ventricle**. • Many defects are detectable by 2D echocardiography. • **Doppler echocardiography confirms the diagnosis.**
CARDIAC CATHETERIZATION & ANGIOGRAPHY	• All pressures are normal with small defects. • Increase in **oxygen saturation** from right atrium to right ventricle and pulmonary artery. • The defect is visualized by left ventricular contrast injection.
TREATMENT	• No therapy is indicated for small defects. • Surgical correction of larger defects requires cardiac bypass. • Surgical palliation by **banding** of the pulmonary artery reduces left-to-right shunting by increasing right ventricular systolic pressure.
PROGNOSIS	• Excellent for small defects. • With larger defects and obvious cardiac enlargement, the long-term prognosis is guarded due to the development of congestive left heart failure and occasionally pulmonary hypertension.

ATRIAL SEPTAL DEFECT

ASD is a right-sided volume overload. Thus, signs are similar to those seen with tricuspid insufficiency.

TYPICAL BREEDS	• Rare
PATHO-PHYSIOLOGY	ASDs often go unrecognized unless they are large. Normally, the right ventricle is more compliant (thinner walled) and shunting occurs in a left-to-right direction mainly during diastole. Any condition that raises right atrial pressure (e.g. tricuspid regurgitation, right ventricular hypertrophy from pulmonic stenosis) can cause right-to-left shunting through an ASD. ASDs may also occur as part of more complex defects such as endocardial cushion defects (AV canal defect).
CLINICAL SIGNS	Usually absent, but right heart failure may develop (jugular distention, ascites).
PHYSICAL EXAM FINDINGS	• Characteristic soft to medium-intensity, early to **mid-systolic pulmonic ejection murmur** that is best heard at the **left heart base**. Split S2 is sometimes present. • Normal arterial pulses.
ECG	• May demonstrate right ventricular hypertrophy type pattern (deep S waves) usually due to right bundle branch conduction abnormalities (partial or complete RBBB).
THORACIC RADIOGRAPHS	• Normal or predominantly **right-sided cardiomegaly** with **pulmonary hypervascularity.**
ECHOCARDIOGRAM	• **Right atrial** and **right ventricular dilatation** occurs with larger defects. • The defect can sometimes be visualized by 2D echo or with contrast injection (bubblegram).
CARDIAC CATHETERIZATION & ANGIOGRAPHY	• Pressure studies and angiography may be normal. • **Oxygen saturation** in the right atrium and ventricle are higher than in the vena cava. • Shunt may be visualized by pulmonary artery contrast injection.
TREATMENT	Usually none. Surgical repair is indicated only for large defects and usually requires cardiac bypass.
PROGNOSIS	The prognosis is good except with large defects.

Cardiology

RIGHT-to-LEFT PATENT DUCTUS ARTERIOSUS

TYPICAL BREEDS	Rare: Any breed predisposed to PDAs (Refer to p. 3.36)
PATHO-PHYSIOLOGY	PDAs occur when the fetal ductus arteriosus fails to close soon after birth. In contrast to the left-to-right PDA, with the right-to-left PDA, pulmonary vascular resistance is greater than systemic vascular resistance. As a result, blood flows from the pulmonary artery to the aorta. This usually occurs because fetal pulmonary vascular resistance has failed to drop after birth. So, as with fetal circulation, blood travels from the right ventricle to the pulmonary trunk and a large amount bypasses the lungs. Blood is then diverted through the PDA into the lower pressure aorta and out to the body. This unoxygenated blood enters the aorta at a point caudal to the brachiocephalic trunk. The oxygenated blood from the left ventricle flows out the brachiocephalic artery and oxygenates the cranial half of the body, while less-oxygenated (shunted) blood goes to the caudal half of the body resulting in **differential cyanosis** (cyanosis of the hindlimbs).
CLINICAL FEATURES	• **Exercise intolerance** (hind end only) • **Differential cyanosis** • **Hind limb weakness** and hind limb collapse with exercise are classic signs. Exercise decreases systemic vascular resistance and enhances the right-to-left shunt. • History of **fatigue, tachypnea,** or **syncope** • Polycythemia occurs in response to the low oxygenation of the blood.
PHYSICAL EXAM FINDINGS	There is no murmur but is usually a split S_2 due to pulmonary hypertension.
ECG	A right ventricular hypertrophy pattern (deep S waves) is evident in dogs with pulmonary hypertension.
THORACIC RADIOGRAPHY	• Right heart enlargement pattern. • **Pulmonary vascularity** is usually normal or slightly diminished. • **Dilation** of the **pulmonary artery segment** and localized **dilation** of the **ductal or post-ductal aorta** (DV view) strongly indicates presence of a right-to-left PDA.
ECHOCARDIOGRAM	• Severe concentric and eccentric hypertrophy of the right ventricle is common. The left ventricle is usually volume underloaded (smaller than normal). • Right ventricular and right atrial pressures are elevated. • Bubblegram shows bubbles in the caudal aorta.
CARDIAC CATHETERIZATION & ANGIOGRAM	With severe pulmonary hypertension, pulmonary arterial pressure is greater than aortic pressure which leads to right-to-left shunting. If the pressures are equal, bi-directional shunting may occur. Angiography is contraindicated in right-to-left PDAs.
TREATMENT	In dogs with pulmonary hypertension and right-to-left shunting, correction of polycythemia may palliate some signs temporarily (if PCV is above 60), but ligation of the ductus is contraindicated (fatal).
PROGNOSIS	Prognosis is poor. Cyanosis and polycythemia increase in severity and the animals rarely survive more than 2-3 years.

TETRALOGY OF FALLOT

Consists of pulmonic stenosis (PS), a large VSD, dextropositioning of the aorta over the interventricular septum, and right ventricular hypertrophy (in response to the PS).

TYPICAL BREEDS	• This is the most common congenital defect with cyanosis due to right-to-left shunting in all species. • Most common in the Keeshond, where a polygenic mode of inheritance has been demonstrated.
PATHO-PHYSIOLOGY	• Valvular and/or subvalvular **pulmonic stenosis** combined with a large ventricular septal defect located in the upper septum. The **root of the aorta is variably displaced** to the right (dextropositioned), over-riding the interventricular septum and VSD. • **Right ventricular hypertrophy** occurs secondarily and is usually severe. • The degree of right-to-left shunting and cyanosis depends on the severity of the pulmonic stenosis and the difference between systemic vascular resistance and pulmonary vascular resistance. Any activity that increases cardiac output and/or reduces systemic vascular resistance increases the right-to-left shunt.
CLINICAL SIGNS	• Affected dogs are usually smaller than their littermates and have a history of exercise intolerance, dyspnea/tachypnea, or syncope. • Symmetrical cyanosis may be evident at rest and is accentuated with exercise.
PHYSICAL EXAM FINDINGS	• A **systolic murmur** over the pulmonary valve area is usually present (due to pulmonic stenosis). The murmur may occasionally be absent with pulmonary artery hypoplasia. • Normal arterial pulse (usually) • No signs of heart failure • Polycythemia may be present (injected, dark membranes)
ECG	A marked right ventricular hypertrophy pattern is present and rhythm is usually normal.
THORACIC RADIOGRAPHS	• Right ventricular enlargement is present • The **main pulmonary artery segment** is usually not visible due to pulmonary artery hypoplasia • **Pulmonary hypoperfusion** (diminished arteries and veins), often with large, lucent, hyperinflated lungs reflecting chronic hyperventilation
ECHOCARDIOGRAM	• Right ventricular hypertrophy, VSD, PS, and the overriding aorta may be seen on both M-mode and 2D studies. • Non-selective contrast injection shows right-to-left ventricular shunting.
CARDIAC CATHETERIZATION & ANGIOGRAPHY	• There is a systolic pressure gradient between the right ventricle and the main pulmonary artery (due to pulmonary stenosis). • Right ventricular and left ventricular systolic pressures are usually identical (due to large a VSD). • Oxygen saturation in the right atrium, right ventricle, pulmonary artery, and left atrium is normal; it is reduced in the left ventricle and aorta (due to the right-to-left shunt). • Left ventricular or aortic angiograms often demonstrate increased bronchoesophageal or other collateral circulation to the lungs (compensating for decreased pulmonary flow).
TREATMENT	• **Phlebotomy** to manage the polycythemia. Keep the PCV below 65. • **Surgery** • **Palliative.** There are a variety of procedures to increase pulmonary blood flow via a systemic artery to pulmonary artery anastomosis (creates a compensatory left-to-right shunt). • **Total correction** requires cardiac bypass.
PROGNOSIS	Poor prognosis for long-term survival. The usual sequelae include progressive polycythemia and progressive cyanosis. Dogs and cats rarely survive more than 3-4 years.

Cardiology

CANINE DILATED CARDIOMYOPATHY

TYPICAL BREEDS	1) Doberman Pinscher, 2) Boxer, 3) Giant breeds (e.g. Irish Wolfhound, Great Dane), 4) Cocker Spaniel. 90% occurs in Boxers and Doberman Pinschers.
PHYSIOLOGY	A decrease in myocardial contractility results in decreased stroke volume. The body compensates in several ways to increase cardiac output. Sympathetic nerve stimulation and withdrawal of parasympathetic tone causes the heart rate to increase. The kidneys retain salt and water under the influence of aldosterone, increasing end-diastolic volume in the ventricles. This increase in end-diastolic volume increases the stroke volume towards normal. Mitral regurgitation is a common complication of dilated cardiomyopathy. Left ventricular chamber dilation causes abnormal orientation of the papillary muscles, resulting in faulty coaptation of the mitral valve leaflets. In the patient that has died suddenly from arrhythmias, a biopsy of cardiac muscle may be needed to diagnose DCM. The histological changes diagnostic for DCM include deposition of fibrous tissue, fatty tissue, or inflammatory cells within the myocardium, as well as microfiber necrosis. These changes contribute to the decreased myocardial contractility seen in DCM.
CLINICAL SIGNS	• In Boxers and Dobermans, the only sign may be sudden death or syncope due to arrhythmias. VPCs and ventricular tachycardia are the most common arrhythmias in Boxers and Dobermans. • Signs of congestive heart failure: lethargy, exercise intolerance, coughing, tachypnea, etc.
PHYSICAL EXAM	Some animals show no abnormalities but arrhythmias can often be heard. Other findings include: • Soft systolic murmur • Normal to decreased arterial pulses • S3 gallop
FINDINGS ON RADIOGRAPH	• With significant chamber dilation, radiographs reveal an enlarged, round heart filling the chest. This generalized cardiac enlargement is seen in most breeds; it is less frequently noted in the Doberman Pinscher as heart size may appear relatively normal due to a deep chest. • Left ventricular and left atrial enlargement are common findings. • Pulmonary congestion and edema (left heart failure) • Pleural effusion, hepatosplenomegaly, and ascites occur rarely due to right heart failure.
ECG	• VPCs occur most commonly in Dobermans and Boxers. • Atrial fibrillation occurs most commonly in giant breeds.
CARDIAC ULTRASOUND	Echocardiography yields a definitive diagnosis. Characterized by **increased end-diastolic diameter** and a low shortening fraction (< 25%).
TREATMENT	• Treat the cardiac arrhythmias. • **Digoxin** (0.004 mg/m2 PO BID) is used to increase contractility and slow the heart rate. When the heart rate won't slow any further with digoxin, add propranolol (initially at a low dose, TID) and gradually increase the dose until heart rate slows to 140 – 160 bpm. Digoxin has a small therapeutic range. Measure the serum digoxin levels in 4-7 days and watch for side effects (vomiting and anorexia). • **Furosemide** is given to alleviate signs of congestion. Start with SID-TID dosing. • **ACE inhibitors** help alleviate signs of congestion. Cardiologists often place animals on ACE inhibitors at the same time or shortly after starting furosemide rather than waiting to see if the furosemide alone works. This can be done if the patient is not dehydrated. • In acute therapy, **dobutamine** (a positive inotrope) may be used to increase contractility. • **L-Carnitine:** BID-TID in Dobermans, Boxers, and occasionally Cocker Spaniels. (Amino Acid Division of Ajinomoto USA Inc. www.ajichem.com). Because it's expensive, test serum levels first and supplement if levels are low. If levels are normal, the owner may still opt to supplement since serum carnitine levels don't always reflect myocardial carnitine levels. • **Taurine:** Check taurine levels in any DCM patient and supplement if indicated.

FELINE CARDIOMYOPATHY
Hypertrophic Cardiomyopathy (HCM)
Restrictive Cardiomyopathy
Dilated Cardiomyopathy (DCM)

Unlike dogs, where valvular disease is the most common form of cardiac disease, myocardial disease is the most common form of heart disease in cats. Primary myocardial diseases are those due to intrinsic abnormalities of the myocardium. Cats also develop myocardial disease secondary to systemic conditions such as hypertension and hyperthyroidism.

Hypertrophic Cardiomyopathy (HCM)
HCM is the most common cardiac disease in the cat.

SIGNALMENT	Occurs in purebred and mixed breed cats. Predisposed breeds include the American Shorthair, British Shorthair, and Maine Coone. HCM can be hereditary, so breeders of purebred cats with HCM require genetic counseling. The mutation varies by breed and familial lines.
PHYSIOLOGY	In one line of Maine Coone cat, HCM has been shown to be caused by a sarcomere mutation in the myocardial cells. The mutation leads to dysfunctional myofilaments; consequently, other muscle filaments hypertrophy to compensate and the result is concentric hypertophy of the ventricle. The abnormal myofilaments degenerate and are replaced by scar tissue, thus the thickened ventricle contracts well but doesn't relax properly during diastole. In addition, the thickening of the ventricles results in skewed orientation of the AV valves so the cat can develop mitral regurgitation as well as **dynamic aortic outflow obstruction** secondary to systolic anterior motion (SAM) of the mitral valve. The other form of obstruction commonly seen with HCM is dynamic right ventricular outflow tract obstruction.
CLINICAL SIGNS	Most cats present in **acute heart failure** even though they have had cardiac disease for years. Cardiac disease develops slowly without the owner noticing obvious clinical signs. When pulmonary edema or pleural effusion develop, the cat becomes progressively more dyspneic. Thromboembolism to one or more limbs may be the first clinical sign that occurs in some cases.
PHYSICAL EXAM	Murmur: HCM cats commonly have a **holosystolic murmur**, usually on the left side or right sternal region. Not all cats have a murmur, and the murmur can vary in intensity. A **gallop rhythm** occurs in many cats but it can be difficult to detect if the cat is tachycardic. Cats with moderate to severe atrial enlargement may also **present with a saddle thrombus**. A cat with a saddle thrombus often presents on emergency in extreme pain and distress with a history of acute onset paralysis to one or both hind limbs. The affected limb is typically cool, lacks a pulse, and the pads may be bluish from lack of blood supply.
RADIOGRAPHY	It can be challenging to determine with radiographs alone whether dyspnea is due to pneumonia, asthma, or heart failure, unless severe cardiomegaly is seen. An echocardiogram is generally needed for a definitive diagnosis of HCM. Changes that may be seen on radiographs include: • Atrial enlargement. Note that biatrial enlargement appears as a valentine-shaped heart on the DV view and a tall heart on the lateral. • Pulmonary edema or pleural effusion if in heart failure.
CARDIAC ULTRASOUND	**Thickening of the left ventricular wall (diastole) > 6 mm** indicates HCM. Rule out systemic hypertension or hyperthyroidism as the cause of the hypertrophy by measuring blood pressure, performing a fundic exam, and measuring T4. • **If left atrium: aortic diameter is > 1: 1.5** then the left atrium is enlarged. If enlargement is marked, check radiographs for signs of heart failure. ratio of 1:2.0 indicates severe atrial enlargement. **Systolic Anterior Motion (SAM):** Anterior mitral valve leaflets can block aortic outflow leading to pressure overload and worsening of the ventricular hypertrophy.

Cardiology

Hypertrophic Cardiomyopathy continued

TREATMENT	Refer to p. 44 for treatment of acute heart failure. The mainstay drugs in heart failure are furosemide and ACE inhibitors such as benazepril. There is controversy as to whether to start ACE inhibitors and other drugs prior to— or after— the onset of clinical signs. • **ß blockers** such as **atenolol** (6.25 - 12.6 mg PO/cat SID-BID) or propranolol (1.0 mg/kg PO TID) decrease heart rate, allowing the heart more time to fill during diastole. They also decrease contractility and blood pressure. Try to keep HR < 160. Avoid ß blockers in asthmatic cats. Although atenolol is a ß1 blocker, at higher doses it causes ß2 blockade as well, leading to pulmonary bronchoconstriction. Also use ß blockers if there is significant SAM. • **Calcium channel blockers** decrease heart rate and relax the heart during diastole, allowing the heart to fill better and increasing stroke volume. In cats, try **diltiazem** (7.5 mg per cat PO TID) or **Cardizem CD** (SID administration, but must be formulated for cats). • **ACE inhibitors: Benazepril** (0.25 - 0.5 mg/kg SID to BID; usually SID) or **enalapril** (0.25 - 0.5 mg/kg SID-BID; usually BID) • **Prevent clot formation:** Aspirin (1/2 of an 81 mg tablet PO q 3 days) has variable efficacy. Low molecular weight heparins such as **lovenox** (enoxaparin: 1-1.5 mg/kg SC SID-BID) shows promise for cats that already have clots. Known atrial clots should be re-evaluated after several months of treatment. **Exercise in the patient with cardiomyopathy:** Exercise precipitates clinical signs but does not increase the progression of clinical signs. Owner need not restrict their pet from exercising because the cat will do this by itself.

Dilated Cardiomyopathy (DCM)

BACKGROUND	DCM in cats is usually caused by **taurine deficiency** although some cases appear to be idiopathic. In DCM, the heart undergoes eccentric hypertrophy and contractility decreases, resulting in decreased cardiac output. DCM is rare now that commercial cat foods are supplemented with taurine.
DIAGNOSIS	• Blood: Low plasma and whole blood taurine levels • Radiographs: Enlarged, often globoid heart • Ultrasound: Enlarged atrial and ventricular chambers and decreased contractility ($\leq$ 45% contractility). Usually these changes are severe by the time the cat is symptomatic.
TREATMENT	• **Taurine:** 250 mg/cat PO BID. This can be administered before taurine deficiency is diagnosed since taurine levels have a long turn-around time. Prognosis is good if taurine-responsive. Takes 3 months to see echocardiographic improvement. • **Positive inotropes** such as **digoxin** should be used when the cat is in severe myocardial failure. Digoxin increases myocardial contractility and decreases conduction through the AV node. • Treat congestive heart failure with enalapril and Lasix® (Refer to CHF section p. 44). • **Anticoagulant therapy:** Use with severe left atrial dilation if spontaneous echocontrast is seen, if a thrombus is present in the left atrium, and in cats presenting with thromboembolism.

Restrictive Cardiomyopathy (RCM)

BACKGROUND	**Restrictive Cardiomyopathy** occurs when there is too much fibrous tissue in the endocardium, myocardium, or subendocardial tissues. Endocardial fibrosis is the most common cause. The fibrosis usually leads to both systolic and diastolic dysfunction. The heart becomes too stiff to fill and pump properly; it must fill at a higher than normal pressure which results in a higher diastolic pressure. This leads to increased capillary pressure and edema or pleural effusion.
DIAGNOSIS	**Cardiac Ultrasound:** Enlarged left atrium or biatrial enlargement.
TREATMENT	Treat as for congestive heart failure and HCM. If severe systolic dysfunction exists, don't use beta blockers or calcium channel blockers. Prognosis is grave.

CARDIAC FAILURE

Heart failure is a clinical syndrome caused by any cardiac disease that results in an accumulation of fluid into the lungs, pleural space, or abdomen (congestive failure) and/or low peripheral perfusion (low output failure).

I. **EVALUATING PATIENTS IN CARDIAC FAILURE:**
   A. **CLINICAL SIGNS:** Refer to the cardiac physical exam section (p. 3.7).
      1. **Signs due to congestion** include dyspnea, coughing, exercise intolerance, inability to sleep comfortably.
      2. **Signs due to low cardiac output** include exercise intolerance (e.g. the dog used to be able to fetch for 10 minutes, now it gets tired after several tosses).
   B. **DIAGNOSTICS:**
      1. **Physical exam:** Look for signs of cardiac disease and its sequelae such as heart murmurs, tachypnea, tachycardia, harsh lung sounds, crackles, ascites.
      2. **Radiographs are important** to evaluate the lungs and abdomen for signs of heart failure.
         a. **Cardiac changes:** Enlarged left or right atrium, marked cardiomegaly, etc.
         b. **Pulmonary changes** (due to congestion or cardiac enlargement): Perihilar edema, engorged pulmonary vasculature, pleural effusion, enlarged caudal vena cava, elevated trachea, airway disease.
         c. **Systemic changes:** Ascites or hepatomegaly
      3. **Ultrasound** helps determine whether or not clinical signs are due to cardiac disease, especially when it's difficult to determine whether radiographic lung changes are due to pulmonary disease or heart disease. It is needed to diagnose the specific cardiac disease. Use ultrasound to evaluate the following:
         a. Valvular insufficiencies
         b. Chamber enlargement and wall thickening. Look for eccentric (larger chambers) or concentric hypertrophy (thickened ventricular walls).
         c. Myocardial contractility
         d. Direction of flow and shunts
      4. **ECG** is the best tool for diagnosing arrhythmias.
      5. **BUN, Creatinine, Urine Specific Gravity, and Total protein:** Check renal function and hydration status early in the course of treatment. Urine specific gravity will be meaningless once the animal is on a diuretic.

II. **TREATMENT Considerations:** The immediate goal is to stabilize the animal and get it out of heart failure. Once the patient is stable, perform further diagnostics and determine a course of maintenance drug therapy. Stabilization will probably lead to some dehydration and hypotension. Try to avoid severe dehydration and hypotension because both can lead to renal failure. On the other hand, it is better to dehydrate the animal and rehydrate later then to let it die from heart failure.
   A. **Administer oxygen** via insufflation or cage if the animal is unstable due to dyspnea. If the patient needs oxygen, provide oxygen therapy before performing diagnostics.
   B. **Principles of Drug Therapy:**
      1. Prior to giving any drugs, first determine:
         a. **What are the goals and why?** To control arrhythmias? Increase myocardial contractility? Decrease the systemic resistance that the heart has to pump against (afterload)? Decrease capillary hydrostatic pressure?
         b. **How will you measure the efficacy of the drug therapy?** For instance, if you're trying to decrease pulmonary congestion, you should monitor respiratory rate and perform recheck radiographs.
         c. **What signs will tell you to discontinue a drug?** You may decide to discontinue a drug if it's decreasing heart rate or contractility too much, or if it's causing vomiting or anorexia.
      2. Ideally, start with **one drug at a time.** Give that drug time to work and then assess the effect. If it's not achieving your goals, discontinue it, modify the dose, or add another drug. Make only one change at a time and allow enough time for the change to take effect. Reassess before and after each change.
      3. Avoid polypharmacy if possible because it often leads to anorexia, especially in cats. However, in severe cardiac failure, you may need to start with more than one drug.

III. **SPECIFIC DRUGS:**
   A. **DIURETICS are the first line for congestive heart failure:**
      1. Clinicians most frequently start with the **diuretic furosemide** (2 - 8 mg/kg IV or SC). Dosage depends on the animal's condition. Furosemide is a fairly safe

The Small Animal Veterinary Nerdbook ™

Cardiology

drug. Unfortunately in cardiac failure, forward flow is decreased so the kidneys are not well perfused. As a result, furosemide may not work as well as in animals with normal renal perfusion. Monitor treatment success with recheck radiographs and by observing respiratory rate and character as well as urine outflow.

a. **In severe cases, be aggressive.** If possible, administer drugs IV for the fastest response (within 5 minutes). IM or SC routes can take 30 minutes (or more if perfusion is severely impaired) to see effect. Expect to cause dehydration in these animals. Dogs will start to eat and rehydrate once you have decreased the preload. Cats may need to be rehydrated before they will start eating and drinking on their own. If the animal is already dehydrated and in heart failure the prognosis is poor.

b. Once the animal is controlled on furosemide, gradually decrease the dose to the lowest maintenance dose possible. You may need to add another drug such as benzapril or enalapril. ACE inhibitors combined with diuretics can cause renal failure, even in animals with normal baseline values— so use caution.

B. **BALANCED VASODILATOR: Angiotensin converting enzyme inhibitors** (ACE inhibitors) such as enalapril, benazepril, and lisinopril work by inhibiting the RAAS system (Refer to page 3.6). Their net effect is to decrease water retention and cause **vasodilation.** Thus, they work to **decrease preload as well as afterload.** ACE inhibitors take about 6 hours to have an effect but are commonly used in cardiac failure.

1. Avoid enalapril in animals with renal disease. Perform a chemistry panel prior to administering the drug and then 7 days after starting drug administration. Most animals that develop renal disease when on ACE inhibitors do so within 7 days.

C. **Venodilators** increase venous capacitance thereby decreasing preload.

1. **Nitroglycerine increases venous capacitance (decreases preload).** The ointment can be rubbed on the ears or inguinal region. Dose: 1/4 inch per 15 pounds every 4-6 hours. Only administer using gloved hands, and don't send it home with the owner! Tolerance to this drug occurs rapidly, so it's not usually used long-term.

D. **POSITIVE INOTROPES** increase myocardial contractility and are valuable if the animal is in myocardial failure (determined by measuring shortening fraction. Normal shortening fraction is **30-40% in dogs and > 45% in cats**). Often with volume overload the shortening fraction is initially normal or increased due to the need to maintain cardiac output in spite of eccentric hypertrophy.

1. **Digoxin** is a weak positive inotrope. It works much better as an anti-arrhythmic. It decreases conduction velocity through the AV node resulting in decreased heart rate.

2. **Pimobendan** (used in dogs) is a positive **inotrope** and **vasodilator** (i.e. an inodilator). It enhances myocardial cell sensitivity to intracellular calcium, which leads to the inotropic effects. The vasodilator effect and a portion of the inotropic effect are due to inhibition of phosphodiesterase III. Pimobendan causes both arterial and venous dilation.

3. **Dopamine** (5 - 10 μg/kg/min) and **dobutamine** (2 - 10 μg/kg/min) are good positive inotropes, but are only moderately effective when used in myocardial failure. These catecholamines are better than epinephrine and isoproterenol (ß agonist) at treating heart failure because both isoproterenol and epinephrine increase heart rate. Dopamine and dobutamine can also increase heart rate when given in high doses. Dopamine is much cheaper than dobutamine (dobutamine also lowers pulmonary venous pressure). All catecholamines have short half-lives and must be given by constant rate infusion.

E. **Arteriolar dilators are used to decrease afterload.** They can cause severe hypotension and are not recommended in cases of pressure overload (e.g. subaortic stenosis).

a. **Nitroprusside** and **oral hydralazine** can cause severe systemic hypotension. Use only if direct blood pressure monitoring is available. Many cardiologists avoid using them.

b. **Amlodipine** is a calcium channel blocker like diltiazem and nifedipine. It is a good arteriolar dilator.

F. **Antiarrhythmic drugs** (e.g. digoxin, propranolol, atenolol, lidocaine) should be used only if an arrhythmia is present that is causing hemodynamic compromise.

IV. **Diet:** Animals in cardiac failure should be on salt restricted diets. Treats should also be low in sodium.

DRUGS COMMONLY USED in TREATMENT of ITP and IMHA

DRUG	DOSE in DOGS
Azothioprine (Imuran®) 50mg tabs	2 mg/kg/day PO
Cyclophosphamide (Cytoxan®) 25, 50 mg tabs	(50 mg/m2 in the AM q 48 hours or for 4 days on and 3 days off.
Cyclosporine (Atopica)	5-10 mg/kg/day divided BID-TID PO.
Dexamethasone 0.25, 5 mg tabs 2 mg/mL, 4 mg/mL	• For treatment of ITP or AIHA: 0.15-0.45 mg/kg PO BID (most potent) • To pre-treat prior to blood transfusion: (2 mg/kg IV)
Diphenhydramine (Benadryl®) 10 mg/mL	0.5 mg/kg IV
Doxycycline	For intracellular parasites: 10 mg/kg IV BID
Heparin	100 U/kg q 6 hours in acute stages to avoid DIC
Prednisone (5, 20 mg tabs)	1-2 mg/kg PO BID
Methylprednisone 2,4,8,16,24, 32 mg tabs	1-2mg/kg PO BID (more potent than prednisone)
Tetracycline 100,250,500 mg, 100mg/ml	For intracellular parasites: 22mg/Kg PO TID
Vincristine (1 mg/mL)	0.50-0.75 mg/m2 IV weekly

Clinical Path

CANINE AND FELINE CBC NORMALS
These values are taken from the University of California, Davis
Veterinary Medical Teaching Hospital.
For a blank version to fill out with your own lab's normals go to www.nerdbook.com/extras.

CANINE AND FELINE CBC NORMALS		
	CANINE	FELINE
RBC	5.5-8.5 M/μL	6-10 M/μL
Hemaglobin	14-19 g/dL	9-15.1 g/dL
Hematocrit	40-55%	29-48%
MCV	65-75 fl	41.5-52.5-55 fl
MCHC	33-37 g/dL	30-33.5 g/dL
MCH	21.5-26.5 pgm	13-17 pgm
% retics	0.5-1.0%	0-0.8
WBC	6,000-17,000/μL	5,000 - 15,000/μL
Bands	0-300/μL	rare
Neutrophils	3000-11,500/μL	2,500 - 11,300/μL
Lymphocytes*	1000-4800/μL	1400-6100/μL
Monocytes	150-1350/μL	100-600/μL
Eosinophils	100-1250/μL	0-1500/μL
Basophils	Rare	0-100/μL
Platelets	200K-500K/μL	200-600K/μL
Icterus index	2-5	2-5
Plasma protein**	6-8g/dl**	6.8-8.3g/dL
Plasma fibrin.	200-400 mg/dL	<100-300mg/dL
Prot: fibrin.	>15:1	> 20:1

* Lymphocyte numbers are highest in young, growing animals. Counts
  decrease with age.
** Values are frequently decreased in newborn and young animals. In dogs
   less than 6 months of age, the values can range from 5-6g/dL

DEFINITIONS
1. **Anisocytosis:** variation in size
2. **Polychromasia:** RBCs with increase in blue color
3. **Poikilocytosis:** variation in shape

4. <u>Corrected white blood count</u>

$$\frac{100 \times WBC}{100 + nRBC} = \text{Corrected White Blood Cell Count}$$

5. **Mean corpuscular volume (MCV)** = RBC size (usually measured by instrument)
   Macrocytic
   Normocytic $\frac{HCT \times 10}{RBC (10^6)} = MCV$
   Microcytic

6. **Mean corpuscular hemoglobin conc.**
   (MCHC)
   Hyperchromic
   Normochromic $\frac{Hb \times 100}{HCT} = MCHC$
   Hypochromic

7. **Mean corpuscular hemoglobin (MCH)**
   $$\frac{Hb \times 10}{RBC \times 10^6} = MCH$$

CANINE & FELINE CHEMISTRY PANEL VALUES

These values are taken from the University of California, Davis Veterinary Medical Teaching
For a blank version to fill out with your own lab's normals go to www.nerdbook.com/extras

	DOG	CAT
A/G Ratio	0.6-1.2	
BUN/Creatinine Ratio	6-26	
Anion Gap (mmol/L)	12-25	
Sodium (mmol/L)	145-154	151-158
Potassium (mmol/L)	4.1-5.3	3.6-4.9
Chloride (mmol/L)	105-116	113-121
CO2 Total (mmol/L)	16-26	15-21
Calcium (mg/dL)	9.9-11.4	9.4-11.4
Inorganic phosphate (mg/dL)	3.0-6.2	3.2-6.3
Creatinine (mg/dL)	0.8-1.6	1.1-2.2
BUN (mg/dL)	8-31	18-33
Glucose (mg/dL)	70-118	73-134
ALT (SGPT) (IU/L)	19-70	28-106
AST (SGOT) (IU/L)	15-43	12-46
Alkaline Phosphatase (IU/L)	15-127	14-71
Total Protein (g/dL)	5.4-7.4	6.6-8.4
Albumin (g/dL)	2.9-4.2	1.9-3.9
Bilirubin Total (mg/dL)	0.0-0.4	0-0.2
Globulin (g/dL)	2.3-4.4	
Cholesterol (mg/dL)	135-345	89-258

	CANINE	FELINE
Ammonia (µg/dL)	0-92	
Amylase (µg/dL)	19-120	
Bilirubin		
direct (mg/dL)	0.0-0.1	0
total	0.0-0.4	0-0.2
Clotting Parameters		
PT	6.2-8.2 sec	7.0-12.7 sec
PTT	9-12 sec	10.0-17.4 sec
PIVKA	15-18 sec	20-24 sec
ACT	60-95 sec	< 65 sec
AT-III	≥ 80% < 60% risk for thrombosis	
FDPs	< 10	
CO2-pCO2 (mmHg)	38	36
Cortisol (µg/dL)	1-6	
Creatine kinase (U/L)	46-320	73-260
Digoxin (ng/mL)	1-2.5	
Fibrinogen	200-400	<100-300
Gamma GT (U/L)	0-6.0	0-4
Insulin (µU/mL)	2-21	0-18
Iron (µg/mL)	33-147	33-135
Lactate Dehydrogenase (U/L)		
Lipase (U/L)	0-500+	0-200+
pH	7.31-7.42	7.24-7.4
Phenobarbital (µg/mL)	15-40	
Sorbital Dehydrogenase (U/L)		
Thyroxine-T4 (µg/dL)	1.6-3.2	2.2-4.7
TIBC (µg/dL)	311-462	189-364
Triiodothy-T3 (ng/dL)	78-144	48-92
Triglycerides (mg/dL)	19-133	8-80

Clinical Path

INTERPRETING THE CHEMISTRY PANEL
Electrolytes
Enzymes
Organic and Inorganic Molecules

I. **ELECTROLYTE PHYSIOLOGY**

   A. **BICARBONATE:** On the chemistry panel, decreased bicarbonate indicates metabolic acidosis, and increased bicarbonate indicates metabolic alkalosis. The kidneys and the respiratory system help maintain acid-base homeostasis. If blood pH drops below normal, the kidneys remove hydrogen ions from the blood and excrete a more acidic urine; the pulmonary system compensates by increasing minute ventilation to help blow off carbon dioxide. If blood pH rises above normal, the kidneys remove bicarbonate from the blood and excrete a more alkaline urine. Minute ventilation may decrease.

   B. **CALCIUM AND PHOSPHORUS:** Both calcium (Ca) and phosphorus (P) are absorbed from the diet, stored in the bone, and excreted in the urine. Because calcium is so vital for nervous, skeletal and cardiac muscle function, it is tightly regulated. Phosphorus is more loosely regulated.

      1. Calcium and phosphorus levels are regulated by three hormones: parathyroid hormone (PTH), vitamin D3, and calcitonin (See p. 9.23). When plasma Ca concentrations fall, the parathyroid gland secretes PTH which stimulates Ca and phosphorus resorption from the bone and calcium resorption but phosphorus excretion by the kidneys. The net effect is that serum calcium levels rise where as phosphorus does not.

      2. In addition, PTH stimulates formation of dihydroxyvitamin D3 from the kidney. Vitamin D3 lead to increased Ca and P uptake from the diet and increased Ca and P resorption from the bone and kidney. When plasma Ca concentration returns to normal, the release of PTH into the plasma decreases.

      3. If plasma Ca levels rise above normal, calcitonin levels increase, CAUSING decreased Ca and P resorption from bone and kidney—consequently lowering the level of both.

      4. About 50% of Ca travels bound to albumin and 50% is in the active ionized form. In the past, correction factors were used to estimate total Ca levels in the face of varying albumin levels, but his method has been found to be non-predictive. Consequently, if total Ca is elevated, then measure ionized Ca.

	INCREASED VALUES	DECREASED VALUES
Calcium	• Neoplasia (e.g. PTH-like hormone) • Chronic renal failure • Hypoadrenocorticism • 1° Hyperparathyroidism (parathyroid tumor—rare) • 2° Hyperparathyroidism (triggered by low dietary Ca or loss of Ca) • Hypervitaminosis D (rodenticide, supplements) • Toxin (e.g. Vit D rodenticide) • Non-malignant skeletal disorder (due to osteoclast activity—rare) • High calcium diet (rare) • Lipemia (artifact) • Young, growing dog (osteoclast activity) • Hyperalbuminemia (increased total but not ionized calcium)	• Eclampsia • Hypoparathyroidism • Low calcium diet • Lymphangiectasia • Malabsorption • Pregnancy and lactation • Chronic renal failure (due to low vitamin D3 formation) • Acute pancreatitis • Hypoalbuminemia (ionized calcium is normal)
Phos-phorus	**Increased absorption** • High-phosphorus diet • Vitamin D toxicity **Decreased excretion or increased bone resorption** • Hypoparathyroidism • Renal disease (1° renal disease) • Renal secondary hyperPTH • Young, growing dogs (osteoclast activity)	**Decreased absorption** • Diet (rickets— low vitamin D3) **Increased renal excretion or decreased bone resorption** • Hyperparathyroidism • Osteomalacia (less present in bone) • Neoplasia (PTH-like substances)

   C. **Chloride:** Chloride and sodium usually travel together. As a result, processes causing hyponatremia cause hypochloremia and processes causing hypernatremia cause hyperchloremia. For instance, chronic severe vomiting can lead to hypochloremia and hyponatremia.

D. **SODIUM AND POTASSIUM:** Aldosterone (a mineralocorticoid produced by the zona glomerulosa of the adrenal cortex) regulates Na^+ and K^+ balance in the blood. Na^+ and K^+ levels are controlled primarily at the distal tubules and collecting ducts of the kidney. Aldosterone is responsible for the reabsorption of Na^+ and excretion of K^+, resulting in increased plasma Na^+ and decreased plasma K^+ levels. In cases of hypoadrenocorticism caused by destruction of the zona glomerulosa, the resulting decrease in aldosterone leads to hyperkalemia and hyponatremia (i.e. decreased Na^+/K^+ RATIO).

	INCREASED VALUES	DECREASED VALUES
Sodium	Water loss > electrolyte loss • Dehydration • Hypodypsia or adypsia • Diabetes Insipidus—central or nephrogenic • Osmotic diuresis (e.g. Diabetes Mellitus, renal failure, mannitol) Excess sodium retention • Primary hyperaldosteronism • Iatrogenic (e.g. salt ingestion, NaCl infusion)	Excess Sodium loss • End stage renal disease • GI loss (vomiting, diarrhea) • Overhydration (e.g. primary Diabetes Insipidus) • Congestive heart failure (increase ANF) Excess water conservation
Potassium	• Acidosis • Dehydration • Hypoadrenocorticism • Renal failure (acute) • Urethral obstruction	• Alkalosis • Hyperaldosteronism • Hyperadrenocorticism • Intestinal obstruction • Insulin therapy • Polyuria • Vomiting, diarrhea, diuresis

1. **The body regulates water by regulating sodium concentration.** Sodium concentration is carefully regulated by the renin-angiotensin-aldosterone system (RAAS), which is triggered by hypovolemia and increased sympathetic tone.

2. **pH affects K^+ levels.** H^+ travels in a direction opposite of K^+. When an animal is acidotic, H^+ flows down its concentration gradient from the plasma and ECF into the cells, and K^+ flows out of the cells. This leads to a K^+ depleted cell and a hyperkalemic patient. Correction of acidosis leads to a decrease in plasma K^+ levels.

3. **Osmotic diuretics, loop diuretics,** and **abnormally high water intake** can increase K^+ excretion. The increased fluid flow through the distal tubules results in an increased gradient for K^+ secretion.

II. **ENZYMES**

	INCREASED VALUES
Alkaline phosphatase (ALP)	• Cholestatic disease (dog or cat) • Cushing's disease (dog) • **Drugs:** Glucocorticoids, barbiturates, and other anti-seizure drugs (dog) • Hyperthyroidism (cat) • Puppies have higher ALP (bone)
ALT	• Liver disease/ hepatocellular damage
AST	• Liver disease (hepatocellular) • Muscle inflammation or necrosis • RBC hemolysis
GGT	• Biliary stasis and steroid hepatopathy

A. **ALT (Alanine aminotransferase)** is the most liver specific enzyme in dogs and cats; Elevated ALT indicates hepatocellular damage. Even in the absence of clinical signs, liver disease is likely and further diagnostics should be performed if a) ALT is $\geq$ AST, b) ALT remains elevated 3-4x normal for 2-3 weeks, or c) ALT remains moderately elevated for 6-8 weeks. In general, elevated liver enzymes in cats should be treated as abnormal.

1. **Increased ALT:** Active hepatocellular damage results in increased ALT but end-stage liver disease does not (No hepatocellular damage occurring). ALT can also

Clinical Path

be mildly increased in GI disease with mild associated liver inflammation or transient bacterial infection.

B. **ALP (Alkaline phosphatase)** is produced in the bone, liver, placenta, gut, and kidney and is elevated in young growing animals. In the liver, ALP is produced by cells lining the bile canaliculi and is consequently **elevated** with biliary obstruction in both cats and dogs. In dogs, the most common cause of elevated ALP is **excess glucocorticoid levels** because glucocorticoids induce an ALP isoenzyme with high activity. ALP can also be elevated due to non-hepatic sources listed previously. In general ALP is nonspecific and often high values are not associated with disease.

C. **AST (SGOT or Aspartate transferase)** is present in hepatocytes, muscle, and red blood cells. As a result, AST levels can be elevated with muscle inflammation or necrosis (e.g. IM muscle injection, exercise), red blood cell hemolysis, or with liver disease. If AST > ALT, check for hemolysis.

D. **AMYLASE and LIPASE:** Both amylase and lipase are made in the pancreas and are excreted by the kidney; both are also synthesized in other locations. Sensitivity of amylase and lipase for pancreatitis is generally low in both dogs and cats. Amylase specificity is low. **Pancreatic lipase immunoreactivity (PLI)** is the test of choice for pancreatitis in dogs and cats0. It is highly sensitive and specific.

III. **ORGANIC COMPOUNDS**
QUICK REFERENCE TO CHEMISTRY PANEL ABNORMALITIES

	INCREASED VALUES	DECREASED VALUES
Albumin	Dehydration	Decreased production • Liver disease Increased loss • Blood loss • GI disease • Glomerulonephropathy • 3rd space loss
Bilirubin	• **Prehepatic** (hemolysis) • **Hepatic** (intrahepatic cholestasis) • **Post-hepatic** (bile duct obstruction— e.g. pancreatitis, pancreatic or proximal GI mass)	
BUN	• **Pre-renal** (dehydration, hypovolemia) • **Renal failure** • **Post-renal** (urinary obstruction) • **Extrarenal** (muscle catabolism, recent protein meal)	Decreased production • End-stage liver disease • Low protein diet Increased loss • Polyuria/diuresis
Cholesterol	• Cushing's disease • Diabetes Mellitus • Hypothyroidism • Glomerular nephropathy • Schnauzer (hyperlipidemia)	• Liver failure (decreased production) • Lymphangiectasia (increased loss)
Creatinine	• Pre-renal disease (dehydration) • Renal disease • Post-renal (urinary obstruction)	• Decreased muscle mass
Globulin	• Chronic immune stimulation (FIP) • Dehydration • Lymphoma or multiple myeloma	• Neonates • Protein-losing enteropathy • Blood loss
Glucose	• Cushing's disease (anti-insulin effect) • Diabetes mellitus • Excitement (cats)	• Insulinoma • Insulin overdose • Liver disease (end-stage) • Sepsis • Toy breeds
Total Protein	• Dehydration • Chronic immune stimulation	Increased loss • Protein-losing gastroenteropathy • Glomerulonephropathy • Acute or chronic hemorrhage Decreased formation • Liver disease • Malnutrition or neoplasia • Lower in young animals

A. **ALBUMIN** is made by the liver and can be lost in the gut, kidney, or 3rd space (e.g. abdominal or thoracic effusions).
  1. **Decreased albumin** occurs with
     a. **Liver disease**– resulting in decreased production
     b. **Glomerulonephropathy** (Mild glomerulonephropathy results in the loss of small, negatively charged proteins such as albumin. In severe glomerulonephropathy, larger proteins including globulins are lost
     c. **GI disease**– resulting in generalized protein loss (both albumin and globulins).
  2. **Increased albumin** is almost always due to dehydration and hemoconcentration.

B. **BILIRUBIN** is a breakdown product of heme. It's carried to the liver by albumin where it is conjugated and excreted into the bile. Elevation can be:
  1. **Pre-hepatic** (hemolytic crisis)
  2. **Hepatic:** due to decreased ability to handle and excrete bilirubin
  3. **Post-hepatic:** due to bile duct obstruction causing an accumulation of bilirubin.

C. **BUN** is synthesized by the liver and excreted in the urine. A constant fraction is excreted in the urine.
  1. **BUN decreases** with decreased production (hepatic insufficiency) or increased loss (polyuria).
  2. **BUN increases** due to **prerenal** conditions (dehydration, hypovolemia), **renal** failure, **postrenal** conditions (urinary obstruction), and extrarenal causes such as GI bleeding and catabolism of muscle (fever, massive muscle trauma, corticosteroid treatment).

D. **CHOLESTEROL** is produced by the liver and absorbed by the gut into the lymphatics.
  1. **Increased with Cushing's** disease and **diabetes mellitus** due to mobilization of fat stores in the liver. It's also elevated in **hypothyroidism** and with **glomerulonephropathy** when the liver responds to protein loss by producing more of everything it makes.
  2. **Decreased with** lymphangiectasia (due to loss via the lymphatics) and liver failure (due to decreased production).

E. **CREATININE** is a metabolic breakdown product of **muscle creatine**. Muscle releases a constant amount of creatinine every day. Its excretion is handled almost exclusively by the kidney via glomerular filtration, so you can use the serum creatinine concentration to evaluate glomerular filtration (a function of the amount of good kidney tissue). Mild prerenal and postrenal elevations in creatinine can occur. Creatinine levels may decrease with muscle wasting (rare).

F. **GLOBULINS** are proteins primarily involved in the immune defense system.
  1. **Monoclonal increase**: Multiple myeloma, lymphoma
  2. **Polyclonal increase**: Chronic immune stimulation (e.g. FIP, Ehrlichia, heartworm disease)

G. **GLUCOSE:** Glucose is produced in the liver via gluconeogenesis and is obtained via the diet. Insulin causes uptake of glucose into the cells.
  1. **Hyperglycemia** occurs in cats due to stress or excitement. In both cats and dogs it can also be caused by **Diabetes mellitus** (insulin release, down-regulation of insulin receptors, or blocked insulin receptors results in decreased uptake of glucose from the blood into the cells).
  2. **Hypoglycemia** occurs due to **decreased production** (hepatic disease) **or decreased intake** (e.g. fasting animals, especially puppies and small dogs). It's also caused by **increased insulin** release which drives glucose into cells (insulinoma or iatrogenic insulin) as well as **increased use**, as with sepsis.

H. **TOTAL PROTEIN:** albumin + globulin
  1. **Decrease**
     a. **Protein-losing gastroenteropathy** results in non-specific loss of protein (albumin plus globulin = total protein).
     b. **Lymphangiectasia:** The GI lymphatics reabsorb water and proteins. They also absorb long-chain fatty acids and triglycerides. With lymphangiectasia,

Clinical Path

the lymphatics are dilated so that these substances cannot be absorbed. In addition, vitamin D and vitamin K are not absorbed.

    c. **Glomerulonephropathy:** Even early in the course of disease, before BUN and creatinine have increased, the animal may exhibit a decrease in total protein from loss through the urine. With mild glomerulonephropathy, small, negatively charged proteins such as albumin are lost. With severe glomerulonephropathy, large proteins such as globulins are lost too.

    d. **Liver damage** results in decreased albumin production.

2. **Increase**
    a. **Chronic immune stimulation or acute inflammation** (increased globulins)
    b. **Multiple myeloma,** lymphoma
    c. **Dehydration**

IV. RATIOS

A. **ANION GAP:** In order to maintain electrical neutrality, the amount of cations in the serum should equal the amount of anions. The electrolytes that are commonly measured are Na^+, K^+, Cl^-, and HCO_3^-, but there are a number of other anions and cations in the serum. Na^+ and K^+ make up 95% of the total serum cations while Cl^- and HCO_3^- make up 85% of the total serum anions. Thus, the concentration of measured cations is greater than the concentration of measured anions. As a result, when you subtract measured anions from measured cations, you get a positive number which is referred to as the **anion gap.** Normal anion gap in dogs and cats is 15-25 mEq/L. This value represents the difference between measured cations and measured anions. It also represents the difference between **unmeasured** cations and unmeasured anions. Anion gap is used to help evaluate the causes or presence of metabolic acidosis.Metabolic acidosis in the presence of increased anion gap indicates a loss in HCO3- with no subsequent increase in Cl-. Causes include ethylene glycol toxicosis, salicylate toxicosis, ketoacidosis, lactic acidosis. Metabolic acidosis with normal anion gap occurs when Cl- increases thus maintaining the normal gap when HCO3 is lost. This acidosis is referred to as hyperchloremic acidosis. Diarrhea, renal tubular acidosis, and acidifying agents such as NH_4Cl are among the causes.

$$(Na^+ + K^+) - (Cl^- + HCO_3^-) = \text{Anion Gap (mEq/L)}$$

ALTERED VALUES	
Anion Gap	• Elevated with an increase in unmeasured anions (e.g. ethylene glycol metabolites, ketone bodies, salicylates, phosphates, sulfates, etc.). • Decreased with an increase in unmeasured cations (e.g. calcium, magnesium, globulins) or decrease in unmeasured anions (albumin). Decreased anion gap is rare.

B. **BUN/CREATININE RATIO** can help predict how the non-renal factors are affecting BUN. The BUN/creatinine ratio factors out the renal cause of ratio changes. (Note: Most people feel the BUN/creatinine ratio is not very useful, but since the ratio is included in many chemistry panels, its possible implications are still considered here).

1. **Normal BUN/Creatinine ratio in small animals is 20-25.** Usually BUN and creatinine go up in the same ratio during renal disease, so that the BUN/creatinine ratio remains the same. If the ratio doesn't stay the same, you must determine why BUN has increased more than creatinine (it's usually the BUN that increases more).

    a. **Diet:** For a given diet (i.e. a set amount of protein/diet), the animal has a fixed BUN/creatinine ratio.
      i. Use the BUN/creatinine ratio to determine whether giving a lower protein diet to a dog in renal failure will make the dog feel better (i.e. calculate whether decreasing protein will decrease BUN enough to make the dog feel better).

2. **Catabolic process** (i.e. fever, sepsis) results in increased nitrogen metabolism.
3. **GI bleeding** acts like an increased protein diet.
4. **Liver damage** leads to decreased BUN production.

C. **OSMOLAR GAP**: Osmolality refers to the number of particles in a solution. These particles do not necessarily have to exert osmotic pressure (if they are freely diffusable).

$$\text{CALCULATED \quad OSMOLALITY} = 2\,(Na^+ + K^+) + \frac{\text{Glucose}}{18} + \frac{\text{BUN}}{2.8}$$

OSMOLAR GAP = Measured serum osmolality - Calculated serum osmolality

1. **Increase in osmolar gap**: The osmolar gap increases with the presence of ethanol, methanol, ethylene glycol, or other unmeasured metabolites in the serum.

REFERENCES

Duncan JR, Prasse KW: *Veterinary Laboratory Medicine: Clinical Pathology*, 4th edition Ames, Iowa, Blackwell Publishing, 2003.

Williard MD, Tvedten H: Small Animal Clinical Diagnosis by Laboratory Methods. 4th edition. Philadelphia, W.B. Saunders, 2004.

Clinical Path

HYPOPROTEINEMIA
Pan-hypoproteinemia
Hypoalbuminemia

There are only a few causes of hypoproteinemia. They include decreased protein production (primarily albumin) due to liver disease and increased loss due to renal disease, blood loss, and gastroenteropathy. Regardless of the cause of the hypoproteinemia, the signs are similar. Signs of severe hypoproteinemia include **ascites, pleural effusion,** or **edema** (Albumin is the main determinant of oncotic pressure). These signs usually don't present until the albumin is <1.5g/dL.

I.   **HYPOALBUMINEMIA vs. PAN-HYPOPROTEINEMIA:** The diseases that cause hypoalbuminemia are different from those that cause pan-hypoproteinemia. Distinguishing between the two conditions is the first step in establishing a diagnosis.

A.   **PAN-HYPOPROTEINEMIA:** Decrease in total protein (albumin and globulins)

ETIOLOGY and DIAGNOSIS of PAN-HYPOPROTEINEMIA

ETIOLOGY	DIAGNOSTIC FINDINGS
BLOOD LOSS	CBC: • **Acute blood Loss:** Macrocytic, hypochromic, regenerative anemia (or non-regenerative if loss occurred within 48 hours). • **Blood loss resulting in iron deficiency:** Microcytic, hypochromic anemia with thrombocytosis. CHEMISTRY PANEL: hypoproteinemia
GI DISEASE Protein-losing gastroenteropathy: e.g. Malabsorption (lymphangiectasia) Maldigestion (exocrine pancreatic insufficiency) Neoplasia Inflammatory bowel disease.	CHEMISTRY PANEL • **Cholesterol is decreased** with lymphangiectasia, a condition in which the lacteals dilate and lymph leaks out. Because animals absorb triglycerides and fatty acids through the lymph system, animals with lymphangiectasia have low cholesterol and vitamin D (fat soluble vitamin). Leakage of lymph also leads to low total protein and lymphocytes. • **Calcium is decreased** with lymphangiectasia because vitamin D, the fat soluble vitamin that regulates serum calcium levels, can't be absorbed by the lacteals. Total calcium is also usually low due to low albumin levels, thus ionized calcium should be measured. • **Calcium may be elevated** with lymphoma, although hypercalcemia is usually not seen with GI lymphoma. • **Globulins are sometimes elevated** with GI or other chronic disease. As a result, the animal may only be hypoalbuminemic due to down-regulation in the liver. CBC • **Anemia** occurs if there's blood loss from the GI tract. • **Eosinophilia** is possible in GI disease associated with allergy or parasites. • **Lymphopenia** accompanies **lymphangiectasia** because lymph is lost in lymphangiectasia, and this lymph contains albumin and lymphocytes. OTHER • **TLI:** Measure trypsin-like immunoreactivity in order to test for exocrine pancreatic insufficiency. • **Dietary trial:** Novel protein diet or highly digestible diet. • **GI biopsy:** Endoscopic or full-thickness

B. HYPOALBUMINEMIA

HYPOALBUMINEMIA

ETIOLOGY	DIAGNOSTIC FINDINGS
DECREASED PRODUCTION **Liver disease:** The liver makes albumin and some globulins. Globulins usually are increased or normal with liver disease.	**URINALYSIS:** • **Bilirubinuria** may occur in liver disease. Trace amounts (1+) may not be significant in dogs with concentrated urine because the renal tubules can conjugate bilirubin, whereas bilirubin is **always significant in cats** due to their higher renal threshold for excreting bilirubin. Increased serum bilirubin, however, is always abnormal in both dogs and cats and indicates liver disease or hemolysis. **CBC:** anemia of chronic disease $\pm$ icteric serum. **CHEMISTRY PANEL:** • $\pm$ **elevated ALT, AST, ALP:** Typically, the liver enzymes are not elevated because the liver must be severely and chronically damaged in order for albumin production to decrease; thus, in the case of severe, chronic liver damage, liver enzymes may not be elevated. • **Bilirubin is elevated** because the diseased liver cannot conjugate and excrete bilirubin. In cases in which bilirubin is not elevated, serum bile acids may be evaluated to detect liver dysfunction. • **Cholesterol, glucose and BUN** are low because the liver synthesizes all three of these compounds. • **Total calcium** is usually low because albumin is low. Ionized calcium levels should be normal. **ELEVATED BILE ACIDS, FASTING AMMONIA and AMMONIA TOLERANCE TEST:** Only necessary in cases when bilirubin is not elevated. Increased bilirubin with no evidence for hemolysis indicates there is cholestasis; therefore, there is no additional value to measuring bile acids or ammonia. **LIVER BIOPSY** is required for a specific diagnosis.
INCREASED LOSS **Glomerular Nephropathy** results in decreased permselectivity which leads to albumin loss by the glomeruli. In extremely severe disease, globulins are lost, too. By this stage, the kidney nephrons are severely damaged resulting in isosthenuria.	**NEPHROTIC SYNDROME consists of** hypoalbuminemia, proteinuria, hypercholesterolemia, and ascites/edema. **URINALYSIS:** reveals increased protein in the absence of a reactive sediment. Be sure to take the specific gravity, and presence of WBC or RBCs into consideration when determining whether the protein elevation is significant. If needed, perform a protein: creatinine ratio to determine whether the elevation in protein is significant. A ratio of < 0.5 mg/dL for dogs and 0.4 mg/dL for cats is normal. **CHEMISTRY PANEL** • **Elevated BUN, creatinine, phosphorus** and acidosis: These parameters are not elevated until a later stage in the disease when the renal tubules are affected. Most dogs with glomerulonephropathy start off with glomerular disease but have normal nephron function, so that in early glomerulonephritis the BUN and creatinine are normal. This occurs because the glomerulus is damaged so that the pores are larger (decreased permselectivity) and proteins can leak into the glomerular filtrate. The renal blood flow and thus glomerular filtration rate are normal though. A dog can have massive glomerulonephropathy but have normal BUN and creatinine. As the disease progresses, the kidney becomes fibrotic resulting in decreased renal perfusion. As a result, the BUN and creatinine increase. • **Hypercholesterolemia** occurs because the liver responds to decrease in proteins by making more of everything. • **Total calcium** is usually low due to low albumin. Ionized calcium should be normal **CBC:** normocytic, normochromic, nonresponsive anemia of chronic disease.

INTERPRETING THE HEMOGRAM
White Blood Cells (WBC)
Red Blood Cells (RBC) and Anemia
Platelets and Thrombocytopenia (ITP)

I. **INTERPRETING the WHITE BLOOD CELL PARAMETERS:** Inflammation is a protective tissue response to damage or injury. It involves migration of white blood cells out of the capillaries into the damaged region where they phagocytize debris and pathogens or attack parasites. Injury that triggers inflammation can be septic (caused by bacteria or fungi) or non-septic (caused by mechanical or chemical trauma, viral infection, neoplasia, immune-mediate diseases and any cause of tissue damage or necrosis). If the damage is localized, the WBC response is localized, but if the inflammation is diffuse or widespread, then we see a systemic inflammatory response/leukocytosis. Usually the CBC does not reveal the specific cause of the inflammation, unless a specific organism is seen on the smear. Nevertheless, the CBC can be useful in identifying systemic disease, determining prognosis, and monitoring progress.

A. **FUNCTION of INFLAMMATORY CELLS**
   1. **Neutrophils** phagocytize debris and bacteria.
   2. **Monocytes/macrophages** phagocytize necrotic debris, foreign particles, abnormal red blood cells, neoplastic cells, and certain organisms such as virus particles and fungi. Expect to see a monocytosis whenever one of these components is high. For example, in hemolytic anemia, monocytosis may occur due to the need to phagocytize the abundant abnormal red blood cells.
   3. **Lymphocytes** indicate a chronic immune stimulus due to infection or immune-mediated disease. B-lymphocytes are responsible for producing antibodies.
   4. **Eosinophils** are responsible for the regulation of IgE-mediated hypersensitivity reactions and are important in killing parasites. Eosinophils attach to parasites and release substances that damage the parasite or parasite egg walls. Parasites must be present or have migrating stages in the tissue in order to incite a strong eosinophilic reaction.

B. **MORPHOLOGIC FEATURES of LEUKOCYTES in DISEASE**

MORPHOLOGIC FEATURES of LEUKOCYTES in DISEASE	
TOXIC NEUTROPHILS (Change are all in the cytoplasm)	To assess toxicity look at the cytoplasm. These toxic changes occur while the neutrophils are still in the bone marrow. Toxic changes indicate bacterial infection. • Foamy, basophilic cytoplasm. The foamy appearance is due to increased vacuolization presumably due to increased lysosomes. Basophilia is due to increase in mRNA. • Dohle bodies (rough endoplasmic reticulum remnants)
LYMPHOCYTES	**Reactive lymphocytes**, lymphocytes responding to antigen, have blue cytoplasm and are called immunocytes.
MONOCYTES	Very vacuolated in infectious disease (not pathognomonic)

C. **TYPES of RESPONSES in INFLAMMATION:** The typical inflammatory response begins with increased release of **segmented neutrophils** from the marginal pool. In dogs, 50% of mature neutrophils and other leukocytes are stored in the marginal pool. They wait in the endothelial lining of capillaries, especially of the spleen. The remaining 50% are in circulation. In cats the marginal pool is 2-3x larger than the circulating pool. Fear, excitement, and strenuous exercise cause splenic contraction leading to increased release of mature neutrophils from the marginal pool. This release can occur within minutes to hours. As this store is depleted, **bands** are released from the bone marrow. In more severe disease processes, younger neutrophil precursors such as metamyelocytes, myelocytes, promyelocytes, and myeloblasts are released in increasing numbers from the bone marrow. An **elevation in immature neutrophils** (a.k.a. immature neutrophils or N-segs) in the presence or absence of neutrophilia is called a **left shift**. The severity of the left shift is determined by the total number of N-segs and their state of maturity (bands vs. more immature forms). The presence of N-segs younger than bands indicates an increasingly severe left shift. It takes up to 6 days to produce mature neutrophils from the bone marrow myeloblast.
   1. The **presence of bands** in cats and presence of increased bands in dogs should increase the index of suspicion for bacterial **infection** as the cause of inflammation, especially if these bands show toxic changes.
   2. A **regenerative left shift** (usually just called left-shift) is a left shift in which the mature neutrophils outnumber N-segs. The N-seg elevation occurs in an orderly fashion.

3. **A degenerative left shift is a left shift** in which N-segs outnumber mature neutrophils. It indicates that neutrophils are consumed faster than they are produced. The bone marrow can't produce them at a sufficient rate to allow for enough time for their full maturaton. Usually bands comprise most of the N-segs. The more immature the N-segs, the more serious the disease.

4. **Leukemoid response (also called extreme neutrophilic leukocytosis)** is a marked leukocytosis ($\geq$ 50,000 WBC/μL) which involves immature N-segs and a left shift. The progression of cells is orderly with the most mature present in higher numbers than the more immature cells. This order is in contrast to granulocytic leukemias, where younger blast cells may outnumber the more mature cells. A leukemoid response can be seen with severe inflammatory disorders including pyometra, pyoabdomen and pyothorax, as well as with immune-mediated hemolytic anemia (mechanism uncertain).

ETIOLOGIES of LEUKOCYTOSIS, LEUKOPENIA

	INCREASE	DECREASE
Leukocyte (Neutrophils are the predominant cell involved)	Leukocytosis refers to increased WBC count which can be due to neutrophilia or, less commonly, increases in other cell types. **Age:** Younger animals have more leukocytes, especially lymphocytes, than adult animals. **Exercise, epinephrine, and acute stress cause** lymphocytosis and neutrophilia.due to the splenic contraction releasing leukocytes from the marginal pool. **Chronic stress** (24-48 hrs) results in bone marrow release of leukoyctes	
Neutrophil	**Acute stress/epinephrine-mediated stress** (Refer to leukocytosis section above) **Chronic stress/glucocorticoid mediated stress:** leads to an increase in corticosteroid release by the adrenal cortex which results in neutrophilia, lymphopenia, monocytosis (dogs), eosinopenia. **Septic inflammation** **Non-septic inflammation:** e.g. tumor, response to hemolysis or blood loss.	**Severe infection:** Production can't keep up with consumption **Toxins,drugs** (e.g. estrogen, chloramphenicol) **Chemotherapy** **Primary bone marrow disease** **Viral** or **rickettsial infections** (e.g. FeLV, Parvo, *E. canis*)
Lymphocyte	**Lymphocytic leukemia** **Acute stress,** especially in cats (+ neutrophilia) **Response** to antigen (e.g. chronic infection/inflammation) **Young** animals > 2000 lymphocytes	**Glucocorticoids**/chronic stress **Lymphangectasia** **Viral** infections **Congenital** immunodeficiency syndrome
Monocyte	**Response to glucocorticoids** (dog) **Acute** or **Chronic infection** or inflammation with tissue damage **Infarction and neoplasia**	**Bone marrow disorder** **Viral** or **rickettsial** infection (FeLV, Parvo, *E. canis*)
Eosinophil	Migrating **parasites** **Allergic** diseases Eosinophilic leukemia, mast cell **neoplasia** and paraneoplastic diseases Disease of the respiratory tract, skin, GI tract, urogenital system	**Glucocorticoid**/stress (Cushing's disease or steroid treatment) **Bone marrow disorder** (rare hypoplasia, dysplasia, aplasia as well as leukemias)
Basophil	Some respiratory and skin disease Mast cell tumors Granulocytic leukemia Heartworm disease or other systemic parasites	

Clinical Path

POOR PROGNOSTIC INDICATORS

- **Degenerative left shift**: This indicates that the demand for neutrophils is higher than the production speed. Immature neutrophils are released from the bone marrow before they can fully mature.
- **Leukopenia** indicates that demand for neutrophils is higher than production.
- **Leukemoid response**: Demand for neutrophils is so high that extremely young N-segs are released from the bone marrow.
- **Toxic neutrophils**: usually indicate bacterial infection. Left shift plus toxicity indicates infection. Toxicity with degenerative left shift usually indicates overwhelming infection.
- **Severe or persistent lymphopenia** indicates severe or persistent stress.

II.   **ANEMIA** is defined as a decrease in red blood cell mass (reflected as a low PCV, low hemoglobin concentration or low red blood cell count). Anemias can be classified into three categories based on etiology.

GENERAL CATEGORIES of ANEMIA

- **Blood loss**
- **Hemolysis** can be intra or extravascular and can have immune-mediated or non-immune-mediated causes.
- **Decreased production** occurs due to space-occupying bone marrow neoplasias, immune-mediated conditions affecting RBC progenitors, conditions causing decrease in erythropoietin, chronic disease causing sequestration of iron, etc.

A. **GENERAL WORK-UP of ANEMIA**
1. **Measure PCV and total protein** in order to **identify anemia** and to determine whether anemia is due to **blood loss vs. hemolysis or decreased production.** Decrease in total protein supports blood loss. Normal or increased total protein levels indicate hemolysis or decreased production. Protein changes may also occur with anemia due to decreased production, so don't automatically assume there is hemolysis or blood loss just based on protein changes.
   a. Also look at **serum color** since with hemolysis, serum color can help determine whether the hemolysis is intravascular or extravascular.
      i. **Red serum** indicates **intravascular hemolysis**. It occurs when RBCs are destroyed within the blood vessels causing a release of hemoglobin into the vessels. These animals may also have hemoglobinuria.
      ii. **Icteric serum** indicates **extravascular hemolysis (or cholestasis)**. The damaged RBCs are removed by the reticuloendothelial system (e.g. spleen and liver) and the heme is metabolized to bilirubin. These animals may also have bilirubinuria.
   b. With a regenerative anemia (see below) and evaluation of protein and serum color, at this point we know whether the patient has blood loss vs. hemolysis. If there is hemolysis, we may have an idea as to whether it's intra or extravascular.
2. **Look at the reticulocyte numbers** in order to characterize the anemia as **regenerative or non-regenerative** and to monitor response to therapy.
   a. **Regenerative anemias** are caused by **blood loss or hemolysis.**
   b. **Non-regenerative anemias** are usually due to **decreased production.** Because it takes 2-3 days to generate a reticulocyte response and 5-6 days for maximal bone marrow response to anemia, **early blood loss** and **hemolytic anemias** are non-regenerative. In addition, there are cases of immune-mediated hemolysis that are directed at reticulocytes and earlier precursors and this type of hemolytic anemia may also appear non-regenerative.
   c. Anemia is considered regenerative if the absolute reticulocyte count is > 50,000/μL or the reticulocyte production index (RPI) > 1.0 (only applies to dogs). RPI takes into consideration the reticulocyte lifespan and the extent of anemia in order to determine the amount of RBCs the bone marrow is producing. Normal RBC lifespan in dogs and cats is about 100 days.
   d. Also look at **RBC size and color**: Regenerative anemias have increased numbers of macrocytic, hypochromic erythrocytes with increased polychromasia.

ETIOLOGY of NON-REGENERATIVE ANEMIA
(Classified by RBC Morphology)

- **Macrocytic, normochromic RBCs** are seen with myelodysplasia (most common in cats with FeLV). In theory, could be seen with folate or cobalt deficiency, but rarely documented in animals.
- **Microcytic, hypochromic RBCs** are due to iron deficiency (e.g. chronic blood loss in dogs such as with GI neoplasia or GI parasites).
- **Normocytic, normochromic RBCs** occur with early blood loss anemia and early hemolytic anemia but also occurs due to decreased production, e.g.
  - **Erythroid aplasia** can be caused by neoplasia (space-occupying lesions in the bone marrow) or immune-mediated destruction of erythrocytes (may be associated with FeLV in cats).
  - **Renal failure** leads to decrease in erythropoietin.
  - **Anemia of chronic disease** occurs due to sequestration of iron in the bone marrow as well as other factors.
  - **Estrogen toxicity** can cause bone marrow destruction leading to pancytopenia.
  - **Hypothyroidism** (dogs)

3. **Look at RBC morphology** and identify changes that could indicate the cause of the hemolytic anemia. Hemolytic anemias can be immune-mediated or non-immune-mediated. Those that are immune mediated may be primary or may be secondary to other conditions. When IMHA is diagnosed, search for an underlying cause.

HEMOLYTIC ANEMIAS CAN BE IMMUNE MEDIATED or
NON-IMMUNE MEDIATED
(Usually are regenerative starting several days after onset)

IMMUNE-MEDIATED CAUSES CAN BE PRIMARY or CAN BE SECONDARY to the FOLLOWING CONDITIONS:
- **Infectious:** Ehrlichia is a blood parasite that is found in granulocytes or monocytes. It can cause IMHA or bone marrow destruction. Heartworm disease or any other infectious disease that causes chronic immune stimulation can cause IMHA via the bystander effect. FeLV and *Mycoplasma hemofelis* are also thought to occasionally cause a 2° IMHA.
- **Tumors** such as hemangiosarcoma, lymphosarcoma, malignant histiocytosis and some myeloproliferative diseases can trigger IMHA.
- **Drug reactions:** Sulfa drugs, penicillins, and cephalosporins have been implicated in IMHA.
- **Vaccination:** In one study 30% of dogs with IMHA had been vaccinated within a month prior to presentation.
- **Envenomation:** There have been a few cases of AIHA following bee stings.
- **Neonatal isoerythrolysis** occurs primarily when pregnant queens with type B blood have offspring with type A blood
- **Transfusion reactions**

NON-IMMUNE-MEDIATED CAUSES of HEMOLYSIS:
- **RBC parasites** can directly damage the RBC (*Babesia, Mycoplasma hemofelis*, etc) leading to extravascular hemolysis.
- **Hereditary diseases** such as phosphofructokinase deficiency (PFK) or pyruvate kinase (PK) deficiency. PFK causes signs primarily after intense exercise and occurs most commonly in English Springer spaniels. Dogs can survive well if activity is limited. With PK, symptoms are severe and recurrent and most develop bone marrow myelofibrosis by 3-4 years of age. Dogs most commonly affected include Beagles, West Highland terriers and Basenjis. PK deficiency has also been described in cats (Abyssinian, Somali, DSH).
- **Microangiopathic disease** (small blood vessel disease). These are diseases where fibrin is deposited in small vessels. The RBC passing through are sheared leading to schistocytes (RBC fragments). E.g. splenic torsion, heartworm disease with caval syndrome, splenic hemangiosarcoma, DIC.
- **Oxidative damage** caused by ingestion of onion, garlic, tylenol, zinc, propylene glycol, etc. These oxidize the hemoglobin sulfhydryl groups leading to cross-linking and consequently precipitation of hemoglobin. These precipitates are visible on New Methylene blue stain as Heinz bodies. Note that zinc causes oxidative damage but may also cause intravascular hemolysis. Oxidative damage to RBC membranes may also occur resulting in formation of eccentrocytes.

Clinical Path

      a. **Heinz bodies** indicate oxidative damage (e.g. onion, garlic, tylenol, zinc). The history should reveal evidence suggesting the cause. Zinc toxicity can often be diagnosed on radiographs (or via history of ingesting zinc-containing creams). Heinz bodies may be seen in cats related to metabolic disease and not necessarily indicative of exposure to oxidants.

      b. **Ghost cells**: With IMHA, antibodies attach to the RBCs and complement is activated. Holes are punched in RBCs causing the contents to spill out leaving just the membrane shell.

      c. **Spherocytes** occur in approximately 80% of IMHA cases. They occur because antibodies attach to the RBCs and macrophages then ingest portions of the membrane thus causing the cell to become rounder and smaller. Spherocytes cannot be reliably identified in cats.

      d. **Schistocytes** are RBC fragments. They suggest microangiopathic disease (DIC, splenic torsion, hemangiosarcoma, heartworm disease with caval syndrome, etc.).

      e. **Nucleated RBCs** are seen with severe anemia as well as with splenic hemangiosarcomas, lead poisoning, and bone marrow disease.

      f. **Parasites** Look for *Mycoplasma felis* (epicellular dots), *Babesia* (little teardrops- common in racing greyhounds and in fighting dogs as it may be transmitted by bite wounds).

4. **Look at the other cell lines**

      a. **Neutrophilia** does not correlate with infection. It may be an indicator of prognosis.

      b. **Platelet count:** Look for concurrent ITP or DIC. The most common reason for low platelets is consumption. Platelet counts of 50K-100K suggest that animals are actively forming little clots and may require anticoagulants.

5. **Slide Agglutination test:** Mix one drop of isotonic saline with one drop of blood on a microscope slide. RBCs clumped due to rouleaux will disperse whereas with IMHA, the cells remain clumped together (due to antibody cross-linking).

6. **Perform a Coomb's test** if the slide agglutination test is negative because there may be antibodies on the RBCs but not enough to cause autoagglutination in the saline test. The Coomb's test uses rabbit or goat antiserum that's specific for dog antibodies and complement. When they bind they cause cross-linking of antibodies and thus agglutination. Sensitivity of this test is only 60-70% so it does not rule out IMHA nor does it determine whether it's primary or secondary.

7. **If IMHA is diagnosed but an underlying cause has not been found, continue to look for an underlying cause** based on history as well as further diagnostics. If IMHA has been ruled out (no spherocytes, coomb's negative), then pursue non-immune mediated causes.

      a. Perform Rickettsial titers

      b. Perform PCR or titer for *Babesia* in greyhounds, fighting dog breeds and where otherwise suspected. *Babesia* can be treated with azithromycin and atovaquone.

      c. Test for FeLV in cats since *M. haemofelis* is more common in FeLV positive cats. Additionally FeLV is associated with immune-mediated attack on erythroid progenitors.

      d. **Look for cancer** on thoracic radiographs and abdominal ultrasound. If IMHA has been ruled out (no spherocytes, coomb's-negative), then pursue non-immune-mediated causes.

8. Run a **coagulation panel** because many of the dogs are already in a hypercoagulable state and are forming clots. The panel can be used to decide whether to start anti-coagulants and to monitor progress. Also perform a blood type if transfusion may be needed and the animal is not autoagglutinating.

9. **Perform bone marrow aspirate +/- biopsy if:**

      a. There's a persistent, severe, non-regenerative anemia.

      b. You suspect neoplasia for any reason.

      c. Other cell lines are affected.

B. **TREATMENT of IMMUNE MEDIATED HEMOLYTIC ANEMIA (IMHA) in DOGS:**
IMHA is the most common cause of hemolytic anemia in dogs. It's caused by antibody and complement-associated destruction of red blood cells. It is often associated with immune-mediated thrombocytopenia (ITP). Once IMHA is identified, be sure to check for ITP as well as for evidence of other immune-mediated diseases (e.g. glomerulonephropathy and polyarthritis). Concurrent IMHA and ITP is called **Evan's syndrome.** IMHA occurs most commonly in Standard Poodles, Cocker Spaniels, and Old English Sheepdogs.

IMMUNE-MEDIATED HEMOLYTIC ANEMIA

CLINICAL FINDINGS	The clinical signs are signs of anemia • Acute lethargy, depression, anorexia and fever • Pale mucous membranes, cyanosis, icterus • Heart murmur occurs due to increased blood viscosity. • Hepatomegaly and splenomegaly occurs due to increased red blood cell (RBC) clearance associated with extravascular hemolysis.
CLINICAL FEATURES	Antibodies attach to RBCs and attract complement resulting in complement attack and lysis of the cells (**INTRAVASCULAR HEMOLYSIS**) or they attract macrophages which phagocytize the tagged RBCs (**EXTRAVASCULAR HEMOLYSIS**). Partial phagocytosis where macrophages remove only part of the RBC membranes produces **spherocytes** (smaller, spherical RBCs). **Hemolysis can be chronic and stable or can be rapid** resulting in a dramatic drop in PCV within the first 24-48 hours. It can drop to below 10% within 72 hours. Affected dogs are often lethargic and have a fever for 1-3 days prior to the actual hemolytic episode.
TREATMENT	**BLOOD TRANSFUSION:** If the PCV is critically low, then administer whole blood. Perform a crossmatch first and pretreat with dexamethasone (2 mg/kg IV) and benadryl (0.5 mg/kg IV) to help prevent transfusion reactions. Animals with IMHA are more likely to reject blood transfusions than donor animals. If the dog's blood autoagglutinates, it's likely to destroy donor cells, too. Since transfusion reactions are common, don't transfuse unless it's necessary. **GLUCOCORTICOIDS** are the first line of defense. About 5-10% of dogs are refractory to glucocorticoid treatment. • **Prednisone**: 1-2 mg/kg BID PO (usually 1 mg/kg). • **Methylprednisone**: 1-2mg/kg PO BID (more potent than prednisone) • **Dexamethasone**: 0.15-0.45 mg/kg PO BID (most potent) After about one month of control start tapering slowly in 2-4 week blocks for a total of about 3-4 months by decreasing 20% each time. With cases of chronic, stable IMHA, start with prednisone alone and try it for up to one month before adding anything else. If disease is acute and severe, use prednisone in conjunction with azathioprine (or cyclosporine). Avoid azathioprine in cats. **AZATHIOPRINE:** 2 mg/kg q 24 hours until clinical response. Then q 48 hours (Dogs only). **CYCLOSPORINE (ATOPICA):** 5-10 mg/kg/day divided BID-TID PO. **VINCRISTINE** can be used if the dog has concurrent ITP and is showing signs from the thrombocytopenia. Administer 0.50-0.75 mg/m^2 weekly until you get a reponse. Vincristine works if the dog has functional megakaryocytes. **DOXYCYCLINE** (10 mg/kg IV BID) or **TETRACYCLINE** (22mg/kg PO TID) can be used to treat for *M. hemofelis* and tick-borne diseases prior to getting titer results. **IV FLUIDS** at 1-1.5x maintenance to maintain vascular volume. This will cause the PCV to drop further so be careful not to fluid overload. **HEPARIN** 100 U/kg q 6 hours in acute stages to avoid DIC **SPLENECTOMY for primary IMHA is controversial.** It decreases antibodies produced by removing B-cells and primed macrophages; consequently a lower dose of steroids is needed after splenectomy.
DISEASE COURSE	• Gradual improvement **may** start 48-96 hours after treatment is instituted. The PCV may rise slowly over the next weeks and full restoration of the PCV can take 1-3 months or longer. The platelet count in recovering animals should return to normal and autoagglutination should subside. • Recovered dogs do not usually have recurrent bouts of this disease.
PROGNOSIS	Prognosis is unpredictable. Unlike other forms of IMHA, the prognosis for peracute disease is poor. If not treated appropriately, almost all animals will die. The prognosis is worse if the animal has hemoglobinuria, severe thromboembolic signs, or no compatible donors can be found. If the dog survives the first three days of optimal treatment, the prognosis improves.

Clinical Path

III. **IMMUNE-MEDIATED THROMBOCYTOPENIA (ITP)** is caused by increased destruction of or decreased production of platelets due to antibodies and complement attacking platelets or platelet precursors. It can occur alone or in association with IMHA.
   A. **BREEDS:** German Shepherd, Standard Poodle, Cocker Spaniel

   B. **CLINICAL SIGNS:** Epistaxis, petechia, ecchymosis

   C. **DIAGNOSTIC APPROACH:**
      1. **First determine** whether the animal is thrombocytopenic. **Platelet counts** of > 20,000 platelets/μL are usually not associated with bleeding. One platelet per oil immersion field is equivalent to about 20,000 platelets/μL (varies with microscope).

      2. **Next,** determine whether thrombocytopenia is related to blood loss or to a specific problem in the platelet line.
         a. **Check the PCV, serum bilirubin and total protein** to assess for concurrent anemia and if present to determine whether it is due to blood loss or hemolysis. If the dog has a macrocytic, hypochromic anemia with normal total protein level, then it likely has concurrent hemolytic anemia.
         b. **Perform a clotting panel** (APTT, PT, and FDPs or d-dimer in dogs) to rule out coagulation abnormalities and DIC.
         c. If the platelet count is normal or not low enough to be associated with bleeding and the coagulation profile is normal, then perform a **von Willebrand's factor analysis** to assess for von Willebrand's disease.
         d. **Bone marrow aspirate or biopsy:** Estimate the number of megakaryocytes and assess for the presence of anti-megakaryocyte antibodies. The bone marrow exam also helps rule out other causes of ITP such as neoplasia.

      3. Rule out other causes of thrombocytopenia

INCEASED DESTRUCTION	DECREASED PRODUCTION
• Blood loss (mild thrombocytopenia) • *Rickettsia* and *Ehrlichia* • DIC	• Bone marrow neoplasia • Estrogen toxicity • Rickettsial disease

      4. If all of these etiologies have been ruled out, then the dog has ITP. Next, determine whether the ITP is primary or secondary to another disease such as neoplasia, *Rickettsia* or *Ehrlichia* infection, drug reaction, etc.

HEMOSTATIC ABNORMALITIES
The Hemostatic System
Localizing the Defect
Platelet Disorders/Evaluation
Coagulation Factor Evaluation
Disseminated Intravascular Coagulation

I. THE HEMOSTATIC SYSTEM

A. PLATELETS: When damaged, the normal blood vessel is initially sealed by a platelet plug. Platelets come in contact with collagen located beneath the endothelium of the damaged blood vessel and begin to aggregate, forming the plug.

B. The COAGULATION CASCADE is stimulated by collagen, tissue thromboplastin, and platelets. The end result of the series of coagulation steps is the formation of insoluble **fibrin** strands which form a meshwork at the site of vascular damage, thereby stabilizing the existing platelet plug and forming a thicker, stronger plug. Coagulation can be divided into the **intrinsic** and **extrinsic** pathways which converge onto the **common pathway** (Refer to p. 4.23 for a diagram).

1. **The intrinsic pathway** is activated by collagen, fibrin or platelets. Factor XII is activated first and it activates factor XI which in turn activates factor IX. Factor IX interacts with factors VIII and PF3 to initiate the common pathway.

2. **The extrinsic pathway** is activated by tissue damage (**thromboplastin, aka Factor III**). Thromboplastin interacts with factor VII to activate the common pathway.

3. **The common pathway:** Factors X, V, and PF3 interact to convert prothrombin (factor III) to thrombin which in turn converts **fibrinogen** to **fibrin**.

4. Vitamin K and calcium ions are essential in a number of these coagulation steps. Factors II, VII, IX and X are all vitamin K dependent. As a result, lack or antagonism of vitamin K and chelation of calcium ions prevent coagulation from occurring.

C. FIBRINOLYSIS: Blood clots are not permanent. Once hemorrhage is controlled and vascular repair has begun, the clot is degraded so that the vessel lumen can re-open. Clot lysis/fibrinolysis is facilitated by antithrombin-III (AT-III).

1. Plasminogen proactivator is converted to tissue plasminogen activator (tPA) which, in the presence of AT-III, converts plasminogen to plasmin. Plasmin in turn degrades the fibrin in the clot to **fibrin degradation products (FDPs)**.

Plasminogen Proactivator

Tissue Plasminogen Activator

AT-IIIa

Plasminogen   Plasmin

Fibrin   FDPs

D. ANTICOAGULANTS

1. **Antithrombin III** is involved in preventing excess coagulation as well as promoting fibrinolysis. As an anticoagulant, it prevents formation of thrombin from prothrombin. AT-III is made by the liver and excreted by the kidney. Liver disease and glomerulonephropathy can lead to deficiencies in AT-III resulting in excess coagulation (hypercoagulability) within the body.

2. **Heparin** activates AT-III.

3. **Sodium citrate and EDTA** chelate calcium, an ion that's essential in the clotting cascade. We use these compounds in blood collection tubes to prevent clotting.

4. **Coumarin,** a product used in rodenticides, interferes with the action of vitamin K, thus it inhibits production of vitamin K dependent coagulation factors.

Clinical Path

II.   LOCALIZING THE DEFECT: The hemostatic defect can be localized based on clinical signs/physical examination and a hemostatic profile.
  A.   CLINICAL SIGNS and physical examination indicate that there's a hemostatic defect. They are not as specific as lab tests in localizing the defect, though, and cannot be used to rule out a specific type of hemostatic defect.

BLEEDING CHARACTERISTICS	DEFECT
Petechia, ecchymosis, epistaxis (Vascular problems are often accompanied by edema.)	Platelet or vascular problem
Large hemorrhage, hematoma	Coagulation factor problem

  1.   Platelet or vascular problems: Petechia and ecchymosis indicate a platelet or vascular problem. They occur when an adequate platelet plug doesn't form and as a result, a little blood leaks out of the vessel. Before the hemorrhage becomes too large, the normal coagulation factors in contact with collagen around the vessel form a fibrin clot to stop the hemorrhage. Epistaxis is often associated with platelet defects, too.
  2.   Coagulation defects are characterized by large areas of hemorrhage such as hematomas. In coagulation defects, a platelet plug forms, but since it's not stabilized by fibrin strands, it breaks down, which allows bleeding. Any defect or deficiency of one or more coagulation factors slows clot formation down and allows a variable amount of hemorrhage to form before the fibrin clot or pressure of adjacent tissues stops the bleeding.

  B.   HEMOSTATIC PROFILE: A hemostatic profile of five or six tests can be used to determine the cause of significant bleeding. These tests include platelet count, buccal mucosal bleeding time, vWF analysis, activated partial thromboplastin time (APTT), prothrombin time (PT), fibrin degradation products (FDPs) (or d-dimer) analysis and antithrombin -III (AT-III) analysis. If these tests are normal, a biopsy for vascular disease (vasculitis) should be performed.

PARAMETER TESTED	PREFERRED TEST
Platelet quantity	Platelet count (if count < 20,000/μL = at risk for bleeding)
Platelet function	Buccal mucosal bleeding time
von Willebrand's disease	Factor VIII-Ag
Intrinsic/common path	Activated partial thromboplastin time (APTT) or activated clotting time (ACT)
Extrinsic/common path	Prothrombin time (PT)
Fibrinolysis	FDP, AT-III

  1.   Blood Vessel Evaluation: Blood vessels are difficult to evaluate except with histology. In certain diseases, enough information is available to predict vasculitis or other vascular defects. Examples of vascular disease in small animals include the rare connective tissue diseases (i.e. Ehlers-Danlos syndrome or feline epitheliogenesis imperfecta). Immune-mediated vasculitis in dogs isn't common. Vascular disease is often diagnosed by exclusion of other possibilities or at necropsy. Skin biopsies for diagnosing vasculitis are rarely performed.

III.   PLATELET DISORDERS/EVALUATION: Platelet problems are the MOST COMMON CAUSE of BLEEDING.
  A.   PLATELET MORPHOLOGY
  1.   Platelet clumping indicates the sample must be carefully redrawn and the platelets counted again.
  2.   The presence of many large platelets suggests active thrombopoiesis and an active bone marrow. Larger platelets are more functionally active than small platelets.
  3.   Sometimes platelets on a smear will have pseudopods or an irregular shape. These irregularities may be artifacts, possibly caused by platelet activation during handling.

  B.   PLATELET COUNT is useful in classifying the severity of thrombocytopenia and in monitoring the course of the disease and response to treatment.
  1.   Platelet estimate from a stained blood smear is quicker than an actual platelet count and is reasonably accurate. First scan the smear to be sure that

the platelets are evenly distributed and that there's no platelet clumping. Then count the average number of platelets in 10 oil immersion fields (100x).

a. Normal **dogs** have about **8-29 platelets** and **cats** have **10-29 platelets** per oil immersion field (100x).

b. If the dog has about **20,000 platelets/μL** (severe enough to cause bleeding), we may see only about **1 platelet** per oil immersion field.

C. ETIOLOGY

ETIOLOGY of PLATELET DISORDERS	
Thrombocytopenia	**EXCESSIVE PLATELET REMOVAL** • **Blood loss** (± mild thrombocytopenia) • **Immune-mediated**: antibodies against platelets lead to platelet destruction (PF-3). (*Rickettsia, Ehrlichia*, autoimmune, etc.). • **DIC** • **Splenic sequestration** (anesthesia, hemangiosarcoma- see next page). **DECREASED PLATELET PRODUCTION** • **Bone marrow disease** (e.g. infiltrative neoplastic diseases, myelofibrosis) • **Immune-mediated**: antibodies against megakaryocytes (Rickettsia, Ehrlichia, autoimmune, etc).
Thrombocytosis (rare and may not be a problem)	• **Infection/inflammation**: generalized bone marrow stimulation • **Splenectomy** may cause a temporary thrombocytosis • **Iron Deficiency** • Rebound effect from treatment with **vincristine** (treatment of immune-mediate thrombocytopenia) or from regenerative response from blood loss. • **Neoplasia** (megakaryocyte line) • **Cushing's Disease**
Function Problems	• **Lymphoproliferative disease** such as multiple myeloma (Circulating abnormal paraproteins bind to platelets thereby impeding function.) • **Drugs**: aspirin, ibuprofen, phenylbutazone, indomethacin, corticosteroids • **Hereditary disease** (e.g. vWD, rare disorders in Otterhounds, Foxhounds, Scottish terriers).

D. DIAGNOSTIC APPROACH

DIAGNOSTIC APPROACH to THROMBOCYTOPENIA

1. Confirm the presence of thrombocytopenia (platelet count)
 2. Classify the severity
    a. **Normal**: 200,000/μL - 500,000/μL
    b. **Severe**: < 20,000/μL
 3. Bone Marrow aspirate (± anti-megakaryocyte antibody)
 4. Rule out DIC (look for increased FDPs or d-dimers, increased clotting times, decreased fibrinogen).
 5. Look for immune-mediated causes such as *Ehrlichia* or Rickettsial infections.
 6. Check for history of toxins, drugs or radiation therapy.

1. First, confirm that the thrombocytopenia is not a result of collection error, sample handling, or the test itself. Note that the spleen stores 30% of the platelets so anything increasing **splenic size** (such as hemangiosarcoma and some anesthetic agents) can lead to **splenic sequestration of platelets** and thrombocytopenia.

2. Next, **classify the severity** of the thrombocytopenia. Normal reference range is 200,000/μL - 500,000/μL.

a. **Severe**: < 20,000/μL puts the animal at risk of bleeding. Factors such as platelet size, functional activity, blood vessel/endothelial support, and severity of the challenge to the hemostatic mechanism also contribute to the presence or absence of bleeding.

Clinical Path

b. If you document a consistent decline in platelet count over time, you can define the animal as being in a thrombocytopenic process even if it has a normal platelet count.

3. **BONE MARROW ASPIRATE:** By judging megakaryocyte numbers and maturity, you can determine whether there's a decrease or compensatory increase in platelet production.
   a. If megakaryocytes are present, perform an **antimegakaryocyte antibody test** to look for an immune-mediated cause of the thrombocytopenia.
   b. Classically, immune-mediated thrombocytopenia involves megakaryocytic hyperplasia.
   c. Rule out **space occupying lesions** such as neoplasias affecting the bone marrow.

4. DIC can be ruled out by the rest of the hemostatic profile (decreased fibrinogen, increased fibrin degredation products, prolonged clotting times).

5. **IMMUNE-MEDIATED thrombocytopenia**: We often diagnose immune-mediate thrombocytopenia by ruling out bone marrow problems and DIC. We can further confirm this diagnosis by a positive response to immunosuppressive therapy. More direct diagnostic methods are of variable efficacy.

6. **EHRLICHIA TITERS** for *E. canis* and *E. equi* (now Anaplasma **phagocytophila**). Ehrlichiosis can be difficult to recognize although a **positive serologic titer** is a sensitive and specific test. A history of tick infestation, especially in endemic areas, plus hematologic findings such as a non-regenerative anemia (about 90% of cases), and leukopenia (about 50% of cases) with a severe neutropenia may suggest *E.* canis. Some dogs with Ehrlichiosis have bone marrow with normal to increased cellularity despite pancytopenia. In endemic areas (e.g. Arizona, Texas, and Florida), perform *E. Canis* titers on any dog with thrombocytopenia, an unusual anemia, pancytopenia, or evidence of a chronic infection. *E. equi* generally causes less severe hematologic abnormalities but should also be considered particularly if there is also joint disease.

7. **RICKETTSIA RICKETTSII TITERS** (Rocky Mountain Spotted Fever)

8. **RADIATION THERAPY OR DRUG THERAPY** (e.g. chloramphenical, chemotherapy agents, estrogens)

E. **PLATELET FUNCTION PROBLEMS**: Platelet numbers may be low or normal.

DIAGNOSING PLATELET FUNCTION PROBLEMS
1. Bleeding time or clot retraction test
2. Take the animal off any drugs that can alter platelet function and after 5 days, repeat the platelet function test.
3. Check for history of vWD and perform a vWD test. (VIII-Ag)

1. **BUCCAL MUCOSAL BLEEDING TIME** (BMBT) is a useful and sensitive test of platelet function.
   a. Significant thrombocytopenia as well as abnormal platelet function may cause prolonged bleeding time.

   b. The bleeding time is considered normal in coagulation defects because the bleeding stops initially in the expected time due to formation of a platelet plug. Since the platelet plug is not stabilized by fibrin strands, the incision often starts to bleed if it is traumatized later. When this occurs, you should qualify the test by stating that the bleeding time was normal but bleeding recurred later.

2. **CLOT RETRACTION TEST** is a crude but simple and easy test of platelet function. It's based on the concept that platelets contract with time and pull the fibrin strands together to form a firm clot.

3. If the platelet function is decreased and the animal has been on a drug that decreases platelet function, **take the animal off the drug** and repeat the platelet function test after about 5 days. If the platelet function is still abnormal, the dysfunction must be caused by another factor.

4. Check for a history of platelet function diseases such as von Willebrand's disease. Von Willebrand's disease is a common disease in some breeds. Dogs with vWD usually have normal platelet numbers, although some dogs with concurrent hypothyroidism have a mild thrombocytopenia and more severe signs of vWD.

   a. **Factor VIII consists of two parts:** The larger part is factor VIII-related antigen (VIII-Ag). This portion is von Willebrand's factor (vWF) and it allows platelets to function normally. The smaller part (factor VIII coagulation activity; VIII-C) functions in the coagulation cascade. Factor VIII can be evaluated to determine whether there's a disorder involving either vWF or VIII-C (hemophilia A).

      i. The APTT will be prolonged if there is a significant decrease in VIII-C.

      ii. VIII-Ag test immunologically measures the quantity of the larger part of the molecule. The amount of vWF the dog has is not a good predictor of how likely the dog is to bleed. BMBT is a better indicator of bleeding susceptibility.

      iii. BMBT measures the ability of vWF to aid in formation of the platelet plug. BMBT is normally < 4 minutes.

   b. **Clinical signs** of vWD are often mild and variable (e.g. more sponges may be needed for hemostasis than expected during surgery). Some types of vWD can cause severe bleeding and require plasma transfusion.

   c. **Animals can have vWD and hemophilia separately (both involve factor VIII).**

TEST	vWF disease	Hemophilia A
BMBT	Prolonged	Normal
Factor VIII-Ag (vW Factor)	Decreased	Normal or high
APTT	Usually normal	Increased

Modified from Williard MD, Tvedten H: Small Animal Clinical Diagnosis by Laboratory Methods. 4th edition. Philadelphia, W.B. Saunders, 2004.

IV. **COAGULATION FACTOR EVALUATION:** Coagulation factors are divided into three areas: the intrinsic system, the extrinsic system, and the common pathway. Note that the extrinsic pathway consists of factor VII, thromboplastin and calcium. Deficiencies in tissue thromboplastin are extremely rare and calcium is never low enough in a living animal to inhibit clotting; therefore, problems with the extrinsic pathway are usually caused by factor VII deficency.

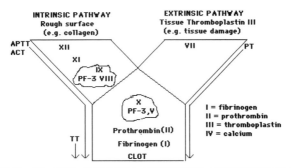

Modified from Williard MD, Tvedten H: Small Animal Clinical Diagnosis by Laboratory Methods. 4th edition. Philadelphia, W.B. Saunders, 2004.

Clinical Path

A. SPECIFIC TESTS FOR COAGULATION PROBLEMS

TEST	PURPOSE
PIVKA	PIVKA tests the vitamin K-dependent clotting factors (II, VII, IX, X). It's a very sensitive test for the early detection of vitamin K antagonism (e.g. in warfarin toxicity). In the later stages of warfarin toxicity, the prothrombin time (PT) is also prolonged. If PT is prolonged, PIVKA will usually be prolonged.
PROTHROMBIN TIME (PT)	The prothrombin time evaluates the extrinsic and common pathways. Since factor VII has the shortest half-life, it is the most likely to initially cause clinical problems (e.g. vitamin K antagonism).
ACTIVATED PARTIAL THROMBOPLASTIN TIME (APTT)	APTT is the most sensitive and specific test of the intrinsic pathway and the common pathway. It tests for all the coagulation factors except factor VII. As a result, the APTT is an important test to have available to screen for a decreased activity of one or more coagulation factors. Routine APTT is not sensitive enough to reveal **carriers** of hemophilia A (factor VIII deficiency) or hemophilia B (factor IX deficiency).
ACTIVATED CLOTTING TIME (ACT)	ACT is used in much the same way as the APTT for defects in the **intrinsic or common pathway.** It's a cruder but quicker test. It's less sensitive and less specific than the APTT and it may be elevated in cases of severe thrombocytopenia. The major advantage of the ACT is that it's cheap and easy to use. It requires a special vacutainer tube.
THROMBIN TIME (TT)	TT tests the amount and activity of fibrinogen. Do not confuse it with the **modified** TT. The modified TT can be used to monitor the anticoagulant activity of heparin and fibrin degradation products. The modified TT is simply a specific and sensitive way to quantitate fibrinogen. It has excess thrombin added to the reagent, so that it is insensitive to anticoagulants. The modified TT is more commonly available than is the TT.
Factor VIII-related antigen	Diagnose von Willebrand's disease.
SPECIFIC FACTOR ANALYSIS	Specific factor analysis can only be performed in a few laboratories. It may be used when a problem has been narrowed down to a likely factor or group of factors (e.g. intrinsic pathway factors).

A 5 second increase in the PT or a 7 second increase in the APTT is significant in dogs and cats. Smaller increases may be significant if they are consistent and coincide with appropriate clinical signs and additional laboratory findings.

B. DIAGNOSTIC APPROACH TO COAGULOPATHIES:

ETIOLOGIES
Multiple Factor Deficiencies
•   Warfarin (vitamin K-dependent factors) or other warfarin-like rodenticides
•   Liver disease (decreased production of multiple factors)
•   Glomerulonephropathy (increased loss of multiple factors)
•   DIC
Single Factor Deficiencies: Hemophilia and other specific factor deficiencies.

1. If you suspect **RODENTICIDE POISONING** with a **coumarin**-type product, perform the **PIVKA test** because it is the most sensitive test for detecting vitamin K dependent factor deficiencies. Coumarin rodenticides interfere with vitamin K epoxide reductase, which returns vitamin K epoxide to an active form. This inhibition results in a functional vitamin K deficiency and reduced hepatic synthesis of factors **II, VII, IX, and X.** All tests except the TT are eventually prolonged in warfarin toxicity, since the vitamin K factors are deficient, creating defects in the intrinsic, extrinsic, and common pathways, while the quantity of normal fibrinogen should be adequate. The **PIVKA** test is the most sensitive test for diagnosing warfarin toxicity. The **prothrombin time** or **PIVKA** (if available) is preferred for monitoring the toxic effect of warfarin. The factor with the shortest half-life becomes deficient earliest. In dogs, factor VII has the shortest half-life (2-4 hours).

2. In other cases where you suspect a coagulation problem, perform an APTT or ACT to evaluate the intrinsic and common pathways and a PT to evaluate the extrinsic pathway. If APTT is prolonged but PT is normal, then the intrinsic pathway is defective. If APTT is normal but PT is prolonged, then the extrinsic pathway is defective. If both are prolonged, then the common pathway or more than one factor is defective.

   a. **When multiple factors are involved**, suspect decreased production of clotting factors by the liver, loss of clotting factors (glomerulonephropathy), consumption of factors (DIC) or rodenticide poisoning.

3. **Thrombin time and specific factor analysis:** In cases where PT and APTT are elevated, TT can be measured to determine whether the common pathway is involved. Usually other information is available to help one make a good clinical judgment prior to specific factor analysis. Clinical signs, breed incidence, sex, and other information, in addition to the hemostatic profile, will allow a fairly accurate diagnosis without the need of the TT or specific factor analysis.

IV. **DISSEMINATED INTRAVASCULAR COAGULATION (DIC):** DIC is the phenomenon in which massive coagulation is triggered resulting in consumption of coagulation factors which leads to an inability to clot. It is one of the more common hemostatic disorders. It occurs secondary to a wide variety of diseases characterized by the formation of necrotic tissue and rough surfaces.

A. **ETIOLOGY:** DIC may be considered to include a variety of situations causing excessive clotting in the vascular system, even if it's localized or chronic and not disseminated and peracute. Consumptive coagulopathy is an alternate term when various factors are consumed in a relatively localized process.

   1. **Inflammatory diseases** create areas of necrosis and exposed collagen, which stimulates clotting. Many infections, such as canine infectious hepatitis, kill the animal through DIC-type episodes.

   2. **Neoplasms** (e.g. hemangiosarcoma) often have necrotic, inflamed areas, and treatment of neoplasms (e.g. chemotherapy) may create additional necrosis and increase the likelihood of DIC.

   3. **Hemolytic anemias** produce abundant RBC necrotic debris which can lead to excessive clotting.

   4. **Obstetric disorders:** Amniotic fluid induces clotting, thus it can lead to DIC.

   4. **Vasculitis** may induce DIC because inflamed vessels are devoid of endothelial cells. Endothelial cells act to inhibit platelet aggregation. If DIC and edema are concurrently present, a skin biopsy may document vasculitis.

B. **PATHOGENESIS and SERIES OF EVENTS in DIC**

   1. **Activation of Clotting:** Primary and secondary hemostatic plugs form simultaneously in many small vessels. If unchecked, this plug formation leads to ischemia. During this process, coagulation factors and platelets are consumed in large quantities leading to thrombocytopenia and decreased ability to form clots.

   2. **Activation of the fibrinolytic system** results in clot lysis, inactivation/lysis of clotting factors, and impaired platelet function.

   3. **Antithrombin III (AT-III)** is consumed in its attempt to halt intravascular coagulation. That is, normal anticoagulation factors are exhausted.

   4. **Formation of fibrin** within the microcirculation leads to hemolytic anemia as the red blood cells are sheared by fibrin strands. Fragmented red blood cells are called **schistocytes**.

C. **DIAGNOSING DIC: The Clotting profile is needed in order to diagnose DIC.** DIC consumes platelets and coagulation factors during formation of excess clotting. The breakdown of these clots causes increased fibrin degradation products (FDP) which act as anticoagulants to interfere with platelet function and clotting. Thus, any of the hemostatic tests may be abnormal. Since production of coagulation factors and platelets can variably compensate for consumption, one test is always abnormal. **If three of the six tests in the hemostatic screening profile are abnormal the animal is diagnosed as having DIC.** The diagnosis is more definitive when thrombocytopenia and coagulation factor deficiency are identified concurrently.

Clinical Path

MOST IMPORTANT LAB TESTS FOR DIAGNOSING DIC
• Platelet Count
• Activated Partial Thromboplastin Time (APTT)
• Prothrombin Time (PT)
• Fibrinogen
• Fibrinogen Degredation Products (FDPs) (or d-dimer)
• Antithrombin-III (AT-III)

Hemogram, chemistry and urinalysis results raise our clinical suspicion that DIC is present, but they do not yield a diagnosis of DIC. The following are the CBC, chemistry and urinalysis findings that may suggest DIC.

DIAGNOSTIC FINDINGS that indicate DIC

TEST	DIAGNOSTIC FINDINGS
HEMOGRAM	• Regenerative or non-regenerative anemia with schistocytes • Thrombocytopenia • Neutrophilia ± left shift
CHEMISTRY	• Hyperbilirubinemia secondary to hemolysis or to hepatic thrombosis • Azotemia or increased phosphorus secondary to severe renal microemboli • Increased liver enzymes due to hepatic microemboli • Decreased total CO_2 due to metabolic acidosis • Hypoproteinemia due to severe bleeding
URINALYSIS	• Do not do a cystocentesis on an animal that you suspect is in DIC. • Hemoglobinuria and bilirubinuria • ± Proteinuria

D. **Treatment**: Goals of treatment are to stop intravascular coagulation, to maintain good organ perfusion, and to prevent secondary complications.
1. **Eliminate the precipitating cause**. This is rarely possible.
2. **Halt intravascular coagulation.**
   a. Heparin
   b. Aspirin
   c. Plasma: to replace the coagulation and anticoagulant factors
3. **Supportive therapy** (fluids, antibiotics, oxygen, etc).

VI. Summary

	Bleeding Time	Platelet count	APTT	PT	FDP
Thrombocytopenia - severe	increase	decrease	normal	normal	normal
Platelet dysfunction	increase	normal	normal	normal	normal
von Willebrand's	increase	normal	normal/high	normal	normal
DIC	increase	decrease	increase	increase	increase
Intrinsic pathway defect	normal	normal	increase	normal	normal
Factor VII deficiency	normal	normal	normal	increase	normal
Common pathway defect	normal	normal	increase	increase	normal
Multiple factor deficiency	normal	normal	increase	increase	normal

Modified from Williard MD, Tvedten H: Small Animal Clinical Diagnosis by Laboratory Methods. 4th edition. Philadelphia, W.B. Saunders, 2004.

URINALYSIS
Visual Inspection
Chemical Analysis
Microscopic Examination
Culture

Urinalysis provides information on renal disease and lower urinary tract disease as well as other disorders such as diabetes mellitus, hepatic disease and hemolytic disorders. Urine can be collected by cystocentesis, catheterization or midstream free-catch. Catheterization and midstream samples are contaminated with materials from the distal urinary tract making interpretation of cell count, protein content, and culture misleading. **Cystocentesis is the best sample when analyzing for bacteria and cell counts.** Collect 10-12mLs so there's enough for other tests such as urine protein:creatinine and so there's a standard amount for sedimentation each time. Read the sample within 15-30 minutes of collection (bacteria can double in 30 minutes and pH can change) or, if refrigerated, read it within 12 hours (extensive refrigeration may kill bacteria resulting in false negative cultures).

I. **VISUAL INSPECTION:** Inspect the sample shortly after collecting it.

URINE COLOR and TRANSPARENCY

	NORMAL	ABNORMAL
Color	Darker urine is usually more concentrated and light urine is usually more dilute. Color can be misleading though, so measure urine specific gravity to determine whether the urine is truly concentrated or dilute.	**Reddish/brown:** Blood or hemoglobin in the urine **Brown:** Bilirubinuria
Transparency	Clear	**Cloudy** due to increased cells, bacteria, fat, crystals, mucus.

II. **CHEMICAL ANALYSIS:** Centrifuge 6-10 mL of urine at 2000 - 3000 rpm for 5 minutes. Perform chemical analysis on the centrifuged supernatant since turbidity can change some results. Ignore nitrate, urobilinogen and leukocyte readings on urine dipstick since values are not accurate for animals.

CHEMICAL ANALYSIS of URINE

	INFORMATION	INTERPRETATION
Urine Specific Gravity (Usg)	1.008-1.012 is the specific gravity of blood. Urine within this range has not been concentrated or diluted by the kidneys, thus it is isosthenuric. Don't use the urine dipstick value. It's not accurate for animals. Interpret the specific gravity in light of the PCV, total protein and BUN values. If the PCV and TP indicate hemoconcentration and the Usg isn't adequately elevated, then the kidneys are not concentrating the urine enough.	**Decreased specific gravity:** < 1.008 can be due to: • Excessive drinking, fluid administration, corticosteroids • Central diabetes insipidus (Decreased ADH production) • Nephrogenic diabetes insipidus (decreased renal response to ADH): Cushing's, Addison's, hypercalcemia, liver disease, etc. **Isosthenuria** indicates renal inability to concentrate or dilute the urine. Evaluate several urine samples to conclude isosthenuria unless the animal is clinically dehydrated or azotemic. In these cases a single urine specific gravity has meaning. **Increased specific gravity** indicates that the kidneys are able to concentrate the urine. Cats should have a Usg > 1.030 and dogs should have a Usg > 1.025. If the animal is dehydrated with or without azotemia, the specific gravity should be concentrated.

Chart continued on next page

Clinical Path

CHEMICAL ANALYSIS of URINE continued

	INFORMATION	INTERPRETATION
pH	pH varies with the diet and metabolic state. High protein diets (especially animal protein) lead to a lower pH while low protein (vegetarian) diets lead to an alkaline pH. Catabolic states in which body proteins are being broken down lead to an acidic pH.	**Etiology of decreased pH (acidic urine)** • Catabolic state (starvation, fever, prolonged heavy exercise, where muscle proteins breaks down) • High protein diet • Acidifying diet • Urinary acidifiers (ammonium chloride, methigel, methionine) • Metabolic or respiratory acidosis (e.g. vomiting) **Etiology of increased pH (alkaline urine)** • Bacterial cystitis due to urease producing bacteria (*Staphylococcus*, *Proteus*, *Klebsiella*) • Metabolic or respiratory alkalosis • High fiber, high vegetable diets • Citrate or bicarbonate administration • Alkaline tide: four hours after a meal
PROTEIN	Proteins are usually not filtered through the glomerular membrane. Very concentrated urine may have 3+ protein, but dilute urine should have trace or 0 protein. When in doubt about the significance of the protein, do a **urine protein: creatinine ratio (Upc)**. Ratio ≤ 0.5 mg/dL for dogs and 0.4mg/dL for cat is normal. **Urine dipstick** is good for screening but it requires 30 mg of albumin/dL and does not detect other proteins (e.g. Bence Jones proteins). Thus, it's not very sensitive. Additionally, it yields false negatives too. **Detection of enzymes** such as gamma glutamyltransferase (GGT) and N-acetyl-ß-D glucosaminidase (NAG)— enzymes from the proximal tubule cells— are sensitive indicators of early renal tubular damage because they are too large to be filtered by healthy glomerular membranes.	**Etiology of increased protein** • **Transient increase** with fever, heavy exercise, seizure. • False elevation in **alkaline urine.** • Increased glomerular permeability (glomerulonephritis, amyloidosis) • **Hematuria**, Hemoglobinuria, Myoglobinuria • Inflammation (cystitis) leads to increase in WBCs and inflammatory proteins in the urine. • **Multiple myeloma** results in Bence Jones proteins in the urine. The sulfosalycilic acid test for protein is elevated but the dipstick test is normal. **Urine Dipstick** If an animal's urine protein is **negative** and the animal has a disease process that predisposes it to proteinuria (hypertension, renal disease, neoplasia) use a more sensitive test such as **sulfosalicylic acid test** (SSA) which picks up 5 gm/dL of protein or ELISA. If the urine is positive on dipstick, regardless of Usg or inflammation, confirm with SSA or ELISA or Upc. . **Enzymes:** When animals are on nephrotoxic drugs it's good to get a baseline measurement. Increase in GGT or NAG by 2-3x during treatment indicates nephrotoxicity. **Urine enzyme:creatinine ratios** can also be measured. False negatives can occur after severe tubular damage depletes tubular enzyme stores.

Chart continued on next page

CHEMICAL ANALYSIS of URINE continued

	INFORMATION	INTERPRETATION
Glucose	Glucose is filtered through the glomeruli and then completely resorbed in the proximal tubules. It's usually absent in urine.	**Etiology of glucosuria** • **Diabetes mellitus**: blood glucose is elevated too. • **Ascorbic acid** causes false elevation when the clinitest is used and false decrease when urine dipstick is used to determine glucose levels. • **Renal glucosuria**: is characterized by normal blood glucose levels but glucosuria. It occurs because the tubules can't reabsorb urine glucose. • **Note**: In cats, transient **hyperglycemia** induced by acute stress should not result in glucosuria because the glucose levels in the blood usually are not high enough to spill into the urine plus the blood glucose does not spill into the bladder instantaneously or in high enough concentrations to be detected in urine. It only enters the bladder at the rate that urine is formed.
Ketones	Ketones are not normally present in the urine. Can get false negatives if the primary ketone is ß hydroxybutyric acid.	**Etiologies of Ketonuria** • **Diabetes Mellitus**: Marked ketonuria occurs with ketoacidosis due to diabetes mellitus. Evaluate ketonuric animals for hyperglycemia and acidemia. • **Malnourished**/starved animals can have ketonuria (rare in small animals).
Bilirubin	A small amount of bilirubin in canine urine is normal since bilirubin is conjugated by renal tubular cells and excreted into the urine. (e.g. SG > 1.020 then 1+ bilirubin is ok). Any bilirubin in the urine of cats is abnormal.	**Bilirubinuria indicates:** • Prehepatic (hemolytic anemia) • Hepatic disease • Posthepatic disease • Bilirubinuria is a more sensitive indicator of liver disease than bilirubin in the blood. • When animals have bilirubinuria, check the liver enzymes (ALP, ALT) and the PCV level to distinguish between prehepatic etiologies vs. hepatic causes. If the PCV is decreased by 10-15%, then suspect pre-hepatic.
Blood	Red blood cells, hemoglobin, myoglobin	If after centrifugation the supernatant is reddish, then the urine has hemoglobin or myoglobin. Hemoglobinuria is due to intravascular hemolysis. If after centrifugation the supernatant is clear and the pellet is red, then the urine contains blood.
WBC	Do not trust the dip stick WBC reading. It's not accurate in animals.	If the urine was collected via catheter or free catch, the WBC can be from the lower urinary tract as well as from the bladder and kidney. Increased WBCs indicate inflammation (infection, neoplasia, urolith, nephritis).

Clinical Path

III. **MICROSCOPIC EXAMINATION:** A standard amount of urine (6-10 mLs) must be centrifuged each time because the normal values are determined for a standard volume of urine. Pour the supernatant off and resuspend the pellet in one drop of urine. Examine an unstained sample (to avoid stain precipitate, or bacteria/yeast from the stain). Lower the condenser. Note: if the sample was collected via free catch or catheter, some of the cells may be from the urethra and more caudal structures rather than from the bladder.

FINDINGS	INTERPRETATION
Neutrophils 0-3/hpf	> 3/hpf indicates inflammation Urinary tract infection Feline urologic syndrome Urolith Neoplasia
Red Blood Cells < 0-3/hpf	> 3/hpf indicates hemorrhage • From the trauma of the cystocentesis • Other trauma • Tumor • Urinary tract infection • Urolith • Sterile cystitis • Urine parasites • Nephritis • Coagulopathy
Epithelial Cells	Increase with cystitis and neoplasia.
Neoplastic Cells	Transitional cell carcinoma (use new methylene blue or Wright's stain)
Casts < 2/lpf of hyaline < 1/lpf granular casts	Casts are formed in the renal tubules • Hyaline casts (protein) are elevated with diuresis following dehydration, with proteinuric patients, and with renal disease. • WBC casts indicate renal inflammation (pyelonephritis). • RBC casts indicate renal hemorrhage. • Renal tubular casts indicate severe tubular disease (e.g. acute renal failure). • Granular casts are comprised of degenerating cells and proteins. They occur with rehydration and with renal disease. • Waxy casts are old granular casts.
Bacteria	The bladder is usually sterile. Any bacteria seen are abnormal.
Fungal/yeast (e.g. *Mycoplasma*)	In fungal/yeast infections, few organisms are present in the urine, making them difficult to examine on a urinalysis. They need to be cultured in special media.
Crystals vary with the urine concentration and pH.	• Calcium oxalate precipitates in acidic urine. • Struvite precipitates in alkaline urine. • Ammonium biurate indicates liver disease. • Cystine may be associated with cystine calculi.

IV. **CULTURE:** The culture should be performed within 15 minutes of sample collection or within 12-24 hours of sample refrigeration. Culture can be collected on the unspun sample because bacteria do not collect in the urine pellet (Refer to p. 21.2 for more information on urinary infections).

WHEN to CULTURE for BACTERIA
• Bacteria are seen • > 3 WBC/hpf • Specific Gravity < 1.015 (won't see bacteria if the urine is this dilute)

CHAPTER 5: **Cytology**

Suggested References:

Cowell RL, et al: Diagnostic Cytology and Hematology of the Dog and Cat, 2nd ed., St. Louis, Mosby, 1999.

Meyer DJ et al: Veterinary Laboratory Medicine: Interpretation and Diagnosis 3rd ed. Philadelphia, WB Saunders, 2004.

Raskin RE, et al: Atlas of Canine and Feline Cytology, Philadelphia, WB Saunders, 2001.

Willard, MD, et al (ed): Small Animal Clinical Diagnosis by Laboratory Methods. 4th ed. Philadelphia, WB Saunders, 2004.

Cytology

CYTOLOGY of INFLAMMATION
Types of Inflammation
Hematomas, Seromas, and Cysts

Inflammation is a reaction of the body to injury. It can be classified in different ways based on duration (acute, chronic), histology, cytology (purulent, pyogranulomatous, granulomatous), etiology (septic, nonseptic).

TYPES of INFLAMMATION

NEUTROPHILIC INFLAMMATION	Samples containing ≥ 85% neutrophils are termed neutrophilic, purulent or suppurative inflammation. Etiology: Neutrophils are the first inflammatory cells to reach an injury site (including chemical or mechanical injury such as those caused by perivascular leakage of anesthetic agents, bile, tumors, and other mechanical irritation). Neutrophils phagocytize **bacteria** and some **fungi**. With purulent inflammation look for bacteria within the neutrophil cytoplasm. Free bacteria in the sample can be from stain or other contamination. Bacteria on the surface of epithelial cells may be normal flora (if sample is from mucosal or skin surface). Cell Characteristics: • **Degenerative neutrophils** indicate a relatively toxic environment and may indicate **septic inflammation**). Intact degenerate neutrophils display **karyolysis**—swelling of the nuclear lobes and a decrease in staining intensity. Bacteria or fungi may be found in the cytoplasm. • **Non-degenerative** neutrophils **indicate a relatively non-toxic** environment (e.g. immune-mediated disease, neoplastic lesions, and sterile lesions caused by irritants such as chyle, bile, and urine). The lack of degenerative changes does not rule out sepsis. Non-degenerative neutrophils may have **hypersegmented** nuclei, which indicates that the cell has been in the tissue for a long time and has not been subjected to insult. The nucleus may shrink and the lobes may coalesce into a single, darkly stained mass, termed pyknosis (pyknotic nuclei). This stage of cell death in neutrophils is called **karyorrhexis.**
PYOGRANULOMATOUS OR GRANULOMATOUS INFLAMMATION Look for an infectious agent and culture even in the absence of organisms on cytology.	Granulomatous and pyogranulomatous lesions are characterized by inflammation involving primarily **macrophages** or **neutrophils and macrophages,** but lymphocytes, plasma cells, and multinucleated cells may be present too. Etiology: Macrophages phagocytize **foreign bodies, cellular debris, fungi** and **higher bacteria** (e.g. *Actinomyces*, *Nocardia*) and chronic tissue injury. When granulomatous or pyogranulomatous inflammation is present, look for phagocytized material in the macrophage cytoplasm. In cats, FIP may cause suppurative to pyogranulomatous inflammation. Cell Characteristics • The **macrophages** have abundant cytoplasm, which is usually vacuolated or foamy. They may be multinucleated and may have prominent nucleoli. • The **neutrophils** are usually not degenerative. They may be hypersegmented.
LYMPHOCYTIC OR PLASMACYTIC INFLAMMATION	**Plasma cells** are terminally differentiated B-cells. Lymphocytic and plasmacytic inflammation is associated with allergic or immune reactions, viral infections, and chronic inflammation. Other inflammatory cells are usually present, too. A monomorphic population of lymphocytes rather than a mixed population (one including small and intermediate lymphocytes as well as other inflammatory cells) may indicate lymphoid neoplasia.

TYPES of INFLAMMATION continued

EOSINOPHILIC INFLAMMATION	Characterized by the presence of > 10% eosinophils (species-dependent). Etiology: Eosinophilic infiltrates are associated with: • Allergic responses • Parasitic migration • Necrotic tissue • Neoplasia (e.g. mast cell tumor) • Fungal infections Cell characteristics: Sometimes it's difficult to recognize the cells as eosinophils because they often shrink and their nuclei become pyknotic. Usually a few cells with eosinophilic granules are recognizable.
DEBRIS	Debris is present in most cytologic preparations but is more common in purulent and necrotic regions. Debris can also be caused by artifact such as with overhandling of the preparation leading to cell rupture and smearing of the nucleus. Cytologically we see strands of eosinophilic or basophilic material. Don't mistake this nuclear streaming for fungi or mucus. Cutaneous cysts (e.g. inclusion cysts) typically have abundant thick accumulations of keratin debris.

HEMATOMAS, SEROMAS and CYSTS

On physical examination, **hematomas**, **seromas**, and **cysts** may be misidentified as inflammatory lesions. Cytologic examination of these lesions can correctly identify them.

HEMATOMA	Hematomas can be distinguished from hemorrhage due to blood contamination based on the absence of platelets and the presence of macrophages containing engulfed erythrocytes (in acute hemorrhage) or degraded blood pigment (chronic phase) such as blue-green hemosiderin granules or yellow-rhomboid hematoidin crystals. These breakdown products of heme indicate that hemorrhage occurred > 24 hours ago. Some tumors (eg, hemangioma and hemangiosarcoma) may have large vascular spaces that on cytology are indistinguishable from hematomas.
SEROMA	Seromas can be a sequalae of aging hematomas (due to lysis of the erythrocytes) or can be caused by injury or chronic irritation (bruising, post-surgery) independent of hematoma formation. In the latter case, plasma leaks from immature capillaries, which are created during granulation tissue formation. Seromas are usually **xanthochromic** (amber-colored) like serum and contain few cells. The predominant cell type is the macrophage. In cases where the seroma has formed from a hematoma, the macrophages may undergo **erythrophagocytosis** in which they've ingested erythrocytes or they may contain degraded blood pigments.
CYSTS	Fluid from cysts is usually colorless and has a low specific gravity. It also contain few cells. Sebaceous (inclusion) cysts often contain abundant grey greasy material that on cytologic examination consists of thick accumulations of sky blue-staining material (keratin debris).

Cytology

EFFUSION FLUIDS
Classifications
Pathogenesis/Etiology
Laboratory Examinations
Characteristics of Effusions

An effusion is an excessive accumulation of fluid in a serous body cavity (pericardial sac, pleural cavity, peritoneal cavity).

I. **CLASSIFICATIONS:** Effusions can be classified on the basis of laboratory findings into the following groups: Inflammatory vs. non-inflammatory, exudates vs. transudate, benign vs. malignant. Other specific effusions include hemorrhagic and chylous effusions.

   A. **INFLAMMATORY vs NON-INFLAMMATORY**

      1. **Non-inflammatory Effusions** are low in protein and low in cell content. They include transudates and modified transudates.

      2. **Inflammatory Effusions** contain high protein and high cell numbers, primarily neutrophils. They are exudates. They can be septic or non-septic.

         a. **Septic effusions** are caused by bacteria or fungi and the neutrophils may be degenerate.

         b. **Non-septic effusions** are negative for bacteria or fungi. The neutrophils are non-degenerate.

   B. **TRANSUDATES vs EXUDATES:**

      1. Transudates and modified transudates are non-inflammatory effusions

      2. Exudates are inflammatory effusions.

	PROTEIN	TOTAL CELL COUNT (nucleated)	CELL TYPES
Transudate	$\leq$ 2.5 g/dL	< 1000 cells/μL	Mononuclear cells (mesothelial cells)
Modified Transudate	2.5-3.5 g/dL	< 5000 cells/μL	Mononuclear cells (mesothelial cells)
Exudate (septic or non-septic)	> 3.0 g/dL	> 5000 cells/μL	Neutrophils > 80%

   C. **BENIGN vs MALIGNANT EFFUSIONS:**

      1. **Benign effusions:** Tumor cells are absent.

      2. **Malignant effusion** are caused by neoplastic processes. Tumor cells may be present. Malignant effusions can be inflammatory or non-inflammatory.

   D. **OTHER TYPES OF EFFUSIONS:**

      1. **Chylous effusion:** Grossly appears milky; caused by lymphatic leakage.

      2. **Hemorrhagic effusion:** Grossly appears bloody; caused by vascular leakage.

II. **ETIOLOGY and PATHOGENESIS OF EFFUSIONS**

TYPE	ETIOLOGY
Transudate	• Hypoproteinemia: liver disease, glomerular disease, GI maldigestion, malabsorption, malnutrition • Lymphatic or venous obstruction • Heart failure
Modified Transudate	• Portal hypertension • Right heart failure
Exudate	• Infectious agent (bacteria, fungi, FIP in cats) • Foreign body (bile, chyle, urine) • Neoplasia • Recent trauma (within weeks)
Chylous	• Obstruction or disruption of lymphatic vessels
Hemorrhagic	• Leaky blood vessels due to vascular obstruction/stasis (diapedesis) • Fulminant hemorrhage due to coagulopathy, trauma or ruptured hematoma, granuloma or tumor

   A. **NON-INFLAMMATORY EFFUSIONS:** Any condition that produces edema can also produce a non-inflammatory effusion. Normally, more fluid is filtered out of the capillaries into the interstitial space than re-enters the venules. The excess interstitial fluid is picked up by the lymphatics and delivered back to the bloodstream via the thoracic duct. Fluid can accumulate in serous cavities and interstitial space when:

1. **Increased capillary pressure** leads to excess fluid leaking out of the capillaries. This can occur with the following:
   a. **Congestive heart failure**
   b. **External pressure on veins from a space-occupying lesion**
   c. **Portal hypertension:** Because lymph vessels in the hepatic parenchyma have higher protein lymph, portal hypertension usually results in a modified transudate.
2. **Plasma oncotic pressure is low due to low plasma protein (especially albumin).** Effusion can occur when the total plasma protein is < 3.5-4.5 g/dL and albumin is < 1.5-2.0 g/dL. Hypoproteinemia can be caused by intestinal malabsorption or maldigestion, renal disease, liver disease (Refer to hypoproteinemia section p. 4.10).
3. **Blockage or obstruction of lymphatic drainage** results in increased fluid in the interstitial tissue and serous cavities (e.g. space-occupying lesion of the thoracic duct or lymph vessels).

B. **INFLAMMATORY EFFUSIONS (Exudates)** are characterized by increased capillary permeability, which allows both fluid and proteins to leak into the fluid. Neutrophils and other inflammatory cells leak into the cavity too.
   1. **Septic effusions** are caused by invasion of the serous cavities by organisms (bacteria, fungi, etc).
   2. **Non-septic effusions** are often caused by foreign material in the serous cavities. Such materials include: bile, chyle, urine, foreign bodies, etc.

C. **MALIGNANT EFFUSIONS** (Effusions containing tumor cells) are usually inflammatory or exudative, but can be non-inflammatory. Tumors can produce effusions due to external pressure on veins and lymphatics or due to invasions of these vessels.

III. **LABORATORY EXAMINATION**
   A. **COLLECTION:** Collect effusion fluids in the following three containers:
      1. A vial with EDTA anticoagulant (lavender top tube) for cytologic evaluation: This is only necessary in extremely bloody fluids or fluids otherwise likely to clot.
      2. A vial with no anticoagulant (red top tube) for chemistry tests
      3. A sterile vial (another red top tube) for culture and additional chemistry tests suggested by the initial lab exam (e.g. amylase, BUN, bilirubin).

   B. **STANDARD FLUID ANALYSIS**

EXAMINE	INTERPRETATION
Turbidity	Cloudiness indicates increase in cells or protein.
Color	Red or pink tinge indicates blood. White/opaque (milky)character may indicate chylous effusion.
Clot Formation	Inflammatory or hemorrhagic effusions may contain fibrin and may clot.
Specific Gravity	Specific gravity is elevated with inflammatory effusions. It's falsely elevated with chyle and blood.
Total Protein	Total protein is falsely elevated with chyle and samples with hemolysis.
Nucleated Cell Count	Use a hemocytometer to measure nucleated cell numbers. Alternatively, cell numbers may be estimated from a direct smear.
Red Blood Cell Count	Use a hemocytometer to measure red blood cell numbers. Alternatively, a spun hematocrit may be done on fluid samples as an indicator of the amount of blood present.
Differential	You may need a cytospin to concentrate the cells. Stain with Wright's stain to look at WBC morphology and to look for organisms. Non-inflammatory effusions contain primarily large mononuclear cells (mesothelial cells and macrophages). Neutrophils, lymphocytes, eosinophils and mast cells are rare. Inflammatory-Septic: Neutrophils comprise 80% or more of the total count. They may be degenerate and may contain bacteria. Inflammatory-Non-septic: These exudates contain a pleomorphic population with varying numbers of neutrophils, macrophages, eosinophils, lymphocytes, plasma cells, mesothelial cells, and mast cells. The neutrophils are usually not degenerative.

Chart continued on next page

Cytology

STANDARD FLUID ANALYSIS continued

EXAMINE	INTERPRETATION
Cytology	**Exfoliated cells:** Cells (including mesothelial cells and tumor cells if they have seeded the wall) may exfoliate from the serosal walls. **Mesothelial cells** are mononuclear cells of variable size with round or oval nuclei. Their cytoplasm is basophilic. They may be found as single cells or in pairs or small clusters. They are easily mistaken for tumor cells. **Macrophages** are phagocytic and often contain neutrophils, RBCs and iron. **Neutrophils** are present in low numbers in most serous fluids and are present in high numbers in the acute stage of inflammatory effusions. In sterile effusions they are well-preserved, whereas in septic effusions they are often degenerative. **Lymphocytes, plasma cells, basophils, and mast cells** appear with similar morphology as when in the blood. **Red blood cells** are often present in effusions due to contamination during sample collection or due to hemorrhage. Erythrophagia and the presence of iron and heme breakdown products in macrophages usually indicates true hemorrhage (unless there's been a delay in sample handling). Neutrophils may also ingest erythrocytes. **Platelets** are only found immediately following the entrance of fresh blood into the cavity.

C. CHARACTERISTICS of INFLAMMATORY vs. NON-INFLAMMATORY EFFUSIONS

EXAMINE	NON-INFLAMMATORY	INFLAMMATORY
Turbidity	Clear	Clear, cloudy, opaque
Color	Straw-colored unless blood is present from a traumatic tap (will clear on centrifugation)	Varies from light yellow to amber to reddish brown. May be gray or white.
Odor	Little or no odor	May be foul-smelling
Total Protein	Usually < 2.5 g/dL. The protein is primarily albumin.	Usually > 2.5 g/dL. It can approach plasma levels.
Coagulation	Usually will not clot	May clot occasionally
Glucose	Equal to blood glucose concentration	Often 30-40% below blood level. This suggests bacterial infection and/or increased WBC numbers.
Organisms	Absent	May be present. They can often be detected on Wright's or NMB-stained smears. Culture is the best method for identification. Inflammation can also be due to causes other than infection.

D. ADDITIONAL TESTS TO RUN if INDICATED

TEST	WHEN to RUN the TEST
Creatinine	Measure creatinine if you suspect bladder rupture. Compare the value to blood creatinine levels. Fluid creatinine concentration is the same or higher compared to serum creatinine with bladder rupture.
Bilirubin	Measure bilirubin if you suspect portal hypertension or gall bladder rupture. Compare the values with blood bilirubin measurement.
Amylase	Measure amylase if you suspect a pancreatic cyst or pancreatic-induced inflammation. Compare the results with serum amylase. If the abdominal fluid amylase is higher than the serum amylase, the pet may have non-septic pancreatic inflammation.
Cholesterol and triglycerides	If chylous effusion needs to be confirmed then consider comparing fluid triglyceride and/or cholesterol to serum values. If the fluid triglycerides > cholesterol or if triglycerides in the effusion is 3x > triglycerides in the serum, the effusion is chylous in origin. Chylous effusions are caused by leakage of lymphatic vessels from trauma or obstruction (e.g. due to neoplasia, lung torsion, fungal granulomas, etc). These effusions are classically milky in appearance with slightly increased numbers of nucleated cells that are predominantly small lymphocytes. In anorectic animals, the milky quality may go away due to a lack of chylomicrons. In addition, over time, this type of effusion may elicit a suppurative reaction due to the irritative nature of chyle.

LYMPH NODE CYTOLOGY

Lymph node aspiration and/or biopsy is indicated when local or **generalized lymph node enlargement** occurs. Enlarged nodes always suggest the possibility of a neoplastic process, either primary or metastatic. Examination of needle aspiration biopsies may reveal the cause of enlargement. When sampling large nodes, aim tangentally to avoid possible necrotic areas which are more likely to exist in the center.

I.   **CELL-TYPES NORMALLY FOUND IN LYMPH NODES**
   A.   **MATURE LYMPHOCYTES:** 90-95% of cells in normal nodes are mature lymphocytes. They are similar to the lymphocytes of the blood except they may have a more coarsely clumped chromatin. These cells are small (a little larger then RBCs) and usually have sparse cytoplasm. The lymphocytes may have dark-staining compact nuclei or less condensed, lighter nuclei.
   B.   **LYMPHOBLASTS or STEM CELLS** are much less common. These cells are 2 - 3x larger than lymphocytes, contain fine, diffuse nuclear chromatin and may have a distinct nucleolus. Both pale and dark types are found.
   C.   **MACROPHAGES (or histiocytes)** make up a small percentage of the cells of a node. Their job is to phagocytose foreign material reaching the node as well as present antigens to lymphocytes. Macrophages have round, oval or oblong nuclei with a net-like or widely stippled chromatin pattern in which there may be one or two nucleoli. The cytoplasm stains pale blue or gray and is often vacuolated. The cytoplasmic borders may be indistinct.
   D.   **PLASMA CELLS** are found in aspirates in varying numbers. They have a dark staining, moderately condensed nucleus which is usually eccentric. The cytoplasm is very basophilic and usually has a perinuclear clear area.
   E.   **CELLS of INFLAMMATION** include neutrophils, eosinophils, mast cells, erythrocytes, and monocytes.
   F.   **LYMPHOGLANDULAR BODIES** are cytoplasmic fragments of lymphocytes or lymphoblasts. They usually stain blue-gray and vary in size from that of a small platelet to that of an erythrocyte.
   G.   **SMUDGED or LYSED CELLS** (i.e. free nuclei) should not be interpreted. Free nuclei frequently have a prominent nucleolus and could lead to a misdiagnosis of lymphoma.

II. **CLASSIFICATIONS OF LYMPH NODE ASPIRATES:** Lymph node aspirates can be classified based on the distribution and morphology of cells in them. On many occasions, this is just a general classification and does not offer a specific diagnosis. In some cases, though, a specific diagnosis can be reached on the basis of the cytologic exam.

NORMAL (Note: an enlarged lymph node is not normal)	Mostly **mature lymphocytes** (90-95% of the cells) Blast cells make up most of the remaining cells. Inflammatory cells are present in small numbers. Blood cell numbers can be elevated due to trauma from the aspirate.
REACTIVE or HYPERPLASTIC	Primarily mature cells but we usually see an increase in blast cells, plasma cells and possibly other inflammatory cells. A few mitotic figures may be seen and the cells may be more basophilic. These nodes are reacting to some foreign antigen presented to the node (i.e. they're draining an area of inflammation, neoplasia, etc.).
LYMPHADENITIS (Inflamed lymph node)	Inflammation can be purulent, pyogranulomatous, or granulomatous. **Purulent** lymph nodes contain many neutrophils which are often degenerative. Macrophages may be elevated too.
LYMPHOSARCOMA	Monomorphic population of intermediate to large-sized lymphoblasts (> 50%; look on 10X for homo or heterogeneity) with few normal cells. The neoplastic cells may vary in size and may have variably sized nuclei, multiple or large nucleoli, and increased numbers of mitotic figures. The morphology of malignant cells can vary markedly between cases. Some cases have cells that are unmistakably lymphoid in nature but are primarily very immature lymphoblasts and prolymphocytes. Other cases may have lightly staining, abundant cytoplasm, which is often vacuolated or foamy. They may have irregular nuclei as well. Occasionally, extremely undifferentiated cells are found. The cells are usually difficult to identify as having a lymphoid origin. These cells have nuclear irregularities and a deeply basophilic cytoplasm that may contain a few distinct vacuoles. There are also well-differentiated, small-cell lymphomas. When in doubt, send the sample to a lab or do a biopsy.
METASTATIC TUMORS	Since many tumors metastasize via the lymphatics, cells of various types of metastatic tumors can be found in lymph node aspirates.

Cytology

TRACHEOBRONCHIAL CYTOLOGY

I. **SAMPLING TECHNIQUES**

    A. **TRANSTRACHEAL ASPIRATION or TRANSTRACHEAL WASH:** Anesthetize the skin over the trachea and surgically prep it. Then make a small incision over the trachea and place a cannula in the trachea by passing it between cartilaginous rings. Next place a catheter through the cannula and thread it down the trachea until it reaches the level of the bifurcation. Infuse the saline rapidly via syringe. Within 3-10 seconds, aspirate the saline and material back into the attached syringe. This method has the advantage that it doesn't require general anesthesia, which is potentially dangerous in animals with respiratory disease. Since the method bypasses the mouth and oropharynx completely, contamination of the material by organisms and by nasal, mouth, and pharyngeal cells is usually eliminated. Minor complications in animals following this procedure include subcutaneous emphysema and superficial skin infection.

    B. **BRONCHOALVEOLAR LAVAGE:** This method is often performed via bronchoscopy with the collection catheter introduced through the larynx (ie, must transit the oropharynx). The washing technique is similar to that of the transtracheal method. Use this method when examination suggests that a lesion is localized to a specific area of the lungs. The drawbacks to this method include the requirement for general anesthesia, and the fact that aspirates obtained during bronchoscopy are frequently contaminated by mouth organisms.

II. **TESTS TO RUN ON THE SAMPLE**

    A. **CULTURE:** The specimen can be cultured if it is not contaminated with nasal, oral or pharyngeal organisms.

    B. **SMEARS:** Bronchial aspirates should be concentrated when possible by centrifugation (500 rpm for 5 minutes) and smears of the sediment should be made. Smears made from the sediment obtained after centrifugation will often have many broken, disrupted cells. Better preparations can be obtained using a **cytofuge** (a special centrifuge designed to concentrate cells in a 0.5mL sample of fluid directly onto the surface of a slide during centrifugation).

III. **CELLS FOUND:** Samples from healthy lung tissue are sparsely cellular and contain primarily macrophages and respiratory epithelial cells.

FINDING	INTERPRETATION
Neutrophils	Normally, the sample contains few (< 5%) neutrophils. With inflammation, the PMNs increase dramatically. Neutrophils increase in both acute and chronic diseases of infectious and non-infectious etiologies. They can also degenerate after the sample is collected. Thus, presence of karyolysis does not confirm infectious disease. Samples with neutrophilic inflammation should be cultured (including for *Nocardia* or *Actinomyces* if filamentous rods are seen). Viral and protozoal infections are also associated with neutrophilia. Eosinophilic inclusion bodies are sometimes seen in the PMNs and epithelial cells in dogs with distemper.
Eosinophils	Healthy cats reportedly have up to 25% eosinophils. Greater than 5% in dogs is abnormal. Levels are elevated with allergic or parasitic (e.g. heartworm, lungworm) pulmonary diseases. Eosinophils may be challenging to ID since they often look different than blood eosinophils. They may be non-segmented and their granules may not stain well.
Mast Cells and Basophils	Mast cells and basophils are usually present in low numbers only. They can be elevated in allergic pulmonary disease.
Granulomatous or pyo-granulomatous	Increased macrophages and multinucleate giant cells, which are often present in small aggregates, indicates granulomatous infection. This type of response is seen with **fungal infections** (blastomycosis, coccidiodomycosis, and aspergillosis), **foreign bodies** or **mycobacteria**. This type of inflammation may also be seen in cases of chronic lung disease associated with inhalant material (eg, silicosis in horses). Perform fungal titers or fungal culture if the causative agent is not apparent.
Red blood cells	Erythrophagocytosis indicates chronic vascular congestion.
Foreign material	Examples include: bacteria, fungi, lungworm larvae, pigment, crystals, plant substances (pollen, etc). Increase in foreign substances, especially in a macrophage reaction, suggests compromised mucociliary clearance.

CEREBROSPINAL FLUID ANALYSIS

Cerebrospinal fluid (CSF) is the fluid that bathes the brain and spinal cord. It can change due to pathology affecting the outer surface of the brain and spinal cord but not of deeper tissue (e.g. not due to granuloma or tumor in the cerebral cortex). CSF analysis is frequently normal even with central nervous disease, but is important in determining whether inflammatory disease is present. Perform CSF titers to distemper, RMSF, ehrlichiosis and toxoplasmosis if these diseases are suspected. PCR testing on CSF can also be performed. Occasionally, neoplastic cells or infectious organisms can be found.

I. GENERAL INFORMATION
   A. **INDICATIONS for CSF TAP.** CSF tap is indicated any time CNS disease is suspected, even if the CBC/chemistry are normal. It is not indicated if the animal's neurologic disease is likely attributed to trauma, metabolic disease, obvious disk disease or congenital abnormality (e.g. hydrocephalus). It's appropriate to perform CSF taps to evaluate an animal's progress. It's good to do the CSF tap when the animal is anesthetized for a myelogram (Collect the CSF prior to the myelogram).
   B. **CONTRAINDICATONS:** CSF tap is contraindicated if there's evidence of increased intracranial pressure or tentorial herniation. These are suggested by decreased mentation, head pressing, anisocoria. If CSF tap must be performed in these cases, hyperventilate the animal and then put it on isoflurane. Premedicate with dexamethasone 0.25 mg/kg (< 20 min. prior to collection doesn't change the CSF count). Alternatively, administer 20% mannitol 1-3g/kg over 30 minutes.
   C. **CONSIDERATONS**
      1. Steroids decrease the nucleated cell count and the protein.
      2. Blood contamination increases the RBC and nucleated cell count. Some clinicians correct for this by assuming anywhere from 1 WBC/1000RBC/μL to 1 WBC/100 RBC/μL. Be conservative when making corrections. Note that blood often appears as a swirl in the collection tube. Also, if the blood decreases as you're collecting the fluid, it was due to contamination.

II. **EVALUATING the SAMPLE:** Evaluate the appearance, cell number, differential count, and morphology. Read the cytology (or prepare the slide) within one hour. Alternatively, refrigerate it and read within several hours or prepare it and send it for evaluation. The CSF can be prepared for cytology using an in-house sedimentation technique or the lab can prepare the slide using a cytocentrifuge; however, it is typically not useful and, in fact, wasteful to prepare direct smears of CSF for cytology (not enough cells).

EVALUATION	NORMAL CSF	ABNORMAL CSF
APPEARANCE	Clear, colorless (Cloudiness + > 500 cells/mL)	• **Pink** indicates increased RBC due to contamination or hemorrhage. • **Xanthochromia** is a yellow discoloration due to prior hemorrhage (days to weeks).
CELL COUNT Use a hemocytometer and count **RBC** and **nucleated cells separately**. Differential count is very important too, even if the cell count is in the normal range.	0-3 cells/ μL In cases of blood contamination, factor in 1 WBC per 100 RBC/μL or per 1000 RBC/μL Mononuclear cells predominate.	• > 5 WBC/μL. Numbers may increase mildly post-seizure • > 10% neutrophils = neutrophilic inflammation. > 10% eosinophils = eosinophilic inflammation.
PROTEIN: Crude test via urine dipstick. Then send to the lab. This test uses up a relatively large amount of fluid and may not be very accurate, so you may elect to forego this step.	< 30 mg/dL > 1+ on dipstick is significant	• > 25 mg/dL Any CNS tissue injury can lead to increased CSF protein (e.g. tumor, FIP, degenerative disk)
CYTOLOGY Perform cytology even if the cell count is normal. It almost always must be done on concentrated smears, preferably cytofuge smear.	Primarily **small mononuclear cells.** Neutrophils are absent in non-contaminated samples.	• **Neutrophils**: degeneration suggests sepsis. • **Eosinophils**: allergic or parasitic. • **Malignant cells** are rare but sometimes we see them with lymphosarcoma. • **Microorganisms** are rare but can be seen, including bacteria, *Cryptococcus* and *Ehrlichia*.

Cytology

EXAMINATION of SYNOVIAL FLUID
General Information
Laboratory Exam
Diagnosis/Etiology

I. **INTRODUCTION:** Synovial fluid is a viscous, protein-containing fluid that lubricates joints and provides nutrients to the chondrocytes in the joint cartilage. Blood flow through the synovial tissue's looped, anastomosing vessel system is high and the body uses the synovium as a phagocytic tissue (> 50% of synovial cells are macrophages and the rest are hyaline-producing cells). The result is that joints are involved in many systemic diseases, especially primary and secondary immune-mediated diseases.

A. WHEN TO PERFORM JOINT TAPS
    1. Swollen joints of unknown etiology—not linked to specific trauma
    2. When an animal has a vague history of lethargy, intermittent lameness, fever
    3. When the joints show erosive or proliferative lesions

B. SAMPLES to COLLECT
    1. A tube with anticoagulant for cytology and cell count (lavender top tube)
    2. A sterile tube for culture and gross examination (red top tube)

II. LABORATORY EXAMINATION OF THE JOINT FLUID

TEST	NORMAL	ABNORMAL
Color	Colorless or straw-colored	Red/pink: indicates bleeding due to trauma, coagulopathy, or contamination Xanthochromia (yellow-tinged) indicates previous hemorrhage.
Turbidity	Clear	Cloudy: indicates increased cell count.
Viscosity	Thick due to synovial mucin: This can be estimated by seeing how far a drop of fluid can be stretched between the thumb and index finger before breaking. Normal mucin strings out several inches.	Decreased viscosity indicates inflammation. Effusions dilute mucin. Bacteria produce hyaluronidase which degrades mucin.
Mucin Clot Test	Good Results are usually similar to those of the viscosity test except that this test specifically test the amount and quality of the mucin.	Poor Infectious: Some bacteria degrade mucin. Rheumatoid arthritis and other immune mediated arthritides result in poor mucin. EDTA may degrade hyaluronic acid.
Clot formation	None Normal synovial fluid doesn't clot because it has no fibrinogen.	Clot indicates inflammation or hemorrhage. If the synovial membrane is damaged enough, it can allow fibrinogen into the joint.
Total cell number Count RBC and nucleated cells separately.	1-3/hpf (< 3000/uL) To estimate, make a smear and count the number of cells/high dry field and multiply x 1500 = cells/μL. This varies between microscopes. You can calibrate your microscope by comparing your cell count to the lab's.	> 3000 indicates a lesion. It can be inflammatory (infectious or non-infectious) or non-inflammatory (less elevation). Increase in RBC may be found with trauma (degenerative disease), coagulopathy or blood contamination.
Differential counts	Mostly large and small mononuclear cells. < 10% neutrophils	Increased neutrophils indicates inflammatory joint disease. The degree of inflammation does not necessarily differentiate between infectious or non-infectious causes. The PMNs are rarely toxic even with infectious arthritides.
Microbe Exam	None	Bacteria or fungi
Protein	< 2.5 g/dL	Increased or decreased

LABORATORY EXAMINATION OF JOINT FLUID

TEST	NORMAL	ABNORMAL
Culture	Negative	Culture can be positive with bacterial or fungal infections but it's often negative. If you suspect bacterial infection, run a blood culture or urine culture. Blood culture > urine culture > synovial fluid culture.
Rheumatoid factor	Negative	Positive: The sensitivity and specificity of this are poor, so this test is often not done.

III. DIAGNOSTIC STEPS: Joint effusion can be divided into inflammatory and non-inflammatory. The inflammatory diseases can be further divided into infectious or non-infectious diseases. The first step is to have the lab determine whether the sample is inflammatory or non-inflammatory.

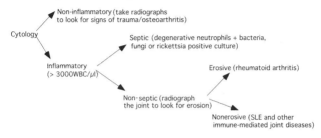

A. **Non-inflammatory** joints have low nucleated cell counts. If the fluid is non-inflammatory, then take radiographs or otherwise examine the animal for evidence of **osteoarthrosis, joint instability or trauma.**

B. **Inflammatory joint disease** is characterized by **increased neutrophils.** Submit samples from multiple joints (even normal-appearing joints) and repeat sampling may be required because cytologic evidence of inflammatory joint disease waxes and wanes. If the fluid is inflammatory, next determine whether it's septic or non-septic.

1. **Rule out septic etiologies:** Presence of degenerate neutrophils suggests sepsis but neutrophils in septic joints are usually not degenerate.

    a. **Bacterial (and fungal) cultures** should be performed to help rule out sepsis. Unfortunately, joint cultures are often negative even with sepsis (bacteria may be confined to synovium) and blood or urine cultures must be performed instead. Thus, culture blood > urine> joint fluid to rule out infection (bacterial, fungal).

    b. **Perform serologic tests for agent that don't grow in culture**
        i. Lyme titer (*Borellia burgdorferi*)
        ii. Rocky Mountain Spotted Fever titers (need paired titers)
        iii. *E. canis* and *E. equi* (*Anaplasma phagocytophilum)* titers (one titer is adequate)

2. **Rule out non-septic etiologies** such as immune-mediated disease if cultures are negative. First, take radiographs of affected joints to determine whether the inflammation is erosive or non-erosive.

    a. **Erosive:** If the joints look erosive, consider rheumatoid arthritis.
    b. **Non-erosive:** If joints are non-erosive, test for primary or secondary causes of immune-mediated diseases.
        ii. **Check the history of drug therapy.** Some drugs can induce immune-mediated disease
        ii. **Rule out SLE** by running an ANA and looking for evidence of multisystemic immune-mediated disease (hematocrit, platelet levels, skin, urinalysis for protein).
        iii. Look for any underlying disease, which can lead to **secondary immune-mediated arthritis** such as infection elsewhere in the body, heartworm disease, neoplasia, GI disease (enteropathic arthritis).

Cytology

CYTOLOGY of MALIGNANT CELLS

I. **DIAGNOSING MALIGNANCY:** Tumors are comprised of cells whose growth escapes normal regulation. As a result, the cells proliferate at an accelerated rate. Because of the rapid, uncontrolled growth rate, the malignant cells are often immature in appearance and poorly differentiated. This poor differentiation is what allows us to distinguish tumor cells from normal cells.

    A. **MONOMORPHIC POPULATION OF CELLS:** Look for a **monomorphic population of cells** (moderate to large increase in one type of cell).

    B. **CELL CLASSIFICATION:** Look at the cell shape and classify the cell as a discrete round cell, an epithelial cell, or a mesenchymal cell.

CELL CLASSIFICATION

CELL TYPE	CHARACTERISTICS	ASSOCIATED TUMOR CLASSIFICATION
Discrete round cell	Individual round cells	Discrete round cell tumors (e.g. mast cell tumor, lymphoma)
Epithelial cell	Round to oval to polygonal cells found in clusters	Carcinoma (e.g. squamous cell carcinoma, transitional cell carcinoma)
Mesenchymal cell	Spindle-shaped cells found in disorganized clusters or as individual cells	Sarcoma (e.g. fibrosarcoma, osteosarcoma)

    C. **DETERMINE WHETHER THE CELLS ARE MALIGNANT**

        1. **Nuclear and cell size variation**
            a. Malignant cells vary in size and tend to have a large nucleus.
            b. They may have a variable or high nucleus to cytoplasm ratio (N:C ratio) due to rapid cell growth and division.
            c. We may see bizarre nuclear shapes (e.g. pseudopods).

        2. **Look for changes in the nucleoli**
            a. Irregular shape (e.g. jagged)
            b. Variation in number of nucleoli (1-5), plus multiple nucleoli
            c. Increased nucleoli size
            d. Numerous mitotic figures suggest increased cell proliferation.

        3. **Look for changes in the cytoplasm.** The cytoplasm may be basophilic due to high **nucleic acid** (RNA) content which reflects the active protein synthesis of these cells. Some normal cells with high protein synthesis abilities such as plasma cells have very basophilic cytoplasm.

    D. **DETERMINE THE TUMOR CLASSIFICATION**

CHARACTERISTICS OF TUMOR CLASSES

	CARCINOMAS	SARCOMAS	DISCRETE CELL
Exfoliate	Readily	Not readily (Scraping may yield moderate cell numbers.)	Readily
Clusters	Usually dense clusters or sheets	Often loosely aggregated rather than in clusters	Usually individual cells
Differentiation	Differentiation may be evident (e.g. acini or ducts, secretory products).	Differentiation may be evident (e.g., azurophilic material in osteosarcomas and chondrosarcomas).	Differentiation may be evident (e.g. mast cell granules).
Cell Shape	Cells are round to oval to polygonal. Borders of cells may be indistinct, but not always.	Cells may be spindle-shaped. Individual cells may have wispy borders but not always.	Cells are round to oval; borders of cells are distinct.

    E. **OTHER AIDS IN MAKING A DIAGNOSIS**

        1. List the tumors that can occur at that site.
        2. Generally, tumor cells retain some of the activities characteristic of their tissue of origin. Look for suggestions of differentiation that can help identify the tumor type.
            a. Formation of ducts or acini indicate an adenocarcinoma.
            b. Secretory products or distinct, even-sized vacuoles indicate adenocarcinoma.

ANTIBIOTICS COMMONLY USED in DENTISTRY

DRUG	DOSAGE
Ampicillin or Amoxicillin	20 mg/kg IV 30 minutes prior to the start of the dental to prevent bacteremia. Follow by 10 mg/kg 4 hours later. Cephalosporins may also be used.
Clavamox	10-20 mg/kg amoxicillin fraction PO BID
Clindamycin	Dog: 5-10 mg/kg PO BID Cat: 50 mg/cat PO SID or 25 mg/cat PO BID
Metronidazole	Dog: 30 mg/kg PO SID Cat: 10 mg/kg PO SID

Clavamox, clindamycin, or metronidazole may be used orally 2 hours pre-operatively to prevent bacteremia. Administration starting 48 hours prior to dental does not prevent bacteremia.

TIMING OF PERMANENT TOOTH ERUPTION

PERMANENT TOOTH	INCISORS	CANINES	PREMOLARS	MOLARS
Puppies	3-5 months	4-6 months	4-6 months	5-7 months
Kittens	3-4 months	4-5 months	4-6 months	4-5 months

SUGGESTED READING

Holstrom, SE., et al. AAHA Dental Care Guidelines for Dogs and Cats. *Journal of the American Animal Hospital Association* (41) 2005: insert.

Dentistry

EXAMINATION of the ORAL CAVITY

Owners often don't recognize serious oral disease in their pets— instead, it is often discovered on routine veterinary examination. Occasionally, animals present with noticeable signs of oral disease such as halitosis, facial swelling, draining tracts, intraoral masses, or difficulty chewing food. Signs of oral disease are often subtle and can be overlooked by the owner. These "subtle" changes may include ptyalism, decreased appetite, the inability to open or close the mouth, and oral bleeding. A complete oral examination includes evaluation of A) hard tissues (teeth, bone, maxillofacial structures), B) soft tissues (lips, cheeks, tongue, palate, gingiva, oral mucosa, mandibular lymph nodes), and C) intraoral radiographs taken under general anesthesia.

I. **EXAMINATION OF THE AWAKE PATIENT:** Perform the oral examination in a systematic manner using adequate illumination (e.g. halogen penlight or a bright, flexible-neck floor lamp). Animals with oral pain are often difficult to examine and may require anesthesia. Additionally, anesthesia is used for periodontal charting and intraoral radiographs.
    A. **EXTERNAL EXAMINATION:** Observe the patient and look for facial asymmetry (e.g. facial swelling), abnormal head carriage, and external draining tracts (suborbital, maxillary, or mandibular). Next, palpate the maxilla, mandible, mandibular lymph nodes, and infraorbital area for swelling, sensitivity, or lesions. Finally, retropulse the eyes using gentle digital pressure.
    B. **EXAMINATION OF THE CLOSED MOUTH:** Retract the lips and evaluate the teeth and gums.
        1. **Check for odor and grade it** as normal, mild, moderate, or severe. Evaluate whether the odor is due to lip fold pyoderma or periodontal disease; also consider metabolic causes such as renal or hepatic disease. Periodontal disease is the most common cause of halitosis in dogs and cats. Other causes include oral neoplasia, uremia, GI disease, and infection or neoplasia of the respiratory tract.
        2. **Assess the gingival and oral mucosa:** Evaluate the gingiva for color and capillary refill time. Look for fistulas in the alveolar mucosa (indicating a periapical abscess) and ulcers on the buccal mucosa. Examine the gingiva for hyperemia, swelling, hyperplasia, or gum recession. All oral masses should be biopsied. Obtain a deep biopsy since superficial biopsies often reveal nothing more than inflammation.
        3. **Look at the teeth:**
            a. Check for **missing** and **loose** teeth, **retained deciduous** teeth, and **supernumerary** or **split teeth/gemination**. Split teeth and supernumerary teeth are considered hereditary if found in the permanent dentition. Also look for malpositioned teeth. Crowded teeth are more likely to develop periodontitis.
            b. Look for fractures, furcation exposure, root canal exposure, exposed dentin, and **resorptive lesions** (a common finding in cats).
            c. Evaluate for **calculus** deposits.
            d. Look for **yellow staining** of the teeth. This can be caused by **tetracycline** administration in pregnant bitches or puppies with growing teeth.
            e. Check for **enamel hypoplasia** which occurs when certain viruses (e.g. distemper) infect the patient during growth. These viruses attack ameleoblasts which leads to the enamel damage. Treatment includes fluoride administration, composite bonding, and regular dental prophylaxis.
            f. Check for discoloration of the teeth indicative of trauma. Purple or gray discoloration indicates endodontic disease (the pulp is dead).
        4. **Check occlusion:** The normal pattern is for all of the upper incisors to be just in front of the lower incisors in a **scissor bite** and for the midlines of the maxilla and mandible to be aligned. The mandibular canines should interdigitate between the maxillary third incisors and maxillary canines. The mandibular premolars should interdigitate with the maxillary premolars in a "pinking shears" effect with the mandibular first premolar rostral to the maxillary first premolar. The upper fourth premolar should be buccal to the lower first molar. The following malocclusions are all considered hereditary due to an autosomal dominant gene that's expressed more dramatically in some animals than others.
            a. **Prognathism** (abnormally long mandible), **brachygnathism** (abnormally short mandible), **level bite** (a form of prognathism where the incisors come together on top of each other instead of the maxillary incisors articulating rostral to the mandibular incisors).
            b. Do the midlines of the mandible and maxilla match, or does the patient have a **wry bite**?
            c. **Base narrow mandibular canine teeth:** Do the mandibular canine teeth strike the hard palate?

    d.   **Anterior crossbite:** Are any of the lower incisors rostral to their counterpart upper incisors?

5.   Evaluate specifically for periodontal disease. **Periodontal disease** is caused by bacteria but also has a hereditary component. The accumulation of bacteria and its glycoprotein matrix is called **plaque**. Calcified portions of plaque are called **calculus**. Plaque first accumulates supragingivally and then spreads subgingivally which lead to periodontitis. Tissues affected in periodontitis include the gingiva, cementum, periodontal ligament (which connects the cementum to the alveolar bone), and alveolar bone. Periodontal disease includes gingivitis and periodontitis.

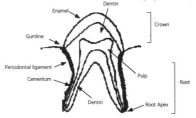

    a.   **Gingivitis is reversible** inflammation of the gingiva with no loss in periodontal attachment. It usually resolves with mechanical/chemical plaque control (e.g. dental prophylaxis and tooth brushing). It is characterized by erythema and blunting of the gingival edges.

    b.   **Periodontitis** is progressive inflammation and destruction of the periodontal tissues. It is characterized by gingivitis, gingival recession, deep periodontal pockets due to breakdown of the gingival attachment (> 3mm in dogs and > 1 mm in cats), loose teeth, and bony alveolar loss seen on radiographs. We can control progression of periodontitis with dedicated home oral hygiene and nonsurgical and surgical therapy (e.g. antibiotics, periodontal debridement, flap surgery, bone augmentation, etc.), but we can't reverse the process.

GRADING PERIODONTAL DISEASE

Grade	Description
I Healthy	The gingiva is light pink or pigmented and the gingival margins have feathered edges. There is no bleeding on examination with a periodontal probe and no calculus. The animal's breath is not offensive.
II Mild periodontitis (gingivitis/early periodontitis)	The gingiva is erythematous and inflamed, especially at the gingival margins. Plaque (bacteria, saliva, and food) and calculus (calcified plaque) has formed on the tooth surface above and below the gum line. On probing, the gums may bleed but the pockets are minimal (< 3 mm in dogs). The pet has minor gingival recession and mild halitosis.
III Moderate periodontitis	Periodontal pockets become deeper and gingival recession may be present. The pet has moderate plaque and calculus formation and marked halitosis. The gums may bleed easily on probing. The animal may have up to 50% bone loss and some teeth may be slightly mobile.
IV Advanced periodontitis	Periodontal pockets are deep and the pet may have extensive gingival recession. Plaque and calculus are heavy, and halitosis may be severe. The gums bleed on probing. The pet may have more than 50% bone loss.

C.   **EXAMINATION of the OPEN MOUTH:** While opening the mouth, assess jaw tone and evaluate for pain. Check the dental arches, hard palate, soft palate, and tonsillar crypts for symmetry, lesions, and foreign bodies. The soft tissue caudal to the last maxillary molar is normally depressed or concave. Always check for sublingual lesions (linear foreign bodies, granulomas, neoplasia). The oral cavity is one of the most common sites for tumors in the dog and cat.

DENTAL PROPHYLAXIS and HOMECARE

I. **DENTAL PROPHYLAXIS:** Because severe periodontal disease can serve as a nidus for infection elsewhere—especially in the kidney, liver, and myocardium— animals should undergo dental prophylaxis and homecare on a regular basis.

   A. **PRE-DENTAL CONSIDERATIONS:** Use pre-operative antibiotics if the pet has moderate to severe periodontal disease, is at high risk of systemic complications from dental bacteremia (e.g. cardiac valve defect, renal or hepatic infection, hyperadrenocorticism), or is having an additional surgical procedure. Starting antibiotics 48 hours prior to the dental has not been shown to prevent bacteremia; however, administering amoxicillin or ampicillin (20 mg/kg IV, 30 minutes prior to dental and then 10 mg/kg 4 hours later), or clavamox, clindamycin, or metronidazole orally 2 hours prior to dental has been shown to prevent bacteremia. Continue antibiotics for 7-10 days post-op. Flush the teeth with chlorhexidine rinse prior to scaling to help keep bacterial numbers down.

   B. **CHART:** Before performing periodontal debridement, perform a complete oral examination. Chart the information before or after the prophylactic procedure (sample chart on next page).
   1. Count the teeth and note any missing teeth.
   2. Note any loose or fractured teeth.
   3. Note gingivitis, gingival recession, and exposed furcations.
   4. Using a periodontal probe, measure the gingival sulci and look for periodontal pockets.

   > Normal sulcus depth in dogs: < 3mm
   > Normal sulcus depth in cats: < 1mm

   C. **RADIOGRAPH** the teeth (intraoral radiographs) as part of a regular dental and when:
   1. Clinical evaluation of a tooth shows signs of gum or bone loss.
   2. Probing depth is abnormal.
   3. You want to evaluate soft or hard tissue enlargements or you want to determine the pattern of bony involvement of a neoplastic process.
   4. Before tooth extraction
   5. Before, during, or after any endodontic or restorative procedure on a tooth
   6. The tooth is discolored or fractured or you suspect a crown fracture, root fracture, or resorptive lesion.
   7. You want to detect the presence or developmental stage of permanent tooth buds (especially if you are extracting a deciduous tooth).

   D. **SCALE:** A thorough periodontal debridement includes scaling and polishing the teeth. Hand scaling the awake animals is not adequate because it creates enamel gouges and a head-shy pet. Additionally it is does not clean below the gum line.
   1. Use an ultrasonic or air driven **scaler**.
   2. Use an **explorer** to assess tooth surfaces to feel for roughness.
   3. **Curettes** can be used above or below the gumline; **hand scalers** are for supragingival use only.

   E. **POLISH:** Polishing smooths the tooth surface making it difficult for bacteria to adhere. Without polishing, plaque and calculus accumulate quickly because plaque adheres readily to irregular surfaces.

   F. **PERFORM EXTRACTIONS and ENDODONTICS** after the teeth have been cleaned. This decreases the likelihood that the animal will develop sepsis from oral bacteria entering the bloodstream. Endodontics should be performed by a veterinary dental specialist.
   1. **When to extract teeth:**
       a. When the pet has an abscessed tooth or loose tooth secondary to periodontitis
       b. In cases of severe tooth root exposure and radiographic evidence of < 1/3 alveolar bone support
       c. When an adult tooth and a deciduous tooth are erupting in the same place (The deciduous tooth should be removed.)
       d. When a cat has a resorptive lesion
       e. When a puppy is brachygnathic: Removing the incisors and canines from the mandible may allow the jaw to grow to its normal potential. This is effective about 50% of the time. It is accepted as an ethical procedure by the American Veterinary Dental College and allowed in animals competing in AKC

6.4

conformation trials. Interceptive orthodontics should be performed by a veterinarian with extensive dental training.

2. **Handling retained roots**: Retained roots are a common problem in dogs due to fractures or poor extraction techniques. In cats, most retained root tips are secondary to resorptive lesions. Root fragments in cats may remain quiescent or they may be resorbed. Retained roots in dogs generally become infected. Intraoral radiographs are essential. Patients with retained roots can be referred to a veterinary dentist for definitive treatment.

3. **How to treat fractured teeth**: Treatment depends on whether or not the pulp is vital. If the pulp is dead or infected, it should be removed even if it's not exposed. **Dead pulp is a nidus for infection.** If you examine the whole tooth surface using an explorer and it doesn't fall into a divot, the pulp may not be exposed. The only way to know for sure that the pulp is healthy is with **intra-oral radiographs. Endodontics should be performed by a veterinary dental specialist.**
    a. **Vital teeth**: For dogs < 18 months of age, send home antibiotics and anti-inflammatory agents and refer to an endodontist for partial coronal pulpectomy within 2-3 weeks. The owner may also opt to wait and observe for changes. If so, they should treat with analgesics and observe for subtle signs of pain and abscess. For dogs > 18 months of age, refer for endodontics within 48 hours or extract the tooth if the owner does not want salvage procedures.
    b. **Non-vital teeth**: The owner may elect to extract the tooth, refer for a root canal, or wait and observe.

F. **POST-OPERATIVE CARE**: Rinse the teeth and gums with CHX Oral Cleansing Solution before, during, and after the dental cleaning. Some dentists feel that placing a dental sealant followed by weekly application of CHX by the owner may slow the development of periodontitis. If teeth have been extracted, place CHX Guard Gel into the extraction site. If the animal has severe periodontal disease, place it on antibiotics (e.g. clindamycin) for 10 days and on an oral antibacterial rinse for 14 days. Recheck the animal in 14 days and start the patient on a daily homecare program. Without daily homecare, periodontitis will progress.

II. **HOMECARE**: Daily homecare is essential. Without it, gingivitis will return and periodontitis will progress after the professional periodontal debridement (teeth cleaning). Homecare can extend the period of good oral health dramatically. For a list of Veterinary Oral Health Council accepted products, go to www.VOHC.org.

A. **BRUSHING**: Daily tooth brushing remains the most effective method for preventing periodontal disease. The mechanical action disrupts accumulated plaque. A soft bristle toothbrush and a pet dentifrice can be used. There are numerous palatable dog and cat toothpastes on the market that help make the experience more pleasurable for the pet. They are safe for pets to swallow and often contain enzymes and abrasives to help retard plaque accumulation.

1. Owners often won't brush their pet's teeth because the animal is uncooperative. Training dogs and cats to accept having their teeth brushed is easy, and when done correctly, should take only several 5-minute sessions.
    b. a. Start by getting the animal used to having its mouth handled. Have the pet sit in your lap (small dogs and cats) or on the floor in front of you with his back against you so that he's facing away from you. In order to teach him to associate mouth handling with pleasurable experiences, place a bite-sized treat in his mouth in such a way that he does not have to reach for it but rather keeps his head stationary. For cats, you can use wet cat food or tuna on a spoon. For dogs, use a bite-sized treat such as kibble, small pieces of semi-moist treats, etc. While the pet is eating the treat, touch the areas around his lips and mouth. For dogs, control the rate at which they eat as well as their head position by holding the treat for several seconds while the dog is taking it from you. When he finishes the treat, immediately stop handling his face and mouth. This timing is important so that he understands the association between the two. Repeat the same exact handling several times in a row. If the animal responds by trying to move his head away, handle him for a shorter period of time or more lightly the next time. The goal is that the pet does not respond aversely to the handling. If he accepts the handling several times in a row, then start handling more assertively (e.g. lift lips, pull commissures back

Dentistry

further, open the mouth for an instant and then close it before the dog or cat tries to pull away). This procedure is termed desensitization and counter-conditioning. (To see videos go to www.drsophiayin.com/resources/videos or view the videos from the *Low Stress Handling, Restraint and Behavior Modification of Dogs & Cats* DVD or online book at www.lowstresshandling.com.)

   c. A variation of this procedure is to handle the animal's head and mouth for a few seconds and then give a treat as a reward for holding his head still. The treats must arrive in his mouth within 1 second for him to learn the association between the behavior and the treat quickly. Start with short, gentle handling and gradually work towards more assertive, longer handling. (To see videos go to www.lowstresshandling.com/online chapter 18.)

   d. Graduate to a toothbrush with flavored pet toothpaste. Start by letting your pet taste the toothbrush. If he does not enjoy the flavor, try a different brand. The flavor should be a reward for him. Once he licks the toothpaste indicating that he likes the flavor, lift his lips and start brushing.

B. **DENTAL DIETS:** While regular dry pet food does have some mechanical cleaning action over canned foods, prescription dental diets do provide significant improvement in oral health. For a list of products approved by the Veterinary Oral Health Council, go to (www.VOHC.org).

C. **CHEW AIDS** such as the proprietary products approved by the VOHC serve as an adjunct to homecare techniques.

D. **CHLORHEXIDINE GLUCONATE** in dogs and **ZINC ASCORBATE** in cats also serve as an adjunct. Neither penetrates plaque or calculi though.

E. **DENTAL SEALANTS** (e.g. Orovet®) may a barrier between the supra and subgingival regions. Efficacy is questionable at this time.

F. **AVOID CERTAIN CHEW TOYS/BONES:**
1. **Avoid chewing on hard objects** such as chew hooves, raw or cooked bones, and hard plastic toys as they can lead to fractures and premature wear of the teeth, especially if they're given frequently.

2. **Avoid allowing prolonged chewing on tennis balls** and cloth toys as doing so can also lead to premature tooth wear. For prolonged chewing, provide soft, durable rubber toys such as Kong toys, Canine Genius food puzzles (www.caninegenius.com), and similarly soft but firm rubber.

FELINE GINGIVOSTOMATITIS

Feline gingivitis/stomatitis is characterized by severe inflammation of the gingiva, buccal mucosa, sublingual tissues, palatoglossal arches, and occasionally the oropharyngeal tissues. The etiology remains unclear though immune system dysfunction is suspected.

TREATMENT

Treatment should be aggressive even if the cat is not showing clinical signs of disease yet. Disease can flare up acutely causing sudden anorexia and other signs of oral pain.

PATHOGENESIS	While etiology is unknown, the presence of bacteria and resorptive lesions stimulate inflammation.
CLINICAL SIGNS	Halitosis, drooling, pain on eating, or anorexia and weight loss. These cats may have an unkempt haircoat due to oral pain during grooming or general lethargy due to pain.
DIAGNOSTICS	Test for FIV and FeLV first. Infections with these viruses may affect the duration of corticosteroids or other immunomodulatory therapy that may be used. Perform a routine CBC, chemistry panel, and urinalysis to rule out other systemic disease. Also assess for Bartonellosis (serology).
MEDICAL TREATMENTS	• **Antibiotics:** Clindamycin (25 mg/cat PO BID or 50 mg/cat PO SID), clavamox, cephalexin, clindamycin, or enrofloxacin are good choices. Sometimes enrofloxacin (5 mg/kg PO BID) and metronidazole (15 mg/kg PO BID) are administered together long-term as they work synergistically. • **Tooth brushing and topical oral antimicrobials** such as chlorhexidine gluconate rinse: Cats are often too painful to allow these treatments. • **Diet:** Warm gruel such as a mixture of cat food and baby food. • **Prednisone or prednisolone:** 2-4 mg/kg for 7 days followed by half this dose for another 7 days. • **Methylprednisolone acetate** (Depo-Medrol®): 20 mg/cat SC every 14 days for up to 6-8 weeks until clinical improvement is seen. Use this if the cat will not tolerate oral prednisone due to oral pain. • Schedule the dental procedure in 5-7 days. • Referral to a veterinary dentist for other medical therapies.
DENTAL PROCEDURES	Perform intraoral radiographs and periodontal debridement and extract any teeth with resorptive lesions, periodontally compromised teeth (severe recession, loose teeth) or retained roots. Results of extraction are variable: • 60% of cats with full-mouth extraction show complete remission of clinical signs. • 20% have occasional flare-ups of clinical signs. • 13% require continued medical management. • 7% show no improvement.
POST-OP CARE	• Continue antibiotics for 5-7 days • Continue or initiate topical oral antimicrobials and start brushing teeth if/when the cat will allow it. • Continue warm gruel diet. • Recheck in 2 weeks and then recheck regularly at intervals determined by patient response to treatment. • Some cats need repeat methylprednisolone acetate injections. • Referral for other medical adjunctive therapies.

Dentistry

DENTAL CHARTS

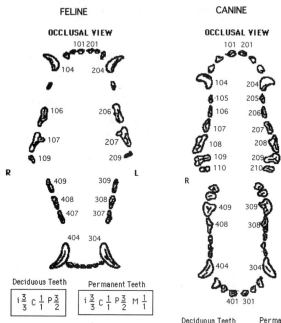

FELINE

OCCLUSAL VIEW

101 201
104 204
106 206
107 207
109 209

R   L

409 309
408 308
407 307

404 304

Deciduous Teeth	Permanent Teeth
$i\frac{3}{3}$ C $\frac{1}{1}$ P $\frac{3}{2}$	$i\frac{3}{3}$ C $\frac{1}{1}$ P $\frac{3}{2}$ M $\frac{1}{1}$

CANINE

OCCLUSAL VIEW

101 201
104 204
105 205
106 206
107 207
108 208
109 209
110 210

R

409 309
408 308

404 304

401 301

Deciduous Teeth	Permanent Teeth
$i\frac{3}{3}$ C $\frac{1}{1}$ P $\frac{3}{3}$	$i\frac{3}{3}$ C $\frac{1}{1}$ P $\frac{4}{4}$ M $\frac{2}{3}$

CODE KEY

AF	Amalgam Filling	**D**	Retained Deciduous
C	Calculus	**E**	Enamel Lesion
CA	Caries Cavity	**F**	Furcation Exposed
CF	Composite Filling	**G**	Gingivitis
CR	Crown Restoration	**GR**	Gingival Recession
CFX	Complicated Crown Fracture	**GH**	Gingival Hyperplasia
UCFX	Uncomplicated Crown Fracture	**M**	Mobile (Loose) Tooth

O	Missing Tooth
P	Plaque
PP	Periodontal Pocket
R	Rotated Tooth
RC	Root Canal
RL	Resorptive Lesion
WF	Wear Facet
X	Extracted Tooth

Three-Rooted Teeth: Upper PM4, M1, M2

Buccal: The tooth surface facing the cheek
Labial: The tooth surface facing the lips
Lingual: The tooth surface adjacent to the tongue
Mesial: The tooth surface facing midline
Distal: The tooth surface facing away from midline
Apical: Toward the root tip
Coronal: Toward the tooth crown
Occlusal: The biting surface of the tooth

6.8

DIAGNOSING SKIN DISEASE
History
Clinical Examination
Diagnostic Tests in Dermatology

I. HISTORY

SIGNALMENT	• **Species and breed:** Many dermatologic conditions have a hereditary component. Consequently, familial history of dermatologic problems is important. • **Age:** Determine both the age of onset and the current age.
ANIMAL'S ENVIRONMENT	• **Geographic location:** Many diseases such as coccidioidomycosis and histoplasmosis have a specific geographic distribution. Remember to determine where the animal has been recently (including travel) as well as where it has lived in the past. • **Home environment:** A multitude of factors—ranging from housing and bedding to sources of contact irritants or chemical allergens—may yield important clues as to the etiology. Additionally, information about other animals in the household may be important. For instance, if a new kitten has recently been adopted from a shelter, and shortly thereafter the adult household pets show patches of alopecia, ringworm should be suspected. • **Other animals affected:** The presence of similar skin conditions in other animals (including the owners and their children) that have been in contact with the patient is particularly valuable in some transmissible diseases such as dermatophytosis and sarcoptic mange, as well as in nutritional and toxic dermatoses. • **Use or type of activity:** The types of activities an animal engages in can predispose it to dermatologic conditions. For instance, hunting dogs are frequently in fields, which predisposes them to trombiculids, fleas, and ticks.
SEASONALITY	• Some dermatologic conditions occur more frequently during specific times of the year. For instance, atopy involving an allergic response to pollens most commonly causes clinical signs in spring or other periods when the specific pollens are high. Flea infestation occurs most often in warm months, and photosensitive diseases are most common in the sunny months.
LESION DESCRIPTION	• **Initial lesion:** Frequently the initial lesions have drastically changed in appearance by the time the animal is presented, so it's important to get the owners to describe the initial lesion in detail. • **Lesion progression:** Try to determine how quickly and broadly the lesion has spread and the **role of various factors** (such as environmental change, self-trauma, treatment) on the progression. • **Pruritus:** Determine whether the lesion is pruritic or non-pruritic.
PREVIOUS TREATMENTS	• **Response to previous treatments** helps rule out specific conditions; however, make sure that the treatment used was **reliable** and that it was administered in an appropriate manner and for a **sufficient period of time.** Often treatment failure is due to inadequate administration of the treatment. Many **topical medications are potential contact irritants**, and in certain animals they cause allergic contact dermatitis (rare). The history usually provides a clear indication as to whether certain medications make the condition worse and which medications these are.
PREVIOUS SKIN DISEASE	Many cases present as a recurrence of a previous skin disease due to the owner's inability to notice subtle differences in the lesions. It's extremely important to know whether the present condition is truly a recurrence, or whether it represents a completely unrelated condition. Usually this decision can only be made on the basis of history.

II. **CLINICAL EXAMINATION:** Examine the skin under good light; direct sunlight is ideal. Look at the entire skin surface; otherwise you may miss the full pattern of the disease. Sometimes you must clip the overlying hair to adequately visualize the lesions. A magnifying glass can help in visualizing small lesions.

A. TYPES of LESIONS

ALOPECIA	Alopecia refers to hair loss.
MACULE	A macule is a flat circumscribed change in the color of the skin (< 1 cm in diameter). The discoloration can result from several processes; erythema is the most common cause, usually from allergy. Other causes include an increase in melanin pigment, depigmentation, and hemorrhage. • A **patch** is a large macule (over 1 cm in diameter).
PAPULE	A **papule** (a.k.a. pimple) is a solid, **erythematous**, circumscribed elevation of the skin up to 1 cm in diameter. It's usually caused by inflammatory cell infiltration of the dermis and is most commonly due to flea allergy. It can also be caused by intraepidermal edema or epidermal hypertrophy. • **Plaque:** Papules can coalesce to form a larger, flat-topped, erythematous elevation (> 1 cm in diameter). If the coalescing plaques form a bumpy elevation, it's called a **vegetation.** Vegetations are frequently covered by crusts. • **Nodule:** A papule (erythematous elevation) that extends into the deeper skin and is > 1 cm is called a nodule. Nodules usually result from massive infiltration of inflammatory or neoplastic cells into the dermis or subcutis. • **Tumor:** A tumor is a large nodule or obviously neoplastic mass. Tumors can involve any structure of the skin or subcutaneous tissue. • **Cyst:** A cyst is an epithelium-lined cavity containing fluid or a solid material. It's a smooth, well-circumscribed, fluctuant to solid mass. Skin cysts are usually lined by adnexal epithelium (hair follicle, sebaceous, or apocrine) and filled with cornified cellular debris or sebaceous or apocrine secretions. • **Wheal:** A wheal is a special type of papule—a solid, sharply circumscribed, flat elevation of the skin produced by edema of the dermis. Clusters of wheals are termed urticaria.
COMEDO	A comedo is a dilated hair follicle filled with cornified cells and sebaceous material. Bacteria may multiply in the sebaceous material causing the surrounding tissue to become inflamed. Inflammation near the surface leads to a pustule. Deep inflammation leads to a papule. If oil breaks through to the surface a **whitehead** forms. If the oil is oxidized, it changes from white to black and is called a **blackhead.**
VESICLE	A **vesicle** is a circumscribed elevation of the epidermis filled with serum. Vesicles are very fragile, so in dogs and cats they usually rupture leading to an **epidermal collarette**, a circular arrangement of loose keratin, which represents the "roof" of the vesicle. • **Bulla:** A vesicle > 1 cm is called a bulla. • **Pustule:** A pustule is a vesicle containing inflammatory cells (neutrophils and/or eosinophils, with or without bacteria).
SCALE	A **scale is an accumulation of fragments of the stratum corneum (cornified epidermal cells).** Skin normally undergoes turnover of the epidermal cells and stratum corneum, but with altered keratinization this process is accelerated. This leads to excessive scaling and the presence of larger scales (clumps of 20 or more cells), which are visible as **dandruff.**
CRUST	Crusts are the residue of dried serum, blood, pus, epithelial cells, keratin, and bacterial debris. Unlike scales, they adhere to each other. They are frequently a product of ruptured pustules.
EROSION	An erosion is a superficial denudation of the skin that does not penetrate the basal laminar zone and consequently heals without scarring. • **Ulcer:** A defect of the skin extending at least into the dermis • **Excoriation:** An erosion produced by self-trauma and usually covered by a crust
FISSURE	Fissures are cracks in the skin secondary to loss of tone associated with inflammation.
LICHEN-IFICATION	Lichenification is a thickening of the skin with an exaggeration of superficial skin marks (wrinkles), giving the skin a tree bark-like character. The skin can look like elephant skin.
HYPERKER-ATOSIS	Hyperkeratosis refers to an increase in thickness of the stratum corneum of the skin. Examples include callus formation, nasodigital hyperkeratosis (hardpad), or primary seborrhea in the Cocker spaniel.

Dermatology

   B. **DISTRIBUTION OF LESIONS:** Lesions can be bilaterally symmetrical, diffuse, generalized, or focal. The pattern can help determine the diagnosis.
III. **DIAGNOSTIC TESTS in DERMATOLOGY**
   A. **SKIN SCRAPINGS** should be performed when you suspect **ectoparasites** such as mites. Make the scraping at the **center of the lesion** and scrape deep enough to draw blood demodex. The scraping should include epidermis, some dermis, and hair. Suspend the sample in **mineral oil,** place a coverslip, and examine it under a microscope. Scrape several lesions of different ages. Generally 3-4 scrapings are adequate to visualize demodectic mites, but 5-10 are required for the elusive mites such as sarcoptes.
   B. **A WOOD'S LIGHT** is used in diagnosing dermatophytosis. Only two species of dermatophytes fluoresce, *Microsporum canis* and *M. audouini.* In veterinary medicine we are only concerned with *M. canis,* and only about 50% of the *M. canis* infections fluoresce. They fluoresce **yellow-green** whereas scales and dandruff fluoresce white. Some topical medications (such as ointments containing tetracyclines) fluoresce too.
   C. **A FUNGAL CULTURE** is the most accurate method of diagnosing dermatophytosis.
   D. **MICROSCOPIC EXAMINATION of HAIR (trichogram)** for fungal elements: Pluck hairs at the border of the lesion and place them in mineral oil (or suspend them in **15% KOH** to clear debris). Also examine the hairs for fungal elements.
   E. **WRIGHT'S STAIN of PUSTULE CONTENTS and EXUDATES** is used to diagnose pyodermas. Smear the contents of a pustule or exudate on a microscope slide, stain it, and then examine it. Pustules can contain infectious agents, or they may be sterile (e.g., pemphigus foliaceus).
      1. Look for **three** things: (1) **neutrophils** (degenerative or hypersegmented), (2) number and type of organisms present, and (3) presence of intracellular organisms.
   F. **BACTERIAL CULTURES and SENSITIVITY TESTS:** While cultures are sometimes contaminated by normal skin flora, they can be an important diagnostic tool. A stain of the exudate can be simple, rapid, and inexpensive, and may reveal engulfed bacteria; therefore, it is occasionally superior to culture. In general, any moist lesion older than 24 hours, especially in the dog, will produce coagulase-positive staphylococci. To interpret a culture, as far as the pathogenic role the bacteria are playing, it's necessary to know exactly how the culture was taken and the **number** of organisms involved.
      1. **When to culture:** Perform a culture and sensitivity when the pyoderma looks significantly atypical, when the smears show organisms that are not typical staphylococci, when the pyoderma fails to respond to ordinary therapy, and when the infection is a deep pyoderma.
   G. **A BIOPSY** can be a useful diagnostic tool when collected correctly, examined by a veterinary pathologist (preferably with a dermatologic interest), and interpreted in light of the clinical signs and history. Findings are not always pathognomonic for recognized entities. Often they are used to either support your gross diagnosis or to help rule out conditions. Diagnosis frequently still rests on gross findings.

BIOPSY the FOLLOWING:

- All obviously neoplastic or suspected neoplastic masses
- All persistent ulcerations
- Any cases that are obviously unusual, quite serious in the clinician's experience, or life-threatening
- A disease that isn't responding to rational treatment
- Any suspected diagnosis in which the treatment is very expensive, potentially harmful to the animal, or time consuming enough to demand a definitive diagnosis before starting

      1. **Types of biopsies**
         a. **An excisional biopsy** can be performed when the lesion is small enough. Generally take at least 3 samples. It can provide both a diagnosis and a cure in the case of single lesions.
         b. **An elliptical biopsy** should include all areas of the lesion (normal skin, edge, and center).
         c. **A punch biopsy** should be taken if the other two options are not appropriate. The sample should include the most developed portion of a lesion that has the least amount of secondary changes. No normal skin should be included, so that if the tissue is trimmed the pathologist won't be confronted with normal skin.
      In all methods the biopsy should be deep enough to include the subcutaneous tissue. With multiple lesions, take the most developed primary lesions.

ALLERGY
Flea Allergy Dermatitis
Food Allergy Dermatitis
Atopic Dermatitis
Allergic Contact Dermatitis

I. FLEA ALLERGY DERMATITIS (FAD)

FAD is a pruritic dermatitis that occurs in animals sensitized to flea saliva. It's the most common hypersensitivity skin disorder in dogs and cats. In general, FAD tends to worsen as the animal gets older—clinical signs begin a little earlier in the season, persist a little longer, and tend to become progressively more severe.

LIFE CYCLE	Adult fleas spend most of their time on the animal, where they eat, mate shortly thereafter (within 24-48 hours), and start producing eggs. Females can produce up to 2,000 eggs in a span of up to 120 days. The eggs fall off the animal into the environment (carpeting, furniture, soil) and hatch within 2-10 days. The resulting larvae gravitate to dark, humid areas, where they feed off flea feces and then pupate within 5-11 days. Adult fleas emerge from their highly resistant cocoons in 5-140 days. The whole life cycle can last from 2 weeks to almost 1 year. The average is 3-4 weeks. Factors that influence life cycle duration include temperature, humidity, and CO_2 levels (e.g., presence or absence of the host). Fleas thrive best under warm, moist conditions and will not emerge from their cocoons when conditions are unfavorable. This explains the fact that when the season changes from cold to warm, or when a pet arrives home after an extended leave, the flea population may suddenly increase.
CLINICAL FEATURES	• **Pruritus with papules and crusts:** Lesions are typically located in the dorsal lumbosacral area, caudomedial thighs, ventral abdomen (umbilicus region), flank, and neck. In cats, the lesions are usually on the dorsal neck, ventral abdomen, and back. • Signs are usually **seasonal** (summer and fall) except with household infestations and warm climates. • Animals that develop hypersensitivity do so after 6 months of age.
DIAGNOSIS	• **Morphology and distribution of lesions** • **Visualization of fleas and flea dirt:** Run a flea comb through the animal's fur. Dogs and cats may be pruritic for 2 weeks after the last flea bite. A single bite can make some FAD animals extremely pruritic. • **Intradermal skin test or ELISA** (refer to atopy): 80% of flea hypersensitivity in dogs is both immediate and delayed. A dog with a positive immediate skin test reaction, has skin sensitizing antibody, but does not necessarily have clinical allergy. The test results must coincide with signs before the animal is declared to have FAD. • **Eosinophilia** is sometimes present in pets with FAD. • **Response to therapy** • A skin biopsy is non-diagnostic but supports allergy.
THERAPY	• **Flea control:** Pupae (cocoons) are resistant to desiccation and insecticides, while ova are vulnerable to desiccation and to some adulticides. Therefore, treatment is aimed at the adults and larvae. Because the adult flea lives on the host and is dependent on the host for food, much of the treatment can focus on the host. Use both an adulticide plus a compound to prevent egg or larvae development [insect growth regulators (IGRs), ovicides, and insect development inhibitors (IDIs)]. The adults are attracted to animals and killed once on the pet. Adults already present are also killed, made unable to reproduce, or their eggs can't develop. If all animals in the household are treated, the flea life cycle can be stopped within one generation. The duration of one generation varies depending on the environment but on average owners should expect to take 8 weeks to clear the infestation. In cases of moderate to severe infestations, cases involving FAD, and those where humans are being bitten, the environment should be treated, too. All animals in the household must be treated. • **Systemic medications to control pruritus:** Use prednisone for 5-7 days followed by alternate-day therapy. Antihistamines and eicosapentaenoic acid-containing products can be used, too, but are generally not helpful. In cats, chlorpheniramine is a particularly useful antihistamine but is inferior to corticosteroids.

FLEA ALLERGY DERMATITIS (continued)

FLEA CONTROL	FLEA CONTROL on the ANIMAL
	Systemic medications • **Lufenuron** (Program®) is a once-a-month oral chitin synthesis inhibitor that prevents flea eggs from hatching. It does not kill the adult fleas, so if the pet is currently infested, an adulticide should also be used. Lufenuron is also combined with milbemycin oxime for canine heartworm control (Sentinel®). • **Nitenpyram** (Capstar®) blocks the nicotinic acetylcholine receptor in fleas. It's given daily or q 48 hours and is very effective. • **Spinosad** (Comfortis™) targets Ach receptors that are different from those targeted by other neonicotinoids and that are very specific to insects. It's starts acting as soon as 30 minutes and has a 100% knockdown in 4 hours. It's effective for a month. **Topical Treatments** • **Fipronil** (Frontline®) is a topical medication that kills both ticks and fleas in cats and dogs. It acts on insect GABA as a non-competitive blocker. It's administered once a month when used to control ticks and fleas on cats and dogs. (It can be used once every 3 months for fleas only in dogs.) Do not bathe 2 days prior to or after application. • **Imidacloprid** (Advantage®) is a topical medication that kills adult fleas in both cats and dogs. It's a competitive inhibitor of the nicotinic acetylcholine receptors in fleas (but not ticks). It's administered once a month. If dogs swim or are bathed frequently, then apply imidacloprid more frequently. Advantix® treats ticks as well for dogs. It contains permethrin and imidacloprid ((Avoid in cats) • **Selamectin** (Revolution®) is like ivermectin in that it inhibits the glutamate-gated Cl channels in neuronal cells, leading to flaccid paralysis. It works on flea, non–demodectic mites, and as heartworm prevention. It's safe in sensitive collies at up to $\geq$ 4x the recommended dose. • **Bathing:** Pets can be bathed weekly to get rid of fleas, flea dirt, and eggs, but the shampoos do not have any residual effect, so bathing must be paired with other treatments. Flea shampoos should contain pyrethrins or permethrins. Avoid permethrins in cats though. • **Flea spray or powder:** Pets can be sprayed 2-3x a week with a spray containing both an adulticide and an insect growth regulator (IGR) such as methoprene or pyriproxifen. Microencapsulated products have the most residual effect. **TREAT THE ENVIRONMENT** if the animal has FAD or if the infestation is moderate to severe. • **Vacuum** all carpets and **wash** all pet bedding. • **Area spray:** Spray the carpets and cracks (hardwood floors) with a combination adulticide and microencapsulated IGR (such as methoprene or pyriproxifen). • **Sodium polyborate** can be applied to all carpets instead of an insecticide, but it should be applied professionally (e.g., Fleabusters®). • **Spray the yard:** Treat the shaded areas of the yard, especially the areas pets frequent the most. Use insecticides such as the organophosphate malathion, or a combination adulticide and microencapsulated IGR, which is longer lasting. Another option is the application of beneficial nematodes (*Steinernema carpocapsae),* which parasitize a variety of insects including fleas. These nematodes die off once the area becomes too dry or the flea larvae and other hosts die off. They may need to be reapplied periodically because they are less heat and moisture tolerant than flea larvae.
PROVEN INEFFECTIVE TREATMENTS	Electronic flea collars, brewer's yeast, garlic, vitamin B tablets, sulfur, thiamine, and extracts of eucalyptus, are **not flea repellent** and provide no protection for the pet. Flea collars have poor efficacy.
OTHER FACTORS	**Avoid organophosphates** in dogs less than 6 months of age, in **cats**, and in households with **small children, pregnant women, or compromised individuals.** Pyrethrins and IGRs can be used in these situations. As a reasonable precaution, pregnant women and small children should not be involved in the application of the chemicals.

II. FOOD ALLERGY DERMATITIS

While food allergy is commonly listed as a cause of pruritus, some dermatologists in private practice feel that food allergy is rarely a cause of dermatologic signs.

PATHOGENESIS	Food allergy in man is primarily IgE-mediated (type I hypersensitivity) or an arthus (type III) response. Pathogenesis in animals is not completely understood.
CLINICAL FEATURES	**Pruritus** is the primary manifestation, although some animals may develop hives. Pruritus leads to self-trauma (alopecia, excoriation). Food allergy in cats has a predisposition for the head and neck. Both young animals and adults can be affected. Some clinicians believe that food allergy is more likely if signs of diarrhea, vomiting, or anal pruritus are seen along with dermatologic signs.
DIAGNOSIS	**History:** A gradual or sudden onset of symptoms involving only one animal on the premises. The animal has usually been on the diet for at least 3 months. The pruritus is non-seasonal. **Variable steroid responsiveness** (less responsive to steroids than is atopy) **An elimination diet for 8 weeks is the gold standard for diagnosing food allergy:** The test diet should contain only one novel protein and one novel carbohydrate source (1 pound protein:6 cups carbohydrates). Cats don't need a carbohydrate source. Novel proteins may include fish (unless fishmeal was in the diet), venison, duck, rabbit, pinto bean, or tofu (unless soy meal was in the diet). Novel carbohydrates may include potato and sweet potato. Once signs have resolved, the pet should be challenged with the potential allergen. The problem with homemade diets is that compliance is poor, and the diets are expensive. Thus, a commercial prescription hypoallergenic diet (e.g., IVD) or hydrolyzed protein diets can be used. Frequently, multiple diets must be tested sequentially. When on a test diet, no other proteins/carbohydrates should pass the pets lips. Avoid oral heartworm medications, vitamins, pig ears, treats, etc. Also, if the pet is on medications, ask the owners whether they hide the medication in food.

III. ATOPIC DERMATITIS

is an inherited condition in which the dog or cat is allergic to environmental allergens such as pollens, molds, and house dust mites that are inhaled, ingested, or absorbed percutaneously. An estimated 10% of dogs have atopy. The condition is lifelong, requiring lifelong management.

PATHOGENESIS	Susceptible animals produce more IgE or IgG antibody than normal ones. The animal comes into contact with or inhales the allergen, and B cells make allergen-specific IgE.
CLINICAL FEATURES	**Pruritus** or salivary staining occurs in light colored dogs due to licking pruritic areas. Lesions are distributed in the facial, pedal, axillary, and groin areas. Occasionally, the animals exhibits reverse sneezing, conjunctivitis, or rhinitis. **Age:** Animals over 6 months of age are most commonly affected, with pruritic symptoms usually beginning between 1-3 years. Occasionally, spontaneous remission occurs. Sudden worsening of signs may be caused by a secondary pyoderma, malassezia infection, or fleas.

Dermatology

ATOPIC DERMATITIS continued

DIAGNOSIS	**Steroid responsive:** Pets are less pruritic when on corticosteroids.
	Intradermal skin testing: Inject aqueous antigens intradermally and compare results with saline (- control) and histamine (+ control). Positive skin tests are graded from +1 to +4 based on size and thickness of the wheal and amount of erythema.
	A positive result only shows that the animal has skin-sensitization (IgE, IgG) antibodies and not necessarily that the skin problem is due to atopy. Interpret the result in light of the history and clinical signs. In addition, wait 3 weeks after oral steroid administration or 3 months after the effects of IM steroid administration have worn off to perform the skin testing. Wait one week after antihistamine administration before testing. A **radioallergosorbent test (RAST)** or ELISA measures relative levels of allergen-specific IgE in the serum of atopic dogs.
THERAPY	The goal of therapy is to keep the dog comfortably pruritic. We may not be able to get rid of all of the pruritus. Treat concomitant disease (flea allergy, pyoderma, etc.).
	Avoid the allergens: This is difficult, but any decrease may be helpful. If the animal has multiple allergies and you decrease one of the allergens, it may be enough so that the animal shows no signs. This is called the **threshold phenomenon.** Also treat for fleas and consider a hypoallergenic diet, as both can be a contributing factor due to the threshold phenomenon.
	Hyposensitization: In theory, with hyposensitization we present allergens SC so that IgG instead of IgE is made; thus, IgG can bind allergen before it reaches IgE in the skin. It's been speculated that success may be achieved by the production of T suppressor cells. Hyposensitization works in **60%** of affected animals, and if it does work, effectiveness is lifelong with continued therapy.
	MEDICAL THERAPY **Corticosteroids** are very effective. Use short-acting (prednisone and methylprednisolone) drugs on an alternate-day basis. When using corticosteroids, perform a urinalysis with urine culture every 6 months. When discontinuing long-term corticosteroids, make a slow withdrawal (i.e., over several weeks).
	Antihistamines are only about 10% effective but may decrease the need for corticosteroids. Examples of antihistamines used include: • Hydroxyzine (Atarax®): 2.2 mg/kg PO TID • Diphenhydramine (Benadryl®): 2.2 mg/kg PO TID • Clemastine (Tavist®): 0.05 mg/kg PO BID • Chlorpheniramine: 2 mg/cat PO BID and 0.5 mg/kg PO TID in dogs • Trimeprazine or trimeprazine/prednisone (Temaril® or Temaril-P®): Trimeprazine is a phenothiazine antihistamine.
	Most antihistamines given at high doses are mast cell stabilizers. Most—except for Tavist®, which does not cross the blood-brain barrier—cause drowsiness.
	Cyclosporine (Atopica®): 5 mg/kg PO SID (Follow labeled dosing recommendations). Atopica® is very expensive; thus, hyposensitization is often used first.
	Omega-3 and -6 fatty acids (Derm Caps®, 3V Caps®, EFA-Z®, etc.): Fish oils and linolenic acid are anti-pruritic. Omega-6 fatty acids (safflower oil, linoleic acid, evening primrose) promote healthy skin, but can supposedly cause pruritus at high doses.

III. ALLERGIC CONTACT DERMATITIS (ACD) is very rare.

INTRODUCTION	ACD is a delayed hypersensitivity reaction (type IV) in which a sensitized animal reacts to a non-irritating concentration of an offending agent.
ETIOLOGY and PATHOGENESIS	Offending agents are usually simple chemicals (haptens that come into contact with epidermal or other proteins). They're taken up by Langerhans cells and are carried to local lymph nodes. Antigen-specific lymphocytes are attracted to the site of future contact with the hapten, and within 12-72 hours of exposure the animal becomes pruritic due to release of mediators.
CLINICAL FEATURES	The animal's coat usually protects the body against many common contact allergens unless the allergens are applied as shampoos, rinses, dips, or perfumes. Lesions are usually in **the hairless regions** such as the muzzle, ears, under the tail, groin, genitals, axilla, and between the toes. **Acute lesions** result in erythema, pruritus, and papules or vesicles **Chronic lesions** result in alopecia, lichenification, hyperpigmentation, etc.
PREDISPOSING FACTORS	• Moisture (decreases the normal skin barrier and increases the contact surface) • Dose, concentration, duration of contact • Skin irritation or trauma
COMMON CONTACTANTS	**Dogs:** Medications, cedar chips, fertilizers, plants (jasmine, wandering jew, etc.), hair spray, vinyl resins (food dishes) **Cats:** Kitty litter, coal tar products, sulfur compounds, carpet fresheners, cement, medications (neomycin)
DIAGNOSIS	**Clinical signs and history:** A detailed history is extremely important. Ask about the animal's bedding, daytime areas, and direct contact substances (shampoos, collars, medications, etc.). Ask whether the onset was gradual or immediate. Many allergies occur to substances that aren't new in the animal's environment. **Patch testing:** Use open or closed patch testing with original or standardized extracts. Apply potential allergens to the skin surface for 48-72 hours. Monitor signs of delayed hypersensitivity. **Isolation and provocative testing:** Gradually remove substances or change the environment. You can hospitalize the animal for 5-15 days and then reintroduce the animal into different sections of its normal environment. **Histopathology** is consistent with allergy. You may find acanthosis, hyperkeratosis, or perivascular and perifollicular infiltrates of lymphocytes and macrophages ± neutrophils and eosinophils. **Irritant contact dermatitis results in the same types of lesions but occurs in all animals that have been exposed.**
THERAPY	Avoid the offending agent if possible. Apply topical or systemic corticosteroids (palliative only).

Dermatology

MITES AFFECTING DOGS and CATS
Canine Demodicosis
Canine Scabies (Sarcoptic Acariasis)
Feline Scabies (Notoedres)
Cheyletiellosis
Otodectosis

I. CANINE DEMODICOSIS

AGENT	Demodectic mites are part of the normal fauna of canine skin. It's thought that animals develop demodectic mange when they are immunosuppressed or immunodeficient. The immunosuppression may allow the mites to increase in number.
PREDILECTION	**Hereditary:** Demodicosis is seen more commonly in certain breeds and certain lines of dogs. Do not breed dogs that have had generalized (and possibly localized) demodicosis. **Immunosuppressed animals** • Young and old dogs • Dogs on anti-neoplastic drugs or high doses of corticosteroids • Dogs with Cushing's disease or hypothyroidism • Dogs with cancer
TRANSMISSION	Demodicosis isn't contagious. The bitch transfers the mites to the puppies within the first 3 days of life. Stillborn and cesarean puppies are mite free.
CLINICAL SIGNS	**LESIONS** • **Alopecia, crusting, erythema** ± pruritus, comedones, and pain. • **Comedones** (blackheads) are comprised of the mite bodies, epithelial cells, sebum, and inflammatory cells. If you squeeze out the debris onto a drop of mineral oil and then put it on a slide, you may observe mites. **SITES** • Sites for **LOCALIZED demodex:** head, forelegs, groin, and trunk. Some dogs only have paw (**pododemodicosis**) or ear (**otodemodicosis**) involvement. • In **GENERALIZED cases** lesions may span the body, in which case the dog should also have **lymphadenopathy** (otherwise he is not mounting an immune response). **PYODERMA** • **Secondary pyoderma:** If you see pyoderma in odd regions, consider demodex. If the folliculitis develops into furunculosis, you will feel nodules (granular or pyogranulomatous).
DIAGNOSIS	**Skin scraping:** Take a deep skin scraping in the middle of the lesion. Look for eggs, nymphs, and adult mites. When the mite dies, the skeleton persists for a week. Presence of only one mite or one egg may indicate the disease is clearing up, or if appropriate clinical signs are lacking, it may represent normal flora. **A biopsy** reveals mites within hair follicles. It may also show a mononuclear perifollicular response and evidence of pyoderma (folliculitis/furuncuolosis).
PROGNOSIS	**Localized:** Prognosis is good. Most cases of localized demodicosis spontaneously clear, but 5-10% of cases become generalized. **Generalized:** Most dogs respond to treatment. Some breeds of dogs are known to have slowly developing immune systems, so that they may self-cure at an older age.

CANINE DEMODICOSIS (continued)

TREATMENT of LOCALIZED DEMODICOSIS	**Benign neglect:** Although localized demodicosis usually spontaneously clear, you may elect to treat so that the owner will feel like he/she is doing something. It also prevents the owner from using harsher products on the animal and from blaming you later if the problem gets worse. **Benzoyl peroxide** shampoo and ointment provide good follicular flushing action and prevent secondary bacterial infection. **Rotenone ointment** (Goodwinol®): Rub the ointment in a circle larger than the lesion until you can no longer see the ointment. Any ointment visible is not doing any good. The animal will lose some hair in the area you rub due to local irritation. **Corticosteroids are contraindicated** **Amitraz dips (Mitaban®) and systemic treatment are not recommended** unless the demodex becomes generalized. Do not spot treat with Mitaban® because, while the concentration of amitraz will be high at the area of contact, it will be more dilute as it gets further away from the site of application. The dilution may induce resistance or select for resistant mites.
TREATMENT of GENERALIZED DEMODICOSIS	• **Corticosteroids are contraindicated.** • **Clip long-haired dogs** (once a month) to allow the medication (shampoo or Mitaban dip) to penetrate into the hair follicles. • **Shampoo** with **benzoyl peroxide shampoo** to kill the bacteria, clean debris, and flush keratin and mites out of the hair follicle prior to dipping the dog with miticidal. Soaks or whirlpool baths may be used. • **Antibiotics:** Use systemic antibiotics in cases of secondary pyoderma. • **Ivermectin** (400-600 μg/kg PO SID): Use ivermectin until monthly skin scrapes are negative on two consecutive tests. Do not use ivermectin in sensitive collies or Shetland Sheepdogs. Some carry a mutation of the multidrug resistance (mdr1) gene. The gene encodes for p-glycoprotein, which transports drugs from the brain back into the blood, thus preventing levels from accumulating in the brain. A commercial test is available for detecting the mutation (Washington State University Clinical Pathology Lab). • **Milbemycin oxime** (0.5-2.0 mg/kg/day) can be tolerated in some ivermectin-sensitive dogs but is expensive. • **Moxidectin and doramectin** are other drugs that can be used. • **Amitraz** (Mitaban®) **miticidal dip** is still used but less frequently than oral treatments. Dip the dog approximately every 7-14 days using 1 vial of amitraz per 2 gallons of water. (250 ppm = .025%. This is the manufacturer's recommended dose.) In refractory cases, 1 vial/gallon (500 ppm) can be used every 7 days. Amitraz is a monoamine oxidase inhibitor (yohimbine is the antidote) with the following side effects: • Depression, sleepiness • Anorexia, PU/PD, urinary incontinence • Ataxia and other neurologic signs • Death (more likely in dogs under 20 pounds) • Transient pruritus Combining amitraz with ivermectin or milbemycin is not more effective than either treatment alone. **End-point for treatment:** Treat 2 months beyond negative skin scrapings for juvenile onset and 3 months beyond for adult onset. **Long-term follow up:** 1 year minimum

Dermatology

II. CANINE SCABIES (SARCOPTIC ACARIASIS)

AGENT	*Sarcoptes scabei* affects primarily dogs and rarely cats. Infestation in humans is uncommon and self-limiting. The mites are transmitted by direct contact. Fomites are of minimal importance.
CLINICAL SIGNS	• Acute onset of intense pruritus caused by hypersensitivity to burrowing mites. • Erythematous maculopapular rash, ± alopecia, crusting: The areas most often affected include the **ventral chest and abdomen** as well as the **lateral elbows, hocks, and pinnae**. Rubbing **ear margins** often elicits a scratch response. Presence of severe pruritus and papules without alopecia is reason to suspect scabies because scabies mites do not affect the hair follicles. That is, animals with scabies may or may not have alopecia whereas with demodicosis the animal is alopecic because the demodex mites affect the hair follicles.
PATHOGENESIS	Mite eggs are laid in epidermal tunnels made by the fertilized female mite. After 3-5 days, the larvae crawl onto the skin surface and burrow into the superficial layers of the skin where they molt to nymphs and then to adults. The adult mites return to the surface to breed. As the mites burrow into the epidermis, they cause mechanical and chemical damage (from salivary secretion). The host may develop a **hypersensitivity** reaction to the allergens. The lesions are often due to self-trauma.
DIAGNOSIS	History of acute onset of **severe pruritus** in a dog recently exposed to other dogs (kennel or pet store situation), or onset of pruritus in **both dogs and humans in a household.** Multiple superficial skin scrapings (e.g. 10) of various regions. Scrapings can be placed on one slide containing mineral oil. A few mites can cause severe disease and can be difficult to observe in skin scrapings; thus, sarcoptic acariasis is often misdiagnosed as food allergy, atopy, or FAD. The location of lesions, severity of the pruritus, and history of coming from a kennel situation strongly suggest scabies. Diagnosis is often based on **response to treatment.**
TREATMENT	Corticosteroids: A short course of corticosteroids can be used to relieve the pruritus and inflammation caused by trauma and hypersensitivity. In dogs, 1.0 mg/kg per day for 1-2 weeks may be needed as there is a 1-2 week lag period in treatment success. Systemic antibiotics: Use in cases of 2° bacterial infections. Shampoo: Use cleansing shampoos (benzoyl peroxide) to remove debris. You may need to clip long-haired dogs. Acaricidal compounds: Treat all dogs in the environment with acaricidal compounds such as: • Ivermectin: Administer 300 µg/kg PO or SC every 1-2 weeks for four treatments since the life cycle lasts 6-21 days. The pruritus should decline quickly. Avoid ivermectin in collies, Shelties, and other dogs with the mdr-1 mutation (For more info refer to parasitology p. 17.10, section C.1.a). • Lime sulfur: Soak in 2-3% solution and repeat weekly x 4 weeks. • Organophosphate dip: Treat weekly for 4 weeks. • Amitraz rinse (0.025%): Dip every 2 weeks for 3 treatments.

III. FELINE SCABIES (*NOTOEDRES*) is rare.

AGENT	*Notoedres cati* is a sarcoptid mite that is highly contagious in cats (primarily sick, adult cats). Dogs rarely develop disease, but humans can become infested (self-limiting).
LOCATION	The mite burrows into the skin on the ears, head, and back of the neck.
CLINICAL SIGNS	Extreme pruritus ± severe self-trauma Lesions: Scaling, thick, yellow-gray crusts; alopecia; lichenification of the skin on the ears, head, back of the neck, and distal extremities
DIAGNOSIS	History of contact with affected animals, strays, boarding kennel Skin scraping: Mites are easily seen in high numbers.
THERAPY	• Corticosteroids: Short course to relieve the pruritus and inflammation • Antibiotics for secondary bacterial infection • Ivermectin: 300 µg/kg SC or PO every two weeks for two injections. This can be used in cats 4 weeks and older. • Clean the environment thoroughly and treat all cats in contact with the affected cat.

IV. CHEYLETIELLOSIS

Cheyletiella is a species of mite that can cause contagious infestations in cats, dogs (rare), and rabbits (occasionally). The mites are readily transferred from pets to humans.

LOCATION	Primarily on the fur, but the mites visit the skin to feed. They only invade the **stratum corneum**.
CLINICAL SIGNS	• Pruritus • **Walking dandruff:** The mites look like powdery skin scales that are shed into the hair or fur. • Occasionally, in severe cases that involve large areas of skin, there may be **crust** formation and hair loss.
DIAGNOSIS	• Consider Cheyletiellosis whenever a dog or cat has excessive dandruff. Part the hair along the back over the sacrum and comb the scruff onto dark paper. See if the **"dandruff"** walks. You may have to wait a long time to see them walk. • **Scraping** is usually not necessary since the mites are always on the skin surface or in the coat, but you can do a superficial skin scraping to find *Cheyletiella*. • **Scotch tape** may be necessary to obtain mites.
TREATMENT	• Mites are easily destroyed by most **insecticides** such as flea sprays or dip (pyrethrins and lime sulfur dips are safe on cats and rabbits). Treat 3x/week with sprays or 1x/week with dips. • **Ivermectin** SC (300 µg/kg), repeated in 2 weeks, is effective in cats and dogs. • Treat all pets in the environment, clean the premises, and improve sanitation (Mites can live up to 10 days in the environment).
ZOONOSIS	May be the most readily transferable mange mite from domestic animals to humans. The mites can penetrate clothing and are easily transferred even with short periods of contact. Humans get severe irritation and intense pruritus. Cases in humans invariably clear up when the animal source is treated.

V. OTODECTOSIS (Ear Mites)

Otodectes cynotis, a mite that feeds on blood, lymph, and debris in the ear canal, is responsible for 50% of the otitis externa cases in cats (mostly kittens) and a small percentage of cases in dogs. The mites irritate the ceruminous glands of the aural skin and cause a dark brown crust comprised of excessive cerumen, epidermal scales, and inflammatory exudates. These signs are most likely due to hypersensitivity; therefore, in some cases (primarily with dogs), mites may be difficult to identify on ear cytology. *Otodectes* mites can occasionally leave the inflamed ear canal and then inhabit ectopic sites. In cats, ectopic infestations are seen occasionally on the neck, head, distal limbs, and lumbosacral region.

CLINICAL SIGNS	• Intense irritation and thick crusts in the ears of dogs and cats. The ears fill with crusts and cerumen. • **Sites:** Mites are commonly found in the external ear canal, neck, rump, and tail. Some cases resemble flea bite hypersensitivity.
DIAGNOSIS	**Smear of otic exudate:** Visualize mites and mite eggs. Because signs are due in part to hypersensitivity, we don't always find mites in the smear (especially with dogs).
TREATMENT	• **Corticosteroids:** You may need to use a short course of corticosteroids to make the animal comfortable. • Treat affected animals and contact animals with **insecticides** (flea powder, dip, spray, such as pyrethrins) repeatedly for 4 weeks. • **Clean the environment.** • **Clean the ears daily and then treat affected ears** once with a miticide such as Acarex® (pyrethrins). Recheck in 1-2 weeks. • **Ivermectin** [200-400 µg/kg (0.2 -0.4 mg/kg)] works for otodectic mange in dogs and cats. Treat all household animals.
ZOONOSIS	Ear mites are highly contagious and especially prevalent in the young. Many species of carnivores can be infested since the mites are not host specific.

Dermatology

IMMUNE-MEDIATED SKIN DISEASES

Bullous Immune-mediated Skin Diseases
Pemphigus Foliaceus
Pemphigus Vulgaris
Bullous Pemphigoid
Non-Bullous Immune-mediated Diseases
Discoid Lupus Erythematosus (DLE)
Systemic Lupus Erythematosus (SLE)

I. BULLOUS and PUSTULAR IMMUNE-MEDIATED SKIN DISEASES (pemphigus foliaceus, pemphigus vulgaris, and bullous pemphigoid): Bullous immune-mediated skin diseases are comparatively rare, blistering diseases in which the animal develops auto-antibodies against various skin antigens. All of these diseases are erosive and/or ulcerative. Vesicles and bullae form but are transient in animals. **The only one of these diseases that we see with any frequency is pemphigus foliaceus.**

	PEMPHIGUS FOLIACEUS	PEMPHIGUS VULGARIS	BULLOUS PEMPHIGOID
SIGNALMENT	Most common immune-mediated skin disease in the dog and cat	Severe but very rare. Affects old and middle-aged dogs and cats.	Very rare
CLINICAL FEATURES	Pustules, vesicles, erosions. Pustules may span many hair follicles. May involve only the feet. Seldom has oral or mucocutaneous lesions but often has footpad hyperkeratosis. Lesions may involve just the nail bed.	Erosions, ulcerations of the oral mucosa, mucocutaneous junctions, and skin. 90% of dogs and cats affected have oral lesions. Lesions are very painful.	Vesicles, erosions, and ulcers of the mucocutaneous junction and skin.
DIAGNOSIS	Biopsy: Subcorneal pustules and acantholysis. IgG, C3 IFA honeycomb pattern due to antibodies against the antigens of the keratinocyte desmosomes. Sometimes lesions are localized to the upper epidermis.	Nikolsky's sign* Biopsy: suprabasilar acantholysis leading to intraepidermal clefts. Infiltration of dermis with plasma cells and lymphocytes. IgG, C3 honeycomb pattern (antigens of the keratinocyte membrane are affected).	Biopsy: Subepidermal clefts and vesicle formation. IgG and IgM or C3 IFA-positive at the basement membrane.
PROGNOSIS	Guarded but better than pemphigus vulgaris. Many animals recover.	Grave. This disease is very difficult to treat.	Grave. This disease is very difficult to treat.

* Nikolsky's sign: Transverse pressure on the lesions can make the epidermis slip off.

A. TREATMENT
1. If you suspect pemphigus foliaceus, **stop all medications first.** Pemphigus foliaceus can occasionally be drug-induced. If it is, the lesions will start to heal within 2 weeks.
2. **Shampoo treatment** can be used to help remove the crusts.
3. **Treat secondary pyoderma** with systemic antibiotics for a minimum of 4 weeks. Treat until the immunosuppressive therapy is controlling the disease.
4. **Glucocorticoids:** Use immunosuppressive doses. 2.2-4.4 mg/kg prednisolone or prednisone PO SID for dogs and 4.4-6.6 mg/kg orally SID for cats (theoretically, prednisolone should be used in cats). Start with a 2-week course of corticosteroids. In many animals, complete remission of signs occurs during this time, but it may take up to 8 weeks. Once the animal is in complete remission, taper the corticosteroid dose over 2-3 months until you reach the lowest possible dose (e.g. q 48 hours). Recheck the animal in 1 month. If the lesions don't respond to corticosteroid treatment, add another immunomodulator. It's best to use other immunomodulators in combination with prednisone for long-term therapy to avoid the long-term effect of prednisone. Other glucocorticoids such as triamcinolone and dexamethasone can be used, too (primarily in cats).

5. Other **immunomodulators:**
    a. **Azathioprine** (Imuran®) 2.2 mg/kg PO SID for 14 days then every 48 hours in dogs only. Azathioprine causes diarrhea, vomiting, and myelosuppression (leukopenia, thrombocytopenia, anemia), which is irreversible in cats. Monitor the CBC monthly for 3 months and then once every 3 months. Most bone marrow suppression occurs within the first 3 months.
    b. **Chlorambucil** (Leukeran®) 0.1-0.2 mg/kg PO SID, then every 48 hours (usually for cats).
    c. **Aurothioglucose** (Solganol®) is rarely effective.
    d. **Cyclosporine** in dogs and cats: 2.5-5 mg/kg PO BID.
6. Treat for **secondary bacterial infection** with antibiotics for 3-6 weeks. Consider performing a culture.

II. **NON-BULLOUS CANINE IMMUNE-MEDIATED DISEASES:** Discoid lupus erythematosus (DLE) and systemic lupus erythematosus (SLE). DLE is seen by some as a more benign variant of SLE.

	DISCOID LUPUS ERYTHEMATOSUS	SYSTEMIC LUPUS ERYTHEMATOSUS
PREDILECTIONS	Animals living in sunny areas Collie, German Shepherd, Husky, Australian Shepherd, Sheltie	Same as with DLE
CLINICAL SIGNS	Symmetrical lesions primarily of the face (dorsum of the muzzle, planum nasale, periorbital regions, and ears) **Depigmentation**, erythema, alopecia, crusting, ± oral mucosa involvement and mucocutaneous involvement Photoaggravated dermatitis	Same cutaneous lesions as with DLE, but the animal also has signs of systemic auto-immune disease such as thrombocytopenia, AIHA, polyarthritis, glomerulonephritis, etc.
DIAGNOSIS	Biopsy: Liquefaction degeneration of the basal layer. Pigment incontinence, thickened basement membrane zone. Lymphoplasmacytic dermal perivascular infiltrate. IFA: Positive basement membrane zone in the involved areas only (IgG, C3), **"lupus band"**	Same as with DLE **ANA positive** **LE preparation positive** 50% of the time. This test is difficult to interpret.

A. **SKIN BIOPSY:** It's best to take a non-nasal biopsy. When biopsying, sample an area that is just beginning to depigment (starting to grey; i.e., an area of pigment incontinence).

B. **THERAPY** is palliative. Often our goal is just to make the animal feel 80% better because the amount of therapy needed for 80% improvement is much lower (5x lower) than that needed for 100% recovery. For mild cases in which the damage is only cosmetic, we may not even need immunosuppressive drugs. In most cases, therapy is lifelong.
    1. **Discoid lupus erythematosus**
        a. **Avoid sunlight.**
        b. **Topical and systemic corticosteroids:** Start with low doses and as the lesions heal, decrease the dose even more.
        c. **Vitamin E:** 400-800 units BID (No data supports this.)
        d. **Water-resistant sunscreens** (guide number > 20). Apply the sunscreen just before feeding or playing so that the dog won't lick it off. Apply it 15-20 minutes before the dog goes outside.
        e. **Topical tacrolimus (Protopic®)** is an immunosuppressant.
    2. **Systemic lupus erythematosus:** Use systemic corticosteroids at immunosuppressive doses. If the animal just has nasal depigmentation, you don't need to use immunomodulators such as Imuran®.

Dermatology

OTITIS EXTERNA

Otitis externa—inflammation of the epithelium of the external auditory meatus ± the pinna of the ear— usually involves infection with mites, bacteria, or yeast. While mites are often a primary cause of otitis (cats), bacterial and yeast infections usually occur secondary to some predisposing factor or disease (e.g., allergy, ear conformation). The predisposing factor alters the ear canal environment allowing opportunistic infections and pathologic changes that often complicate resolution of the ear inflammation.

CLINICAL SIGNS	Clinical signs are caused primarily by pruritus and pain, which lead to self-trauma. • **Head-shaking** and scratching the ears • **Erythema, alopecia, excoriations, lichenification** of the pinnae and periauricular region • **Ear exudate:** may be dry and crusty or wet, and may vary in color from yellow/green to brown/black
PREDISPOSING FACTORS	**EAR CONFORMATION and EXCESSIVE MOISTURE:** Stenotic ear canals, dense hairs within the ears, and floppy, hanging ears decrease the air flow and increase humidity within the ears. The result is excessive moisture, which can lead to maceration of the otic epithelium predisposing the ear to opportunistic microbial colonization and infection. Swimming/bathing or increased environmental humidity can also contribute to excessive moisture within the ear canals. **HYPERSENSITIVITY** • **Atopy:** Up to 73% or more of atopic dogs develop otitis externa. In the early stages, the inner ear and pinna may be only mildly erythematous with little or no exudate. This often develops into a prominent bacterial or yeast infection. Sometimes otitis externa is the only clinical sign of atopy. Atopy is not curable; rather, management is lifelong. Thus, the ears may need lifelong management. • **Food allergy** is also associated with otitis externa but less commonly. • **Contact allergy** is an uncommon cause of otitis externa. Suspect contact allergy when a patient's ears get dramatically worse shortly after treatment with a topical ear medication. **PARASITES** (mites and ticks—also refer to p. 7.13 on mites) • *Otodectes cynotis,* a mite that feeds on blood, lymph, and debris in the ear canal, is a common cause of otitis in kittens (It rarely affects dogs.). • *Otobius megnini,* the spinous ear tick of dogs, can be found on dogs and less commonly on cats. Clinical signs include acute, severe pruritus. • **Other parasites that may occasionally infect the ear canal include:** *Sarcoptes scabei, Notoedres cati, Demodex canis,* and *D. cati* **FOREIGN BODY** (e.g., foxtail), **POLYP** (inflammatory or epithelial), OR TUMOR **IMMUNE-MEDIATED DISORDERS** (Pemphigus, discoid or systemic lupus erythematosus, drug reactions): These disorders usually involve other parts of the body too. **CORNIFICATION DEFECTS** are characterized by an increased epidermal turnover rate. Changes in otic glandular secretions occur in certain seborrheic diseases, resulting in ceruminous otitis externa. **ENDOCRINE DISORDERS** (e.g., hypothyroidism): Some of these animals also have seborrhea.
BACTERIAL and YEAST INFECTIONS	**BACTERIAL OTITIS EXTERNA:** In dogs, *Staphylococcus* is the most common bacteria involved in acute infections, while *Proteus, Pseudomonas,* and other Gram-negative bacteria are the most common bacteria found in chronic infections. In cats, *Staphylococcus* and *Pasteurella* are the most common isolates. **YEAST:** *Malassezia pachydermatis* is isolated from the ear canals of 50-70% of dogs with otitis externa. Pure infections with *Malassezia* result in the development of copious, dark brown, sweet-smelling exudate. Other fungal organisms (e.g., *Candida)* are rarely involved.

OTITIS EXTERNA (continued)

APPROACH to OTITIS EXTERNA	History: Look for evidence of predisposing factors.
	Examine the external pinnae. Look for masses, ticks, alopecia, erythema, and discharge.
	Otoscopic exam: Look for **foreign bodies, polyps, tumors,** and exudate within the ear canals and evaluate the tympanic membrane. Often the tympanic membrane is obscured by debris, in which case the ear must be cleaned first and then re-examined.
	Cytologic exam: Take a smear of the exudate and/or any crusts, and stain for bacteria and fungi. Also look for ear mites.
	Skin scrape: If the pinna is lichenified, or it's erythematous and the animal is very pruritic in other areas of its body, too, perform a skin scrape for mites.
	Remove foreign bodies (e.g., foxtail).
	
	Clean the ears: If the ears contain a lot of waxy-thick debris, apply a ceruminolytic agent such as:
	  • Dioctyl sodium sulfosuccinate (DSS)
	  • Squalene
	  • Detergent (e.g., triethanolamine polypeptide oleate)
	  • Carbamide peroxide
	Once the debris is softened, irrigate the ear with an otic cleansing agent or one of the following:
	  • **Warm water** and isotonic (0.8%) or hypertonic (3%) **saline** are non-irritating and should be used when the animal has a **ruptured tympanic membrane** (saline is less irritating).
	  • **Povidone iodine** (5% or 0.5%) titratable iodine (Betadine solution) is often used as a flushing solution. Its antimicrobial activity lasts 6-8 hours.
	  • **Chlorhexidine** (0.5%-1%) provides better results as an antiseptic than povidone iodine and does not elicit a hypersensitivity response. It's a good antibacterial, but may cause delayed epithelialization. It may be ototoxic.
	Once the ear is cleaned and dried, you should be able to evaluate the tympanic membrane.
	Treat the ear for the specific problem (e.g., bacteria or yeast infection or mites) and look for underlying etiologies.

CLEANING (HOME-CARE)	CLEANING and DRYING AGENTS for IRRIGATING the EAR: With many ear infections, the owner must clean the ears 1-2 times per day for several weeks using a solution that contains a cleaning agent ± a drying agent. The following irrigating solutions are acidifying agents. Acidification is good against yeast and Gram-negative bacterial infections.
	  • Chlorhexidine and povidone iodine are **antibacterial and antimycotic.**
	  • Alcohol is a good cleaning and drying agent for the removal of waxy or oily debris, and it has short-term antibacterial properties. In it's pure form, however, it can be irritating.
	  • Lactic and salicylic acids are good keratolytics or keratoplastics.
	  • Boric acid has some astringent properties.
	  • Acetic acid is an **antibacterial** that kills *Pseudomonas* (2% solution) and Staphylococcus (5% solution).
	
	Be sure the owner massages the horizontal canal to loosen up wax buildup and then tilts the ear or lets the dog shake its head before swabbing cleaner from the external ear. Owners can also be taught to clean using a bulb syringe with water/saline (1:1) after the cleanser or ceruminolytic is used. To demonstrate correct pressure, have the owner squeeze air out of the bulb. They should not hear air hissing out of the bulb. To ascertain that they are cleaning the ear effectively, have them bring their dog in the same day they clean the ear. If the ear canal is not clean, reinstruct them on the technique or change techniques. Some dogs may need intermittent hospital cleaning. In cases of chronic otitis externa, once the infection is cleared the cleaning schedule can be decreased to weekly until the ear's normal self-cleaning ability returns. To determine when this has occurred, recheck the ears 2 weeks after the last cleaning. If it's still clean, recheck again in 6-8 weeks.

Dermatology

Dermatology: **Otitis Externa:** Page 3 of 3

OTITIS EXTERNA (continued)

TREATMENT	**TOPICAL ANTI-INFLAMMATORY AGENTS:** Use corticosteroids when there's a lot of inflammation, especially when the ear canal is obstructed by inflammation. They can be used alone in uncomplicated ceruminous or allergic otitis externa. • **Mometasone furoate** (Mometamax®) • **Fluocinolone acetonide** (Synotic™) • **Betamethasone valerate** (Otomax®) Start with SID-BID treatment. In case of atopy, once signs are controlled, go to SID. If long-term treatment is required, then switch to a lower strength corticosteroid such as 1% hydrocortisone. In severe cases of chronic, hyperplastic otitis externa, intralesional triamcinolone (0.05-0.1 mL/injection) can be used under anesthesia before opting for surgery. Injections are placed in a ring (2-3 injections/ring) at multiple levels (approximately 1 cm apart) in the ear canal. Recheck in several days and repeat in regions that have not responded well. Repeat in 2 weeks when the triamcinolone effects wear off. Oral corticosteroids for 2-4 weeks can be used too. **TOPICAL ANTIBACTERIAL AGENTS** • **Gentamicin/neomycin** is broad-spectrum and kills Gram-negative bacteria. It is ototoxic when used in dogs with ruptured tympanic membranes. Ototoxicity has also occurred within short periods of time in dogs with intact tympanic membranes. • **Enrofloxacin** is also broad-spectrum. • **Polymyxin B** works on **Gram-negative bacteria.** • **Chloramphenicol** works on **Gram-positive bacteria** and most **Gram-negative bacteria** are susceptible, too. **TOPICAL ANTIFUNGAL AGENTS** • **Imidazoles:** Miconazole (Conofite®), thiabendazole, and clotrimazole are good broad-spectrum antifungal agents. • **Amphotericin B** 3% (Fungizone® cream or lotion) is effective against *Candida* and *Aspergillus spp.* **TOPICAL ANTIPARASITIC TREATMENTS** • **Otodectes cynotis:** Use otic **pyrethrin** preparations or give one injection of **ivermectin** (300 µg/kg SC). Recheck in 2 weeks and re-treat if needed. • **Tick infestations in the ears:** Mechanically remove the ticks and then use topical anti-inflammatory medications. Treat all household animals with total body insecticidal dips or with Frontline® (or in dogs only, Advantix®¹). Also treat the premises.
OTITIS MEDIA	Otitis media most commonly results as an extension of otitis externa. When a tear is seen in the tympanic membrane, assume otitis media is present. It may also be present with intact tympanic membranes if infection was present and the membrane ruptured and then healed. Ruptured tympanic membranes are common with chronic otitis. They require deep cleaning and long-term antibiotics, often for more than 4 months. **CLEANING** can be performed using an ear flushing machine or a feeding tube (5, 8, or 10 french) and a 12-mL syringe. Infuse saline or water and aspirate the fluid out repeatedly. Vestibular syndrome can occur even when ototoxic drugs are not used; however, this complication is rare with deep ear cleaning. **SYSTEMIC ANTI-INFLAMMATORIES:** Otitis media requires systemic anti-inflammatories. Start with an induction dose for the first 4-7 days, and then go to a maintenance dose. • Prednisolone: 1-2 mg/kg • Methylprednisolone: 0.8-1.8 mg/kg • Dexamethasone: 0.025-0.1 mg/kg • Triamcinolone: 0.1-0.2 mg/kg

7.18

PYODERMA in DOGS
General Information
Features of Pyoderma
Diagnosis and Treatment

I. **GENERAL INFORMATION:** Pyoderma is a bacterial infection (with pus-producing bacteria) of the skin. It is characterized by pustules and crusted papules; however, pustules need not be seen to diagnose pyoderma. Pustules are often not visible because they may be microscopic in size (identifiable only on histopathology) and because they rupture easily, producing a crust. Furthermore, the presence of pustules is not pathognomonic for pyoderma. Pustules may be seen in other situations, too, including infections with demodex or dermatophytes and auto-immune skin diseases. More than 90% of pyodermas are caused by *Staphylococcus intermedius.* Those with Gram-negative organisms usually contain *Proteus* and *Pseudomonas.* Pyodermas with *Proteus* and *Pseudomonas* can be secondary to infections with *Staphylococcus.*

A. **PREDISPOSING FACTORS:** A number of factors can predispose an animal to developing pyoderma and can make it difficult to cure. Some predisposing factors include:
    1. **Inflammation** from any cause, even if the inflammation is not visible as erythema
    2. **Pruritus** from any cause (e.g., flea allergy dermatitis), especially in the groin and axillary region
    3. **Poor grooming,** especially in long-coated dogs
    4. **Seborrhea** is a disorder of cornification. Areas of seborrhea containing *S. intermedius* are pyodermas waiting to happen.
    5. **Endocrine diseases** such as hypothyroidism and Cushing's disease
    6. **Immunologic defects,** especially defects in T-lymphocyte function
    7. **Medications,** especially glucocorticoid therapy. This is more likely in animals injected with long-acting corticosteroids such as methylprednisolone acetate (Depo-medrol®) to decrease their allergy-induced pruritus.

B. **CLASSIFICATION of PYODERMAS:** Pyodermas can be classified by their depth of involvement. This is a clinically useful classification.

CLASSIFICATION of PYODERMAS

SURFACE PYODERMA	SUPERFICIAL PYODERMA	DEEP PYODERMA
Acute moist dermatitis (hot spot) **Intertrigo** (skin fold pyoderma) • Lip fold • Facial fold • Vulvar fold • Tail fold	**Impetigo** (superficial pyoderma consisting of non-follicular pustules) **Superficial folliculitis** (follicular pustules) **Superficial spreading pyoderma** (spreads beneath the stratum corneum)	**Deep folliculitis and furunculosis** • Canine acne • Nasal pyodermas • Pressure point pyoderma • Interdigital pyoderma • Generalized furunculosis **Cellulitis** –(deep infections dissect deep tissue layers)

1. **Surface pyodermas** are bacterial infections that don't invade living tissue. That is, the infections are limited to the non-living portion of the epithelium (stratum corneum).
2. **Superficial pyodermas** are bacterial infections located within the skin below the stratum corneum down to and including the intact hair follicle. Most canine pyodermas are superficial pyodermas.
3. **Deep pyodermas** are bacterial infections located deeper than the hair follicles. They may involve furunculosis (cases where the bottom of the hair follicle ruptures allowing bacteria to invade deep layers of the skin). The deeper the pyoderma, the more likely that it's secondary to something else and the more difficult it is to treat. Dogs may die from the septicemia that results from deep pyodermas.

Dermatology

II. **FEATURES of PYODERMA** (Treatments are considered later in this section.)
   A. **SURFACE PYODERMAS** are bacterial infections that are limited to the surface and stratum corneum of the skin. The two categories of surface pyoderma include acute moist dermatitis and intertrigo.

SURFACE PYODERMAS

	FEATURES	MANAGEMENT CONSIDERATIONS
ACUTE MOIST DERMATITIS (hot spot)	These surface lesions are produced by self-trauma as the patient tries to alleviate pain or pruritus from an underlying etiology (e.g., flea allergy). **Lesions:** The typical lesion is alopecic, red, moist, and exudative. The lesion and the surrounding non-affected area are sharply delineated. A true hot spot (surface pyoderma) is fairly flat and ulcerated or eroded. Lesions that are thickened and contain papules or pustules at their borders may indicate a **superficial pyoderma** rather than just a surface pyoderma. The lesions have a **rapid onset** and may be located in areas near the primary problem (e.g., in animals with flea allergy dermatitis, the hot spots may be located on the dorsal rump).	Hot spots that are thickened and contain papules or pustules around their borders most likely involve **superficial pyodermas** and should be treated as such (with systemic antibiotics). Hot spots usually have an underlying etiology. **Flea allergy dermatitis** is the most common, but other causes include poor grooming, skin irritants, and pruritus of any cause (atopy, food allergy, etc.). If the underlying etiology is not determined and treated, the hot spots will be difficult to treat successfully. In cases of persistent or recurrent hot spots with no underlying cause, you may elect to perform a skin scraping, fungal and bacterial cultures, and a biopsy to rule out: • superficial or deep pyoderma • demodicosis • dermatophytosis • neoplasia
INTERTRIGO	Intertrigo occurs from skin constantly rubbing against skin, causing irritation and increased glandular secretions. The area is warm, dark, and moist—an ideal environment for bacterial growth. The affected areas may be excoriated, erythematous, and odiferous.	While the initial infection can usually be easily controlled with antibacterial shampoos (except in vulvar fold pyoderma, which is usually too painful to treat topically), surgery may be required for a lasting cure.
Lip Fold	**Predilection:** Springer and Cocker spaniels **Lesions** are characterized by bad odor. To prove to the owner that the halitosis is from the lips rather than the inside of the mouth, swab the lips and the throat and let them compare the smell of the two swabs.	It can be treated with topical and sometimes systemic antibacterial products.
Face Fold	**Predilection:** brachycephalic breeds	Treat with topical antibacterials. Surgically correct the fold.
Vulvar Fold	**Predilection:** older, obese bitches that were spayed before their first estrus **Lesions** can be very painful.	Topical antibacterial shampoos or cleansers would be beneficial, but the area is usually too painful. DES may be useful in treatment if the pet's vulvar fold is continuously moist due to urine leakage from incontinence. Weight loss is also beneficial. Vulvoplasty (episioplasty) is curative. These dogs may have urinary tract infections, too.
Tail Fold	**Predilection:** dogs with corkscrew tails (e.g., Bulldogs, Boston Terriers).	Surgical repair (by a surgeon) is often required.

B. **SUPERFICIAL PYODERMAS** involve the skin down to and including the hair follicle. They may involve the non-haired areas as with impetigo or the haired areas as with superficial folliculitis.

SUPERFICIAL PYODERMAS

	FEATURES	MANAGEMENT CONSIDERATIONS
IMPETIGO (puppy pyoderma)	**Signalment:** young dogs (< 1 year old) **Lesions:** Subcorneal pustules that do not involve the hair follicles are present in the groin or axilla ± alopecia and pruritus. The pustules are usually small. Impetigo may just be an incidental finding.	In **young animals,** topical treatment is usually sufficient because the infection is typically self-limiting. Underlying causes such as parasitism and a dirty environment should be considered.
SUPERFICIAL FOLLICULITIS	The pustules are confined to the superficial portion of the hair follicle. **Lesions:** papules, pustules, crusts, and alopecia. These signs may be obliterated by self-trauma.	It's difficult to distinguish superficial folliculitis from impetigo unless you see a hair emerging from a pustule.
SUPERFICIAL SPREADING PYODERMA	**Lesions:** pustules, pruritus, crusts, alopecia, and collarettes. Epidermal collarettes occur when epidermal abscesses spread beneath the stratum corneum, causing the stratum corneum to peel off. We see similar lesions with other disease processes, too (e.g., bullous impetigo).	Rule out: • dermatophytes (ringworm) • demodex Superficial spreading pyodermas often have an underlying cause (e.g., atopy, allergy, hypothyroidism, seborrhea) and recur.

Dermatology

C. **DEEP PYODERMAS** are bacterial infections deep to the hair follicles. They often involve ruptured hair follicles (furunculosis). In general, deep pyodermas are more likely to involve secondary infection with *Proteus*, *Pseudomonas*, and *E. coli* than other pyodermas; thus, a culture and sensitivity must be performed. Clinically, deep pyodermas are characterized by pustules, crusts, ulcers, thickened skin, and fistulous draining tracts. German Shepherd pyoderma is a recurrent and sometimes refractory deep pyoderma that often appears as a hot spot over the hip.

DEEP PYODERMAS

	FEATURES	MANAGEMENT CONSIDERATIONS
CANINE ACNE	Canine acne is deep folliculitis and furunculosis of the chin and lips. **Predilection:** short-haired dogs (e.g., Doberman Pinschers) Often self-limiting Often occurs in young, prepubescent dogs **Lesions:** pustules, crusts, papules, draining nodules, alopecia, and hemorrhage	This can be treated topically. In severe cases, systemic antibiotics should be used. They can decrease the likelihood of scarring, although it's still possible.
NASAL or MUZZLE PYODERMA	Nasal or muzzle pyoderma is characterized by a somewhat symmetric, painful, and swollen furunculosis of the dorsal muzzle.	Other similar-looking diseases that must be ruled out include: • auto-immune skin disease • ringworm • demodex • drug eruptions Skin scraping, cytology, and fungal and bacterial cultures should be performed initially. If the condition does not respond to therapy, then a biopsy and immunofluorescent staining should be performed.
INTERDIGITAL PYODERMA	**Lesions:** erythema, pustules, crusts, nodules, and draining tracts Most interdigital pyodermas are secondary to other diseases and are therefore difficult to treat unless the primary condition is controlled.	Rule outs include: • foreign body • atopy or food allergy • psychogenic disorder • immune-mediated disorder • neoplasia Perform skin scraping, cytology, and bacterial cultures. If the condition doesn't respond to appropriate treatment, then radiograph to look for bony changes or radiopaque foreign bodies, and perform a biopsy, histopathology, and immunofluorescent staining.
PRESSURE POINT PYODERMA	Pressure point pyoderma is a deep furunculosis of pressure points (e.g., elbow, hocks). **Predilection:** large-breed, short-coated dogs; mature dogs; hypothyroid dogs	The dog should be kept off hard surfaces while it has pressure point pyoderma. Special elbow/pressure point pads may be devised to protect affected elbows/pressure points.
GENERALIZED DEEP PYODERMA (CELLULITIS)	**Cellulitis** is a deep infection dissecting through tissue planes. The skin may be edematous, darkly discolored, devitalized, and friable. The tissue should be handled with care.	Demodex should always be ruled out with a skin scraping. Cellulitis is always very serious and can result in sepsis. If possible, devitalized tissue should be removed.

III. DIAGNOSIS and TREATMENT
   A. OVERVIEW of DIAGNOSIS and TREATMENT

OVERVIEW of the DIAGNOSIS and TREATMENT of PYODERMA

1. **Physical exam/clinical evaluation: Observe appropriate lesions** such as crusts, pustules, papules, or draining tracts. Try to determine the depth of the involvement (i.e., surface, superficial, or deep). Also observe the animal for evidence of **predisposing factors** such as deep skin folds, flea dirt, obesity, or evidence of Cushing's disease or hypothyroidism.

2. **Sample collection:** Aspirate, swab, smear, and stain the sample and evaluate it for the presence of bacteria. In cases of deep pyoderma, a culture and sensitivity should be performed. With surface pyoderma, the animal may just be treated empirically (Note that hot spots may involve deep pyoderma as well as surface pyoderma). In cases such as muzzle folliculitis or pododermatitis, in which the lesions look similar to those caused by other disease processes, other appropriate diagnostics should be performed (e.g., skin scraping for demodex, fungal cultures, etc.).

3. **Treatment:** If Gram-positive cocci are seen—confirming the diagnosis of pyoderma—treat the animal appropriately. Use systemic antibiotics ± adjunctive shampoos and soaks for most superficial and deep pyodermas. Use topical medication for surface pyodermas ± corticosteroids for hot spots. Also control any obvious predisposing factors and perform a systemic evaluation if indicated (e.g., if the animal appears hypothyroid or cushingoid).

4. Recheck all animals that are on antibiotics within 7-10 days and modify therapy appropriately. Animals with deep pyodermas will have to be on long-term antibiotics (up to several months). Continue antibiotics 7 days past clinical cure.

5. For recurrent or uncontrolled pyoderma, follow-up steps may include further diagnostics to rule out underlying predisposing factors such as atopy, food allergy, and immune suppression (Cushing's, hypothyroidism). Perform a biopsy and reevaluation of the diagnosis (rule out other similar-looking diseases if you haven't already done so, by taking skin scrapings, fungal cultures, etc.).

   B. DIAGNOTIC TESTS for PYODERMA
      1. Make a **swab or impression smear** of pustule contents or draining tracts, and stain the contents using a hematologic stain such as Dif Quik or Giemsa stain. The presence of intracellular cocci in pairs or groups indicates *Staphylococcal* infection. If rods are visible in addition to cocci this usually indicates that the rod bacteria have invaded secondary to the cocci. The presence of only extracellular cocci may suggest an immunodeficiency (no phagocytosis of the bacteria) or indicate contamination. Empirical therapy based on the visualization of cocci in initial cases of superficial pyodermas is generally acceptable. In cases of deep pyodermas, the animal should initially be placed on empirical therapy, but a culture should be submitted and antibiotic therapy should be modified according to the culture and sensitivity results.

      2. **A culture and sensitivity** is usually not indicated in simple cases of surface or superficial pyoderma. It should be performed in cases of deep pyodermas or those that are difficult to clear.

      3. **A skin biopsy** is useful in cases that are difficult to treat. Take samples of the primary, active lesions and submit them to a veterinary histopathologist or a pathologist with a specific interest in dermatology.

      4. **Rule out underlying predisposing factors** and **immune incompetence.** In an immunocompetent animal with deep pyoderma, we expect to see neutrophilia and $\geq$ 1000 lymphocytes/mL.

Dermatology

C. GENERAL THERAPIES
1. **Topical therapy:** The purpose of shampoos, soaks, and whirlpool baths is to remove crusts, flush the follicles, prevent matting, decrease pruritus and pain, and encourage re-epithelialization and healing.
   a. **Antibacterial shampoos:** Commonly used antibacterial shampoos contain benzoyl peroxide, chlorhexidine, or ethyl lactate. Benzoyl peroxide is effective, but it exacerbates dry skin and should not be used more than 1-2x per week unless used with an emollient shampoo or unless it contains an emollient. Different brands of benzoyl peroxide-containing shampoos may have different efficacies. Chlorhexidine and ethyl lactate are less drying and thus are good in animals with concurrent seborrhea sicca.
   b. **Whirlpool baths and soaks:** The water should be lukewarm and should contain povidone iodine or chlorhexidine (≥ 8 oz per 20-30 gallon tub). Povidone iodine is less irritating than chlorhexidine. The animal should be soaked up to its neck for 10-30 minutes.

   c. **Topical antibiotics or steroids** have limited use because they are messy, they may block pores, and the animal may lick them off. They are usually reserved for skin fold pyodermas and canine acne.

2. **Systemic antibiotics:** Animals placed on systemic antibiotics should be re-examined in 7-10 days. If no significant improvement is shown within this time, re-evaluate the antibiotic choice and dosage, rule out complicating factors, and re-evaluate the diagnosis. If the animal is immunosuppressed, use bactericidal drugs. In cases of *Staphylococcus*, a ß-lactamase resistant antibiotic should be used. **Antibiotics should be used for a minimum of 21 days or one week beyond clinical cure.**

INITIAL CHOICE of ANTIBIOTICS

GOOD INITIAL CHOICES (but bacteria often develop resistance over time)	POOR CHOICES (resistant strains)
• Chloramphenicol 25-50 mg/kg PO, IM, IV TID • Clindamycin (Antirobe®) 5.5-11.0 mg/kg PO BID • Enrofloxacin 5-10 mg/kg PO SID-BID • Erythromycin 50-20 mg/kg PO TID • Lincomycin 22-33 mg/kg PO BID or 10-15 mg/kg PO TID • Trimethoprim sulfa combinations 15 mg/kg PO BID • Ormethoprimsulfadimethoxine 55 mg/kg PO on day 1 and then 27.5 mg/kg PO SID • Doxycycline 3-5 mg/kg PO BID for 7-14 days	• Ampicillin • Amoxicillin • Penicillin • Other nonpenicillinase-resistant penicillins • Tetracyclines • Nonpotentiated sulfa drugs

LONG-TERM ANTIBIOTICS

GOOD INITIAL and LONG-TERM CHOICES (drug resistance rarely develops)	POOR CHOICES (due to toxicity and other side effects)
• Amoxicillin-clavulanic acid (Clavamox®) 22 mg/kg PO TID • Cephalexin 22-33 mg/kg PO BID • Oxacillin 20 mg/kg PO TID • Enrofloxacin (Baytril®) - good for pseudomonas	• Gentamicin and other aminoglycosides • Trimethoprim sulfa (KCS)

D. **SPECIFIC TREATMENTS:** Surface pyodermas can usually be treated successfully with topical therapy alone. Superficial and deep pyodermas should be treated with systemic antibiotics (except for possibly impetigo and canine acne, which may initially be treated with topical therapy alone). Shampoos, soaks, and whirlpool baths are often helpful ancillary treatments in superficial and deep pyodermas.

SPECIFIC TREATMENTS

CLASSIFICATION	TREATMENT
SURFACE PYODERMAS	**HOT SPOT** • Clip the hair in the area. • Gently cleanse the area. • Consider using topical corticosteroids if it's in an area where the animal won't lick the steroids off. • Administer prednisone (0.5 mg/kg BID) for 5-7 days. • Control the predisposing cause (usually flea allergy dermatitis). • If the hot spot involves deep pyoderma (as indicated by the presence of papules or pustules in the surrounding area or if the hot spot is in an area such as the head or dorsal neck, where it could not have been caused by excessive chewing or licking), place the animal on the appropriate systemic antibiotics and do not use corticosteroids. **SKIN FOLD PYODERMA** Use topical antibacterial shampoo or benzoyl peroxide gel. This is usually not possible with vulvar fold pyoderma, however. With vulvar fold pyoderma, weight loss and moderate doses of DES (if the animal is incontinent) may help. Surgically correcting the anatomic defect is curative.
SUPERFICIAL PYODERMA (impetigo)	In animals less than one year of age, impetigo can usually be treated with topical antibacterial shampoo or benzoyl peroxide gel every 2-3 days for about one month. Impetigo in adult animals should be treated with systemic antibiotics.
SUPERFICIAL PYODERMA (other than impetigo)	• Administer systemic antibiotics (based on cytology results). Systemic antibiotics should be used for at least 3 weeks and should be continued for 7 days beyond apparent cure. • Cleansing with antibacterial shampoo twice a week is helpful in removing crusts and exudates. • After recovery, weekly long-term use of antibacterial or antiseborrheic shampoos may be used in dogs susceptible to pyoderma to help prevent or delay its recurrence.
DEEP PYODERMA	• Administer systemic antibiotics (based on culture results). Initially, use empirical antibiotic therapy based on cytology results, and then modify the antibiotic therapy based on the culture and sensitivity results. Animals with deep pyoderma often need to be on prolonged therapy (up to 2-3 months) and should be kept on antibiotics for 2 weeks beyond apparent cure. • Daily cleansing with antibacterial shampoo ± whirlpool soaks once or twice a day for at least 1-2 weeks. After initial hospitalization, the owner can continue these soaks and shampoos at home if possible. **PODODERMATITIS** (interdigital pyoderma): Fistulous tracts should be explored and devitalized tissue removed. **CANINE ACNE** may be treated initially twice a day with antibacterial shampoo. As the condition improves, the cleansing may be decreased to once every 2-3 days. The dog should be treated for 7-10 days following recovery. Mupirocin antibacterial ointment can penetrate the granulated area to reach the infection.

DERMATOPHYTOSIS (ringworm)

DERMATOPHYTOSIS is a fungal infection most often caused by *Microsporum canis*.

SIGNALMENT	Dermatophytosis occurs most often in young and immunosuppressed animals (such as kittens in an animal shelter).
CLINICAL SIGNS	• **Scaling, crusting, alopecic lesions** in the **haired regions** of the body ± hyperpigmentation: The multifocal lesions are usually sharply demarcated. They do not involve the nasal planum because the nose has no hair follicles. Lesions may be erythemic, but if they look like the typical collarette seen in humans, the animal probably has bacterial pyoderma rather than dermatophytosis. • The animal may be pruritic. • **Kerions** are well-circumscribed, nodular types of furunculosis with multiple draining tracts. They may also involve hypersensitivity to *M. canis*. • Some animals are carriers and have no clinical signs.
DIAGNOSIS	**Wood's light:** *M. canis* is the only animal dermatophyte that fluoresces. The bright yellow-green fluorescence involves the hair shaft. Epidermal scales and dust fluoresce in the blue-white range. **Direct microscopic examination:** Collect hairs from the lesions (especially ones that fluoresce) and place them on a slide with mineral oil. Examine them under a microscope for spores inside and outside the hair shaft (endothrix and ectothrix). **Fungal cultures:** Clean the area with alcohol to kill saprophytes. Pluck hairs at the periphery of the lesion and place them on **dermatophyte test media (DTM)**. Alternatively, animals can be screened by combing their hair with a new, clean toothbrush or a clean gauze wipe. Focus on the face, feet and insides of the ears as well as on any visible skin lesions. Then stab the toothbrush bristles or gauze onto the fungal culture medium. • Examine the media daily. Before use, the DTM is amber colored. With dermatophytes, the media turns red due to alkaline metabolites. This color should occur **at the time the colony first appears.** Dermatophyte colonies should be **fluffy, light-colored colonies.** Any colony that has a green or black coloration should be regarded as a contaminant. **A stained slide preparation** of a wet mount or a Scotch tape preparation of the colony surface may identify the dermatophytes cultured (stain with lactophenol blue or new methylene blue). **A biopsy** is occasionally required.
TREATMENT	• With widespread involvement, the animal may need to be shaved, especially if it's long-haired. • Administer **itraconazole** at 5-10 mg/kg PO SID or 25 mg/adult cat for 21 days; Or SID for 1-4 weeks and then 2-3 consecutive days each week (i.e., pulsed). Other medications include fluconazole, terbinafine (20-40 mg/kg PO SID for dog and cats), ketoconazole (10 mg/kg PO SID, dogs only), and griseofulvin (50 mg/kg/day PO or microsize with a fatty meal, for dogs and cats). • Dip all affected an suspect animals in **lime-sulfur dip** 2x/week (8 oz/gal) until the animal is cured. Apply with a garden sprayer. Do not pre-wet or rinse the animal. This dip is safe on kittens. • **Shampooing** with a chlorhexidine/miconazole or chlorhexidine/ketoconazole shampoo is sometimes useful but generally not needed. Continue treatment and perform weekly fungal cultures until you get 2-3 negative cultures in a row.
OTHER CONSIDERATIONS	• Keep affected animals away from other animals. • This disease is difficult to control. It requires diligent cleaning. Treat the environment with bleach weekly (1:10 dilution) and wash clothes, bedding, etc. with bleach weekly.
PREVENTION	• Isolate all new cats/kittens and perform fungal cultures using the brush technique. • Consider prophylactic lime-sulfur dipping of all new additions to a shelter or cattery, especially kittens, long-haired cats, and those surrendered from a crowded, stressful situation.

ALOPECIA
General Information
Alopecia Associated with Pruritus
Endocrine Alopecia

I. **GENERAL INFORMATION**
    A. **ALOPECIA** in dogs and cats can be caused by several diseases.

DISEASES CAUSING ALOPECIA
• **Allergic:** flea allergy, atopy, food allergy, or contact allergy
• **Infectious:** bacteria, fungal, or yeast
• **Parasitic:** mites or ticks
• **Genetic:** follicular dysplasia
• **Psychogenic** alopecia in cats
• **Endocrine:** hypothyrodism, sex hormone imbalances, growth hormone responsive, hyperadrenocorticism
• **Nutritional:** essential fatty acids, zinc responsive, vitamin A deficiency
• **Immune-mediated:** DLE, SLE, pemphigus
• **Neoplastic**

    B. **FINDINGS**
        1. Look at the **pattern.** Bilaterally symmetric truncal alopecia with hair on the head and legs most likely indicates endocrine alopecia. Alopecia of the dorsal rump indicates flea allergy dermatitis.
        2. Look for **lesions** such as crusts, papules, pustules, and collarettes. Also look for fleas, flea dirt, and mites.
        3. Determine whether the alopecia is caused by **pruritus.** If the hair is broken at the distal end, the alopecia is due to self-trauma. Note that cats with pruritus often groom themselves primarily when the owner is not present. Therefore, the owner may report that the cat is not pruritic.
        4. **Trichogram:** Pluck hairs and examine them under a microscope. Look for signs of breakage (i.e., as with trauma) vs. those that are intact (ends taper gradually). Also note how easy or difficult it is to pluck the hairs.

II. **ALOPECIA ASSOCIATED WITH PRURITUS:** The presence of pruritus rules out many dermatologic conditions.

DISEASE	DIAGNOSIS	TREATMENT
ALLERGY (fleas, atopy, food allergy, contact allergy)	History: seasonality, presence of fleas, diet history Clinical signs: The pattern of alopecia, erythema, and crust may indicate which disease the pet has (e.g., dorsal rump is more likely fleas).	Remove the source. Treat with anti-pruritic medications such as antihistamines, EFA, and corticosteroids.
DERMATOPHYTOSIS (may or may not be associated with pruritus)	• Wood's lamp • direct microscopic examination of hair follicles • fungal culture	Griseofulvin, ketoconazole, or itraconazole Medicated shampoos
PARASITES (mites, ticks)	History of exposure to parasites Skin scrape or visualize the mites or ticks.	Treat for the specific parasites with miticidal dips or ivermectin.
PSYCHOGENIC ALOPECIA in CATS (rare) Compulsive disorders are those in which the behaviors are expressed independent of the original context or need and have no apparent goal.	Signalment: There's usually an underlying etiology or set of factors such as atopy, food allergy, or FAD. Cytology, fungal culture, trichogram, parasiticidal treatment (for fleas), food elimination trial, and response to corticosteroids should be performed to rule out other causes prior to coming to a diagnosis of a compulsive disorder.	Find the underlying cause and remove it. Compulsive disorders are most frequently treated with serotonin reuptake inhibitors such as fluoxetine and paroxetine. Tricyclic antidepressants can also be tried. Amitriptyline is a good choice when dermatologic signs are apparent.
PYODERMA	Clinical signs: Crusts, pustules, collarettes Cytology of a pustule reveals bacteria	Appropriate antibiotics

Dermatology

III. **ENDOCRINE ALOPECIA:** With endocrine alopecia, the hair loss is not due to pruritus. Animals with endocrine alopecia may be pruritic, though, due to secondary bacterial infections or seborrhea.

ENDOCRINE ALOPECIA

DISEASE	DIAGNOSIS
HYPOTHYROIDISM	**Clinical signs:** Overweight, lethargic dog with tragic expression (due to myxedema) **Blood work:** Hypercholesterolemia, mild non-regenerative anemia, low T_4, high TSH, TSH stimulation
CUSHING'S DISEASE (may be iatrogenic)	**History:** If the alopecia is iatrogenic, the pet has a history of being on systemic or long-term topical corticosteroids. **Clinical signs:** PU/PD, polyphagia, pot belly, thin skin, panting **Chemistry:** stress leukogram, elevated alkaline phosphatase, hypercholesterolemia **Urinalysis:** low specific gravity ± urinary tract infection **ACTH stimulation test:** elevated cortisol **Low dose dexamethasone suppression test:** No suppression
ALOPECIA X (formerly known as growth-hormone responsive or castration responsive alopecia) It's due to sex hormone imbalance.	**Signalment:** Adult, male, Chow, Pomeranian, Toy or Miniature Poodle, or Keeshond **Clinical signs:** Bilaterally symmetric alopecia ± hyperpigmentation of the trunk. The head and extremities usually have hair. **CBC/chemistry** are normal. T_4 is normal. **ACTH stimulation test:** Perform this test to help rule out Cushing's disease and also to measure sex hormone levels (17-hydroxyprogesterone, dehydroepiandrosterone, and androstenedione) pre- and post-cortroysn administration. Results vary, but an increase in 17-hydroxyprogesterone (usually around 3x the pre-stimulation value) indicates alopecia X. **Biopsy:** The follicles are in catagen phase. Unlike Cushing's, no epidermal atrophy is present.
HYPER-ESTROGENISM In females, it's due to ovarian cysts. In males, it's caused by Sertoli cell tumors. Treatment is OVH or castration. 10-20% of Sertoli cell tumors are malignant, so also try to rule out metastasis.	**Signalment** • Intact bitches • Intact males, especially if they are cryptorchid. In males, it's due to a **Sertoli cell tumor.** **Clinical signs:** Alopecia starts in the perineal/genital area and extends cranially. • **Females:** gynecomastia and estrus cycle abnormalities • **Males:** gynecomastia (enlargement of the nipples and associated mammary tissue), pendulous prepuce that faces down instead of forward, squatting to urinate, attracting other male dogs, decreased libido, **linear preputial erythema, or a line of comedones** from the testicular area to the prepuce **Diagnosis:** • Abdominal ultrasound may reveal an ovarian tumor/cyst or a cryptorchid mass. • Elevated estrogen levels

SEBORRHEIC DISEASE COMPLEX
Pathophysiology
Classification
Topical Antiseborrheic Therapy

Seborrhea is a chronic skin condition of dogs characterized by a defect in cornification leading to increased scale formation. If the sebaceous glands are involved, it can also be characterized by excessive greasiness of the skin and haircoat, and sometimes by secondary inflammation. Seborrhea has many etiologies. It may be a primary disease, or it can be secondary to another disease (e.g., allergy, nutritional deficiency).

I.   PATHOPHYSIOLOGY: Seborrhea involves the epidermis, hair follicles, and sebaceous glands. Normally, new epidermal keratinocytes are constantly being produced by mitosis of the basal epidermis while cells of the stratum corneum are being sloughed. The sloughing, anuclear, keratinized cells are known as **scales.** Excessive scaling occurs when this process of keratinocyte formation is accelerated. The acceleration causes the desquamating keratinocytes to slough more rapidly and in aggregates.
     A. **EPIDERMAL CELL TURN-AROUND TIME in DOGS** is the time it takes for keratinocytes to travel from the basal cell layer of the epidermis to the stratum granulosum.
         1. **Normal:** 20-27 days
         2. **Seborrheic:** about 1 week

     B. **MAJOR FACTORS AFFECTING NORMAL KERATINIZATION or SEBUM PRODUCTION**
         1. Zinc, copper
         2. Vitamin A
         3. **Hormones:** estrogens, testosterone, corticosteroids, thyroid hormone, growth hormone, and prostaglandins (omega-3 and omega-6 fatty acids are precursors)
         4. **Bacteria:** Seborrheic skin has a high number of coagulase positive *Staphylococcus spp* instead of the coagulase negative *Staphylococcus* that normal skin has.

II. CLASSIFICATION: Seborrheic diseases can be classified based on appearance or etiology.
     A. **CLASSIFICATION BASED on APPEARANCE** helps determine the appropriate topical antiseborrheic therapy, but it does not indicate the underlying etiology. Usually the pet has a combination of these descriptions.

CLASSIFICATION	DESCRIPTION
Seborrhea sicca	Dry scales are the major abnormality
Seborrhea oleosa	Oily haircoat
Seborrheic dermatitis	Involves significant inflammation in the form of erythema, alopecia, and pruritus

     B. **CLASSIFICATION BASED on ETIOLOGY: PRIMARY or SECONDARY SEBORRHEA**

PRIMARY	SECONDARY
FOCAL	Allergy (flea allergy, atopy, food allergy,
Nasal hyperkeratosis	contact allergy)
Digital hyperkeratosis	Pyoderma
Tail gland hyperplasia	Parasites (e.g., mites)
Schnauzer comedo syndrome	Endocrine disorders (e.g., hypothyroid)
	Dermatophytes
GENERALIZED	Nutritional factors
Idiopathic generalized	Immune-mediated disorders
seborrhea	Neoplasia

         1. **Primary seborrhea** has specific breed predilections, specific lesion distribution, and no discernable underlying etiology. You must rule out secondary seborrhea before calling the disease a primary seborrhea. Primary seborrhea can be focal (affecting a small area) or generalized.

Dermatology

PRIMARY SEBORRHEA

	DESCRIPTION	TREATMENT
NASAL HYPER-KERATOSIS	Can occur with digital hyperkeratosis or as a separate disease **Predilection:** older animals **Location:** the most rostral portion of the planum nasale **Lesion:** Lesions are raised, dry, firm, excessive keratin accumulation with randomization of the normal architecture of the planum nasale. Lesions are not painful or pruritic. **Differentiate** this pathologic condition (excessive production of dead keratinocytes) from normal age-related retention of the stratum corneum (physiologic hyperkeratosis).	**Topical tretinoin** (e.g., Retin-A®) is used in conjunction with topical emollients. Tretinoin reduces keratinocyte cohesion and mitosis, which allows the accumulating keratinocytes to slough. **Corticosteroids** may be helpful, too, because they decrease the epidermal turnover rate. **KeraSolv®** is a high concentration salicylic acid ointment that loosens and removes crusts.
DIGITAL HYPER-KERATOSIS	May be an age-related change or may be associated with disease **Predilection:** older animals **Location:** any footpad **Lesion:** painful fissures in the footpad resulting in lameness **Diseases associated** with digital hyperkeratosis include distemper, pemphigus foliaceus, DLE, SLE, zinc-responsive dermatosis, hypothyroidism. **Differentiate** this pathologic condition from normal age-related change. With age-related changes, there's an accumulation of the pad keratin in non-contact areas, while the weight-bearing portion of the pad is normal. All footpads are affected (including the carpal pads). The lesion distribution suggests that the problem is caused by retention of the keratin due to lack of being worn off. These lesions may be accompanied by a mild amount of nasal hyperkeratosis.	Try to find the underlying cause. **KeraSolv®** is a high concentration salicylic acid ointment that loosens and removes crusts. **Surgical removal** of the affected area may provide the most dramatic cosmetic results in idiopathic cases.
SCHNAUZER COMEDO SYNDROME	This condition is characterized by the formation of multiple comedones along the dorsal spine in miniature schnauzers. The lesions are rarely painful or pruritic unless there's a secondary bacterial folliculitis.	The goal is to reduce the seborrheic component of the disease and to express the follicular contents. **Topical benzoyl peroxide** gels or shampoos work well. **Isotretinoin** (Accutane®, Roche, Nutley, NJ) has been used with good response in 3-4 weeks. A generic form is also available.
GENERALIZED PRIMARY IDIOPATHIC SEBORRHEA	**Breeds:** American cocker spaniel, English springer spaniel, Basset hound, West Highland white terrier, dachshund, Labrador retriever, golden retriever, German shepherd. The familial history usually suggests that the disease is hereditary. **Onset:** Usually at less than 18-24 months of age. The disease often progresses throughout the patient's life. **Lesion:** Generalized but usually worse along the dorsum and the intertriginous areas (e.g., axilla, inguinal, interdigital), as well as (around the ear and ventral neck).	Etretinate (a retinoid) is no longer on the market. Acitretin, a metabolite of etretinate can be used.

2. SECONDARY SEBORRHEA

DISEASE	DIAGNOSIS
ALLERGY • Atopy • Flea allergy dermatitis • Food allergy (rare) • Allergic or irritant contact dermatitis	**History:** Ask about seasonality, diet, fleas, and exposure to pollens and other antigens. **Lesion distribution:** Pruritus of the paws, axilla, and inguinal regions may indicate atopy, whereas pruritus primarily of the caudal half of the body (especially the dorsal rump) indicates flea allergy. **Removal** or challenge with the offending agent **Intradermal allergen testing/in vitro allergy testing** Elimination diet
PYODERMA	• Pustules, collarettes, crusts, erythema • **Rancid odor:** Bacteria act on the sebaceous secretions, producing free fatty acid pro-inflammatory products and a rancid odor. • Skin scraping and microscopic examination
ENDOCRINE DISORDERS Hypothyroidism	Onset usually occurs before other classic signs of hypothyroidism such as lethargy; tragic expression (myxedema); normocytic, normochromic, nonresponsive anemia; and hypercholesterolemia. Test for low T$_4$ or high TSH. The TSH stim test is more reliable.
Hyperadrenocorticism	PU/PD, thin skin, other infections, pot belly, organomegaly, bilaterally symmetric alopecia, slow-healing wounds, elevated ALP, **ACTH stim test, dexamethasone suppression.**
Sex hormone imbalance (hyperestrogenism)	Hormone levels, gynecomastia, and other feminine traits in dogs with Sertoli cell tumors
Alopecia X	Rule out other etiologies. Melatonin treatment may rule out seasonal flank alopecia. An ACTH stimulation test can help rule out Cushing's disease and rule in alopecia X if sex hormones are measured (elevated 17-hydroxyprogesterone).
PARASITES Sarcoptic mange, demodex, *Cheyletiella, Otodectes,* pediculosis	**History:** Other animals or people in the house may be affected. **Clinical signs:** May be very pruritic. **Skin scraping**
DERMATOPHYTES (common)	• Wood's lamp • Superficial skin scraping for fungi • Fungal culture
NUTRITIONAL FACTORS Vitamin A Responsive (This may actually be 1° seborrhea.)	**Lesions** are multifocal, well-defined areas of scaling, alopecia, and crusting with prominent, adherent, frond-like keratinous plugs. No ophthalmic changes. **Histopathology:** prominent follicular keratosis in the presence of minimal surface hyperkeratosis **Serum** vitamin A levels are normal. **Treat** with oral vitamin A supplementation (600-2500 IU/kg). See clinical signs of improvement in 3 weeks and complete remission in 5-20 weeks in some cases. Then decrease the vitamin A dose.
Zinc Responsive	**Lesions are usually well demarcated from normal skin.** Crusting involves pinnae, pressure points, periocular and perioral areas, muzzle, and chin. **Histopathology** reveals marked diffuse proliferative parakeratosis ("church spire"). **Oral therapy** with zinc sulfate or zinc methionine results in clinical remission of lesions within 3 weeks.
Essential Fatty Acid Deficiency (EFA) (linolenic, linoleic acids)	This disease is rare. Linolenic, linoleic, and arachidonic acids are necessary for cell membrane structure and function. Their metabolism results in the production of pro- or anti-inflammatory agents (leukotrienes and prostaglandins) and influences immunoregulation. **History:** dogs on poor quality or improperly stored dog food. **Diagnosis** is based on response to EFA supplementation.
IMMUNE-MEDIATED DISORDERS (rare)	Biopsy
NEOPLASIA (eg. mycosis fungoides/ cutaneous lymphoma)	Biopsy

Dermatology

III. **TOPICAL ANTISEBORRHEIC THERAPY** involves shampoos, sprays and rinses.

A. **HOW TO USE SHAMPOOS:** Most shampoos contain two or more antiseborrheic products that have an additive or synergistic effect.
1. **Mix the shampoo with 5-10 parts water,** and then apply the mixture to the animal. Massage the shampoo in, concentrating on the most severely affected areas first so that they get a longer contact time with the shampoo. Leave the shampoo on for **at least 8-10 minutes** (VERY IMPORTANT!). Then rinse the animal, starting with the most severely affected areas. Be sure to rinse thoroughly to minimize irritation from shampoo residues.
2. **Treat** pets 1-3 times per week depending on the severity of the skin disease. Once the animal is improving, you may switch to less frequent bathing with milder products.

B. **TYPES of MEDICATIONS in SHAMPOOS**

CLASSIFICATION	DESCRIPTION
Keratolytic • Sulfur • Salicylic acid • Tar • Selenium sulfide • Benzoyl peroxide • Propylene glycol • Pyridoxine	These agents remove the stratum corneum by causing cellular damage that results in the ballooning of the cells. The cells slough, resulting initially in exacerbated scaling during the first 10-14 days and then decreased scaling. The skin then feels softer.
Keratoplastic • Tar • Sulfur • Salicylic acid • Selenium sulfide	These agents help normalize cornification by slowing basal cell layer mitosis, often by decreasing DNA synthesis.
Antimicrobials • Chlorhexidine • Benzoyl peroxide • Iodine • Triclosan • Ethyl lactate	These agents help control secondary and primary bacterial infections. Benzoyl peroxide also has excellent follicular flushing properties.
Antifungals • Chlorhexidine • Iodine • Ketoconazole, miconazole	These products may help decrease the fungal spores.

C. **WHICH PRODUCT to USE:** In general, the more oily the coat, the more degreasing action is needed. The more scaling, the more keratolytic and keratoplastic action is needed. We can divide the seborrheic patient into four categories and treat according to the category.

SCALING and OILINESS of the HAIRCOAT	APPROPRIATE SEBORRHEIC SHAMPOO THERAPY
Mild scaling, no oiliness	Hypoallergenic shampoos with emollients
Moderate to severe scaling Mild oiliness (the most common presentation)	Sulfur-salicylic acid shampoos are a good choice because they are keratolytic, keratoplastic agents with minimal drying/degreasing ability. Humectants are useful adjuncts.
Moderate to severe scaling Moderate oiliness	Tar and sulfur shampoos with degreasing and keratolytic-keratoplastic effects are most beneficial. Humectants are very useful adjuncts.
Mild scaling Severe oiliness	Benzoyl peroxide is ideal because it has a strong degreasing action with mild keratolytic and keratoplastic effects.

D. SHAMPOO DESCRIPTIONS

SHAMPOO CONTENT	DESCRIPTION
HYPOALLERGENIC	Hypoallergenic shampoos are good for the mildly seborrheic patient, for dogs that are irritated with medicated shampoos, or for clients that have a tendency to over-bathe. Hypoallergenic shampoos cleanse the skin and encourage rehydration. The products often contain emollients, lanolin, lactic acid, urea, glycerine, or fatty acids rather than detergents or specific antiseborrheic agents.
EMOLLIENTS (oils, humectants)	Emollients are products that rehydrate the skin. They should be used in cases of excessive scaling as they are an excellent adjunct following bathing with a keratolytic shampoo. Emollients work best after the skin has been hydrated (after bathing) where they act by reducing water loss from the skin. For best results, use emollient therapy for at least 4 weeks. Between baths, severely affected areas can be treated with emollient sprays. Some emollient products contain EFAs that are well-absorbed topically. These products are beneficial for treating EFA deficiency. Emollients can also be added to flea dips to counteract their drying tendency.
SULFUR, SALICYLIC ACID	These shampoos are good for alleviating scaling in the moderately scaling animal. Both agents are keratolytic and keratoplastic, antibacterial, and antipruritic, and they have a synergistic effect. In addition, sulfur is antiparasitic and antifungal.
TAR	Tar shampoos are both keratolytic and keratoplastic and have degreasing actions. The disadvantage is their unpleasant odor. This odor dissipates as the haircoat dries, though. **Do not use these products on cats.**
BENZOYL PEROXIDE	Benzoyl peroxide shampoos are good for severely oily animals with only mild scaling. Because it has the strongest degreasing action and it's a potent antibacterial agent (better than chlorhexidine, triclosan and iodine) with follicular flushing activity, it's excellent for cases of demodicosis, especially when used prior to amitraz dip treatment. Other antimicrobial products are better suited for patients with pyoderma and only mild oiliness. Use a veterinary 2-3% benzoyl peroxide product. Human products are usually too strong and are irritating to canine patients. You can also alternate with tar, or sulfur salicylic acid shampoos.

REFERENCE:
Shanley KJ: The Seborrheic Disease Complex. Vet Clin N Am. Philadelphia, WB Saunders, November 1990, pp. 1557-1576.

CORTICOSTEROIDS

I. **CORTICOSTEROIDS** are used for their **anti-inflammatory, antipruritic, and immunosuppressive effects.** In the last case, they tend to suppress the abnormal immune response more easily than they suppress the normal immune response, which allows us to use them in immune-mediated skin diseases. Corticosteroids have many potent, adrenocorticoid side effects, especially when administered chronically. Consequently, they must be used carefully.

GUIDELINES for the SAFE USE of CORTICOSTEROIDS

1) Try safer methods of treatment first (antihistamines, flea control, etc.).
2) Use corticosteroids as infrequently as possible. A short course (less than one month) 2-3 times per year is not likely to induce serious side effects.
3) Use the lowest dose possible and go to alternate-day therapy as soon as possible.
4) Start with the least potent form (e.g. topical vs. systemic and prednisone vs. triamcinolone), as it will have less HPA suppression.
5) For long-term treatment, oral medication is preferable because it can be regulated more closely. Even single dose repositol steroid injections cause prolonged adrenocortical suppression.
6) If one glucocorticoid doesn't work or is causing undesirable side effects, try a different one at an equivalent dose (e.g. replace prednisolone with methylprednisolone).
7) If one corticosteroid stops working, rather than immediately increasing the dose, do the following:
    - Check for complicating factors (e.g. flea infestation, pyoderma, hypothyroidism, etc.).
    - Check the owner's ability to give the medications according to schedule.
    - Check that the animal is on an effective maintenance dose.
    - Switch to a different corticosteroid, and use an equivalent dose. You may be able to switch back later.
8) Be careful with topical glucocorticoids because they can have potent systemic effects. With topical medications, if one doesn't work well, try a different one. Generic brands are sometimes less potent than their name-brand counterparts.
9) When possible, use adjunct therapy to decrease the amount of corticosteroids needed.
    - Antihistamines
    - Medicated shampoos (e.g., hypoallergenic shampoos)
    - Omega-3 and -6 fatty acids

A. **SIDE EFFECTS and MONITORING:** Pets on chronic glucocorticoids should be evaluated every 6 months. Although blood work is a good idea, it often does not give us much information. Typically it reveals a stress leukogram plus elevated alkaline phosphatase (in dogs) and other elevated liver enzymes. More practical parameters for evaluating these pets include:
    1. **Evaluation for iatrogenic Cushing's disease:** Look for PU/PD, polyphagia, increased weight, pendulous abdomen, and hepatomegaly.
    2. **Evaluation of control of the skin condition**
    3. **Personality changes**
    4. **Urinalysis and culture** to check for urinary tract infection

---
SIDE EFFECTS of GLUCOCORTICOIDS

- Polyuria, polydipsia, nocturia, polyphagia, panting
- Urinary tract infections
- Secondary pyoderma
- Hepatopathy
- Muscle wasting/weakness
- Depression psychosis: Humans sometimes become suicidal. Dogs and cats may become hyperexcitable or lethargic.
- Insulin antagonism
- Hypertension

B. **CLASSIFICATION of CORTICOSTEROID by POTENCY and ACTION:**
Glucocorticoids work by traveling into the cell nucleus where they alter gene expression and consequently protein synthesis. All work via this mechanism, but some have less mineralocorticoid effect. Ideally, we want the anti-inflammatory effect without the mineralocorticoid effects (e.g., PU/PD, volume overload, hypertension).
    1. The more potent corticosteroids have less mineralocorticoid effect, but they also suppress the HPA axis more profoundly and for longer periods.

Consequently, we usually start with a less potent form such as prednisone, even though it has marked mineralocorticoid activity. Potency is based on the anti-inflammatory ability relative to hydrocortisone.

2. **Formulations:** Corticosteroids are formulated as alcohols, soluble esters, or insoluble esters (which have a longer $t_{1/2}$). Soluble esters such as those with succinate or phosphate added (e.g., prednisolone sodium succinate-Solu-Delta-Cortef®) have the same $t_{1/2}$ as the alcohol form. Formulations with insoluble esters, like acetate, added have prolonged action from days to weeks (e.g. prednisolone acetate). Addition of acetonide, dipropionate, or pivalate prolongs the action even further, for weeks to months (e.g. desoxycorticosterone pivalate (DOCP) is given $\geq$ 4 weeks).

SHORT-ACTING (least potent) $t_{1/2}$ < 12 hr	INTERMEDIATE-ACTING (intermediate potency) $t_{1/2}$ = 12-36 hr	LONG-ACTING (most potent) $t_{1/2}$ = 48 hr
• **Cortisol** (the naturally occurring/circulating corticosteroid) • **Hydrocortisone** (1.0)*	Prednisone (4.0) is converted to the active prednisolone by the liver. Prednisolone Methylprednisolone (Medrol®)	• Flumethasone (15.0) • Dexamethasone (40.0) • Triamcinolone** (40.0) • Methylprednisolone acetate (50.0) (Depo-Medrol®)

*Values in parentheses indicate the relative potency. The higher the number, the more potent the drug.
** Triamcinolone is between intermediate and long-acting.

C. **ANTI-INFLAMMATORY DOSES:** Because these doses are based on metabolic weights, larger dogs should receive slightly lower doses than smaller dogs. Also, use lower doses in older animals.

DRUG	DOG	CAT
Prednisone and prednisolone (5, 10, 20 mg tablets)	Induction: 1.1 mg/kg per day Maintenance: 0.55 mg/kg q 48 hours	Induction: 2.2 mg/kg per day Maintenance: 1.1 mg/kg q 48 hours
Methylprednisolone* (Medrol®) 4, 8, 16mg	Induction: 1-2 mg/kg per day Maintenance: 0.5-1 mg/kg q 48 hrs	
Triamcinolone (Vetalog®) 0.5, 1.5 mg tablets; 2 mg/mL, 6 mg/mL	Induction: 0.22 mg/kg PO SID or 0.1-0.2 mg/kg IM or SQ Maintenance: 0.055 mg/kg PO SID	Induction: 0.1-0.2 mg/kg/cat IM or SC
Methylprednisolone acetate (Depo-Medrol®)	2-40 mg/dog IM	10-20 mg/cat IM
Dexamethasone	0.25-1.0 mg/dog IM	0.125-0.5 mg/cat IM

*Give 80% the prednisolone dose. So 5 mg prednisone = 4 mg methylprednisolone.

1. **Induction:** Start with the induction dose administered SID or divided and given BID. Once-a-day treatment is easier for the client and is usually associated with fewer side-effects. Once the dermatologic signs are controlled (e.g. no more pruritus), then taper the dose.
    a. **Anti-inflammatory use:** 3 to 7-day induction period
    b. **Immunosuppressive dose:** 2-week induction period. The induction dose in dogs is 2.2-4.4 mg/kg/day.

    Injectable glucocorticoids (subcutaneous or intramuscular administration) reach effective levels at the same rate as oral administration. So usually there's no need to start with an injection. If you do start with injectable dexamethasone, wait 4-5 days before giving the first dose of prednisone. Injectables should not be used as the first line of treatment in dogs.

2. **Maintenance:** Use prednisone, prednisolone, or methylprednisolone on an alternate-day basis. First use the induction dose every 48 hours, and then cut the dose in half every 1-2 weeks until you reach the lowest effective maintenance dose. If this dose is lower than 0.5 mg/kg, the pet is not likely to have many side effects, but if the dose is higher, the pet will probably develop chronic glucocorticoid side effects within 1-2 years.

Dermatology

a. If possible, decrease the dose interval to every 3-4 days to help avoid side effects. If the animal is PU/PD on prednisone, or if prednisone does not control the pruritus on the off day, try dexamethasone or triamcinolone. Unless you can taper the dose to every third day, the pet will develop chronic glucocorticoid effects within 1- 2 years.

b. Cats are okay on alternate-day triamcinolone or dexamethasone. They can often be tapered to treatment every 3-4 days.

3. **Injectable glucocorticoids**
   a. **Dogs:** Injectable glucocorticoids are okay for induction but not for maintenance. A single injection can cause prolonged adrenocortical suppression. One injection 2-3x per year is probably safe.
   b. **Cats** can be maintained safely on injectable glucocorticoids given at long intervals. They can receive 20 mg methylprednisolone acetate (Depo-Medrol®) SC or IM (with IM injections, you don't get sterile injection site granulomas) every 2 weeks until their dermatologic signs are suppressed. Then follow with maintenance injections no more then every 8 weeks.

4. **Topical treatments:** In general, more potent steroids are more effective, but this varies with the formulation. Non-prescription 0.5% hydrocortisone is not very effective in dogs and cats. If one topical corticosteroid doesn't work, try a different one. Topical corticosteroids can have potent side effects, so do not overuse them. Triamcinolone and betamethasone used topically for less than a week can cause adrenal suppression for one month.

COMMON DRUG DOSAGES for CARDIAC ARREST

	2 kg	5 kg	10 kg	20 kg	40 kg	50 kg
Atropine 0.4 mg/mL, 0.04 mg/kg IV	0.2 mL	0.5 mL	1.0 mL	2.0 mL	4.0 mL	5.0 mL
Dexamethasone SP 0.5 mg/kg, 4 mg/mL	0.25 mL	0.63 mL	1.25 mL	2.5 mL	5.0 mL	6.3 mL
Epinephrine low dose: 0.02 mg/kg 1:1000=1mg/mL	0.04 mL	0.1 mL	0.2 mL	0.4 mL	0.8 mL	1.0 mL
Epinephrine— high dose: 0.2 mg/kg (may be more effective than low dose) 1:1000=1mg/mL	0.4 mL	1.0 mL	2.0 mL	4.0 mL	8.0 mL	10.0 mL
Furosemide 2 mg/kg of 50mg/mL solution	0.08 mL	0.2 mL	0.4 mL	0.8 mL	1.6 mL	2.0 mL
Lidocaine-2% 0.25 mg/kg (cat)	0.02 mL	0.06 mL	0.12 mL	------	------	-----
Lidocaine-2% 0.5 mg/kg (dog)	0.08 mL	0.2 mL	0.4 mL	0.8 mL	1.6 mL	2.0 mL

COMMON ANALGESICS

	2 kg	5 kg	10 kg	20 kg	40 kg	50 kg
Oxymorphone 0.05 mg/kg of 1.5 mg/mL solution	0.07 mL	0.16 mL	0.33 mL	0.66 mL	1.32 mL	1.65 mL
Hydromorphone 0.05 mg/kg of 4 mg/mL solution	0.02 mL*	0.06 mL*	0.12 mL*	0.24 mL*	0.48 mL*	0.6 mL*
Morphine 0.5 mg/kg of 15 mg/mL solution	0.07 mL*	0.17 mL*	0.33 mL*	0.67 mL*	1.33 mL*	1.67 mL*

*Low end dosage

BASIC EMERGENCY ASSESSMENT and CARDIAC ARREST PROTOCOL

In emergency medicine, it's important to treat the most life-threatening problems first. Once animals go into cardiac arrest, prognosis is poor. Less than 10% of all animals that go into cardiac arrest survive long enough to be discharged from the hospital. Even those that are revived usually die within 24-48 hours. Most of these animals have end-stage disease (e.g. pneumonia, cardiac disease, neoplasia, severe trauma). Only animals that arrest due to anesthetic complications and other accidents have a good chance of survival. **Warning signs of impending cardiopulmonary arrest include:**

- Hypotension, weak pulses, increasingly irregular pulses
- Hypothermia
- Cyanosis, Decreasing respiratory rate and depth
- Sudden unexplained deepening under anesthesia

STEPS for EVALUATING the CRITICAL PATIENT

AIRWAY PATENCY	Check for a patent airway. If the animal is trying to breath but isn't able to get air, place an endotracheal tube or, in the case of upper airway obstruction, perform a tracheostomy. Suction out any fluid and remove any foreign material in the pharynx.
BREATHING	Check to see if the patient is breathing. If not, then ventilate the animal with 100% oxygen. Ventilate at a rate of 20-30x per min.
CARDIOVASCULAR	Evaluate for circulatory shock (See next section). Check the mucous membranes, capillary refill time, pulse quality, and heart rate. Pale mucous membranes, prolonged capillary refill time, weak thready pulses, and elevated heart rate in dogs indicate hypovolemic or cardiogenic shock. Injected mucous membranes, short CRT, and bounding pulses suggest vasodilatory shock. • Catheterize and administer fluids to correct hypotension. Place a Doppler or arterial catheter to monitor blood pressure. Does the animal have a **heart rate or pulse?** If no, then begin **external chest compression** at a rate of 80-120 beats/minute. Ventilate during chest compression at a ratio of 1 breath to every 4 chest compressions. **Compress the abdomen** with a sandbag to decrease caudal diaphragm movement and to increase blood flow to the cranial half of the body. **The goal of chest compression is to** maximize blood pressure and cerebral and coronary perfusion and to get the heart to beat on its own. Consider open-chest cardiac massage in larger dogs with no lethal underlying disease when external compression is ineffective. What is the cardiac rhythm? • **Ventricular asystole:** Administer epinephrine and atropine • **Ventricular fibrillation:** Defibrillate (2-4 Joules) • **Bradycardia:** Give atropine • **Ventricular tachycardia:** Give lidocaine (3 mg/Kg in dogs and 0.5 mg/kg in cats)
LEVEL of CONSCIOUSNESS	**Obtundation** (a decrease in consciousness) may suggest intracranial problems, particularly in a trauma patient. It's important to avoid increasing intracranial pressure in such patients.
LEVEL of PAIN	Assume the critical patient is in pain. Butorphanol is generally safe to use, often in conjunction with valium. For severe pain, use full agonists such as hydromorphone, morphine, oxymorphone, or fentanyl.
POST-ARREST	Keep the animal on oxygen. If it doesn't regain consciousness in 15-30 minutes or if the arrest is > 20 minutes, administer drugs to decrease toxic oxygen radicals and resulting cerebral edema. • Mannitol (0.5 g/kg) • Dexamethasone (0.5 mg/kg) • Lasix (5 mg/kg) • Hyperventilate the animal. • DMSO (1 g/kg) < 10% over 2 hours Take further action if you see: • Mean blood pressure < 60 mmHg or systemic blood pressure < 80 • MM = pale or CRT > 3 sec • Heart rate < 60 or > 200 bpm • **Arrhythmias:** Ventricular or atrial fibrillation and multiform VPCs or presence of arrhythmias that gradually get worse.

CIRCULATORY SHOCK

Shock is a lack of energy production within the cell. This lack of energy, in the form of ATP, leads to cell death and consequently organ dysfunction and failure. In order to produce ATP, cells need oxygen as well as substrates such as glucose. Anything causing low oxygen delivery to the tissues (e.g. pneumonia, severe blood loss, poor cardiac output, vasoconstriction, or anemia), or causing low cellular substrates (e.g. prolonged hypoglycemia) can cause cell dysfunction, shock, and death. The most common type of shock seen in veterinary medicine is **hypovolemic shock.**

I. **PHYSIOLOGIC CLASSIFICATIONS OF CIRCULATORY SHOCK**
   A. **PHYSIOLOGIC COMPONENTS OF THE CIRCULATORY SYSTEM**: The circulatory system is composed of a pump (the heart), pipes to carry the fluid (blood vessels), and fluid (blood) in the system. Failure can occur in any of these levels. For instance, heart failure leads to cardiovascular shock, dilation of the blood vessels leads to vasodilatory shock, and loss of fluid leading to inadequate blood volume results in hypovolemic shock.

TYPES OF CIRCULATORY SHOCK BASED on the
PHYSIOLOGIC SYSTEM THAT'S DAMAGED

Functional Component	Physiologic Component	Type of Circulatory Shock
Pump	Heart	Cardiovascular shock
Pipes	Blood vessels	Vasodilatory shock
Fluid	Blood/fluid	Hypovolemic shock

   B. **ETIOLOGY of CIRCULATORY SHOCK**
      1. **Hypovolemic shock** is the most common type of circulatory shock. It's due to any cause of **inadequate blood volume** such as:
         a. **Hemorrhage**: Blood loss leads to decreased blood volume as well as decreased oxygen carrying capacity.
         b. **Dehydration**: When animals show obvious signs of dehydration such as persistent tenting of the skin or sunken eyes ($\geq$ 10% dehydrated) they are also hypovolemic. Many causes of abnormal fluid loss can lead to dehydration and consequently hypovolemia. They include:
            i. Vomiting, diarrhea
            ii. Persistent panting (e.g. due to hyperthermia)
            iii. Polyuria
         c. **Third space loss** is the loss of fluid into the abdominal or thoracic cavity. It can be due to a number of processes such as hypoproteinemia leading to loss of oncotic pressure, sepsis or toxins leading to increased vascular permeability, or cardiac insufficiency leading to back-up of fluid.

      2. **Cardiogenic shock** occurs when the heart is not pumping adequately and consequently, **cardiac output is decreased.** Causes include:
         a. **Arrhythmias**: Severe tachyarrhythmias of 250-300 bpm diminish ventricular filling, thus there's little blood in the heart to pump forward. With severe bradyarrhythmias (HR $\leq$ 30) or severe 3rd degree heart block, the heart rate is too slow to maintain an adequate cardiac output.
         b. **Obstructive conditions** such as pericardial effusion prevent the heart from filling.
         c. **Valvular regurgitation**: The heart pumps well but variable amounts of blood flows backwards instead of forwards.
         d. **Valvular stenosis** such as aortic or pulmonary outflow tract obstructions.

      3. **Vasodilatory shock** occurs when there's a loss of vascular tone. Vascular tone is usually tightly regulated in order to maintain arterial blood pressure. Loss of tone leads to hypotension. This vasodilation can be caused by:
         a. **Sepsis**: Products of leukoactivation (cytokines) impair normal vascular tone. When these mediators are flushed into the circulatory system they can cause generalized vasodilation. These animals may start to recover from their hypovolemic shock but then go into vasodilatory shock due to release of inflammatory mediators.
         b. **Anaphylaxis**: Histamine release from antigen-antibody complexes causes vasodilation.
         c. **Ischemia** causes hypoxia and accumulation of metabolites, which cause vasodilation.

   d. **Ischemia-reperfusion injury:** When blood flow is reintroduced to
       ischemic tissues, reactive oxygen intermediates are released, causing cell
       damage and vasodilation. The release of high amounts of potassium also
       cause membrane instability.

II. **PHYSIOLOGY of CIRCULATORY SHOCK**

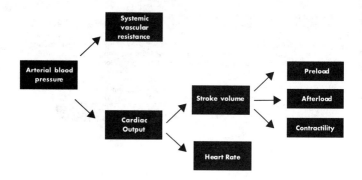

A. **HOW the BODY NORMALLY MAINTAINS PERFUSION:** Arterial blood
    pressure is the most important factor for maintaining cerebral and coronary
    perfusion. Consequently, maintaining arterial blood pressure is a priority of the
    cardiovascular system. (See Cardiac Physiology p. 3.23 for more info).
    1. **Arterial blood pressure** is determined by **cardiac output**—the amount of
        blood pumped out by the heart per minute— and **systemic vascular
        resistance.**
        a. **Cardiac output** is a product of **heart rate x stroke volume** (the
            volume ejected by the ventricle with each contraction). Stroke volume is
            determined by preload (end-diastolic volume), afterload (the pressure the
            heart has to pump against), and cardiac contractility.

        b. **Systemic vascular resistance (SVR)** is controlled by vasomotor tone
            of the vasculature. Vasodilation reduces SVR whereas vasoconstriction
            increases SVR. Even if cardiac output is high, arterial blood pressure can still
            be low if systemic vascular resistance is low (i.e. vasodilation).

B. **PHYSIOLOGIC RESPONSE to SHOCK**
    1. **Response to hypovolemic shock:** When a patient suddenly loses blood
        volume, preload, cardiac output, and arterial blood pressure decreases.
        Baroreceptors respond by triggering an increase in heart rate **(tachycardia)**
        which increases cardiac output to normal. Simultaneously, epinephrine causes
        intense vasoconstriction (SVR). Dogs can lose up to 30% of their blood volume
        and still **maintain arterial blood pressure** due to increased heart rate and
        systemic vascular resistance.
    2. **Response to poor myocardial contractility:** If myocardial contractility
        decreases, heart rate and systemic vascular resistance increase to compensate.

    > Animals in hypovolemic shock and cardiogenic shock look similar.
    > They are both tachycardic and vasoconstricted.

    3. **Response to low systemic vascular resistance** (e.g. sepsis, anaphylactic
        shock): These animals can respond by **increasing their heart rate** but they
        can't increase systemic vascular resistance (i.e. they can't vasoconstrict);
        consequently, they can't compensate adequately and their blood pressure falls.

> Regardless of whether the circulatory insult is due to fluid loss, poor cardiac
> function, or vasodilation, **dogs** respond with tachycardia. Consequently,
> tachycardia is a useful sign for monitoring shock.

C. **INTERPRETING BLOOD PRESSURE:** Normal arterial blood pressure does not mean
the animal is not in shock. If, for instance, an animal presents collapsed and in shock
but with a normal blood pressure, the animal may be maintaining blood pressure
through intense vasoconstriction. It may be in the compensatory stages of
hypovolemic or cardiogenic shock.

> A normal arterial blood pressure does not rule out shock! Animals have
> normal arterial blood pressure when they are in the compensatory stage
> of shock.

1. **Low blood pressure** means the patient is in the non-decompensated stage of
shock—the heart has failed to compensate, too much blood has been lost, and
arterial blood pressure can no longer be maintained.

III. **DIAGNOSING SHOCK:** Shock is a clinical diagnosis.

A. **EVALUATING the CIRCULATORY STATUS:** This should take < 1 minute.

	Hypovolemic or Cardiogenic Shock VASOCONSTRICTION	Vasodilatory Shock VASODILATION
Mentation	Obtunded or depressed	Obtunded or depressed
Mucous Membrane Color	Pale	Red (injected)
Capillary Refill Time	Slow (> 2 seconds)	Fast (< 1 sec)
Heart Rate	Tachycardic (normal or low with decompensation)	Tachycardic (normal or low with decompensation)
Pulse Quality	Weak	Bounding
Extremity Temperature	Cold	Warm

1. **Mentation:** Animals in shock have abnormal mentation (obtunded, stuporous,
or comatose) because low perfusion leads to brain hypoxia.

2. **Mucous membrane (MM) color:** Vasoconstriction leads to pale mucous
membranes.
a. **Hypovolemic** and **cardiogenic shock** animals have generalized
vasoconstriction of capillary beds, leading to pale, often white, MM.
b. **Vasodilatory shock:** These animals have dilated capillaries and low
resistance to blood flow. Their mucous membranes are injected. Some dogs
such as bulldogs and boxers normally have bright red mucous membranes.

3. **Capillary refill time (CRT):** Vasoconstriction causes a slow CRT (> 2 sec).
Vasodilation leads to a fast CRT (< 1 sec).

4. **Heart rate:**
a. **Dogs** in circulatory shock exhibit a tachycardia in an attempt to maintain
cardiac output and tissue perfusion. Once they can no longer compensate
(**decompensated shock**), they become normocardic or bradycardic.
Experiments have shown that dogs remain in compensatory shock with
losses of up to 30% of their blood volume— but beyond this, they suddenly
decompensate as seen with a sudden decrease in HR and blood pressure.
The prognosis is much worse once they decompensate.
b. **Cats** commonly present in shock with a **normal heart rate** (or
bradycardia) rather than tachycardia. In cats, absence of tachycardia is not
a prognostic indicator.

5. **Pulse quality:** Vasoconstriction reduces pulse quality (poor, thready) whereas
vasodilation is associated with tall, wide pulse pressure contours (bounding
pulse).

6. **Extremity temperature:** Animals with generalized vasoconstriction have poor peripheral perfusion leading to cool extremities. Vasodilated animals have increased peripheral perfusion leading to warm feet.

B. **CLINICAL SIGNS of HYPOVOLEMIC AND CARDIOGENIC SHOCK LOOK VERY SIMILAR.** Affected animals are obtunded, have pale MM, prolonged CRT, tachycardia, poor pulse quality, and cool distal extremities. Animals with vasodilatory shock have hyperemic MM, rapid CRT, bounding pulse quality, and normal extremities.

1. Animals in vasodilatory shock sometimes present with concurrent hypovolemia (slow CRT, pale MM, etc). Once they are adequately hydrated, they still remain hypotensive, now with signs of vasodilation (rapid CRT, hyperemic MM, etc.).

IV. **MANAGING SHOCK** (Refer to fluid therapy p. 8.7.)
   A. **START with the ABCs of EMERGENCY CARE** (Refer to p. 3.2 for more info.)
      1. **Airway:** Make sure the animal has a patent airway. Provide oxygen if the animal will tolerate it.
      2. **Breathing:** Evaluate breathing pattern.
      3. **Circulation:** Evaluate for shock. Get an IV catheter in quickly.

   B. **FLUID ADMINISTRATION in SHOCK**
      1. The first goal is to bring blood pressure back to the normal range. Start with **isotonic crystalloids.** Some clinicians use hypertonic solutions, but doing so has not been shown to improve survival rate.
         a. **Hypovolemic and cardiogenic shock animals look clinically similar;** however, if you bolus large amounts of fluid to the cardiogenic shock patient, it will fluid overload. Usually you can determine the animal is in heart failure because it has a heart murmur, distended jugular veins, and perhaps pulmonary edema. This patient will likely require diuretics, a vasodilator, and a positive inotrope. Do not give fluids for the time being.
         b. **Dilated cardiomyopathy dogs** sometimes are not in obvious cardiogenic failure. Consequently, give 5-10 mL/kg at a time while monitoring preload parameters. Such patients may need catecholamines such as dobutamine and dopamine to increase contractility if ultrasound reveals poor contractility.
         c. **Vasodilatory shock:** Because these patients are vasodilated, their blood pressure will remain low despite adequate fluids. These animals may need a vasopressor such as dopamine, phenylephrine, or norepinephrine and their underlying disease (ruptured pyometra, etc.) must be treated.

      2. **Give 25% of the shock dose of fluids and reevaluate:** If the animal looks better and then suddenly starts looking worse (i.e blood pressure decreases and HR increases), first ask if you've given enough fluids. Try more first. Look for evidence of ongoing hemorrhage. If the heart rate is normal or low, the dog may be decompensating or may be in the ischemic perfusion phase. Look for pericardial fluid with ultrasound. Most cases of cardiogenic shock have bad prognoses.

      3. **Cats:** Use warm fluids to help prevent hypothermia. Blood pressure will not rise in the face of low temperature. Warming externally may lead to peripheral vasodilation which may further exacerbate the shock.

   C. **CORTICOSTEROIDS ARE NOT INDICATED IN SHOCK**

FLUID THERAPY
Fluid Compartments
Types of Fluids Used
Fluid Therapy

I.   THE BODY CONTAINS THREE FLUID COMPARTMENTS— the **intravascular** fluid
     compartment, the **interstitial** fluid compartment, and the **intracellular** fluid
     compartment. The intravascular fluid compartment plus the interstitial fluid compartment
     comprise the **extracellular fluid compartment (ECF)**.

     A.   **THE FLUID COMPARTMENTS are INTERCONNECTED:** The body's three fluid
          compartments are separated by semipermeable membranes which are freely
          permeable to water, thus distilled water would diffuse into all three compartments in
          an amount proportional to the size of the respective compartments.
          1.   **Sodium is pumped out of cells** by sodium/potassium-ATPase. As a result,
               the sodium concentration inside the cell is low, while the potassium
               concentration inside the cell is much higher than outside of the cell.
               a.   If you administer a fluid containing a higher concentration of sodium than
                    the ECF (**hypertonic crystalloids**), the fluid will draw water from the
                    cells out into the ECF.
               b.   If you administer a fluid with a lower concentration of sodium than the ECF
                    (**hypotonic crystalloids**), the excess water component will flow into the
                    cells.
               c.   Solutions that have a similar sodium concentration as the ECF (**e.g.
                    isotonic crystalloids**) are distributed only to the ECF.

          2.   The vascular membrane is freely permeable to water, sodium, and other
               electrolytes. It is not very permeable to large molecules such as albumin— the
               main protein involved in **maintaining the plasma colloid osmotic pressure
               to keep fluid in the vascular compartment**. Fluid with large molecular weight
               molecules can't diffuse across cell membranes. These fluids are called colloids
               and can be used to maintain plasma osmotic pressure.

II. FLUIDS USED in FLUID THERAPY
     A.   TYPES of FLUIDS USED in FLUID THERAPY

TYPE	DESCRIPTION	EXAMPLES
COLLOIDS	Colloid fluids are retained primarily in the vascular fluid compartment. They draw water into the intravascular space.	• Plasma • Whole blood • Dextrans • Hetastarch
ISOTONIC CRYSTALLOIDS (ECF replacement fluids) Sodium concentration ranges from 130 mEq/L (LRS) to 154 mEq/L (saline).	Isotonic crystalloids rapidly diffuse into the interstitial fluid space (only 25% remains in the intravascular space after about 30 minutes).	**With bicarbonate-like anion such as lactate or acetate:** • LRS • Plasmalyte 148 • Normosol R **Without bicarbonate-like anion** (Acidifying): • Ringers • Normal saline (0. 9%)
HYPOTONIC CRYSTALLOIDS (Whole body replacement fluids—low in sodium and high in water compared to the ECF)	Hypotonic crystalloids redistribute to both the interstitial and the intracellular fluid spaces.	• Plasmalyte 56 • 2.5%, 5%, 7.5% dextrose • 1/2 LRS in water • Normosol M
HYPERTONIC CRYSTALLOIDS These have a higher concentration of sodium than the ECF so they draw water into the intravascular space.	Hypertonic crystalloids are retained within the ECF and draw in water from the intracellular space. They are used in acute hypovolemia to increase blood volume.	• 7.5% saline

III. FLUID THERAPY is DIVIDED into TWO PHASES

FLUID THERAPY IS DIVIDED into TWO PHASES
1) **Phase 1:** Restore circulating blood volume with crystalloids and colloids. 2) **Phase 2:** Correct acid-base and electrolyte imbalances and restore whole body fluid balance.

A. **STEP 1: BLOOD VOLUME REPLACEMENT:** When the animal has lost significant blood volume or is hypovolemic, administer fluids rapidly to restore the blood volume. Use appropriate amounts of **crystalloids and enough colloids** to prevent excessive hemodilution. The fastest way to get fluids into the animal is through a **short, wide bore catheter** such as an 18 gauge cephalic catheter. Jugular catheters are much longer than cephalic catheters and resistance to fluid flow is higher. If the animal has some type of obstruction of venous return (such as gastric dilatation), the catheters should be placed in the cephalic veins rather than the saphenous veins.

BLOOD VOLUME REPLACEMENT

CLINICAL SIGNS of HYPOVOLEMIA (Refer to chapter on hypovolemic shock)	• Pale mucous membranes, slow capillary refill time, cold appendages • Tachycardia • Weak, thready pulses • Decreased central venous pressure (CVP) • Decreased arterial blood pressure (ABP) ▪ Mean arterial pressure $\leq$ 60 mmHg ▪ Systolic blood pressure $\leq$ 80 mmHg
START WITH CRYSTALLOIDS with bicarbonate-like anion (e.g. LRS)	With severe hypovolemia, you may need to infuse up to one blood volume or more of crystalloids rapidly. Start with 20-25% of the dose and then re-evaluate. Because cats have a smaller blood volume, use a syringe pump or buretrol for good control of fluid dose. One blood volume comes out to: • **Dog:** 80-90 mL/kg (or a little less than 10% of its body weight in kilograms) e.g. one blood volume in a 10 kg dog is a little less than 1 L of fluids. • **Cat:** 55 mL/kg (about 5.5% of its body weight in kg) e.g. 5.5% of a 5 kg cat is 0.275 L or 275mL of fluid When greater than one blood volume is required, use colloids (especially blood) as part of the fluid treatment. Some clinicians like to administer hypertonic crystalloids. The maximum amount to administer is 6 mL/kg in dogs and 4 mL/kg in cats.
ADD COLLOIDS if oncotic pressure is falling due to blood loss or hypoproteinemia	Hypovolemic patients often already have decreased oncotic pressure due to low albumin (and low total protein in the case of blood loss), and administration of crystalloids further dilutes the blood. Consequently, colloids may be needed. **Add colloids when:** • Total protein $\leq$ 3.5 g/dL • Albumin $\leq$ 2.0 g/dL • Anemia with PCV $\leq$ 20% or Hb $\leq$ 7g/dL (Administer whole blood. Refer to the blood transfusion section on p. 8.11.)
MONITOR for SIGNS of FLUID OVERLOAD and response to therapy	Signs of fluid overload are similar to signs of vasodilatory shock. They include: • Bounding pulses • Injected MM • Fast CRT < 1 sec • Increased respiratory rate and effort due to pleural effusion or pulmonary edema. • Distended jugular veins and elevated CVP • Large postcava on thoracic radiograph • Increased end-diastolic diameter (EDD) on cardiac ultrasound

B. **STEP 2: WHOLE BODY FLUID and ELECTROLYTE REPLACEMENT:** Once you've provided an effective circulating volume, the next goal is to design a whole body fluid/ electrolyte replacement which takes into consideration the animal's fluid deficit, normal ongoing losses (maintenance), and abnormal on-going losses.

1. Note that fluids can be given orally, subcutaneously, IV, or intraosseously. In cases of marked dehydration, it's best to give fluids IV since these animals are usually also hypotensive. Otherwise fluids can be given orally or SC.

BASIC OUTLINE for FLUID REPLACEMENT THERAPY

After establishing an effective circulating volume, design a whole body fluid/electrolyte replacement as follows:

1. Determine the **deficit** (by estimating dehydration), **regular maintenance needs** (based on the maintenance charts such as on p. 8.11), and abnormal **on-going losses** (due to vomiting, diarrhea, etc.). Add all three volumes together to determine the amount of fluids to administer over the first 24 hours.

2. Start with an ECF replacement fluid, usually LRS or an equivalent solution. Supplement with potassium and bicarbonate if needed.
   - **Administer bicarbonate** if the pH < 7.2, bicarbonate concentration is < 14 mEq/L or the base deficit is < -10 mEq/L. Administer 0.3 x (weight in kg) x (the amount of base deficit that you want to correct). Give 1/2 of this volume over 30 minutes and then repeat the blood-gas measurement.
   - **Add potassium** to the ECF replacement fluid if the pet is hypokalemic. (Refer to chart on p. 8.10) Do not administer at a rate of more than 0.5 mEq/kg/hr.

3. Monitor the patient's PCV, BUN, total protein, acid/base status, and potassium periodically and adjust the fluid flow rate and composition accordingly.

2. **DETERMINE the AMOUNT of FLUIDS to ADMINISTER:** Administer enough fluids to compensate for the **deficit** (estimated by dehydration), **regular maintenance needs** (based on maintenance needs chart on the following page), and **on-going losses** (due to vomiting, diarrhea, etc.). Try to replace the deficit slowly over 24 hours.

   a. **Estimate the deficit volume** by evaluating skin turgor and dehydration.

ESTIMATING FLUID DEFICIT	
Mild dehydration (skin fold flattens slowly). This is barely noticeable. Assume all patients with diarrhea or vomiting are at least 5% dehydrated	5%
Severe dehydration (skin fold remains standing)	10-12%

   Example: If a 10 kg animal is 10% dehydrated, it has a 1 kg or 1 L fluid deficit. So 1 L of fluids should be administered over 24 hours to replace this deficit.

   b. **Estimate maintenance fluid volume:** Refer to the fluid requirement charts on p. 8.11. According to this chart, a 10 kg dog needs 742 mL of fluid per day.

   c. **Estimate on-going losses by guessing how much vomiting/diarrhea, etc. the animal will produce.** For instance, a 10 kg dog with moderate diarrhea may produce 200 mL of fluid loss through diarrhea in 24 hours.

   d. **Add the deficit, maintenance, and on-going loss volumes together.** A 10 kg dog that's 10% dehydrated and has moderate diarrhea needs about 2 liters per day (1950 mL/day) which is roughly 2.5x its maintenance needs.

Deficit	1000 mL
Maintenance	742 mL
On-going losses	200 mL
	1942 mL = about 2 liters/24 hours

   Administer this volume of fluids over about 24 hours. The fluid composition will need to be adjusted throughout therapy.

3. **ELECTROLYTE REPAIR**

   a. **Acid-base status:** Sick or hypovolemic patients are usually acidemic. Dehydration and hypovolemia lead to decreased peripheral perfusion. Thus, acidic waste-products build up leading to whole body acidemia. Mild

acidemia is corrected just by restoring blood volume. In severe cases of
acidemia, **bicarbonate** should be administered.

CRITERIA for BICARBONATE ADMINISTRATION
• Bicarbonate concentration is < 14 mEq/L
• Base deficit is < -10 mEq/L
• pH < 7.2

Amount of Bicarbonate to Administer
0.3 x (Animal's weight in kg) x (amount of Base Deficit you want to correct)

Administer 1/2 of the calculated amount of bicarbonate over 30 minutes and then
recheck the acid-base status.

b. **POTASSIUM STATUS**
  HYPOKALEMIA and HYPERKALEMIA

HYPERKALEMIA	Hyperkalemia commonly occurs in association with acidemia, renal failure, and urinary blockage.
	Signs of hyperkalemia include bradycardia and an abnormal ECG (tall, tented T waves, small P waves, prolonged P-R intervals, widened QRS complexes, ± bradycardia, premature ectopic beats, or asystole).
	• Rehydrate the pet and correct the acidemia. Correcting acidemia drives potassium into the cells, thereby decreasing serum potassium levels.
	• If there are ECG abnormalities (cardiotoxic range), treat by administering calcium, or insulin (0.1 to 0.25 u/kg IV) and dextrose (0.5 to 1.5 g/kg administered IV over 2 hours).
HYPOKALEMIA	Hypokalemia commonly occurs due to diuresis, vomiting, diarrhea, anorexia (decreased uptake), and dehydration (aldosterone-induced urinary losses).
	Signs associated with hypokalemia include U waves on ECG (positive deflections following the T wave), general muscle weakness, ileus, hypotension, and CNS depression.
	When potassium is low, add potassium to the deficit repair solution (as per the chart below). If it's normal, do not supplement the deficit repair solution. During maintenance fluid administration, the fluids usually need to be brought up to 20 mEq of KCl to keep the potassium levels in the normal range. When administering K^+, monitor for iatrogenic hyperkalemia either via ECG or serum levels. Potassium should be infused at a rate slower than 0.5 mEq/kg/hr.
	Example: A 10 kg dog has a serum potassium level of 2.0 mEq/L; thus, administer fluids with 40 mEq/L potassium at a rate of 100 mL/hr (0.1 L/hr). To calculate the potassium infusion rate: concentration x infusion rate (40 mEq/L) x (0.1 L/hr) = 4.0 mEq/hr. If the maximum safe rate is (0.5 mEq/kg/hr) x (10 kg) = 5.0 mEq/hr, the planned infusion should be safe.
	If the patient has refractory hypokalemia in spite of supplementation, suspect hypomagnesium and supplement with magnesium. Plasmalyte and Normosol contain magnesium. Avoid adding magnesium to LRS, since it may react with the calcium salts.

AMOUNT of POTASSIUM to ADD

ESTIMATED PLASMA $[K^+]$	PLASMA K^+ LEVELS	$[K^+]$ of DEFICIT REPAIR SOLUTION (mEq/L)
Increased	> 5.5	0-4
Normal	3.5-5.5	4
Mildly low	3.0-3.5	20
Moderately low	2.5-3.0	30
Severely low	2.0-2.5	40
	< 2.0	50

FLUID THERAPY REQUIREMENTS in DOGS and CATS

Daily Crystalloid Requirements in DOGS		
BODY WEIGHT (Kg)	TOTAL Kcal/day or water (mL/day)	FLUIDS (mL/hr)
1	132	6
2	222	10
3	301	13
4	373	16
5	441	19
6	506	21
7	568	24
8	628	26
9	686	29
10	742	31
11	797	33
12	851	36
13	904	38
14	955	40
15	1006	42
16	1056	44
17	1105	46
18	1154	48
19	1203	50
20	1248	52
21	1295	54
22	1341	56
23	1386	58
24	1431	60
25	1476	62
26	1520	64
27	1563	65
28	1607	67
29	1650	69
30	1692	71
35	1900	79
40	2100	88
45	2293	96
50	2482	104
55	2666	111
60	2846	119
70	3194	133
80	3531	147
90	3857	161
100	4174	174

132 Kcal*Kg$^{0.75}$; Nutritional Requirements of the Dog, National Research Council, Bethesda, MD., 1995.

Daily Caloric Requirements in CATS		
Body Weight (Kg)	Total Kcal per day or water (mL/day)	Fluids (mL/hr)
1.0	80	3.3
1.5	105	4.4
2.0	127	5.3
2.5	148	6.2
3.0	167	7.0
3.5	185	7.7
4.0	203	8.4
4.5	219	9.1

80 Kcal*Kg$^{0.67}$; Nutritional Requirements of the Cat, National Research Council, Bethesda, MD., 1995.

ION	MAINTENANCE FLUID	REPLACEMENT FLUID
Na$^+$	40-50 mEq/L	130 - 155 mEq/L
K$^+$	15-20 mEq/L	4 mEq/L

BLOOD/PLASMA TRANSFUSION
Indications
Blood Products
Blood Types and Crossmatching
Blood Donors
Performing the Blood Transfusion

I. **INDICATIONS for TRANSFUSIONS:** Blood transfusions are most commonly used in cases of anemia or blood loss. Fresh whole blood contains a number of components including **red blood cells** (RBCs), **white blood cells, proteins** (albumins, globulins, etc.), and **hemostatic factors** (coagulation proteins, antithrombin III); therefore, transfusions can replace a number of blood components. Furthermore, transfusions can be in the form of whole blood, or specific blood components (e.g. packed RBCs, plasma, platelet rich plasma).

INDICATIONS for TRANSFUSION with BLOOD PRODUCTS

INDICATIONS	EXAMPLES	WHEN to TRANSFUSE
REPLACEMENT of RBCs	Decreased RBC production (e.g. chronic renal failure, bone marrow tumor) RBC loss due to: • Hemorrhage • Hemolysis	The point at which you transfuse depends upon cardiovascular status. • With cardiovascular compromise, transfuse when the PCV is ≤ 20-25% • When cardiovascular status is reasonably normal, transfuse when the PCV is < 12%
REPLACEMENT of HEMOSTATIC PROTEINS	Decreased production: • Hemophilia • von Willebrand's disease • **Hepatic disease** leads to decreased production of antithrombin III and coagulation proteins. • **Vitamin K deficiencies** lead to decreased production of vitamin K-dependent coagulation factors. These deficiencies occur with ingestion of rodenticides such as warfarin and broudifacoum. Loss/ destruction: • **Hypoproteinemia** leading to loss of albumin and coagulation factors (e.g. glomerulonephropathy) • **DIC:** consumption of clotting factors	Transfuse if the pet has clinical signs of bleeding, if the clotting tests are very prolonged, or if the animal is anemic
REPLACEMENT of PLATELETS	Decreased platelet production: Bone marrow neoplasia **Increased platelet utiliization:** Rickettsial disease, immune-mediated thrombocytopenia, DIC Platelet dysfunction (aspirin, artificial colloids)	Transfuse when the pet has clinical signs of bleeding, petechiae, or ecchymoses. Usually you don't see clinical signs of thrombocytopenia until the platelet count is < 20,000/μL.
REPLACE ALBUMIN	Decreased production: Hepatic disease Increased loss: • **Parvovirus** or other protein-losing gastroenteropathy • Glomerulonephropathy	Transfuse when the animal has clinical signs of low albumin (e.g. hypovolemia, ascites, edema) or when albumin is down to 1.5-2.0 g/dL.

II. **BLOOD and BLOOD PRODUCTS** can be stored in a number of solutions. The most common ones are **ACD** (acid-citrate-dextrose), **CPD** (citrate-phosphate-dextrose), and **CPDA** (citrate-phosphate-dextrose-adenine). Each of these solutions contains a form of citrate, which acts as an **anticoagulant** by binding calcium. Citrate makes calcium unavailable, thus the calcium-dependent steps in the clotting cascade are inhibited, preventing clotting. Dextrose provides an **energy source** for RBC glycolysis. CPDA also contains a buffer (phosphate) and adenine, which gives blood a **longer lifespan**. The type of anticoagulant and preservatives used as well as the method of storage (e.g. refrigeration, freezing) determine the shelf life of the blood product.

A. **TYPES OF PRODUCTS:** Blood can be administered as whole blood or plasma. Both products can be used fresh or can be stored.

WHOLE BLOOD AND PLASMA PRODUCTS

	PLASMA	WHOLE BLOOD
Contents	**Fresh plasma** contains albumin, globulin, clotting factors, and platelets. Platelets are active if the plasma is used within 6 hours of collection. Fresh plasma stored for over 24 hours lacks factor V, factor VIII, and vonWillebrand's factor. **Fresh frozen plasma** (separated from whole blood within 3-4 hours of collection and then frozen) contains albumin, globulins, and clotting factors. **Frozen plasma** is fresh frozen plasma that's been stored frozen for over one year. It contains albumin and globulins.	**Fresh whole blood** contains red blood cells plus albumin, globulin, clotting factors, and platelets. Platelets are active if the blood is used within 6 hours. **Stored whole blood** (kept refrigerated) contains red blood cells, albumin, and globulins. **Packed red blood cells** contain RBCs separated from the plasma. The PCV is about 80%.
Storage	**Fresh plasma** refrigerated at 4° C lasts 1-2 days. **Fresh frozen plasma** stored below 40°C lasts about one year.	**Whole blood** • In citrate lasts 24 hours • In ACD (cats) or CPDA (dogs) lasts 4 weeks **Packed RBCs** last 42 days
Advantages	• Decreased risk of immune reactions • Provides proteins without providing RBCs	Provides red blood cells and other blood components.
Disadvantages	Expensive	Expensive • The animal may not need the red blood cells. • We can't store RBCs as long as plasma.
Rate	5-10 mL/kg/hr	5-10 mL/kg/hr

B. **WHICH PRODUCT TO USE**

WHICH PRODUCT to USE

NEED	PRODUCTS AVAILABLE
Red blood cells	• Fresh whole blood • Stored whole blood • Packed red blood cells
Platelets	• Fresh whole blood • Platelet rich plasma • Fresh plasma (within 6 hours)
Clotting factors	• Fresh whole blood • Fresh plasma (within 24 hours) • Fresh frozen plasma

III.   BLOOD TYPES and CROSSMATCHING
   A.   BLOOD TYPES: Dogs and cats have different blood types. When recipients receive blood from non-compatible blood donors (donors with different blood types), the recipient's immune system may attack the donor's RBCs resulting in an **acute transfusion reaction**.

   1.   CATS have three blood types—A, B, and AB. Most mixed breed cats are type A. Certain specialty breeds have a higher incidence of type B blood. Cats with type B blood often have antigens against type A blood, thus, on transfusion with type A blood they develop an **acute transfusion reaction** that results in death. When type B cats donate blood to type A recipients, the RBCs have a shorter than normal life span. If the type A recipient has already been sensitized to type B blood, it will have a transfusion reaction.

BREEDS with higher incidence of type B blood	
Abyssinian	Himalayan
Bermese	Persian
British Shorthair	Scottish Fold
Devon Rex	Somali

   2.   DOGS have 8 major dog erythrocyte antigen (DEA) groups designated DEA 1 through DEA 8. Most transfusion reactions involve groups DEA 1.1, 1.2, or 7, so donor dogs should be negative for these groups. Most dogs don't have pre-formed antibodies against these RBC antigens, so you rarely see acute transfusion reactions with incompatible blood on the first transfusion or on subsequent transfusions within the following 4-7 days. Dogs may have transfusion reactions during future transfusions once they have been sensitized to incompatible donor cells.

   B.   CROSSMATCHING detects pre-formed antibodies to foreign cell antigens. It's a less expensive alternative to blood typing. If possible, a crossmatch should be performed prior to all transfusions, even if the donor has a compatible blood type.
   1.   WHEN to CROSSMATCH

WHEN a CROSSMATCH is ESSENTIAL
• Patients with a past history of transfusions
• Cats likely to have B type blood
• Patients with immune-mediated hemolytic anemia or immune-mediated thrombocytopenia
• Pets that may need multiple transfusions

   2.   MAJOR AND MINOR CROSSMATCHES: Two types of crossmatches— a major and a minor crossmatch, should be performed. The **major crossmatch**, which is more clinically significant than the minor crossmatch, detects recipient antibodies to donor cells. The minor crossmatch detects donor antibodies to recipient cells. Minor crossmatches should be performed for plasma transfusions.

   3.   PERFORMING a CROSSMATCH
      a.   Collect one mL of donor blood and one mL of recipient blood and place each in a separate EDTA or heparinized tube. Spin each tube for 10 minutes to separate the serum. Remove and save the serum from each in clean labeled glass or plastic tubes
      b.   Wash the RBCs by taking 0.2 mL of RBCs and diluting in 4.8 mL of 0.9% saline. Spin this for 1 minute, remove the supernatant, and repeat the process 2 more times with the pelleted RBCs and 4.8 mL of 0.9% saline.
      c.   Prepare three tubes by labeling them as Major, Minor, and Recipient Control. Add two drops (50 μL-100 μL) of plasma and two drops of blood to each tube as follows:

      Major Crossmatch: Recipient plasma + donor cells
      Minor Crossmatch: Donor plasma + recipient cells
      Recipient Control: Recipient plasma + recipient cells

      Let the tubes sit at room temperature for 15 minutes and then centrifuge for 15 seconds. Check the supernatant for hemolysis and then gently resuspend the pellet by tapping the tube so that you can check for RBC agglutination. Agglutination or hemolysis of the control indicates immune-mediated disease.

IV. DONORS
   A. CHOOSING a DONOR

CRITERIA for DONOR ANIMALS

DOG	CAT
• **Weight > 25 kg** • PCV > 40% • Females should be spayed (to avoid hormone fluctuations which affect RBC count) • **Negative for blood-borne pathogens** such as Rickettsia, heartworm, Brucella • Ideally negative for DEA 1.1, 1.2, and 7 and normal vWF levels	• **Weight > 5 kg** • PCV > 30% • **Negative** for FeLV, FIV, Hemobartonella, Toxoplasma

   B. **HOW to COLLECT DONOR BLOOD:** Collect donor blood into CPDA (dogs) or ACD (cats) solutions and use it within 24 hours, or, store at 4°C in order to decrease the rate of glycolysis and use within one month. One unit is 500 mL in dogs and 50-60 mL in cats.

	DOG	CAT
AMOUNT	In dogs, collect up to about 20% of their blood volume. Since blood volume is about 8.5% of body weight, dogs can donate about 0.85% of their total body weight in blood (1 kg of body weight = 1 liter or 1000 mL of fluid). Thus, a 30 kg dog has a blood volume of 2500 mL and can donate 500mL of blood.	Cats can donate 10% of their blood volume. Since blood volume is 5.5% of body weight, cats can donate 0.55% of their total body weight in blood (1 kg of body weight = 1 liter or 1000 mL of fluid). Thus, a 5 kg cat has a blood volume of 275 mL and can donate 45 mL of blood.
COLLECTION VOLUMES	Collect 450 mL blood into 50 mL of CPDA.	Collect 45 mL of blood into 10 mL of ACD.

V. PERFORMING the BLOOD TRANSFUSION

PERFORMING a BLOOD TRANSFUSION

MATERIALS	• IV catheter • 1-3 IV extension sets • **Hemo-nate® blood filter** for removing clots: Use this filter when transfusing ≤ 50 mL of blood (i.e. with cats). • **Syringe pump:** Use this if administering blood via syringe. • **Standard blood administration set with clot filter:** Use this instead of the Hemo-nate® when transfusing ≥ 50mL of blood. • **Donor blood:** Discard blood with dark brown or black supernatant because this discoloration indicates bacterial growth. • **Packed RBCs can be diluted** in 0.5-1.0 mL of 0.9% saline per mL of RBCs. Do not mix solutions other than 0.9% saline with RBCs because they may cause clots or cell lysis. • One bag of **0.9% saline**
PRE-TRANSFUSION STEPS	INSERT an INDWELLING CATHETER in the patient. PREPARE the BLOOD PRODUCT: Place the blood or plasma in **lukewarm** water until the blood/plasma is lukewarm. For frozen plasma, let the bag sit at room temperature for 20-30 minutes before defrosting with lukewarm water. Any blood that's been opened or warmed (unrefrigerated for 30 minutes) should be used within 24 hours in order to reduce the possibility of bacterial proliferation in the warmed blood.

PERFORMING A BLOOD TRANSFUSION continued

PRE-TRANSFUSION STEPS	SET up TRANSFUSION LINES: • **For blood/plasma in a bag,** attach the blood transfusion set with at least one IV extension set to the blood or plasma bag. Squeeze the filter chamber so that it's at least half-full of blood or plasma. Open the clamp and start running the blood/plasma into the transfusion set. Once the transfusion set is full, connect the extension set to the patient's IV catheter. • **For blood or plasma in a syringe,** attach the filter with at least two attached IV sets. Attach the syringe to the filter and then attach the extension sets to the filter. Push blood or plasma through the filter and extension lines and connect the lines to the patient's IV catheter. Insert the syringe into the syringe pump. Do not use an IVAC® infusion pump (an IVAC® 530 is okay) for whole blood, packed RBCs, or plasma infusion where platelets are important. IVACs apply direct pressure to the infusion pump lines and this can damage blood product cells. **PRE-TREAT with DIPHENHYDRAMINE** 0.5 mg/kg IV to help avoid transfusion reactions. This step is optional.
TRANSFUSION RATE	**Whole blood or plasma:** Administer at a rate of 10 mL/kg/hr. The maximum rate in the case of hypovolemia is 20 mL/kg/hr. **Packed RBCs:** The maximum rate is 10 mL/kg/hr. If the animal is hemorrhaging, you may need to administer blood at a faster rate. Administer the entire volume over two or more hours. For the first hour, transfuse at half the desired administration rate and watch for transfusion reactions. Cooled blood (refrigerated) has an increased viscosity. Once the blood warms up and starts flowing faster, you may need to adjust the flow.
AMOUNT to TRANSFUSE	**For anemia:** 2 mL of whole blood/kg will raise the PCV by 1%. A more precise method is: **Blood required =** Blood $\times$ $\dfrac{\text{PCV desired - PCV of recipient}}{\text{PCV of the donor}}$ Volume **Plasma:** Administer 10-20 mL/kg/day. Administer even more if the disease involved causes increased protein losses. The animal needs to receive about 45 mL/kg to see an appreciable difference in albumin.

TRANSFUSION REACTION	Check the pet's temperature, pulse, and respiration (TPR) before the transfusion and after 30 minutes. Then check it hourly. The earlier the transfusion reaction occurs, the more severe the reaction. Watch for:
	• **Signs of vascular overload** due to rapid transfusion administration including pulmonary edema and dyspnea, vomiting, and increased CVP.
	• **Signs of immune-mediated reactions/allergic reactions** such as restlessness, fever, nausea, salivation, vomiting, tachypnea, tachycardia, hypotension, urticaria, muscle tremors, seizures, angioedema of the face, and erythematous pinnae.
	
	WHAT to DO in the CASE of a TRANSFUSION REACTION:
	• If the transfusion reaction is mild (restlessness, mild-moderate dyspnea, vomiting), discontinue the transfusion.
	• If the transfusion reaction is severe (urticaria, convulsions, changes in pulse or respiration, decreased arterial blood pressure), discontinue the transfusion and administer:
	  • **Dexamethasone sodium phosphate** at 2 mg/kg IV or **Solu-Delta Cortef** at 10 mg/kg IV.
	  • **Benadryl** 0.5mg/kg IV slowly over 3-5 minutes.
	  • Severe anaphylaxis may require **epinephrine**.

POST TRANSFUSION	**Post-Transfusion:** Once the transfusion is completed, attach a bag or a syringe of normal saline to flush the infusion line. Administer the saline at the same rate the blood or plasma was being administered. Continue to administer saline until the transfusion lines are clear of blood or plasma.

8.16

RESPIRATORY DISTRESS
Emergency Diagnostic Flow Chart
Steps in Handling Respiratory Distress
Etiologies and Treatment of Increased Respiratory Effort

Respiratory Distress
Emergency Diagnostic Flowchart

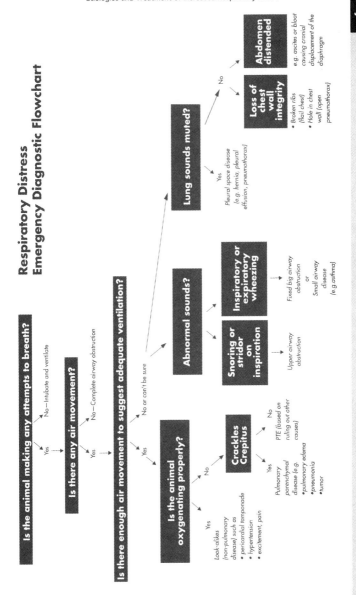

Is the animal making any attempts to breath?
- No — Intubate and ventilate
- Yes

Is there any air movement?
- No — Complete airway obstruction
- Yes

Is there enough air movement to suggest adequate ventilation?
- No or can't be sure
- Yes

Is the animal oxygenating properly?
- Yes
  Look-alikes (non-pulmonary disease) such as
  • pericardial tamponade
  • hypertension
  • excitement, pain
- No
  Crackles Crepitus
  - Yes
    Pulmonary parenchymal disease (e.g.
    • pulmonary edema
    • pneumonia
    • tumor
  - No
    PTE (based on ruling out other causes)

Abnormal sounds?
- **Snoring or stridor on inspiration** → Upper airway obstruction
- **Inspiratory or expiratory wheezing** → Fixed big airway obstruction or Small airway disease (e.g. asthma)

Lung sounds muted?
- Yes
  Pleural space disease (e.g. hernia, pleural effusion, pneumothorax)
- No
  Loss of chest wall integrity
  • Broken ribs (flail chest)
  • Hole in chest wall (open pneumothorax)

  Abdomen distended
  e.g. ascites or bloat causing cranial displacement of the diaphragm

STEPS in HANDLING RESPIRATORY DISTRESS

Quick evaluation and stabilization are the keys to handling respiratory distress successfully. Evaluation consists of determining whether the distress is due to an **obstruction** that must be quickly removed, by-passed (tracheostomy), or treated with medications (e.g. corticosteroids if it's due to inflammation or bronchodilators if it's due to asthma), **pleural space disease** (pleural effusion) which requires emergency thoracocentesis to provide quick relief, **chest wall disorder** (e.g. open pneumothorax) which must be repaired, or **parenchymal disease**. In most cases, the animal needs to receive oxygen via face mask, oxygen cage, oxygen bag (hospital set-up), nasal insufflation, endotracheal tube, or tracheostomy tube. The oxygen may need to be provided while you are assessing the patient and sometimes before the patient can be thoroughly assessed.

STEP 1: ADMINISTER OXYGEN	If there's no obstruction, you can administer oxygen by mask, oxygen cage, nasal insufflation, intubation, or "homemade" set-up. Don't use positive pressure ventilation until you have ruled out a pneumothorax.
STEP 2: CHECK BREATHING EFFORT (INCREASED OR DECREASED)	• If the breathing effort/rate is significantly decreased so that the pet is hypoxemic (cyanotic), then intubate and ventilate using 100% oxygen. • If the respiratory effort is increased, go to step 3, which is to determine whether the animal is moving air and if so, is it moving **enough air.**
STEP 3: LISTEN FOR BREATHING SOUNDS TO DETERMINE WHETHER THE ANIMAL IS GETTING AIR INTO THE LUNGS. THIS STEP EVALUATES FOR AIRWAY OBSTRUCTION	**Observe the chest and abdominal movement while listening for stridor or wheezing.** The absence of sound production indicates a **complete obstruction.** The presence of any of stridor or wheezing indicates a **partial** obstruction. • **With a complete airway obstruction, the chest wall will be drawn in while the abdomen expands outward during inspiration.** • **Presence of stridor** suggests **upper airway disease** (from the nose to the bronchi). Inspiratory stridor indicates extrathoracic disease while expiratory stridor indicates intrathoracic disease. • **Wheezing** indicates lower airway disease such as asthma and bronchitis. • **Lower airway diseases typically cause inspiratory and expiratory difficulty.**
STEP 4: DEAL WITH THE COMPLETE OR PARTIAL UPPER AIRWAY OBSTRUCTION	In cases of complete or partial upper airway obstruction (stridor or snorting), sedate or anesthetize the patient and then administer oxygen and look for the obstruction. Sometimes short-acting corticosteroids such as prednisolone sodium succinate at 10-20 mg/kg IV are useful because they decrease inflammation which may be causing or contributing to the obstruction. In **non-life threatening cases of stridor** or **airway obstruction,** sedation may allow the patient to breathe more easily. If you suspect **laryngeal paralysis,** use thiopental to induce a light level of anesthesia and perform a laryngeal exam. Administer thiopental in 2-4 mg/kg boluses. Usually you don't need to exceed a total of 6-10 mg/kg. On laryngeal exam, the arytenoid cartilages should open (abduct) in a coordinated fashion during inspiration; if not, the animal has laryngeal paralysis. Be careful not to give too much thiopental or it will suppress spontaneous breathing and laryngeal reflexes. In **life-threatening cases,** quickly look in the mouth for an obvious obstruction or laryngeal paralysis. Anesthetize, examine, and remove the obstruction or intubate. If you can't intubate because of an obstruction, you can jet ventilate or perform an emergency tracheostomy to bypass the obstruction. Under anesthesia, perform a thorough oral exam for foreign bodies, laryngeal edema, everted saccules, elongated soft palate, etc. If you suspect a foreign body obstruction which you can't physically reach or see, you can try the Heimlich maneuver.

STEPS in HANDLING RESPIRATORY DISTRESS continued

STEP 5: **THORACO-** **CENTESIS**	If there's evidence of trauma or you suspect air or fluid in the chest, perform a thoracocentesis to remove the fluid or air in order to allow the pet to breathe more easily.
STEP 6: **PERFORM THE** **PHYSICAL EXAM**	**External physical exam:** • Check for loss of chest wall integrity, flail chest (broken rib segments), or abdominal enlargement. Little flails do not cause big dyspnea, so if you see this, look for a different cause of the dypnea (e.g. hemorrhage or pneumothorax). • **Auscult the thorax:** Decreased lung sounds may be due to pleural space disease (e.g. air, fluid, intestines in the pleural space). Crackles in the lung fields indicate fluid in the lungs. • **Percuss the chest** for evidence of fluid or pleural air. • **Abdominal palpation:** If the abdomen feels empty, the animal may have a **diaphragmatic hernia.** If the abdomen is big and taught, the pet may have a **gastric dilatation or torsion.**
STEP 7: **PERFORM FURTHER** **DIAGNOSTICS**	Thoracic and abdominal radiographs and ultrasound help identify whether there's cardiac disease, pleural space disease, pulmonary parenchymal disease, or disease of the pulmonary airways. Be sure to rule out look-alikes such as excitement and pericardial tamponade. BLOOD-GAS measurements: Blood gas measurements help confirm the presence of pulmonary dysfunction. They can tell you whether the animal has a problem with ventilation or oxygenation and whether the pet has venous admixture indicating a problem getting oxygen from the lungs into the circulation. The following is a simplified, short-cut method for determining the above parameters in an animal on room air. (Refer to the anesthesia section on p. 1.35) Normal PCO_2 = 40 (35 - 45) mmHg Hyperventilation = < 35 mmHg Hypoventilation = > 45 mmHg Normal PO_2 = 95 mmHg (80 - 110) Hypoxemia = < 80 mmHg PCO_2 + PO_2 = > 130 mmHg = no admixture < 120 mmHg = yes, admixture 120 – 130 mmHg = maybe If you've ruled out other causes of pulmonary disease and the animal is getting better on oxygen, think **pulmonary thromboembolism** (PTE), especially if the animal has concurrent disease that can lead to PTE (e.g. renal disease, liver disease, Cushing's disease, or DIC).

INCREASED BREATHING EFFORT—ETIOLOGIES AND TREATMENTS

CAUSES OF INCREASED BREATHING EFFORT	DIAGNOSIS	TREATMENT
LOOK-ALIKES: Hypotension, hypovolemia, pericardial tamponade Excitement, pain Hyperthermia Acidemia	Pericardial tamponade is the trickiest of the look-alikes to diagnose because it rarely exhibits cyanosis. Diagnosis requires radiographs or pericardiocentesis ± cardiac ultrasound. On auscultation you hear decreased heart sounds. You may also detect electrical alternans on the ECG and pulsus alternans on pulse palpation.	Correct the underlying problem.
LARGE AIRWAY OBSTRUCTION: Obstruction from the nose to the mainstem bronchi (e.g. foreign body, neoplasia, laryngeal paralysis, laryngeal edema)		Remove or bypass the obstruction. You may need to do a life-saving tracheostomy.
Complete Obstruction: These don't present to the hospital because they die too quickly. You may see iatrogenic causes at the hospital though (e.g. kinked or mucous-occluded endotracheal tube).	These animals present with ineffective attempts at breathing. In other words, they are trying to breath but no sound is heard and they aren't moving any air. Typically the diaphragm expands while the chest wall is sucked inward.	**For the non-life threatening case,** provide oxygen, cool and sedate the animal so that it's relaxed and can breath more easily. Evaluate the obstruction when the animal is stable.
Partial Obstruction (Brachycephalic syndrome, recurrent laryngeal paralysis, foreign bodies, neoplasia, edema).	If the partial obstruction is severe, the animal will make squeaking noises. Otherwise, the animal will make snoring noises.	**For the life-threatening case,** do not use sedatives; anesthetize the animal (any fast intravenous anesthetic) and remove or bypass the obstruction. An emergency tracheostomy is occasionally necessary.
SMALL AIRWAY OBSTRUCTION	Mid-pitched wheezing or breathing sounds Thoracic radiographs reveal hyperinflated lungs, bronchointerstitial pattern if the condition is chronic.	**Non-life threatening case:** Oxygen. Administer aminophylline or theophylline. These are moderately potent bronchodilators that are relatively safe to use. **Life-threatening cases:** Oxygen. Use a more potent bronchodilator such as a β2 agonist (terbutaline) or a β1, β2 agonist (e.g. epinephrine, dopamine, dobutamine, isoproterenol). These drugs also have cardiac and vascular effects.

Condition	Diagnosis	Treatment
LOSS OF CHEST WALL INTEGRITY Open pneumothorax: hole in the thoracic wall	A hole is present in the thoracic wall allowing the intrathoracic space to communicate with the environment.	Close the opening and drain the pleural space. Initially, you can put a tube in the hole, manually close the tissues tightly around it and suck the air out. You can then anesthetize, intubate, and ventilate. Then perform an exploratory thoracotomy and definitively fix the problem(s).
Flail chest is seen when animals have torn intercostal muscles (most commonly torn during dog fights) or fractured ribs (often caused by blunt trauma).	Often you don't see a skin injury. You may just see a flailing depression in the thoracic skin. Little flails do not cause big dyspnea. If you see big dyspnea, the animal may have hemothorax or some other problem in addition to the flail chest.	If it's not too bad, sedation and cage rest. If it's bad, sedation, intubation, positive pressure ventilation (PPV), and surgical repair. Rigidize the chest wall and rest the animal until its ribs heal.
CRANIAL DIAPHRAGM DISPLACEMENT (gastric torsion, ascites, pregnancy, pyometra)	Abdominal palpation/visualization	Oxygen and PPV until the underlying problem can be corrected.
PLEURAL SPACE DISORDERS (fluid, pus, or intestines in the pleural space)	Decreased lung and heart auscultability. Thoracic percussion is hyperresonant for air and hyporesonant for fluid. Obtain radiographs if the animal will tolerate positioning. Perform diagnostic thoracocentesis if dyspnea is severe.	Perform thoracocentesis and chest drainage and treat the underlying problem. Surgical repair for diaphragmatic hernia.
CLOSED PNEUMOTHORAX A hole in the lungs allows air to leak into the intrathoracic space with each breath. The pneumothorax allows the lungs to collapse away from the chest wall.	Thoracic percussion is hyperresonant. Thoracocentesis reveals air. Radiographs are diagnostic.	**Thoracocentesis:** many cases of pneumothorax don't re-develop after you've removed the air. Rest the animal. **Positive pressure ventilation is contraindicated.**
PULMONARY PARENCHYMAL DISEASE Cardiogenic or non-cardiogenic pulmonary edema, neoplasia, pulmonary interstitial emphysema (PIE), pneumonia, contusion, respiratory distress syndrome	Hyperresonant lung sounds. Crepitation, crackles, or bubbling sounds on auscultation. Normal sounding lungs do not rule out pulmonary parenchymal disease. Radiographs	Put the animal on oxygen or positive pressure ventilation as indicated. Treat the underlying etiology (e.g. antibiotics for infection). Perform symptomatic treatment (e.g. fluids, chest coupage, postural drainage).
PULMONARY THROMBOEMBOLISM	Rule out other causes of dyspnea. Look for an underlying disease that causes formation of thromboemboli or DIC. Use imaging techniques such as angiography or nuclear scintigraphy.	**Treatment:** Treat as for DIC (heparin, aspirin, plasma for clotting, and anticoagulant factors if indicated).

GASTRIC DILATATION-VOLVULUS (GDV)

Gastric dilatation-volvulus (GDV) is one of the most common surgical emergencies affecting dogs. It is characterized by excess gastric distention ± displacement and torsion of the stomach. The stomach enlarges so much that it impinges on other abdominal organs and interferes with visceral organ perfusion. It blocks blood flow through the caudal vena cava and portal vein, decreasing venous return to the heart and resulting in decreased cardiac output and hypotension. The enlarged stomach causes anterior displacement of the diaphragm, which interferes with ventilation. GDV occurs most commonly in large, deep-chested dogs, but can also occur in other breeds as well as in cats.

CLINICAL SIGNS	• **Non-productive retching** or regurgitation of saliva from the esophagus. • **Restlessness** due to discomfort • **Distended abdomen** • Respiratory distress • Drum-like hyperresonance with percussion • Signs of **hypovolemic shock**: prolonged capillary refill time, pale mucous membranes, weak, thready pulse, tachycardia
AIRWAY	The upper airway can be partially obstructed with saliva or vomitus and such secretions should be suctioned.
BREATHING	The enlarged stomach pushes the diaphragm cranially, restricting inspiratory reserve capacity; thus breathing is often shallow and fast. These animals often benefit from oxygen.
CARDIO-VASCULAR	These animals are usually in **hypovolemic shock**. The reduced cardiac output results in tissue hypoxia which induces a **systemic inflammatory response syndrome (SIRS)**, a syndrome characterized by vasodilation, increased capillary permeability, and DIC. • **Catheterize and administer isotonic crystalloids and colloids over 5-10 minutes in quantities sufficient to correct hypovolemia and electrolyte imbalances.** Re-evaluate cardiovascular status and adjust treatment accordingly. • **Monitor PCV, TP, electrolytes, pH and blood gases, lactate, BUN, glucose, platelet count, and coagulation.** The pre-fluid values provide a baseline for monitoring progress. Lactate levels > 6 mmol/L have been reported to be associated with a higher incidence of gastric necrosis. EKG: Animals may have **ventricular arrhythmias.** Provide adequate fluid restitution and analgesia. Indications for antiarrhythmic therapy include: evidence of cardiovascular impairment, increasing severity of the arrhythmia, multiform complexes, instantaneous rate > 200 bpm, and ectopic beats overriding the previous R wave ("R-on-T"). • Start with a lidocaine bolus of 1-4 mg/kg slowly. If the arrhythmia converts, put the animal on a CRI of 50-100 μg/kg/min. If the arrhythmia does not improve, try procainamide (1-4 mg/kg). These antiarrhythmics can be hypotensive, so monitor arterial blood pressure. • Tachycardias are important to control because when severe, they decrease diastolic filling and cardiac output, and interfere with subendocardial perfusion— which occurs primarily during diastole.
LEVEL of CONSCIOUSNESS	Circulatory shock, SIRS, and pain can lead to altered mentation.
PAIN	GI distention, ischemia, and inflammation cause pain. Opioids are good analgesics and are reversible. • **Oxymorphone** 0.02-0.05 mg/kg • **Hydromorphone** 0.02-0.05 mg/kg • **Morphine** 0.2-0.5 mg/kg Administer IM or slow IV to avoid hypotensive effects. Avoid alpha-2 agonists (xylazine, medetomidine) in cardiovascularly unstable patients. Avoid NSAIDS because of their tendency to cause GI ulceration and hemorrhage.

DECOMPRESS the STOMACH	The stomach can be decompressed via stomach tube or with trocharization.
	• **Gastrocentesis (trocharization of the stomach):** Percuss a sterilized area of the lateral abdominal wall and trocharize the area that most resonates (pings). Use a 14-16 gauge catheter. One can't predict where the spleen or stomach will be because all the organs are shifted. The insertion point should be based on percussion, although some clinicians recommend inserting the needle in the left cranial abdomen just caudal to the last rib. Insert the catheter and remove the needle. Hold the abdomen so that the stomach does not fall away from the catheter as it decompresses. Most of the time this procedure removes enough air and fluid to significantly decrease pain and allow stomach tube placement.
	• **Stomach tube:** Some emergency clinicians prefer to avoid stomach tubing due to the difficulty of passing the tube, the possibility of perforating the damaged stomach, the likelihood that all of the air cannot be removed, and the stress to the animal. This procedure is best performed under anesthesia using a light, balanced technique (i.e. fentanyl/diazepam, etomidate,.or ketamine/diazepam can be used)
	Decompression of the stomach may be associated with reperfusion tissue injury.
RADIOGRAPHS	Radiographs aren't necessary for diagnosing GDV. Additionally it's not important to distinguish dilatation alone vs. dilatation and volvulus since surgical decompression and gastropexy should be performed regardless. In addition, both cases may be equally difficult to pass a stomach tube.
	Radiographs should be performed to evaluate for concurrent megaesophagus and other intrathoracic lesions that could affect long-term prognosis. They are also useful for demonstrating to the owner the nature of the animal's problem.
	• Take radiographs with the dog in right lateral recumbency. Look for stomach **compartmentalization** (tissue dense line = fold in the stomach) and displacement of the pylorus dorsally. On V/D view it may be left of midline.
SURGERY after STABILIZATION	All GDV patients should undergo surgical decompression and gastropexy to prevent recurrence. Animals should be stabilized as much as possible prior to anesthesia and surgery.
	• The animal should be on antibiotics prior to surgery. A first generation cephalosporin such as cephalexin is a good choice (20 mg/kg IV).
	• Gastropexy the right side of the stomach to the right abdominal wall.
	• Decompression may release toxins/endotoxins from the ischemic/necrotic stomach and/or spleen leading to shock.
	• Resect any unhealthy stomach. You can determine which tissue is dead by cutting it. Dead tissue does not bleed.
FOLLOWING SURGERY	Monitor 3-5 days for signs of DIC, shock, and VPCs.

For information on risk factors for GDV, go to: www.vet.purdue.edu/epi/bloat.htm

Endocrinology

SUGGESTED READING

Nelson RW: Endocrine Disorders. *In* Cuoto CG, Nelson RW (ed): Essentials of Small Animal Internal Medicine. St. Louis, Mosby-Year Book, 2003.

Feldman EC, Nelson RW: Canine and Feline Endocrinology and Reproduction. Philadelphia, W.B. Saunders, 2004

DIABETES MELLITUS
Classification
Diagnostic Findings
Treatment
Diabetic Crises: Hypoglycemia and Ketoacidosis

Diabetes mellitus is a complex metabolic disorder that results when ß cells of the pancreas can't secrete enough insulin or when insulin is ineffective at the peripheral tissues. This disorder results in abnormalities in carbohydrate, lipid, and protein metabolism leading to hyperglycemia, ketonemia, hyperlipidemia, glucosuria, ketonuria, and metabolic ketoacidosis. Concurrent hyperglycemia and glucosuria are the hallmarks of diabetes mellitus.

The presence of hyperglycemia and glucosuria together are the hallmarks of diabetes mellitus. Be sure that both are present because hyperglycemia and glucosuria can occur alone in other diseases.

I. CLASSIFICATION
    A. **INSULIN-DEPENDENT DIABETES MELLITUS (IDDM) OR TYPE I DIABETES** results when pancreatic ß cells are destroyed (or absent) leading to a decrease in insulin production and secretion. IDDM is the most common form of diabetes mellitus in dogs and cats.
        1. **Etiologies** include pancreatitis, immune destruction of ß cells, inherited disorders (e.g., some Keeshonds are born with low numbers of ß pancreatic cells), amyloidosis (cats).

        2. **Ketoacidosis** can occur in severe, unregulated IDDM. It occurs because when glucose isn't taken up into the cells, the liver compensates by burning more fatty acids as fuel. This causes an overproduction of ketone bodies, which are weak acids. As a result, the pet becomes acidotic. An estimated 40% of dogs presenting to university veterinary hospitals with diabetes present with ketoacidosis.

    B. **NON-INSULIN-DEPENDENT DIABETES MELLITUS (NIDDM) OR TYPE II DIABETES** results when the pancreas can secrete insulin (secretion may be abnormal), but there's peripheral resistance to insulin. NIDDM is more common in cats than dogs. While rare in dogs, 30-50% of diabetic cats have NIDDM. Disease is less severe than with IDDM, and cats can go into remission when treated with insulin (glargine) and proper diet. Animals with NIDDM rarely develop ketoacidosis.

        1. **Etiologies** include:
            a. **Down-regulation of insulin receptors:** This occurs in obese pets.
            b. **Insulin receptor antagonism**
                i. **Excessive growth hormone** due to **acromegaly** in cats or **diestrus** and elevated progesterone levels in intact female dogs
                ii. **Excess cortisol levels** as with iatrogenic or spontaneous hyperadrenocorticism, excess **epinephrine** as with acute stress, excess **glucagon**, or deficiency in **thyroid hormone.**
            c. **Obesity** can lead to reversible down-regulation of insulin receptors. In one study, cats allowed free access to food over 10 months increased their body weight by 44.2% and decreased their insulin sensitivity by 50%. Twenty-five percent had insulin sensitivities within the range reported for diabetic cats.

II. CLINICAL SIGNS and DIAGNOSTIC FINDINGS: Once diabetes mellitus is diagnosed, the animal should undergo a thorough work-up to diagnose diseases resulting from DM (e.g., UTI) or diseases that contribute to or alter the therapy of DM (e.g., Cushing's disease or pancreatitis).

CLINICAL SIGNS and DIAGNOSTIC FINDINGS in DIABETES MELLITUS

CLINICAL SIGNS	POLYURIA, POLYDIPSIA (PU/PD): Blood glucose levels rise above the renal threshold, and glucose spills into the urine causing an osmotic diuresis. POLYPHAGIA is due to the decreased intracellular glucose levels. Without insulin, the blood glucose levels are high but the glucose can't get into the cells. As a result, the animal must metabolize protein and fat reserves. This stimulates the hypothalamic feeding or hunger center. Consequently, the animal has a large appetite, yet it remains in a state of negative nitrogen balance leading to **weight loss.** URINARY TRACT INFECTION (UTI) and OTHER INFECTIONS occur due to the catabolic state. Diabetic animals are especially prone to UTIs because of the high glucose levels in their urine and hyperglycemia-related immunodeficiencies. CATARACTS (dogs): Glucose diffuses into the lens where it's converted by aldose reductase to sorbitol, which is then metabolized to fructose. Since neither sorbitol nor fructose can diffuse out of the lens, the osmotic pressure within the lens increases, thereby drawing water into the lens and leading to disorder of the lens fibers. 30% of dogs have reduced vision on presentation, and 80% have significant cataracts at 16 months following diagnosis. Onset and progression of cataracts are often acute (within days or weeks) SIGNS OF KETOACIDOSIS: Animals can exhibit vomiting, diarrhea, anorexia, dehydration, stupor or coma. They may also have **acetone breath.**
HEMOGRAM	The hemogram is usually normal although the PCV may be elevated with dehydration. If the pet has concurrent pancreatitis or infection, the hemogram may reveal a neutrophilic leukocytosis with toxic neutrophils.
CHEMISTRY	HYPERGLYCEMIA: Normal range is 80-120 mg/dL. Stress-induced hyperglycemia in cats can be as high as 275 mg/dL. Diabetic dogs showing clinical signs of diabetes mellitus have plasma glucose concentrations consistently above 200-250 mg/dL; levels may rise as high as 800 mg/dL. HEPATIC ENZYMES ALT and ALP may be ELEVATED (> 500 IU/L) due to secondary hepatic lipidosis (mobilization of fat stores so that fatty acids can be used to provide energy). Liver function may also be impaired for the same reason. HYPERCHOLESTEROLEMIA (300-500 mg/dL) is caused by lipolysis and changes in lipoprotein (VLDL, LDL) metabolism. OTHER SECONDARY CHANGES • BUN and Creatinine are usually normal in uncomplicated cases. They may be elevated in ketoacidotic animals due to dehydration caused by vomiting, anorexia, severe unregulated glycosuria, and acidosis. • Bicarbonate may be low in ketoacidotic animals (< 12 meq/L). • Hyperosmolality can occur in the **ketoacidotic animal** due to the ketone bodies, hyperglycemia, dehydration, and decreased glomerular filtration rate. • Ions: Na^+, Cl^-, K^+ are decreased due to the PU/PD and hyperglycemia. The body tries to maintain normal osmolality. • Lipase may be elevated if the animal has concurrent pancreatitis or decreased glomerular filtration (dehydration, etc.).
URINALYSIS	• GLUCOSURIA: Cats that are stressed develop a transient hyperglycemia without glucosuria. The hyperglycemic state is so transient that the glucose that does spill into the urine does not reach high enough concentrations to be detectable. • SPECIFIC GRAVITY > 1.015: Specific gravity helps differentiate pre-renal azotemia from primary renal failure in the animal with a mildly elevated BUN or creatinine. • UTI: Bacterial infections are common. • PROTEINURIA is usually associated with UTI. • KETONURIA if the animal is ketoacidotic.

Endocrinology

III. **TREATING DIABETES MELLITUS:** The goal of treatment is to control the signs associated with hyperglycemia and glucosuria while avoiding insulin-induced hypoglycemia. It's important to get the hyperglycemia under control quickly because excess glucose and lipids are toxic to ß pancreatic cells. Ideally it's best to monitor blood glucose levels closely and stay within target range, but clinical signs are as important for monitoring. Since it is difficult to keep levels within this range, at least keep it below the levels where chronic diabetic complications, such as cataracts (dogs) and peripheral neuropathy (cats), develop.

PATIENT	TARGET GLUCOSE LEVELS
Dog without cataracts	120-180 mg/dL
Dog with cataracts	120-250 mg/dL
Cats*	120-300 mg/dL

*Renal threshold for cats is higher than for dogs. Cats manage hyperglycemic states better than dogs.

A. **INSULIN POTENCY and DURATION:** Insulin is categorized by its onset, duration, and potency after SC administration. The shorter-acting the drug, the more potent it is. Zinc and protamine (a fish protein) are used to slow down the SC absorption and prolong the effect of the insulin. Insulin should be kept refrigerated and mixed gently prior to injection by rolling gently between the hands. Most insulins are suspensions.

INSULIN/ROUTE	DURATION	USE	CONCENTRATION
Regular (IV, IM, SC)	Short-acting (Peak 0.5-2 hours)	DKA emergency	U 100
NPH (Humulin-N)	Intermediate	Dog	U 100
Lente (Vetsulin™: porcine)	Intermediate	Dog	U 40
PZI	Long	Cats/dogs	U 40
GLARGINE	Long	Cats (First choice)	U 100

1. **Regular crystalline insulin is quick-acting but short-lasting.** It's good for emergencies. It's the only form that can be given IV and IM as well as SC.
2. **NPH and Lente are intermediate-acting insulins** that take action in 0-3 hours and last about 4-10 hours. NPH contains protamine and zinc. Lente relies on zinc content and the size of zinc-insulin crystals to affect absorption. The smaller amorphous insulin (not complexed) peaks quickly and has a short effect. The larger zinc-insulin crystals are absorbed more slowly and have a longer duration of action. Dogs are usually started on lente (Vetsulin™) or NPH insulin.
3. **Glargine** (Lantus®) was first used in veterinary medicine in 2004 and is now the insulin of choice for **cats.** It's an insulin analog that has been synthesized in the laboratory by changing the amino acid sequence slightly in order to change the pharmacokinetics. Rather than providing a "V"-shaped glucose curve, it leads more to a "U"-shaped curve where the glucose drops more slowly and rises more gradually. Glargine has a longer duration of action than other insulins.
   a. Glargine is a 100 U **solution** rather than a suspension. Its pH is 4.0 so that when injected SC into a pH of 7.0, it precipitates out into the tissue and consequently is **slowly absorbed throughout the day.** Because of the pH, it cannot be diluted or mixed with other insulins. Such diluting or mixing causes it to precipitate out in the bottle instead of in the patient. Glargine can be refrigerated for 6 months but should be discarded after one month once opened. Insulin pens should be at room temperature prior to injecting due to the effect of temperature on fluid volume.
   b. **PZI** also contains both protamine and zinc. It has proven efficacy in cats.
B. **TREATING DIABETIC CATS:** With appropriate treatment, up to 90% of newly diagnosed diabetic cats can achieve remission. This recent change in outcome has been brought about by the introduction of longer-acting insulins such as **glargine** (and PZI). They provide better glycemic control in cats than the previous shorter-acting insulins; consequently, glucose toxicity is prevented. These transiently diabetic cats probably start with mildly abnormal pancreatic secretory ability. Then they experience a period of stress (boarding, illness, new cat in the neighborhood), and they become hyperglycemic. Two days of hyperglycemia of > 250 mg/dL is enough to cause glucose toxicity and consequently further suppress insulin secretion. In the early stages, glucose toxicity is fully reversible. Early control of hypoglycemia with diet, insulin, and sometimes oral hypoglycemics allows the glucose

toxicity to resolve such that many cats go into remission as soon as 4-6 weeks after the start of treatment.

1. **Starting dose of glargine:** Start with BID administration. If the owners are overwhelmed with the idea of treating BID, then start with SID treatment to give them a chance to habituate to the routine. (View video on training cats to accept SC injections at www.behavior4veterinarians.com).

STARTING DOSE of GLARGINE in CATS

BLOOD GLUCOSE	GLARGINE DOSE CHANGE
> 360 mg/dL	0.5 U/kg (based on ideal body weight)
< 360 mg/dL	0.25 U/kg (based on ideal body weight)

2. **Monitoring the first 3 days:** For the first 3 days on glargine, hospitalize the cat and perform a 12-hour BG curve by taking measurements every 4 hours (e.g., at 0 hr, 4 hr, 8 hr, and 12 hr) starting just prior to insulin administration to monitor for **hypoglycemia**. While the glargine has almost no glucose-lowering effect within the first 3 days, it can sometimes lead to hypoglycemia, and cats may require that their dose be **lowered by 25%** during this period. Dose should be based on the **nadir or lowest glucose concentration** during this period. **Do not increase the dose for the first week** regardless of how the curve looks, because it takes at least 5-7 days for glucose and insulin levels to equilibrate. Instead, start the cat on insulin, send the cat home on day 4, and recheck at 1, 2, 3, and 4 weeks after discharge.

MAIN POINTS of TREATMENT

- **Do not increase the insulin dose** within the first 10 days regardless of how the blood glucose curve looks.
- **Do not discontinue glargine** within 2 weeks of starting treatment regardless of the curve.
- **Decrease the dose by 25-50%** if the cat becomes clinically or chemically hypoglycemic.

3. **On weekly rechecks, adjust the glargine dose based on the pre-insulin BG levels** (± nadir), as well as daily water intake and urine glucose concentration.

ADJUSTMENT of GLARGINE DOSE BASED on
PRE-INSULIN and NADIR BLOOD GLUCOSE LEVELS

BLOOD GLUCOSE (mg/dL)	GLARGINE DOSE CHANGE
Pre-insulin BG > 216 Nadir > 180	**Increase dose 0.25-1 U per cat.** Check BG curve for hypoglycemia the next day.
Pre-insulin BG = 180-216 Nadir = 90-160	**No change**
Pre-insulin BG < 180 Nadir = < 54	**Decrease by 0.5-1 U/cat** or, if total dose is 0.5-1 U SID, stop insulin and check for diabetic remission.
Clinical signs of hypoglycemia	**Decrease** dose by 50%.
Pre-insulin 198-252	Use clinical signs such as water intake, urine glucose, and next pre-insulin glucose **to determine whether to increase dose.**
Nadir = 54-72	Use clinical signs (water intake, urine output, next pre-insulin glucose) **to determine whether to decrease dose.**

ADJUSTMENT of GLARGINE DOSE BASED on
PRE-INSULIN GLUCOSE LEVELS (no nadir)

BLOOD GLUCOSE	GLARGINE DOSE CHANGE
> 290 mg/dL	**Increase** by 0.25-1 U. Check BG curve for hypoglycemia the next day.
220-290 mg/dL	No change. Recheck BG curve for hypoglycemia the next day.
180-220 mg/dL	**Decrease** by 0.5-1 U/cat.
< 180 mg/dL	**Decrease** by 0.5-1 U/cat.
< 80 mg/dL	**Decrease** by 1 U/ cat.
Signs of hypoglycemia	**Decrease** dose by 50%.

4. **Checking for remission:** Once the cat has been controlled for at least two weeks and pre-insulin blood glucose is < 180 mg/dL, you can start checking to see whether the cat is in remission. Don't discontinue insulin prior to two weeks. It takes the pancreas time to recover from the toxic effects of the hyperglycemia. If you stop the insulin within two weeks, the DM signs often return. If the cat remains on insulin longer, the pancreas has more time to recover and the remission lasts longer.
    a. Gradually decrease the insulin dose by 0.25-1 U/cat/injection until the cat is at 1 U/cat BID.
    b. Then if the pre-insulin BG is < 180 mg/dL, go to SID administration.
    c. The next day, if the pre-insulin BG is still < 180 mg/dL, do not administer insulin. Instead, perform a full 12-hour glucose curve.
    d. If the pre-insulin blood glucose concentration is > 180 mg/dL on 1 U SID, go back to BID. Attempt to wean the cat again in several weeks.

5. **Treatment and Monitoring of Aggressive Cats:** For cats that are aggressive or highly stressed, in-house monitoring may not be possible. For these cats start with **2 U glargine/cat BID** and check the water intake and urine glucose several times a week.

ADJUSTMENT of GLARGINE DOSE BASED on CLINICAL SIGNS

BLOOD GLUCOSE (mg/dL)	GLARGINE DOSE CHANGE
Water intake normal < 20 mL/kg on wet food < 70 mL/kg on dry food	Same dose
Water intake (polydipsic) > 40 mL/kg on wet food > 100 mL/kg on dry food	Increase dose by 0.5-1.0 U/cat
Urine glucose > 3 + (scale 0-4+)	Increase dose by 0.5-1.0 U/cat
Urine glucose negative	Check for diabetic remission

    a. **Monitor urine glucose:** It should be negative or 1+ at any time during the day. If it is 2+ or higher, then keep increasing the glargine dose by 1 U/cat per week until urine glucose is negative or the water intake is less than 20 mL/kg/day when on dry food or 70 mL/kg/day if on wet food. This is an easier way to monitor than measuring **fructosamine**. Urine glucose can be measured using the Purina glucotest.
    b. Any time the dose is changed, maintain it for 2 weeks and then recheck urine glucose again.
    c. When testing for remission, back off by 1 U/ week and monitor urine glucose and water intake. If urine glucose is positive, then go to the previous dose.

6. **Dietary therapy:** Because cats are carnivores, diabetic cats should be on a **low carbohydrate (< 20%), high protein diet** such as Hill's m/d, Purina DM, or Royal Canin diabetic. If during the first few weeks of treatment their appetite is reduced and they refuse the new diet, then they should receive a palatable food that they will eat, preferably high protein and meat-based. They can be gradually switched to the low carbohydrate diet. For those cats with renal disease, restriction of protein takes precedence over dietary management of the diabetes. (Refer to behavior4veterinarians.com for information on training picky eaters to eat their meals).

    Since obesity decreases insulin sensitivity, cats should be on a restricted calorie diet and the total food allotment for the day measured out and divided into two meals. Meals can be fed in a treat ball or some other type of puzzle feeder so that the cat must exercise to obtain their food. Because cats are carnivores, they make glucose primarily through gluconeogenesis rather than needing to obtain glucose from their diets. As a result, feeding schedule has little effect on blood glucose concentrations in normal cats. Even when deprived of food for over 72 hours, cats can maintain normal blood glucose concentrations. Cats that go into remission should remain on the high protein, low carbohydrate diet indefinitely and maintain a healthy body weight.

7. **Oral hypoglycemics** such as **glipizide** (Glucotrol®), a **sulfonylurea drug,** can be used in cats but are only occasionally effective and may be more difficult to administer than insulin since cats can be hard to pill. These drugs stimulate insulin secretion and enhance sensitivity to insulin. The cat must have some pancreatic function for these drugs to be effective. Starting dose is 2.5 mg PO BID with food. If the cat does not develop adverse effects such as vomiting or icterus, and the ketonuria is controlled, the dose of glipizide can be increased to 5 mg PO BID. Effects may not be seen for several months.

C. **TREATING DIABETIC DOGS**
1. **Insulin therapy:** Dogs are usually started on lente or NPH (Humulin-N).
   a. Porcine lente insulin called **Vetsulin™** (Intervet) is FDA approved for use in dogs and may be approved for cats soon (www.vetsulin.com). It is a U-40 insulin and comes in 2.5 and 10 mL vials that can be refrigerated for 2-4 months. The Vetsulin package insert recommends starting SID and increasing to BID if needed. 80-96% of dogs are controlled by 60 days, although over half require BID treatment. Some clinicians start with BID treatments immediately using a dose such as that in the table below.

STARTING DOSE of VETSULIN™ in DOGS

WEIGHT	SID VETSULIN DOSE	BID VETSULIN DOSE
< 10 kg	1 U/kg +1 U	0.5 U/kg +1 U
10-11 kg	1 U/kg +2 U	0.5 U/kg +2 U
12-20kg	1 U/kg +3 U	0.5 U/kg +3 U
> 20 kg	1 U/kg +4 U	0.5 U/kg +4 U

   b. **NPH:** Start by giving 0.5 unit/kg every 24 hours along with dietary therapy. Dogs usually end up needing BID treatment with NPH too.
   c. As with cats, it's a good idea to keep dogs in the hospital for 24 hours to **monitor for hypoglycemia.** Measure blood glucose at the time of insulin administration and then 3, 6, and 9 hours later to check for hypoglycemia (BG < 80 mg/dL). If the patient becomes hypoglycemic, then decrease the insulin dose before sending him home. If the patient remains hyperglycemic, continue the same dose since the purpose of therapy early on is to start reversing the metabolic abnormalities, and get the pet accustomed to the new diet and the owner to the new regimen.
   d. **Re-evaluate patients once a week** with a history and blood glucose curve until they are under glycemic control. Ideally the clinical signs of diabetes resolve, body weight is stable, and if possible, blood glucose is 80-250 mg/dL for dogs. It usually takes a month to reach glycemic control. Once glycemic control is reached, re-evaluate every 2-4 months using PE, body weight, clinical signs, **blood glycosylated hemoglobin** or **serum fructosamine** concentrations (fructosamine is more useful).

2. **Note on blood glucose curves:** Take the first sample early in the morning (8:00 a.m.), feed the dog, administer the insulin, and then measure the blood glucose every 2 hours. If the dog is on BID insulin, perform a 12-hour curve. If it's on SID insulin, do a 24-hour curve. The ideal glucose curve gradually drops after administration of the insulin and then rises close to its starting height before the next dose. If the blood glucose rises too high, too quickly, then try a longer-acting insulin or dose the animal more frequently. If the effect is minimal, then the dose should be increased by 25%.

3. **Monitoring blood glycosylated hemoglobin (gHB) or glycosylated albumin (fructosamine).** Glycosylated proteins form at a rate proportional to blood glucose. So the higher the blood glucose, the higher the glycosylated proteins will be. Glycosylated hemoglobin reflects changes over 2-3 months, whereas fructosamine reflects changes over about 2 weeks. So fructosamine is a better reflection of recent changes in blood glucose. Unfortunately, many well-controlled animals have elevated fructosamine. The specificity of the test for evaluating glycemic control is low. It can be used, though, to differentiate stress hyperglycemia and to monitor trends in blood glucose. Do not change insulin levels based solely on fructosamine, and don't try to normalize fructosamine.

Endocrinology

Rather, treat based on clinical signs and use fructosamine to increase the index of suspicion for deregulation.

4. Diet and exercise
   a. **Diets:** Studies in diabetic dogs have shown that single meals containing increased soluble fiber result in lower postprandial hyperglycemia; however, over a 1-2 month period diets containing increased insoluble fiber resulted in better glycemic control (measured by significantly lowered glycosylated hemoglobin or fructosamine). One study found that in stabilized diabetic dogs, there was no difference in glycemic control between dogs on a high fiber diet vs. a moderate fiber diet. These conflicting findings indicate marked variation among responses of individual diabetic dogs on dietary fiber. This may be due in part to side effects associated with such diets, including flatulence, diarrhea, vomiting, and constipation, as well as poor palatability of the food. Consequently, the number one concern in changing diets is to choose a moderate to high fiber diet low in carbohydrates that the dog will eat and experience few side effects on. **Avoid semi-moist** foods as they are high in disaccharides and propylene glycol, both of which promote hyperglycemia.

   b. **Dogs with concurrent pancreatitis** should be fed a highly digestible, low fat diet divided into multiple small meals. These dogs initially may need to be on a **low fat cottage cheese** and rice diet (1:2 ratio) and then changed to a prescription high fiber diet. If they get recurring bouts of pancreatitis, keep them on a highly digestible, low fat food such as Waltham LowFat or Hills i/d.

   c. **Weight reduction:** Overweight animals should be placed on a weight reduction regimen involving a high fiber diet and an exercise program. Refer to *Obesity and Weight Reduction* p. 13.5 for more information.

   d. **Exercise** helps with weight loss, thus decreasing the insulin resistance induced by obesity. It also improves distribution of insulin from the injection site. Strenuous exercise, on the other hand, can lead to hypoglycemia. Insulin dose should be reduced—for instance, by 50% initially—during sudden bouts of strenuous exercise (e.g., hunting dogs during hunting season) and the dog evaluated by the owner for clinical signs of hyper- or hypoglycemia. The insulin dosage may also need adjusting during the weight reduction program.

D. SYNOPSIS of HOME CARE

HOME CARE

- The owner should administer a **fixed dose of insulin** at a fixed interval and should keep the animal on its specific diet.
- The owner can monitor urine output, appetite, and body weight. If these factors are normal, the animal is usually well-controlled. The animal should not show signs of vomiting, diarrhea, or anorexia.
- Once or twice a week, owners should check the urine for ketone bodies or glucose using a urine stick. If the patient has ketone bodies or recurrent glucosuria in the face of appropriate clinical signs, perform a blood glucose curve and re-evaluate the pet.
- In cases where the animal shows signs of hypoglycemia such as lethargy, weakness, ataxia, or seizures, the owner should rub a small amount of **Karo syrup** on the pet's mucous membranes and then bring the animal in for examination. (Don't do this if the animal is seizuring because the owner may get bitten.) In cases where the pet stops eating well, the owner should give 1/2 the normal insulin dose. This half-dose is safe even in fasting animals.
- Re-evaluate the pet every 2-4 months. Recheck involves a history, physical exam, and review of the urine glucose information. It may also include a serial blood glucose, or if history is normal, fructosamine levels instead.

E. DIFFICULTY REGULATING GLUCOSE LEVELS
   1. Check that the owner is handling and administering the insulin correctly. Is the bottle being shaken or rolled? Is it overheated or outdated? Is the owner using the correct insulin syringe and giving the correct dose? Is the insulin too dilute?

      a. Perform a blood glucose curve using new, undiluted insulin. If the pet does not respond to the insulin adequately, it's either resistant or it's receiving an inadequate dose. If the dosage administered is greater than 2.2 U/kg, the pet likely has insulin resistance.

2. **Check for the Somogyi effect (counter-regulatory effect).** If the insulin dose is too high causing hypoglycemia, counter-regulatory hormones may be causing the glucose to go back up quickly. The next insulin shot then may only produce a small effect since the counter-regulatory hormones are still elevated. A 24-48 hour serial blood glucose curve will reveal this effect. You'll see the glucose levels drop low and then shoot up soon thereafter. Alternatively, you can reduce the insulin dose and evaluate the patient over a 2-5 day period. If its clinical signs worsen, then it's not the Somogyi effect; the animal is insulin resistant. If there's no change or the animal improves clinically, the hyperglycemia is likely due to the Somogyi effect.

3. **Change the type of insulin:** An alternative to glargine in cats is PZI insulin (2 U/cat BID SC to start).

4. **Check for other disorders** when clinically indicated by performing a CBC, chemistry panel, T4, ACTH stimulation test, progesterone assay, CT scan or MRI (to look for a pituitary tumor causing Cushing's disease or acromegaly). Disorders to check for include:
   a. Renal, liver, or pancreatic insufficiency
   b. Acromegaly (increased GH production)
   c. Hypothyroidism
   d. Diestrus in intact female dogs causes elevated progesterone, which stimulates GH production.
   e. Infection (UTI, etc.)
   f. Cushing's disease
   g. Diabetogenic drugs (steroids, estrogen)

IV. **HANDLING the DIABETIC CRISIS: Hypoglycemia or ketoacidosis**

A. **THE HYPOGLYCEMIC CRISIS:** Hypoglycemic crisis occurs when the animal receives excess insulin or when it receives the correct amount but vomits or fails to eat.
   1. **Treatment:** Discontinue all insulin and administer **Karo syrup** orally. Then place the pet on 5% dextrose until it can be fed. The goal is to stop the seizures and weakness, not to normalize the glucose. Do not administer insulin until hyperglycemia returns.
   2. **Transient or persistent signs:** The pet may experience blindness or cerebral edema due to hypoglycemia. These signs are often transient and may resolve within weeks to months, but they can also be severe and permanent.

B. **TREATMENT for KETOACIDOTIC CRISIS:** Animals in DKA crisis exhibit: (1) hyperglycemia, (2) glucosuria, (3) acidosis, and (4) ketonuria. They may be clinically ill and displaying signs of vomiting, anorexia, and lethargy, or they may look healthy and only show standard signs of diabetes. The **goals** of treatment in the severely ill ketoacidotic patient are to **correct the hypovolemia, dehydration** and **acid-base/electrolyte** imbalances, and to **provide enough insulin** to allow adequate uptake of glucose into the cell. These corrections may be made over 36-48 hours.
   1. **Fluid therapy:** Since total body sodium is usually low in ketoacidotic patients, use 0.9% saline.
      a. **Correct dehydration:** Administer based on the degree of dehydration. Patients are commonly started at a rate of 1.5-2x maintenance. Dehydration should be corrected over 24 hours.
      b. **Acid-base balance** will improve with rehydration and increased tissue perfusion. If pH < 7.1 or bicarbonate is < 12 meq/dL, administer bicarbonate in the fluids over 6 hours to correct acidosis. (Refer to *Fluid Therapy* p. 8.7).
      c. **Hypokalemia:** Most DKA patients are hypokalemic and hypophosphatemic due to losses through urine, vomiting, and decreased intake associated with anorexia. The hypokalemia is masked by acidosis and low insulin. With acidosis, potassium is drawn out of the cells when H+ flows into the cells. With treatment for acidosis, H+ flows out of the cell and potassium flows intracellularly causing the serum potassium levels to fall. If K+ concentration is normal, add 20-40 meq K+ to the fluids (1/2 as KCL and

1/2 as KPO4). Avoid rates faster than 0.5 meq/kg per hr potassium. Check K+ concentrations 1-2x per day.

2. **Insulin:** Use **regular insulin** because it's short-acting and has a rapid onset so it can be dosed more frequently based on blood glucose concentrations.

    a. **Method 1:** Administer 0.2 U/kg insulin IM the first hour and perform blood glucose measurements every 1-2 hours. Then administer 0.1 U/kg every 1-2 hours until the blood glucose is < 250 mg/dL. This usually occurs within 10 hours in dogs and 16 hours in cats. When the pet's blood glucose has decreased and it is rehydrated, maintain the pet on SC regular insulin at 0.1-0.4 U/kg every 4-6 hours until the ketosis is resolved and the patient is eating. Start administering 5% dextrose when the blood glucose is < 250 mg/dL. The goal of insulin therapy is to maintain blood glucose between **200-300 mg/dL**. Once the pet is eating, go to a longer-acting insulin.

    b. **Method 2:** Administer regular insulin every 4-6 hours. Give the first 2-3 doses IM in dehydrated animals or else absorption may be uneven. Start with 0.25 U/kg. Take a blood glucose measurement in 4-6 hours and then redose based on the change. Start administering 5% dextrose when the blood glucose is < 250 mg/dL. When the pet starts eating and drinking, discontinue the dextrose and switch to a longer-acting insulin.

3. **Broad spectrum antibiotics:** Most ketoacidotic patients have concurrent infections. Look for UTI and pneumonia prior to administering antibiotics.

4. **Treat concurrent illness.**

9.10

Endocrinology

HYPERADRENOCORTICISM (CUSHING'S SYNDROME)

Cushing's disease is a clinical syndrome caused by chronic excess cortisol in the blood. This excess may be iatrogenic or spontaneous. The disease is much more common in dogs than in cats; furthermore, Cushingoid cats are usually diabetic.

I. **GENERAL INFORMATION**
Normal Adrenal Glands

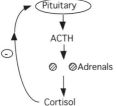

A. **PHYSIOLOGY:** The pituitary gland secretes ACTH, which causes the adrenal cortex to synthesize and release cortisol. Cortisol feeds back to the pituitary gland to regulate ACTH production. If the pituitary gland secretes too much ACTH or if there's a tumor of the adrenal cortex, the adrenals will secrete excess cortisol.

B. **THREE CATEGORIES of HYPERADRENOCORTICISM**

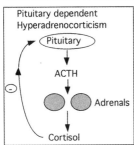
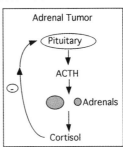

1. **Pituitary-dependent hyperadrenocorticism (PDH):** PDH occurs when the pituitary secretes excess ACTH causing **bilateral adrenocortical hyperplasia**. About 80% of Cushingoid dogs and cats have PDH. 95% of the time this excess secretion is due to a pituitary adenoma. Occasionally it's due to a pituitary adenocarcinoma or to pituitary hyperplasia resulting from a disorder of the hypothalamus leading to increased corticotropin releasing hormone.
2. **Functional adrenocortical carcinoma or adenoma:** About 20% of Cushingoid animals have a **unilateral** adrenal tumor that autonomously secretes excess cortisol. Approximately 50% are adenomas and 50% are carcinomas. The opposite adrenal gland, comprised of non-neoplastic cells, atrophies.
3. **Iatrogenic Cushing's** disease is caused by excessive or prolonged corticosteroid administration leading to atrophy of the adrenal cortices.

II. **GENERAL DIAGNOSTIC INDICATORS OF HYPERADRENOCORTICISM:** Cushing's disease is a clinical syndrome characterized by two or more clinical signs. Signs usually develop slowly over 6 months to 6 years. Thus the owner may not notice the signs until they become a recognizable problem leading to, for instance, urination in the house or raiding of trash cans.
A. **SIGNALMENT:** Middle-aged (over 6 years of age) or older, with 75% of affected animals over 9 years of age
B. **CLINICAL SIGNS:**
1. **PU/PD** occurs in 80% of Cushing's patients. They may urinate 2-10 times more than normal (normal in dogs is under 40-50 mL/Kg/day).
2. **Polyphagia** occurs in about 90% of Cushingoid patients.
3. **Pot-bellied abdomen** occurs due to muscle weakness/atrophy (from the catabolic effects of glucocorticoids), full bladder (due to polyuria),

hepatomegaly (due to steroid-induced hepatopathy), and redistribution of fat to the abdomen. This redistribution occurs in 80% of Cushingoid animals.

4. **Muscle weakness, decreased exercise tolerance, and lethargy** are caused by the catabolic effects of steroids.

5. **Poor wound healing** and increased pyoderma can occur due to immunosuppression.

6. **Hyperpigmentation, calcinosis cutis, bilaterally symmetric hair loss** (due to atrophy of the hair follicle), **poor hair regrowth, thin skin**

7. **CNS signs** can occur in cases where the hyperadrenocorticism is caused by a large pituitary tumor.

8. **Increased vascular fragility** (e.g., purpura) reflects poor wound healing due to decreased tissue granulation.

9. **Panting** is due to increased abdominal and thoracic fat and respiratory muscle weakness, whereas sudden **dyspnea** can be due to **pulmonary thromboembolism.**

C. **HEMOGRAM** is characterized by a **stress leukogram**—leukocytosis, neutrophilia, monocytosis (dogs), lymphopenia, eosinopenia and basopenia. Leukocytosis and neutrophilia are most likely due to release from the marginal pool. Eosinopenia is most likely a result of bone marrow sequestration, and lymphopenia is likely due to destruction of lymphocytes. Dogs may develop polycythemia due to ventilatory problems.

D. **CHEMISTRY PANEL**
1. **Increased ALP** is due to induction of an alkaline phosphatase isozyme with increased activity. Increase occurs in 95% of dogs with Cushing's. It can be mild to severe. Severity does not correlate with disease severity. ALP is a sensitive but not highly specific test and alone should not instigate testing for Cushing's.

2. **Increased ALT** (> 400 IU/dL) is due to hepatocyte damage from swelling and glycogen accumulation.

3. **Hypercholesterolemia** is due to increased fat lipolysis or fat mobilization.

4. **Increased glucose** is due to increased gluconeogenesis in the liver and to insulin antagonism. Blood insulin levels in Cushingoid dogs are elevated relative to the glucose level. Only a small percentage of Cushingoid dogs have diabetes.

5. **Decreased BUN** is due to polyuria, which causes medullary washout.

6. **Decreased T$_4$**: High cortisol levels suppress the pituitary secretion of TSH, leading to decreased secretion of T$_4$ and decreased binding to plasma proteins, which may lead to increased metabolism of T$_4$.

E. **URINALYSIS**
1. **Specific Gravity:** (1.001-1.027; usually < 1.015) Hyposthenuria and isosthenuria are common, but on a water deprivation test, the dog may concentrate the urine to 1.035. Low urine specific gravity and resulting polyuria may be caused by inhibition of ADH at the kidney (nephrogenic diabetes insipidus).

2. **UTI** is common due to immunosuppression. The WBC count in the urine may be lower than normal in cases of UTI since the Cushingoid animal is immunosuppressed. Consequently, in cases where Cushing's disease has been diagnosed, the urine should be cultured even in the absence of elevated urine WBC count.

3. **Glucose:** If the patient has concurrent diabetes mellitus, it will be glucosuric.

4. **Mild to moderate proteinuria** and **high blood pressure** are common (60-70% of cases). Proteinuria is commonly due to glomerular hyperperfusion, glomerular hypertension, glomerulonephritis, and glomerulosclerosis. Urine protein-creatinine ratio is usually ≤ 4.0 mg/dL.

III. **SPECIFIC DIAGNOSTIC TESTS:** Presumptive diagnosis of Cushing's should be made based on history and physical examination. Diagnostics tests are for confirming the diagnosis and determining the cause—pituitary tumor, adrenal tumor, or iatrogenic.

SCREENING TESTS (perform these first)	TESTS to DISTINGUISH PDH FROM ADRENAL CUSHING'S
• **Urine cortisol-creatinine ratio** (< 13 IU/L rules out Cushing's disease) • **ACTH stimulation test** (differentiates iatrogenic from spontaneous Cushing's) • **Low dose dexamethasone suppression test (LDDS)**	• **High dose dexamethasone suppression test (HDDS)** • **Endogenous ACTH levels** • Abdominal **ultrasound** (or brain imaging)

A. **URINE CORTISOL-CREATININE RATIO (UCCR):** Most Cushingoid dogs have elevated UCCR; however, UCCR is elevated with many stress and disease states, too. Consequently UCCR yields many false positives (only 25% specificity). As a result, it is not used to diagnose Cushing's. Rather, low levels (< 13 IU/L) are used to rule out Cushing's disease. Urine should be collected by free catch in the less stressful home environment. UCCR is a good initial screening test to rule out Cushing's disease.

B. **ACTH STIMULATION TEST** is a screening test that shows whether the animal has spontaneous Cushing's disease. It's expensive and less sensitive than the LDDS thus it is often a second choice test. The ACTH stimulation test does not distinguish pituitary-dependent Cushing's from an adrenal tumor, but it does separate endogenous from iatrogenic Cushing's. It is 80% accurate in detecting Cushing's, but 20% of dogs with Cushing's have a normal ACTH stimulation test (20% false negatives). So for dogs that have normal levels with clinical signs of Cushing's, perform further diagnostics to test for Cushing's disease. To run the test, measure the cortisol levels in the morning since they are higher at that time. Then give either 2.2 IU/Kg ACTH gel IM or 0.25 mg synthetic ACTH, such as Cortrosyn® IM (The synthetic ACTH is more readily available). Next measure the cortisol levels 2 hours after ACTH gel administration or 1 hour after synthetic ACTH administration. Cushingoid animals have marked increases (higher than normal) in cortisol. In cats, the dose of synthetic ACTH is 0.125 mg/Kg IM, and blood is drawn prior to administration and at 30 minutes and 1 hour afterward. (An alternate protocol is 0.05 mg/Kg cortrysyn IV with blood samples drawn at 0 and 60 minutes. Excess Cortrysyn® can be stored frozen for up to 3 months.)

	PRE-STIMULATION	POST-STIMULATION
Normal animal	Variable	6-17 μg/dL
Iatrogenic	< 5 μg/dL	< 5 μg/dL (flat line)
Pituitary-dependent	Variable	> 24 μg/dL
Adrenal Cushing's	Variable	> 24 μg/dL

Note: Values in cats are lower, and values vary among diagnostic labs.

1. **Iatrogenic:** The adrenals atrophy due to decreased ACTH release; therefore, they can't respond well to stimulation. Pre- and post-stimulation levels of cortisol may be elevated (but still a flat line) due to prednisone being measured in the blood. For the ACTH stimulation test to be valid, the patient must be off prednisone for more than 3 days.

2. **Pituitary-dependent:** Both adrenals are hypertrophied so they over-respond to ACTH. Cortisol levels are elevated (post-stimulation) in 85% of animals with pituitary-dependent hyperadrenocorticism.

3. **Adrenal tumor:** The neoplastic adrenal over-responds to ACTH. Cortisol levels are elevated (post-stimulation) in 50% of animals with adrenal tumors. Remember that adrenal Cushing's is much less common than PDH.

C. **LOW DOSE DEXAMETHASONE SUPPRESSION TEST (LDDS)** is considered by many to be the test of choice for the diagnosis of hyperadrenocorticism in dogs. It is 95% accurate in determining whether the pet has Cushing's disease. It usually does not differentiate between PDH and adrenal Cushing's, and it does not reveal iatrogenic Cushing's because cortisol levels are chronically low in these patients. In the LDDS test, draw blood prior to administering 0.01 mg/Kg dexamethasone sodium phosphate IV (or dexamethasone polyethylene glycol), and then measure cortisol 4 and 8 hours later. Normal animals have a low cortisol level because the dexamethasone negatively feeds back to the pituitary causing decreased ACTH secretion. Results at 8 hours tell whether the animal is Cushingoid. If 8-hour levels show no suppression, the animal is Cushingoid. If the test shows no suppression at 8 hours but suppression at 4 hours (or partial suppression at 4 and 8 hours) then the pet likely has PDH. In cats, the dose of dexamethasone is 0.01 to as high as 0.1 mg/Kg IV.

	O HOURS	4 HOURS	8 HOURS
Normal animal	Variable	Suppression Cortisol < 1.5 mg/dL or < 50% baseline	
Pituitary - dependent	Variable	± suppression	No suppression Cortisol > 1.5 µg/dL
Adrenal Cushing's	Variable	No suppression Cortisol > 1.5 µg/dL	

1. **Normal animal:** The dexamethasone feeds back to the pituitary, depressing ACTH release. As a result, cortisol levels decrease.
2. **Pituitary-dependent:** No suppression at 8 hours but may have suppression at 4 hours. Animals with PDH have accelerated metabolism of glucocorticoids that leads to the pattern of suppression at 4 hours but not at 8 ("escape" pattern).
3. **Adrenal Cushing's:** The adrenals secrete autonomously. There is no adrenal suppression at 8 or 4 hours with this test. Thus, if there's no suppression at either 8 or 4 hours, the animal has Cushing's disease. If there's no suppression at 8 hours but there is at 4 hours, then it's PDH.

D. **HIGH DOSE DEXAMETHASONE SUPPRESSION TEST (HDDS):** Once the animal has been diagnosed with Cushing's disease, the HDDS test can be used to **rule out PDH.** Perform this test by taking blood prior to administration of **0.1 mg/Kg dexamethasone sodium phosphate** and then again 8 hours later. In cats, the dose of dexamethasone is 1.0 mg/Kg. The high level of dexamethasone causes adrenal suppression in 75% of animals with pituitary-dependent hyperadrenocorticism but does not cause suppression of autonomously secreting adrenals (adrenal Cushing's). If there's suppression, the animal has PDH. If there's no suppression, the animal could have either. So if there's no suppression, perform an **endogenous ACTH**. Note that, usually, if LDDS does not differentiate between PDH and adrenal Cushing's, the HDDS won't either.

	O HOURS	4 HOURS
Normal animal	Variable	Suppression
Pituitary-dependent	Variable	Suppression Cortisol < 1.5 µg/dL or 50% of baseline
Adrenal Cushing's	Variable	No suppression

E. **ENDOGENOUS ACTH** is elevated in animals with PDH vs. adrenal Cushing's. ACTH is susceptible to protease activity that can result in falsely low measured endogenous concentrations.

	ACTH LEVELS*
Pituitary-dependent	> 50 µg/dL
Grey zone	30-50 µg/dL
Adrenal-dependent	0-50 µg/dL

*Values depend on the lab

F. **ULTRASOUND** can help differentiate the cause of Cushing's disease but can't diagnose or rule out the disease. **Bilaterally enlarged adrenals** indicate pituitary-dependent Cushing's. **Unilaterally enlarged adrenals** indicate a primary adrenal tumor but do not specify whether the tumor is functional.

G. **MRI or CT scan** is used to look for and evaluate pituitary tumors.

H. **WHICH TESTS to USE?** The choice depends on whether it's more important to detect possible Cushing's disease or to avoid the likelihood of a false positive (sensitivity vs. specificity).
1. Use UCCR to rule out Cushing's disease. If it's < 13 µg/dL the animal is unlikely to have Cushing's.

2. **LDDS is the test of choice by many for confirming Cushing's in dogs.** It is more sensitive (more likely to detect disease) than the ACTH stimulation test; however, it is less specific (yields more false positives) than the ACTH stim, especially in animals with concurrent disease such as diabetes mellitus. Consequently, use LDDS if the dog has moderate to severe signs of Cushing's, especially proteinuria and hypertension, such that you want to start treating soon, but has no signs of concurrent illnesses.

3. **ACTH stimulation test** has an overall lower sensitivity than LDDS but has a better specificity when the animal has concurrent illnesses. Consequently, use the ACTH stimulation, if the dog has concurrent illness or if the dogs has received exogenous steroids.

4. **Note that** a diagnosis of Cushing's is based on history and clinical signs. Dogs should have marked clinical signs. The screening tests are to confirm the diagnosis. If animals have concurrent illness you may delay testing until they have recovered from the illness.

5. **Once Cushing's is diagnosed**, perform HDDS, endogenous ACTH, or advanced imaging to determine whether it's PDH.

IV. TREATMENT
A. TREATMENT OF PITUITARY-DEPENDENT CUSHING'S

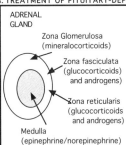

ADRENAL GLAND

Zona Glomerulosa (mineralocorticoids)

Zona fasciculata (glucocorticoids) and androgens)

Zona reticularis (glucocorticoids and androgens)

Medulla (epinephrine/norepinephrine)

1. **Mitotane (o,p'DDD, Lysodren®)** is cytotoxic to the fasciculata layer of the adrenal gland, which makes most of the glucocorticoids. It's used to treat PDH and can also be used to treat adrenal Cushing's in cases where surgery is not a good option.

   a. **Loading dose:** Start with 20-25 mg/Kg BID with meals for better absorption until a response is seen (usually 5-15 days). Monitor the dog for PU/PD and polyphagia. The owner can monitor the dog for polyphagia by feeding only 2/3 of its normal meal size and timing the mealtime.

   The owner can also measure water intake per day (normal dogs drink < 100 mg/Kg/24 hours). When there's a change in signs, stop medication and have the dog come in for an ACTH stim test. If there is no response in 7-10 days, recheck the ACTH stim test. The goal is for post-ACTH stimulation levels of cortisol to be around 2.0-5 μg/dL (mild hypoadrenocorticism). If the animal becomes anorexic or vomits, or levels are ≤ 1.0 μg/dL immediately discontinue and treat for overdose (see below).

   b. If the ACTH stim test results are still high after 10 days, keep medicating every day and then have the dog come back weekly until a low post-ACTH response is achieved or until the dog responds clinically. Owners should be contacted by a technician on a daily basis so that progress can be monitored.

   c. **Maintenance:** Keep the dog on 50 mg/Kg of mitotane orally divided over 2-3 doses per week (e.g., M-W-F or M-F, etc.). Perform a recheck ACTH stimulation test one month after starting the maintenance dose and adjust to keep cortisol levels between 2.0-5.0 μg/dL. Every time dose is changed, repeat the ACTH stim in 6-8 weeks. Once the goal level is reached, repeat ACTH stim every 3-6 months.

   d. **Adverse reactions to mitotane:** Animals can develop GI signs due to toxicity or to sensitivity to mitotane. If signs consistent with **hypocorticism** develop (anorexia, lethargy, vomiting and diarrhea), perform an ACTH stim test to differentiate between hypoadrenocorticism and drug sensitivity. If the dog has drug sensitivity, divide the dose further or increase the interval between treatments. Stop the medications for a few days if needed. If it's hypoadrenocorticism, discontinue mitotane and treat with prednisone or other corticosteroids. At the onset of mitotane treatment, the owner should be sent home with 0.25-0.5 mg/Kg PO prednisone just in case the dog develops acute toxicity. Corticosteroids should take effect within several hours. Continue this dose for 3-5 days before tapering over 1-2 weeks. Once the post-ACTH stim is around 2 μg/dL, mitotane therapy can be started again but at a lower dose, with ACTH stim repeated at 3-4 weeks. Also monitor for changes associated with mineralocorticoid deficiency. **Note:** Mitotane toxicity can cause stupor, circling and ataxia, and behavioral alterations—signs that can also be seen with pituitary tumors.

2. **A safer alternative to mitotane is trilostane**, a competitive inhibitor of ß hydroxysteroid dehydrogenase, which is an enzyme involved in the synthesis of steroids. Trilostane blocks synthesis of both cortisol and aldosterone; however, unlike mitotane, effects are reversible. It is not cytotoxic to the adrenal glands. Trilostane is as effective as mitotane and safer although it can have severe side effects related to induction of hypoadrenocorticism. It's the treatment of choice in Europe but is not approved for use in the U.S. yet.

3. Treating with Trilostane (Vetoryl®).
   a. **Dose:** Start with 0.5-1.0 mg/Kg BID-TID (available in 30, 60, 120 mg tablets) administered with a meal for better absorption. **Side effects include:** decreased appetite, vomiting, diarrhea, shivering, weakness, ataxia or generalized involuntary movements. One study using a starting dose of 3.1 mg/Kg revealed that 25% of the 44 study dogs that were treated for up to two years, exhibited side effects. The 11 dogs exhibiting these adverse effects all had post-ACTH cortisol values < 2μg/dL and half experienced hyperkalemia and hyponatremia. While all responded well to IV fluids and glucocorticoids, trilostane was discontinued indefinitely in 5 of the dogs due to prolonged depression of cortisol values. Four of these dogs no longer needed therapy and one required long-term glucocorticoid and mineralocorticoid supplementation. If the dog develop side effects, stop the medications until the signs subside. Then restart at the same dose but given every other day for a week. Then go to the full dose. Most dogs tolerate it the second time on the full dose.
   b. **Recheck and perform an ACTH stim test at 10-14 days, then at 30 and 90 days,** and then every 4-6 months thereafter. The test should be run 4-6 hours after trilostane administration because by 8 hours the levels are close to zero leading to false impression that the dose needs to be increased . The goal is to keep the levels between 1.0-5 μg/dL. Adjust the dose as needed. Discontinue for 48-72 hours if the dose falls below 1.0 μg/dL and repeat the ACTH stim test prior to restarting treatment. If cortisol levels are in the target range and the animal's clinical signs are controlled, then continue at the same dose.
   c. **Resolution of clinical signs:** PU/PD and polyphagia take 1-4 weeks to resolve, and skin disease may take over 3 months to resolve.

B. **TREATMENT of ADRENAL TUMORS:** Surgery is the primary treatment, but Lysodren® can be used in cases where the owner elects to forego surgery.
C. **TREATMENT of IATROGENIC CUSHING'S:** Wean the animal off corticosteroids.
D. **HYPOPHYSECTOMY:** When performed by experienced surgeons the remission rate can be up to 85% with a 68% 4-year survival time.
V. **PROGNOSIS:** The prognosis for animals that have had their adrenal tumors removed and animals with iatrogenic hyperadrenocorticism is good; however, due to the high incidence of perioperative complications in dogs with adrenal tumors, prognosis in dogs prior to surgery is guarded. Once they survive the surgery and the following weeks, the prognosis is good. The prognosis for animals with PDH depends on other medical complications. On proper medication, they live an average of two years and often die of other diseases such as renal failure. Younger animals with Cushing's tend to have a longer lifespan. Cushingoid animals often develop fatal pulmonary thromboemboli due to hypercoagulopathy.

HYPOADRENOCORTICISM (ADDISON'S DISEASE)

Addison's disease is caused by adrenocortical insufficiency. It can be primary or secondary.

I. **GENERAL INFORMATION**

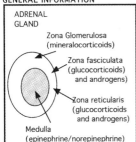

ADRENAL GLAND

Zona Glomerulosa (mineralocorticoids)

Zona fasciculata (glucocorticoids) and androgens)

Zona reticularis (glucocorticoids and androgens)

Medulla (epinephrine/norepinephrine)

A. **CLASSIFICATIONS**
   1. **Primary:** Destruction of the adrenal cortex leads to inadequate levels of glucocorticoids and mineralocorticoids (aldosterone). Mineralocorticoids control sodium, potassium, and water homeostasis. As a result, primary hypoadrenocorticism is characterized by hyperkalemia and hyponatremia. Most dogs with Addison's disease have primary hypoadrenocorticism (e.g., immune-mediated destruction).
   2. **Secondary:** Decreased ACTH production leads to a deficiency in cortisol secretion but not mineralocorticoid secretion. Etiologies include destructive lesions in the pituitary and iatrogenic causes such as glucocorticoid or Ovaban® (estrogen) administration.

II. **DIAGNOSIS**
   A. **SIGNALMENT:** Primarily young or middle-aged females (mean age = 4 years).
   B. **CLINICAL SIGNS,** including vomiting, diarrhea, anorexia, weight loss, and lethargy, initially may present only when the animal is stressed. Other signs include:
      1. **Dehydration and hypovolemic shock:** Loss of sodium by the kidneys leads to hyponatremia and consequently excessive water excretion. This in turn leads to hypovolemia and dehydration. Suspect Addison's disease in animals that present with hypovolemic shock for unknown reasons, especially if they're also bradycardic or they have a history of GI signs. These animals may have a history of appropriate treatment for dehydration followed by representation weeks later for hypovolemia.
      2. **Polyuria and polydipsia** are not as severe as with Cushing's disease.
      3. **Bradycardia** can occur if hyperkalemia is severe enough.
   C. **CBC**
      1. Non-regenerative anemia can be masked by dehydration.
      2. ± Eosinophilia and lymphocytosis occur due to the absence of glucocorticoids.
   D. **CHEMISTRY**

   > Addison's disease must be distinguished from renal disease because both are accompanied by azotemia and hyperphosphatemia.

   1. **Decreased aldosterone** leads to:
      a. **Hyperkalemia,** which is exacerbated if acidosis exists. Note that acute renal failure and post-renal obstruction can cause hyperkalemia too.
      b. **Hyponatremia** leads to intravascular volume loss.
      c. **Hypochloremia** occurs because chloride follows sodium.

      > Normal Na/K = 27:1 - 40:1
      > Addison's Na/K = < 27:1

   2. **BUN increases** due to decreased renal perfusion (prerenal azotemia). It may also increase due to **GI hemorrhage,** which is common with Addison's disease.
   3. **Calcium** increases (**hypercalcemia**). The pathophysiology is unknown.
   4. **Signs similar to that of liver disease:** Addisonian animals often have signs that mimic liver disease, including: microhepatica; decreased BUN, albumin, cholesterol, and glucose; and increased liver enzymes. If the signs are due to Addison's disease rather than primary liver disease, they resolve with treatment for Addison's.
      a. **Hypoalbuminemia** may be due to GI bleeding and decreased synthesis.
      b. **Hypocholesterolemia** can occur due to decreased hepatic synthesis and decreased cholesterol absorption.
      c. **Increased liver enzymes** and microhepatica may be a result of hypovolemia.

Endocrinology

     d. **Hypoglycemia:** Glucocorticoids cause increased gluconeogenesis and increased peripheral uptake of glucose; therefore, a decrease in glucocorticoids has the opposite effect, leading to hypoglycemia.

E. **URINE SPECIFIC GRAVITY** can be normal, increased, or decreased (isosthenuric). With Addison's disease, increased specific gravity is due to hypovolemia and dehydration. Isosthenuria and hyposthenuria are due to sodium loss in the urine. Sodium is needed to establish the medullary gradient for concentrating urine. If urine specific gravity is > 1.030, rule out prerenal azotemia vs. Addison's disease. If specific gravity is isosthenuric, rule out primary renal disease vs. Addison's.

F. **SPECIFIC TESTS** to confirm Addison's disease:

    1. **ACTH stimulation test:** Cortisol levels are most commonly measured in the

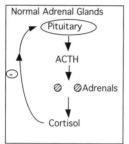

morning because they are higher at that time, but you can perform this test any time of day. In the crisis case, it's important to perform the test immediately. Perform the test as described under Cushing's disease. Addisonian animals have minimal increases (lower than normal) in cortisol. In cats, the dose of synthetic ACTH is 0.125 mg/kg IM, and blood is drawn prior to administration and at 30 minutes and 1 hour afterward. It's best to use syntropin IV since IM injections may not be absorbed well in circulatory shock.

	ACTH STIM	ALDOSTERONE	ACTH LEVELS
Primary Addison's	< 2 µg/mL	Decreased	Increased
Secondary Addison's	< 2 µg/mL	Normal	Decreased

G. **TREATMENT in the ADDISONIAN CRISIS:** Treatment consists of fluid therapy, electrolyte stabilization, control of GI hemorrhage, and glucocorticoid plus or minus mineralocorticoid replacement.

    1. **Fluids:**

        a. **Correct the hypovolemia:** Use 0.9% NaCl at a shock dose (30-90 mL/kg rapidly) to increase the vascular space and provide NaCl. Don't give potassium; the animal is hyperkalemic.

        b. **Restore acid-base balance:** Correction of the hypovolemia and dehydration restores much of the acid-base balance.

        c. **Correct hyperkalemia** by rehydrating the animal and fixing the acid-base balance.

    2. **Administer corticosteroids** once the ACTH stim test has been performed confirming the diagnosis of Addison's disease. Use a rapid-onset steroid such as dexamethasone sodium phosphate or prednisolone sodium succinate. Dexamethasone does not interfere with the ACTH stim test.

        a. Dexamethasone SP: 2-4 mg/kg IV

        b. Prednisolone sodium succinate (Soludelta®): 30 mg/kg IV

        c. Hydrocortisone: 2.4 mg/kg slow IV (has mineralocorticoid action)

    3. **Administer mineralocorticoids** for primary Addison's disease:

        a. Florinef® (fludrocortisone): 0.02 mg/kg PO divided BID

        b. Desoxycorticosterone pivalate (DOCP): 2.2 mg/kg IM every 25 days

    4. **Treat GI hemorrhage** with GI protectants and a blood transfusion if needed.

H. **MAINTENANCE TREATMENT:** Send the pet home on **prednisone** or **prednisolone** (2.5-10 mg per dog PO daily or every other day). If the dose is too low, you will see GI signs. Addisonian animals have a poor response to stress. If you can predict that the animal will be under more stress (i.e., a plane trip), increase the prednisolone dose a little in advance.

    1. **Mineralocorticoids:** Administer Florinef® (fludrocortisone at 0.1 mg/10 pounds body weight PO SID to BID) or DOCP (2.2 µg/kg SC q 25 days).

    2. If it's **iatrogenic** Addison's, taper the dose of prednisolone. The amount of time over which to taper the dose depends on the chronicity of development.

I. **PROGNOSIS** for a normal life expectancy is good as long as the patient is medicated appropriately at the correct intervals. Recheck the patient and perform a chemistry panel about once every 3 months.

HYPERTHYROIDISM in CATS

Hyperthyroidism is the most common endocrine disorder in geriatric cats. It results from excessive production of T_4 and T_3. 95% of hyperthyroid cats have hyperplastic thyroids or adenomas; the other 5% have malignant thyroid adenocarcinomas.

SIGNALMENT	Older cats. 95% are 8 years and older. Test for hyperthyroidism in any sick cat over 10 years of age.
CLINICAL SIGNS	• Polyphagia, PU/PD • Weight loss • **Hyperactivity,** attitude changes, seeks cool places, becomes restless • **Vomiting** and **diarrhea** (increased frequency of defecation; feces are often pale and fatty looking due to steatorrhea, a small intestinal sign) • **Skin changes:** Unkempt coat (common) and patches of alopecia (uncommon) due to psychogenic licking • **Apathetic hyperthyroidism** is characterized by lethargy, anorexia, and dehydration.
PHYSICAL EXAM FINDINGS	• ± dehydration • Thin • **Cardiac:** Sinus tachycardia, a gallop rhythm, or a murmur may be associated with hypertrophic, or less commonly dilative, thyrotoxic cardiomyopathy. Later in disease, other arrhythmias can occur. • **Thyroid nodule:** 90% of cats have a palpable thyroid mass in their ventral cervical region. The thyroid gland is loosely attached to the trachea and may be found as caudal as the thoracic inlet or cranial mediastinum. Both thyroid glands are affected in approximately 75% of cats. When only one gland is affected, the unaffected gland is atrophied and non-functional due to decreased TSH secretion. • **Systemic hypertension** may manifest as retinal hemorrhage or detachment.
CBC AND CHEMISTRY	• Slight **polycythemia,** especially if the cat is dehydrated. This is the opposite of kidney disease where the cat has a non-regenerative anemia. • **Elevated liver enzymes:** Mild increase in ALP and ALT. • Decreased creatinine and BUN due to muscle wasting, or **increased creatinine, BUN and/or phosphate** due to dehydration, leading to pre-renal or renal disease. Older cats may have concurrent renal disease.
SPECIFIC TESTS	**Elevated baseline serum T_4 (T_4):** If T_4 is borderline high in the face of clinical signs, and physical exam findings indicate hyperthyroidism, retest T_4 in 2-4 weeks because T_4 levels sometimes fluctuate in hyperthyroid cats with mild disease. Some thyroid nodules are non-functional though. **TSH stimulation test** is not helpful in cats. **T_3 suppression test** evaluates the responsiveness of the pituitary TSH secretion to suppression by T_3. Measure baseline serum T_4 and T_3 concentration in the morning and then administer T_3 (25 µg/cat) PO TID for 7 treatments. Measure T_3 and T_4 2-4 hours after the last treatment. Because T_3 can't be converted to T_4, measurement of serum T_4 assesses thyroid gland function, whereas measurement of serum T_3 assesses whether the cat received adequate T_3. In the normal cat, T_3 should suppress pituitary secretion, causing a decline in serum T_4 concentration by $\geq$ 50%. Perform this test when baseline T_4 is normal but clinical signs and physical exam findings suggest hyperthyroidism.

HYPERTHYROIDISM in CATS (continued)

SPECIFIC TESTS CONTINUED	**Thyroid Scan:** This involves injecting technetium intravenously and then evaluating its uptake in all functional thyroid tissue. The thyroid gland uptake can be compared with the salivary gland uptake. This scan tells us whether the cat is truly hyperthyroid and whether disease is: • Unilateral • Bilaterally symmetric • Bilateral but asymmetric (the most common) It also tells us where the affected tissue is located and whether there's multiple ectopic thyroid tissue either from embryonic thyroid material or from metastasis of thyroid carcinomas.
TREATMENT Surgery and irradiation are attempts to cure the disease. Oral antithyroid medication is given to control the disease either short term or long term.	**Oral antithyroid medications, such as methimazole** (Tapazol®), **propylthiouracil, and carbimazole,** should be used initially in hyperthyroid cats to reverse the metabolic and cardiac derangements in order to stabilize the animal for anesthesia and to assess the effect of treatment on renal function. These drugs block the synthesis of thyroid hormone but don't block the release of stored thyroid hormone into the circulation, and they don't have antitumor action. Problems with giving them include: (1) pilling hyperthyroid cats is difficult (See instructional video at www.behavior4veterinarians.com, (2) the drugs can cause GI upset (vomiting) and bone marrow suppression (the granulocyte line is suppressed first so you tend to see neutropenia), and (3) cats on oral antithyroid medications often become ANA positive and develop AIHA. Cats on these medications should have a CBC performed once every two weeks initially. **Methimazole has the lowest incidence of adverse effects.** Start with 2.5 mg PO SID and adjust as needed after two weeks. Once an appropriate level is achieved, recheck T_4 levels every 4-6 months. **Surgery** to remove the affected glands can be curative. The disadvantages are: • If the disease is bilateral, the parathyroid glands may be damaged or destroyed during the surgery causing the cat to become hypocalcemic. This problem may be transient due to temporary disruption of the blood supply to the parathyroid glands, or it can be permanent. Supplement with calcium or vitamin D_3 if needed when the serum calcium is less than 7 mg/dL or when the cat shows clinical signs of hypocalcemia. • The cat may develop Horner's syndrome or vocal cord paralysis. • It's difficult to perform anesthesia on hyperthyroid cats. They can die suddenly during anesthesia due to sinus tachycardia. They can be medicated with methimazole (Tapazol®) for several months prior to surgery and/or given propranolol or atenolol starting a week prior to surgery to treat for tachycardia and ventricular arrhythmias. • Hypothyroidism • Cats with unilateral thyroidectomies may develop hyperthyroidism later. **Irradiation with** [131]**I:** This is the treatment of choice in any hyperthyroid cat unless the cat is also in renal failure. The treatment kills functioning cells but not atrophied normal cells, thus the cat can still retain normal thyroid function. This is a low risk, low stress treatment that requires the cat to be hospitalized for several weeks. This treatment can be curative but is not 100% effective (may need repeat treatment). Most cats attain normal thyroid hormone levels within 1 week but some take as long as 6 months.
COMPLICA- TIONS	The cat should be evaluated for the presence of cardiac disease and renal disease and treated appropriately. Furthermore, hyperthyroidism often masks renal disease by increasing cardiac output, thereby increasing glomerular filtration rate. Once the hyperthyroidism is corrected, glomerular filtration rate may decrease dramatically. Prior to surgical or radiation therapy, perform a trial of methimazole and then perform repeat chemistries to monitor for azotemia. Renal decompensation usually occurs within the first several weeks of treatment.
PROGNOSIS	PROGNOSIS depends on the cat's physical condition at the time of diagnosis as well as the cause of the hyperthyroidism (adenoma vs. adenocarcinoma). Surgery and irradiation may be curative while medical therapy is just palliative. Cats with hyperthyroidism due to thyroid hyperplasia can be maintained on **methimazole** for years.

HYPOTHYROIDISM in DOGS

I. THE THYROID GLAND secretes the following:

A. **90% T4,** which when circulating in the blood is 99% bound to serum

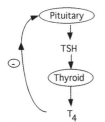

proteins. This bound T4 serves as a storage form. The remaining **free or unbound T4** (fT4) is the biologically active form that can enter the cells and can also feed back to the pituitary to inhibit further secretion. Once in the cells, it's converted to T_3 through deiodinations (leading to a product with 3 iodines instead of).

B. T_3 (3,5,3' triiodothyroxine) is found **intracellulary**. It binds to receptors on mitochondria, the nucleus and the plasma membrane, and exhibits a physiologic effect of stimulating cellular activity.

C. REVERSE T_3 (3,3,5' triiodothyroxine) is physiologically inert. When the animal is in a state of illness where decreased metabolism is beneficial (e.g., heart failure, starvation, other illnesses), it converts **T4** to reverse T_3.

SIGNALMENT	Large breed dogs are more likely to develop hypothyroidism. Certain breeds such as Doberman Pinschers and Golden Retrievers are predisposed.
CLINICAL SIGNS Suspect hypothyroidism when you see a dog with lethargy, weight gain, an endocrine pattern of non-pruritic alopecia and no PU/PD.	Signs due to slow cellular metabolism • Lethargy, obesity, mental dullness Dermatologic signs • Seborrhea and/or hyperkeratosis • Alopecia (usually truncal), hyperpigmentation and lichenification: The guard hairs epilate easily because they are stuck in the resting (telogen) phase of the growth cycle. The alopecic regions take a long time to regrow. Hair loss and lichenification of the tail result in a "rat tail" appearance. • Pyoderma occurs due to impaired T-cell function and decreased lymphocytes. • Dry, brittle haircoat that's lighter in color: The hair may look frizzy like that of a puppy. • Myxedema: Mucopolysaccharide accumulation in the skin and binding of water leads to increased skin thickness. The result is often a tragic facial expression. • Otitis externa Cardiac signs: Bradycardia, decreased contractility Neuromuscular signs are caused by impaired neuronal metabolism leading to segmental demyelination or by compression of neurons due to myxedema. They include: • Seizures • Polyneuropathy: facial paralysis, Horner's syndrome, localized or diffuse weakness Hematologic: It's unclear whether von Willebrand's disease is related to hypothyroidism. Reproductive signs: Infertility and lack of libido Ocular disease such as corneal dystrophy (lipid deposits in the cornea) may occur in association with hyperlipidosis.
CBC/CHEMISTRY	Chemistry: 75% of patients have hypercholesterolemia (usually > 400 mg/dL and sometimes > 1000 mg/dL). If a seizuring dog has hypercholesterolemia, rule out hypothyroidism as an etiology. CBC: Dogs often have a normocytic, normochromic, nonresponsive anemia. They may also have target cells (leptocytes) due to increased cholesterol in the RBC membranes.

HYPOTHYROIDISM in DOGS (continued)

SPECIFIC DIAGNOS-TIC TESTS	Do not measure T_3 levels. T_3 is primarily intracellular. **Serum T4** (includes bound and unbound T4): 95% of dogs with hypothyroidism have a low T4 (95% sensitivity), but this test is only 80% specific, meaning that there's a 20% chance of false positive. Thus **T4 can be used to rule out hypothyroidism;** if the T4 is normal, it's highly likely the dog is not hypothyroid. But T4 cannot be used to definitively diagnose hypothyroidism (due to 20% false positive). T4 is decreased in severely sick patients (such as those in ICU). **Free T4 (fT4)** is the T4 in the serum not bound to protein. Only 0.1% of T4 is fT4 but because it is the biologically active form, the body regulates it tightly. Consequently it's a much better indicator of thyroid function than total T4. It should be measured using the **equilibrium dialysis method.** This method has a 98% sensitivity such that most hypothyroid dogs will have low fT4, and it has a specificity of 93% such that there are only 7% false positives (100%-93% = 7%). If T4 is low then **fT4** should be measured. Half of dogs with severe illness have low thyroid levels (sick euthyroid). **TSH concentration:** With low T4, TSH should be elevated; however TSH is only elevated in 70% of dogs with hypothyroidism. Unlike T4 and fT4, TSH does not change in sick dogs. So if a dog is sick and you want to check for hypothyroidism, TSH concentration is useful. . **Response to empirical therapy** can be used to diagnose hypothyroidism. Truly hypothyroid dogs generally respond in 3-7 days with a dramatic increase in activity and mental alertness. Other abnormalities respond more slowly over weeks or months. Continue trial therapy for at least 4-8 weeks and then wean off medications. If signs return, this indicates true hypothyroidism.
WHICH TESTS	Ideally T4, fT4 and TSH would all be used in diagnosing hypothyroidism, but where limits exist, here is one scheme to try: If T4 is low and the dog has only a few mild clinical signs (such as obesity and poor haircoat), because the serum T_4 yields 20% false negatives, perform an **fT4** to confirm. If the dog has numerous signs of hypothyroidism such as bilaterally symmetric alopecia; rat tail; hypercholesterolemia; normochromic, normocytic anemia; and a low T4, there's no need for an fT4 to make the diagnosis of hypothyroidism.
TREAT-MENT	Therapy is life-long, but all abnormalities are reversible. Treat with **sodium levothyroxine** (Soloxine® or Synthroid®). It's better to use T4 supplements because they can be converted to T_3, whereas T_3 can't be converted to T4. Start with 0.02 mg/kg every 12 hours and measure T4 every 2-4 weeks until the dog is in a normal thyroid range. If the dog is on twice-a-day treatment, then take the blood sample just before it receives a dose and again 4-6 hours later. If it's on once-a-day treatment, take the blood sample just prior to dosing and then 8-10 hours after. This way you get both a peak and a trough value. Peak values should be in the upper 50th percentile of normal range, whereas trough values should be above the low end of normal. If the animal is hypothyroid, improvements occur within the following time frames: • Dramatic improvement in **activity** within the **first week:** The average euthyroid dog on thyroid hormone feels better, too, but the change is not as dramatic. • **Skin improvement** in one month: Skin conditions may not fully resolve for several months. Additionally, improvement in skin condition may not indicate that the dog is hypothyroid. Normal dogs on thyroxine have an increased rate of hair growth. So dogs with alopecia due to causes other than hypothyroidism may also improve on thyroid medications. • **Neuromuscular** improvement in 3 months • Improvements in **reproductive problems** (anestrus): 6 months to 1 year
ANES-THESIA	Take precautions when anesthetizing hypothyroid dogs. These dogs tend to become hypothermic, and due to the decreased cellular metabolism, anesthetic agents may have a more potent and long-lasting effect.

CALCIUM and PHOSPHORUS
Calcium and Phosphorus Regulation
Hypercalcemia

I. **CALCIUM and PHOSPHORUS REGULATION:** Both calcium and phosphorus are absorbed from the diet, stored in the bone, and excreted via urine. Because calcium is so vital for nerve function, skeletal function, and cardiac muscle function, it is tightly regulated. Total serum calcium is generally kept between 9-10 mg/dL. Phosphorus, which serves as an intracellular buffer and a constituent of macromolecules in bone, is not as tightly regulated.

  A. **OVERVIEW of HORMONES:** Three hormones—**parathyroid hormone (PTH), vitamin D, and calcitonin** are involved in calcium/phosphorus regulation.
  PTH and vitamin D function to keep serum calcium levels from falling below normal.
  1. Both **PTH and vitamin D** levels increase in response to hypocalcemia. This increase triggers absorption of dietary calcium by the GI tract, release of calcium from the bone into the blood, and resorption of calcium from the renal tubules back into the blood. Diseases where PTH is pathologically elevated (such as with parathyroid tumor) lead to hypercalcemia.

  2. **Calcitonin** functions to prevent elevated serum calcium. Calcitonin levels increase in response to hypercalcemia and lead to decreased calcium resorption from bone into the blood and decreased calcium resorption at the kidneys. Calcitonin can be administered exogenously as a therapy for hypercalcemia.

  B. **SITES of CALCIUM and PHOSPHORUS REGULATION:** Both calcium and phosphorus are regulated at the level of the gut, bone, and kidney.

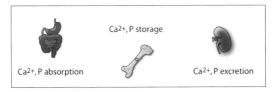

Ca^{2+}, P storage

Ca^{2+}, P absorption

Ca^{2+}, P excretion

  1. **GI Tract:** Dietary calcium and phosphorus are absorbed in the intestinal tract. Absorption is regulated by **vitamin D.** Diets deficient in calcium can lead to hypocalcemia. Diets with excessive calcium can lead to soft tissue calcification/bladder stones.

  2. **Bone** acts as a **storage site** for calcium and phosphorus. Both calcium and phosphorus flow in and out of the bone depending on the amount of remodeling and normal turnover. Remodeling, which is carried out by osteoclasts and osteoblasts, reshapes and reforms bone to meet the changing mechanical needs that occur throughout life. When calcium levels in the blood are low, osteoclasts are activated and both calcium and phosphorus are resorbed into the blood. When calcium levels in the blood are high, osteoblasts are activated and calcium and phosphorus are deposited into the bone.

  3. **Kidney:** The kidney is the primary route of excretion for calcium and phosphorus. Calcium in the blood is either in the **active ionized form** or is bound to albumin. The ionized form (about 50%) is filtered by the glomerular apparatus of the kidneys. 99% is reabsorbed, mostly in the proximal tubule. Since most of the calcium is reabsorbed into the blood, the calcium does not appear in the urine. When glomerular filtration rate (GFR) is decreased (e.g., anuria or oliguric renal failure), less calcium and phosphorus are filtered; therefore, calcium and phosphorus remain in the blood resulting in hypercalcemia and hyperphosphatemia. On the other hand, if an animal is PU/PD, the glomerular apparatus filters calcium and phosphate normally, but because the tubular flow rate is so fast, serum calcium and phosphorus levels drop.

ORIGIN of the PTH, VITAMIN D, and CALCITONIN
1. **PTH** is made by the four parathyroid glands located near the thyroids.
   Calcitonin is made by the thyroid gland.

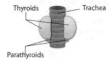

2. Vitamin D is a group of steroid vitamins (synthesized from cholesterol).

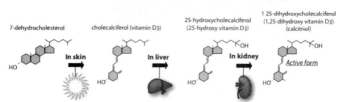

a. Cholesterol is converted to 7-dehydrocholesterol. In the presence of sunlight this compound is converted to vitamin D_3 (a.k.a. **cholecalciferol**) in the skin. Humans who aren't exposed to enough sunlight or who wear sunscreen continuously require vitamin D supplementation such as in vitamin D-fortified foods.

b. Vitamin D_3 is transported bound to vitamin D binding protein within the blood to the **liver.** At the liver it's hydroxylated to 25-hydroxy vitamin D_3 (a.k.a. 25-hydroxycholecalciferol or **calcidiol**).

c. Calcidiol travels to the kidney where it is hydroxylated either to **1,25-dihydroxy vitamin D_3** (a.k.a. 1,25-dihydroxycholecalciferol or **calcitriol**), which is the **active form,** or it is converted to 24,25-dihydroxy vitamin D_3, which is inactive. Vitamin D_3 is converted to the active form when calcium levels are low (thus PTH is high and the body needs higher active D_3 levels to normalize the calcium). It's converted to the inactive form when calcium levels are high and thus less active D_3 is needed.

D. **REGULATION of CALCIUM LEVELS and PHOSPHORUS LEVELS by HORMONES**

Vitamin D: ⇧Ca^{2+}, ⇧P

Vitamin D: ⇧Ca^{2+}, ⇧P resorption
PTH: ⇧Ca^{2+}, ⇧P resorption
Calcitonin: ⇩Ca^{2+}, ⇩P resorption

Vitamin D: ⇧Ca^{2+}, ⇧P resorption
PTH: ⇧Ca^{2+}, ⇩ P resorption
Calcitonin: ⇩Ca^{2+}, ⇩P resorption

1. The goal of **vitamin D$_3$ (a.k.a. cholecalciferol)** is to increase serum Ca^{2+} levels.
   a. **GI:** It increases intestinal absorption of calcium and phosphorus.
   b. **Bone:** It increases bone resorption (release) of calcium and phosphorus into the blood.
   c. **Kidney:** It increases kidney resorption of calcium back into the blood.

   With vitamin D$_3$ excess (as occurs in rats poisoned with cholecalciferol), you'd expect to see hypercalcemia due to increased GI uptake, increased bone resorption and increased kidney resorption of calcium. This could lead to renal failure and ectopic calcification. A deficiency of vitamin D$_3$ leads to rickets and osteomalacia. Note that active vitamin D$_3$ (calcitriol) levels may decrease in chronic renal disease, leading to hypocalcemia.

2. **PTH** is secreted in response to low serum calcium and low active vitamin D$_3$ (calcitriol) levels. Like calcitriol, it serves to increase serum calcium. Additionally, in order to keep the Ca^{2+} x P product below 60-70 mg/dL, a level leading to ectopic calcification, PTH causes lowering of phosphorous levels. While vitamin D$_3$ works at three sites, PTH works directly at two sites—the bone and kidney—to increase resorption of calcium into the blood. It also stimulates the formation of active vitamin D$_3$ by the kidneys.
   a. **Bone:** Because calcium and phosphorus resorption occur together, PTH stimulates both calcium and phosphorus resorption. Thus the main difference occurs at the kidneys.
   b. **Kidney:** PTH increases resorption of calcium but decreases resorption of phosphorus.

3. **Calcitonin** functions to decrease serum calcium. Like PTH, it works at the bone and kidneys. Calcitonin is only involved in fine-tuning calcium and phosphorus levels.
   a. **Bone:** It activates osteoblasts leading to deposition of calcium and phosphorus into the bone (decreasing serum calcium and phosphorus in the blood).
   b. **Kidney:** It decreases calcium and phosphorus resorption at the kidney (leading to decreased serum calcium and phosphorus levels in the blood).

EFFECTS of HORMONES on Ca^{2+} and PO$_4$ METABOLISM

	FUNCTION		INTESTINE		BONE	KIDNEY		SERUM PO$_4$
Vitamin D	$\uparrow$ Ca^{2+}	$\uparrow$ PO$_4$	$\uparrow$ Ca^{2+} absorption	$\uparrow$ PO$_4$ absorption	Increased bone resorption	$\uparrow$ Ca^{2+} resorption	$\uparrow$ PO$_4$ resorption	$\uparrow$
PTH	$\uparrow$ Ca^{2+}	$\downarrow$ PO$_4$	No direct effect		Increased bone resorption	$\uparrow$ Ca^{2+} resorption	$\downarrow$ PO$_4$ resorption	$\downarrow$
Calcitonin	$\downarrow$ Ca^{2+}	$\downarrow$ PO$_4$	No direct effect		Decreased bone resorption	$\downarrow$ Ca^{2+} resorption	$\downarrow$ PO$_4$ resorption	$\downarrow$

II. HYPERCALCEMIA

DEFINITION	Hypercalcemia is defined as: **Dog:** Total serum calcium concentration > 12 mg/dL **Cat:** Total serum calcium concentration > 11 mg/dL About 50% of calcium is in the active ionized form and 50% is bound to albumin. Consequently, total calcium levels are influenced by albumin levels, but ionized calcium is not. Correction factors were once used to get a true idea of ionized calcium levels, but these factors have been found to be non-predictive. Therefore, if total calcium is elevated, then measure **ionized calcium.** If ionized calcium is high, the animal is **hypercalcemic.** Prior to checking ionized calcium, you may first check for lipemia and hemolysis, which can falsely elevate total calcium levels. Then recheck total calcium levels. If they are still high, check ionized calcium levels to confirm hypercalcemia. If total calcium is $\geq$ 15 mg/dL, the ionized calcium will be high and there is no need to measure ionized calcium in this case.
CLINICAL SIGNS	Calcium is vital to bone structure, nerve function, neuromuscular function (important in muscle contraction of skeletal and cardiac muscles), and enzyme activity (e.g., as a cofactor for clotting cascade enzymes). **PU/PD** due to renal damage **Pollakiuria/stranguria** due to calcium oxalate uroliths or renoliths **Weakness** due to decreased CNS and PNS excitability; **seizures** **Vomiting/constipation** due to decreased GI motility
ETIOLOGIES	**NEOPLASIA** such as **lymphosarcoma** and apocrine gland adenocarcinomas can lead to production of PTH-like hormones. These neoplasms may release factors that stimulate osteoclastic bone resorption (hypercalcemia of malignancy). Those involving bone may lead to localized osteolysis. **CHRONIC RENAL FAILURE:** Hypercalcemia occurs in 10-14% of dogs and cats with chronic renal failure. Be sure to determine whether the hypercalcemia is the cause or result of the renal failure. **ADDISON'S DISEASE:** The exact mechanism of hypercalcemia related to hypoadrenocorticism is unknown. 28-45% of dogs with Addison's disease are hypercalcemic. **HYPERVITAMINOSIS D** (cholecalciferol rodenticides) leads to increased calcium and phosphorus levels followed by signs of renal failure. **PRIMARY HYPERPARATHYROIDISM** (rare): The parathyroid gland secretes too much PTH leading to hypercalcemia. Phosphorus is normal or low. If the animal is severely hypercalcemic for a long time, it develops renal failure, which leads to elevation of phosphorus too. Once this occurs, the condition looks like secondary renal hyperparathyroidism. Primary hyperparathyroidism is due to **parathyroid adenoma, adenocarcinoma, or hyperplasia.** **SECONDARY HYPERPARATHYROIDISM** occurs in response to hypocalcemia such as occurs with low dietary calcium intake or chronic renal disease. Note in renal disease, hypocalcemia is due in part to decreased renal formation of calcitriol. • **Secondary nutritional hyperparathyroidism** is triggered by low dietary calcium intake. • **Renal secondary hyperparathyroidism** is triggered by low calcium and low calcitriol levels that occur with chronic renal failure. Release of PTH leads to an increase in calcitriol and increased absorption of calcium from the kidney, gut, and bone. So in addition to an already elevated phosphorus, PTH and calcium increase. If the serum Ca^{2+} x P product are > 60, the animal develops dystrophic mineralization; therefore, with renal secondary hyperparathyroidism, it's important to combat hyperphosphatemia by restricting dietary phosphorus, using phosphate binders, and possibly administering **calcitriol** (vitamin D_3). **GRANULOMATOUS DISEASE** (rare—e.g., blastomycoses): Hypercalcemia is due to increased bone remodeling. **NON-MALIGNANT SKELETAL DISORDER** (rare—osteomyelitis or hypertrophic osteodystrophy): Hypercalcemia is due to increased bone remodeling.

CHANGES in SERUM PHOSPHORUS, CALCIUM and PTH WITH HYPERPARATHYROIDISM

	Serum Ca^{2+}	Serum PO$_4$	PTH
Primary hyperparathyroidism	↑	N or ↓	↑
Malignancy (PTH-like hormone)	↑	N or ↓	N
Secondary hyperparathyroidism (i.e., due to renal failure, etc.)	↑	↑	↑

HYPERCALCEMIA (continued)

DIAGNOSTIC WORK-UP	Check for evidence of **renal failure** by examining the chemistry panel for elevation in **BUN** and **creatinine,** and by checking the urine specific gravity for **isosthenuria.** If the values indicate renal failure, next determine whether the renal failure is primary or secondary to the hypercalcemia. • **Check the PTH levels.** Normal or elevated levels indicate hyperPTH. If kidney function is abnormal this suggests it is secondary to renal disease. If kidney function is normal this suggests primary hyperparathyroidism. A low PTH plus high calcium indicates hypercalcemia of malignancy, bone disorder, or hypervitaminosis D. Serum can be evaluated for calcitriol levels. • Perform an **ACTH stim test** to rule out Addison's disease. (Additionally, low K+, high Na+ suggest Addison's.) • **Ultrasound** the thyroid and parathyroid area to **look for parathyroid tumors.** • **Rule out lymphosarcoma and other tumors or bone conditions.** Perform a rectal and mammary gland exam and a lymph node aspirate (of enlarged lymph nodes). Also take abdominal and thoracic radiographs to look for lymphadenopathy, calcification, and masses to help rule out neoplasia as a cause of the hypercalcemia. Bone marrow aspirate can help identify multiple myeloma or lymphosarcoma. One treatment with L-asparaginase followed by calcium measurement 12 hours later can be used to identify lymphosarcoma as the etiology if other tests have not yet revealed the etiology. With lymphosarcoma, the calcium levels are normal at 12 hours following administration. Perform **radiographs** for bone abnormalities.
TREATMENT	The goal of treatment is to treat the underlying cause. You may have to start treating the hypercalcemia first to prevent severe renal damage. Treat hypercalcemia if the serum **calcium concentration is > 16 mg/dL,** the **serum calcium x phosphorus product is > 60-70** (a ratio that is associated with dystrophic calcification of tissues), or the animal is **azotemic.** TREAT the HYPERCALCEMIA **Rehydrate** and correct acidosis. **Diurese** with saline and furosemide (enhances calcium excretion) once the pet is rehydrated. **Glucocorticoids** inhibit bone resorption. Do not use glucocortioids until lymphoma diagnostics have been performed. **Calcitonin** and **bisphosphonates** (e.g., pamidronate) decrease bone resorption of calcium. Calcitonin also enhances renal excretion of Ca/P. CORRECT the UNDERLYING CAUSE • Treat for renal failure and Addison's disease if present. • **Surgically remove the affected parathyroid glands:** Evaluate all four parathyroid glands before deciding which to remove. Usually it's easy to identify affected glands. If all four are enlarged it's usually due to hyperplasia, so look for a primary cause (renal or nutritional). Removal leads to rapid decrease in PTH leading to hypocalcemia within 24-96 hours following surgery, so you may need to supplement with calcium and calcitriol. Animals with hypercalcemia of > 14 mg/dL are most likely to need supplementation. • Treat **neoplasia** surgically or with chemotherapy or radiation therapy.

Endocrinology

COMMON DRUGS

DRUG	DOGS	CATS
Azothioprine 50 mg tabs	2 mg/kg q 24-48 hours or taper to q 48 hours over 2-4 weeks	Use with caution in cats
Azulfidine	50-60 mg/kg PO TID; max 3g/24 hours	125 mg/cat PO TID for at least 10-14 days
Chlorpromazine 25 mg/ml	0.2-0.4 mg/kg SC or IM, TID	
Chlorambucil 2 mg tablets		Cats<7 lbs: 1 mg PO q3 days Cats>7 lbs: 2 mg PO q3 days
Cisapride (Propulsid®)	0.1-0.5 mg/kg TID	
Dexamethasone 0.25, 0.5, 0.75, 1, 1.5, 2, 4, 6 mg tablets		0.2 mg/kg PO SID to BID
Dimenhydrinate (Dramamine®) 50 mg	8 mg/kg PO TID to QID	
Diphenhydramine (Benadryl®) 25, 50 mg tabs; 10 mg/mL oral liquid	2-4 mg/kg PO or IM, BID to QID	Not an effective antiemetic in cats
Dolasetron	0.6 mg/kg PO SID to BID when vomiting is anticipated; 1.0 mg/kg PO for active vomiting (doses are tested in dogs)	
Famotidine (Pepcid®) OTC 20, 40 mg tabs; 9 mg/mL oral liquid; 10 mg/mL injection	0.5 to 1.0 mg/kg PO, IM, or SC, SID	0.5 mg/kg PO, IM, or SC, SID-BID
Loperamide (Imodium®) 0.2 mg/mL oral liquid; 2 mg capsules	0.08 mg/kg PO TID	
Methylprednisolone acetate (Depo-Medrol®) 20 mg/mL		20 mg SC or IM q 2 weeks. Discontinue after 8-12 weeks of remission
Metaclopramide (Reglan®)	0.2-0.4 mg/kg PO, SC, or IM, QID or 30-45 minutes prior to meals; 1-2 mg/kg a day as CRI	
Misoprostol (Cytotec®) 100µg, 200µg tablets	2-5 µg/kg PO q 6-8 hours	2-5 µg/kg PO q 6-8 hours
Omeprazole (Prilosec®) 20 mg capsules	0.7-1.5 mg/kg PO SID	0.7-1.5 mg/kg PO SID
Ondansetron (Zofran®)	0.5-1.0 mg/kg PO SID to BID 0.5-1.0 mg/kg PO 30 min prior to chemotherapy	
Osalazine (Dipentum®)	10-20 mg/kg PO BID	125 mg/cat PO TID for at least 10-14 days
Prednisone 5 mg, 20 mg tablets	1-2 mg/kg PO BID for 1-2 weeks and then decrease to 0.5 mg/kg BID for 4 weeks and then taper	1-2 mg/kg PO BID. After 2 weeks of remission, decrease to 0.5-1.0 mg/kg.
Prochlorperazine (Compazine®)	0.5 mg/kg SC or IM TID	
Ranitidine (Zantac®) 300 mg tablets; 15 mg/mL oral liquid; 25 mg/mL solution IV	0.5-4.0 mg/kg PO BID	0.5-4.0 mg/kg PO BID
Yohimbine		0.25-0.5 mg/kg SC or IM, BID

GI Disease

REGURGITATION

Regurgitation is the passive expulsion of ingesta from the esophagus or pharynx. The food is usually expelled soon after eating but can occur up to 24 hours later. It is usually undigested and may be tubular-shaped. Because expulsion is passive, there are no prodromal signs as with vomiting (e.g. lip-licking, hypersalivation, restlessness, depression) and no retching or abdominal effort. Often the animal exhibits repeat attempts at swallowing a single bolus and may show difficult or painful swallowing (dysphagia). Contents are usually not acidic or bile stained (as occurs frequently with vomiting) unless gastroesophageal reflux occurs first.

I.   GENERAL INFORMATION on REGURGITATION

ETIOLOGY	Regurgitation is usually caused by esophageal dysfunction but can also be caused by pharyngeal disorders. These disorders include obstruction, abnormal motility, and inflammation. Additionally, immature animals can regurgitate stomach contents because their **gastroesophageal sphincter** is not fully developed. These animals spit up easily when you hold their abdomens (e.g. burping a baby or puppy). **DISEASES ASSOCIATED WITH REGURGITATION** • Cricopharyngeal Dysphagia • Megaesophagus • Esophageal Obstruction • Esophagitis
HISTORY	**Young animals (newly weaned)** may have congenital etiologies such as idiopathic megaesophagus or vascular ring anomaly (persistant right aortic arch). **Adult animal rule outs:** • Recent anesthesia, exposure to caustic chemicals, foreign bodies, toxic agents, or evidence of reflux esophagitis. All of the above conditions can lead to esophagitis and consequently stricture. • Muscle weakness (can indicate neuromuscular disease).
PHYSICAL EXAM	• Check the oropharyngeal cavity (under sedation if necessary) for inflammation or foreign bodies. • Palpate the neck and pharynx for pain, asymmetry, or masses. • **Watch** the animal eat. • **Auscult the chest** and neck for evidence of aspiration pneumonia, a common sequelae of regurgitation.
RADIOGRAPHY	**SURVEY RADIOGRAPHS** • The **pharynx** is usually visible because it is air-filled. **Decrease in size** indicates local inflammation, elongated soft palate, laryngeal edema, or neoplasia. **Increase in size** indicates megaesophagus, pharyngeal dysfunction, or chronic respiratory disease. • The **esophagus** is usually not visible unless it is filled with air. Mild distention can occur with **aerophagia** due to excitement or anesthesia. Marked dilation can occur with **motility disorders** such as megaesophagus or **obstruction** where dilation occurs cranial to the obstruction. **RADIOGRAPHS WITH CONTRAST MEDIA:** Contrast is not normally retained in the pharynx and cranial esophagus. In the dog, the esophagus may deviate ventrally at the thoracic inlet, leading to a mild irregularity in the mucosal pattern. Don't mistake this for an esophageal diverticulum. In the cat, the caudal 2/3 of the esophagus has a herring bone pattern. Don't confuse this with esophagitis. **Pooling of contrast** is abnormal. The pattern of pooling is diagnostic: • Pooling at the **base of the heart** indicates esophageal obstruction caused by vascular ring anomaly. • Irregular mucosal border indicates an intramural lesion. With severe dilation, esophageal function is not likely to be regained. • **Hiatal hernias** can occasionally be seen but must be ruled out using fluoroscopy.
FLUOROSCOPY & ENDOSCOPY	**FLUOROSCOPY** shows the formation of the bolus in the pharynx, constriction of the pharynx, and propulsion of the bolus through the pharyngoesophageal sphincter and into the esophagus. Contrast material should move aborally by progressive peristaltic waves. **ENDOSCOPY** allows visualization of esophageal foreign bodies, strictures, and esophagitis. Biopsies can be taken.

II. CONDITIONS CAUSING REGURGITATION

Cricopharyngeal Dysphagia
Megaesophagus
Esophageal Obstruction
Esophagitis

CRICOPHARYNGEAL DYSPHAGIA (a.k.a. Cricopharyngeal Achalasia)

PATHO-PHYSIOLOGY	Usually when food or fluid is passed to the base of the tongue, a peristaltic wave travels from the cranial pharynx and moves the food towards the esophagus. The epiglottis closes to prevent aspiration of food and the pharyngoesophageal sphincter (PES) relaxes, allowing food to pass into the esophagus. With cricopharyngeal dysphagia, the PES **fails to relax** or there is a **lack of coordination** between PES relaxation and pharyngeal contraction. As a result, food or fluid accumulates in the pharynx and cranial esophagus and is regurgitated during swallowing. Additionally, with uncoordinated opening and closing of the epiglottis, the animal may aspirate food or fluid into the lungs leading to aspiration pneumonia.
ETIOLOGY	• Fibrosis of the cricopharyngeal muscle • Lesions in the nerves going to the oral cavity • Neuromuscular disorders such as myasthenia gravis, polyneuropathies, or polymyositis • Reportedly congenital in cocker spaniels, springer spaniels, and golden retrievers • Hypothyroidism
CLINICAL SIGNS	• **Dysphagia:** The animal must swallow several times instead of just once. • **Regurgitation** occurs during eating or immediately after consuming a bolus. That is, it occurs during swallowing. • **Nasal regurgitation** can occur because the nasal orifice does not always close appropriately. • **Signs of aspiration pneumonia** can occur due to uncoordinated closure of the epiglottis. • **No pain on swallowing** and the animal has a good appetite.
DIAGNOSIS	• **Examination** of the pharynx: Look for other causes of dysphagia such as foreign bodies, abscesses, pharyngitis, or neoplasia • **Radiographs** can be used to help rule out foreign body or mass obstruction in the pharynx. **Thoracic radiographs** are useful to evaluate for aspiration pneumonia and concurrent megaesophagus. • **Positive contrast fluoroscopy** reveals failure of the PES to relax normally and shows reflux of contrast material. This procedure should be performed with liquid contrast as well as a barium soaked kibble as the animal may be able to pass liquids but not kibble, and some materials may make it down into the stomach. Sometimes the study looks normal in abnormal subclinical dogs (especially golden retrievers). In these dogs, viewing the video in slow motion and timing the swallow reflex reveals that the process is slow and food occasionally refluxes.
TREATMENT	• Treatment has been myotomy or myectomy but the outcomes are poor in part because patients often have concurrent neuromuscular conditions such as megaesophagus. For this reason, patients must first be screened for other such conditions. Even in uncomplicated cases, dysphagia may be exacerbated after surgery and aspiration can occur as a complication of surgery. • Some affected animals can be managed with dietary change alone, while others must be managed with gastrostomy devices which greatly reduce aspiration pneumonia.

GI Disease

MEGAESOPHAGUS is a loss of esophageal motor function leading to dilation and lack or peristalsis. Consequently food and fluid accumulates in the esophagus.

CLINICAL SIGNS	• **Regurgitation** most commonly occurs within several hours after eating but can occur up to 24 hours later. Usually there is no dysphagia, however, if an animal develops esophagitis, pain on swallowing and anorexia can occur.
	• **Halitosis:** Food retained in the esophagus may ferment, causing halitosis.
	• **Respiratory problems** can occur from secondary aspiration pneumonia or due to ventral displacement and compression of the lungs and airways by retained food in the esophagus.
ETIOLOGIES	Most often a specific etiology is not diagnosed and the condition is considered **idiopathic**. Primary megaesophagus can be inherited in wire-haired fox terriers, miniature schnauzers, German shepherds, great danes, and Irish setters.
	Megaesophagus can be secondary to:
	• **Neuromuscular problems** such as myasthenia gravis or polymyopathy. Esophageal function is controlled by nerves in the brain stem. The esophagus is striated muscle, so unlike smooth muscle, without extrinsic innervation, it is paralyzed.
	• **Stricture or obstruction** leading to dilation cranial to the stricture
	• **Esophageal foreign bodies** such as fishhooks may damage the esophagus leading to dilation and motility disorders.
	• **Hypoadrenocorticism, hypothyroidism,** or immune-mediate diseases such as SLE
	• **Reflux esophagitis**
DIAGNOSIS	• **Survey radiographs** often reveal a dilation if the esophagus fills with air. The esophagus can be normal distal to an obstruction and dilated cranial to the obstruction. Radiographs do not reveal whether the dilation is due to motility disorders.
	• **Contrast radiographs:** Same as survey radiographs. Proceed with caution due to the chance of regurgitation and aspiration.
	• **Fluoroscopy** will reveal whether there is motility or lack of motility.
MANAGEMENT	• Treat the primary problem (e.g. esophagitis) if possible or treat any secondary signs (e.g. pneumonia).
	• Feed the animal a high caloric liquid diet with its cranial body tilted up so that the food can get into the stomach via gravity.
	• The prognosis for idiopathic or unresolved megaesophagus is guarded because the animal is likely to develop aspiration pneumonia. Many animals, however, can be well managed.
	• Gastrostomy tubes can be placed. The silicon tubing should be replaced yearly.

ESOPHAGEAL OBSTRUCTION

Esophageal obstructions may be **intraluminal** (such as a fishook or bone stuck in the esophagus), **intramural** (such as a stricture caused by esophagitis), or **extraluminal** (such as a persistant right aortic arch).

A. **INTRALUMINAL OBSTRUCTION:** Foreign objects tend to lodge at the thoracic inlet, over the base of the heart, or just before the diaphragm. They can usually be diagnosed on survey radiographs, contrast radiographs, or via endoscopy. A foreign object should be removed endoscopically or pushed into the stomach and removed surgically. If it can't be removed orally without markedly damaging the esophagus, it should be removed surgically to decrease risk of esophageal perforation, further esophagitis, or damage to esophageal nerves, leading to megaesophagus.

B. **INTRAMURAL OBSTRUCTION:** Strictures are often due to trauma from a foreign body, chemicals, reflux esophagitis, or neoplasia. If the etiology is non-neoplastic, then resting the esophagus for an extended period of time may allow the animal to recover. The animal can be fed by pharyngostomy or gastrostomy tube.
   1. **Balloon catheter dilation in dogs and cats:** The balloon is dilated for 1-2 minutes and then deflated. Mucosa is evaluated and re-ballooned if necessary. After successful ballooning, the stricture is largely broken down but hemorrhage and mucosal erosion occur as a result of the procedure. The balloon is inflated

and deflated several times during one anesthetic procedure. The procedure is repeated 4-5 days later in order to prevent restricture. On average, three separate anesthetic procedures with 3-4 balloonings each time are required.

C. **EXTRALUMINAL OBSTRUCTION:** The only treatment is to surgically correct the cause of the obstruction (e.g. persistant right aortic arch). The prognosis for complete recovery is poor.

ESOPHAGITIS and REFLUX ESOPHAGITIS

ETIOLOGY & PATHOPHYSIOLOGY	Esophagitis • Ingestion of chemical irritants or thermal insult • Acute or persistent vomiting • Foreign body obstruction • Drugs that get lodged in the esophagus (water should be routinely given with drugs to minimize the risk of esophageal injury) • Gastroesophageal reflux (reflux esophagitis): It is not known why the GE sphincter loses competency; one theory suggests there is herniation of the abdominal esophagus into the thorax. This can occur with neoplasia, neuromuscular disease, protracted vomiting, or abdominal surgery.
CLINICAL SIGNS	• Regurgitation • Painful swallowing • Anorexia • Dogs with idiopathic reflux esophagitis may vomit a small amount of bile-tinged vomitus in the morning before their meal.
DIAGNOSIS	Radiographs are usually unremarkable. • **Positive contrast fluoroscopy** may show dilation and dysperistalsis in severe cases of esophagitis. • **Endoscopy and biopsy** of the caudal esophagus is the most reliable procedure for identifying esophagitis. Diagnosis is based on finding inflammatory changes when the problem is acute, or thickening of the basal or germinative layer and elongation of the papillae in chronic cases. Chronic inflammatory changes can include infiltration by eosinophils.
TREATMENT	• **Rest the esophagus:** Do not give any food orally for 24-48 hours. Water can be given orally. On resumption of feeding, use bland foods low in fat and protein and feed in small meals. • **Antacids:** Antacids such as amphogel or basogel neutralize gastric acid; however, they need to be given six times a day to prevent rebound hypersecretion of acids. **H2 blockers** such as famotidine and ranitidine decrease hydrogen ion release by parietal cells. **Omeprazole** (1-2 mg/kg), a hydrogen ion pump, is a better antacid than the H2 blockers. • **Metoclopramide, cisapride,** and **bethanechol** increase gastroesophageal sphincter pressure and increase gastric emptying. Cisipride (0.5-1.0 mg/kg TID) is much more effective than metaclopramide but because it only works on smooth muscle, in dogs it only works on the GES. Avoid using it if the dog has megaesophagus because it will cause even more food/fluid retention in the esophagus. • **Sucralfate** coats the esophagus, thereby protecting it from acid secretion. It can be given as a dissolved slurry. • In the case of **hiatal hernias,** the stomach and esophagus should be pexied.

VOMITING
General Information
Working-up Cases
Diagnosis and Treatment

Vomiting is the primary clinical sign associated with gastric dysfunction; however, it can be associated with disease of other parts of the GI tract (including the colon), other abdominal organs, systemic toxins, and CNS disorders. Up to 20-30% of colitis patients vomit.

GOALS in the EXAM ROOM

Step 1: Determine that the animal is **vomiting, not regurgitating.**
Step 2: Determine whether the vomitus contains **blood** (hematemesis).
Step 3: Determine whether the vomiting is **acute and self-limiting** or more
     severe or chronic such that it warrants additional diagnostics.

I. **GENERAL INFORMATION**
   A. **Pathways for vomiting:** The **vomit center** in the medulla receives input from
      two major pathways (humoral and neural pathways) and **four sources**
      overall (vagosympathetic afferents, the chemoreceptor trigger zone (CRTZ), the
      cortex, and the vestibular apparatus). Neuronal output for vomiting travels from the
      vomit center through the spinal and phrenic nerves and initiates retrograde
      contraction of the stomach and duodenum, relaxation of the caudal and proximal
      esophageal sphincters, and contraction of the abdominal muscles and diaphragm.

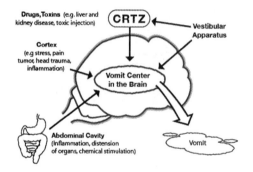

   1. **Humoral pathway:** Blood-borne drugs or toxins (e.g. bacterial toxins, blood
      urea nitrogen, ammonia) trigger the **chemoreceptor trigger zone** (CRTZ)
      which in turn triggers the vomit center. Several types of neurotransmitters are
      involved at the CRTZ. They include D_2 dopaminergic, serotonergic (5-HT),
      histaminergic, M_1 cholinergic, and α_2 adrenergic receptors.

   2. **Neural pathway:** Signals travel through nerves to the vomit center directly or
      through nerves to the CRTZ to the vomit center.
      a. **Abdominal** inflammation, distention of abdominal organs (as occurs with
         GI stasis), and chemical stimulation of the abdominal organs can initiate
         signals that travel from the abdominal cavity, through the vagal and
         sympathetics, to the vomit center.

      b. Signals initiated by head trauma, brain tumors, cerebral inflammation, as
         well as psychogenic factors such as fear and stress can originate from the
         higher cortical area of the brain.

      c. The **vestibular system** can send signals that go directly to the vomit
         center (cats) or to the CRTZ (dogs). In cats, this involves the **muscarinic
         receptors** (mixed M_1/M_2 such as atropine, or pure M_1 such as pirenzepine),
         whereas in dogs it involves **histaminergic receptors.** Thus, atropine

works for motion sickness in cats but not dogs, whereas antihistamines work as an antiemetic in dogs but not cats.

B. **ANTI-EMETICS** work on the vomit pathway

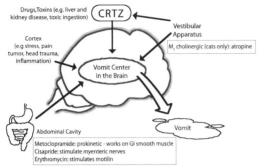

D_2 Dopaminergic: metoclopramide
Serotonergic: Ondansetron, dolasetron
Histaminergic (dogs): diphenhydramine, dimenhydrinate
M_1 Cholinergic (cats only): atropine
α adrenergic: yohimbine, chlorpromazine, prochloperazine

Drugs,Toxins (e.g. liver and kidney disease, toxic ingestion)

CRTZ

Vestibular Apparatus

Cortex (e.g stress, pain tumor, head trauma, inflammation)

M_1 cholinergic (cats only): atropine

Vomit Center in the Brain

Abdominal Cavity

Vomit

Metoclopramide: prokinetic - works on GI smooth muscle
Cisapride: stimulate myenteric nerves
Erythromycin: stimulates motilin

CLASS-IFICATION	DRUG	SITE of ACTION
$α_2$-adrenergic antagonists	Chlorpromazine Prochlorperazine (Compazine®) Yohimbine (Note that xylazine, an α2-adrenergic agonist, is a potent emetic in cats)	CRTZ & vomit center (Moderately effective but cause sedation)
H_1-Histamine antagonists	Diphenhydramine Dimenhydrinate (Dramamine®)	CRTZ in dogs but not the cats. It blocks the CRTZ histamine receptor where vestibular input enters. Decreases vestibular-related vomiting (motion-sickness)
D_2-Dopamine antagonist	Metoclopramide (Note that apomorphine, a D_2 dopamine agonist in dogs is a potent emetic in dogs but not cats)	CRTZ in dogs but not cats GI smooth muscle: Stimulates GI motility so it's a prokinetic
5-HT3 Serotonin antagonist	Ondansetron (Zofran®) Dolasetron	CRTZ Vagal afferent
5-HT4 Serotonin agonist	Cisapride (Propulsid®)	Myenteric neurons: Stimulates motility (prokinetic) thus decreasing GI distension.

1. **Chemoreceptor Trigger Zone (CRTZ)**
   a. **Chemotherapeutic** agents frequently act on the serotonergic receptors at the **CRTZ** or at the visceral and vagal afferents in dogs. Both **ondansetron** and **dolasetron** work as serotonergic antagonists. **Ondansetron** is highly effective but very expensive (0.5-1.0 mg/kg PO BID). **Dolasetron** is less expensive. For patients in which vomiting is anticipated, a dose of 0.6 mg/kg PO SID-BID can be used. For active vomiting, the dose is 1 mg/kg PO BID.
   b. **D_2-dopamine antagonists:** Metoclopramide works at the CRTZ in dogs. It also works as a prokinetic in both dogs and cats (stimulates GI

GI Disease

motility). As a result, it accelerates gastric emptying and intestinal motility and consequently decreases GI distension. In cats, it works primarily as a prokinetic. A number of conditions including pancreatitis cause secondary ileus and stasis making metoclopramide an appropriate drug in some cases in cats. The problem with metoclopramide is its short half-life (60-90 minutes). Thus, if it's used only 3-4 times a day for cats with intractable vomiting, it will probably have little effect. For maximal benefit, it should be given as a constant rate infusion (CRI). It can be helpful when given 30-45 minutes prior to a meal in patients with delayed gastric emptying (e.g. cats with hepatic lipidosis being fed by feeding tube). Other drugs should be used as central-acting anti-emetics in cats.

c. **Histaminergic antagonists:** Antihistamines are effective for motion sickness in dogs but not in cats. Use α_2-adrenergic antagonists for anti-emesis or atropine for motion sickness in cats.

2. **Emetic Center:** α_2-adrenergic antagonists such as chlorpromazine work directly at the emetic center.

3. **Vestibular Apparatus:** Muscarinic receptors in the cat inhibit motion sickness. Consequently, atropine can be used in cats for motion sickness.

4. **Gut Efferents** initiate retrograde contraction of the stomach and relaxation of the esophageal sphincters. **Cisapride** works at the myenteric neurons and is considered a prokinetic rather than a true anti-emetic. It does not cross the blood-brain barrier; rather, it works by promoting gastric emptying and consequently decreases nausea and vomiting (e.g. gastritis can lead to delayed gastric emptying and consequently gastric distention). Cisapride is a stronger motility modifier than metoclopramide. Indications for use include any disorder involving delayed gastric emptying such as gastritis and GDV. **Erythromycin (0.5-1.0 mg/kg PO TID)** stimulates motilin, a hormone that facilitates gastric emptying.

a. **Anticholinergics such as atropine and scopolamine are not effective** in preventing vomiting. They are muscarinic antagonists and consequently affect smooth but not striated muscle. If they did, atropine would paralyze animals (Refer to *Overview of the Neurologic System* at www.nerdbook.com/extras).

C. **Many diseases cause vomiting.** Some are GI diseases and others are not. Most ingested toxins can cause vomiting.

GI DISEASE	NON-GI DISEASE
Reactions to food: Dietary indiscretion, food intolerance, or food allergy.	**Exogenous toxins** (e.g. apomorphine, xylazine, chemotherapy, narcotics, ethylene glycol, antibiotics, insecticides, most toxins)
Pancreatitis or IBD	**Endogenous toxins:**
Obstruction (foreign body, pyloric hypertrophy, intussusception, tumor, e.g. adenocarcinoma or lymphoscarcoma)	• Uremia due to renal or liver disease • Sepsis and endotoxemia • Acidosis
Compression: intra or extraluminal	**Endocrine disease**
Delayed gastric emptying (as with obstruction or gastroenteritis for any reason)	• Addison's disease • Diabetes Mellitus: ketoacidosis • Hyperthyroidism • Hypercalcemia
Infectious	**CNS disease** (intracranial lesions) such as brain tumors, infection, inflammation, head trauma, or vestibular disorders
• Parvo	**Pyometra**
• Distemper gastroenteritis	**Heartworm disease**
• Panleukopenia	**Congestive heart failure**
• Bacterial (Campylobacter)	
Parasites	
• *Ollulanus Tricuspis* (cats)	
• Ascarids	
• Physaloptera	
• Heartworm (cats)	

II. WORKING-UP CASES OF VOMITING

A. **First determine that the animal is vomiting rather than regurgitating.**
Vomiting is characterized by **retching** and bile-tinged fluid. Vomiting animals often
exhibit prodromal signs (e.g. salivation) and vomit digested food. Both vomiting and
regurgitation can occur soon after or many hours after a meal, therefore, time is not
a good distinguishing factor. Bile staining is due to the presence of duodenal
contents and is more likely due to vomiting.

B. **Next determine whether there is blood in the vomitus (hematemesis).**
Hematemesis is always serious. It can be cause by **GI ulceration, coagulopathy,**
or it can be **swallowed from elsewhere** (e.g. nasal bleeding).

ETIOLOGIES of GI ULCERATION

Gastrointestinal Causes
- **Neoplasia:** GI adenocarcinoma is the most common cause in dogs and
  lymphoma is the most common cause in cats. Mast cell tumors can also cause
  ulceration.
- **Foreign body**
- **Inflammatory bowel disease**
- **Gastroesophageal reflux** may lead to esophageal ulcers due to acidity of
  the refluxed material.

Systemic Causes
- **Stress:** due in part to high corticosteroid levels
- **Drugs:** Corticosteroids, NSAIDS (even COX-2 inhibitors)
- **Toxins**
- **Uremia due to hepatic failure:** When liver disease suddenly gets worse, it
  may be from a bleeding ulcer due to uremia.
- **Uremia due to renal failure**
- **Addison's disease** is always on the differential list for vomiting (especially
  with hematemesis and clinical signs that wax and wane).
- **Infectious:** Salmon poisoning, PARVO, panleukopenia, histoplasmosis,
  Clostridium perfringens, *Clostridium difficile*, Salmonella

---

1. If no response to therapy is seen within 10 days, perform endoscopy to look for
   ulcers. Surgical resection may be required (Refer to p. 10.10 for initial
   supportive treatment).

C. **DETERMINE IF IT'S ACUTE and SELF-LIMITING or CHRONIC and/or LIFE-
THREATENING:** Acute vomiting such as that associated with mild dietary
indiscretion frequently improves with empirical therapy such as fluids and a
controlled diet. It often requires minimal diagnostics to check for hydration status
and to rule out early indication of a more serious problem. **Signs of fever,
lethargy, or dehydration indicate a more serious problem requiring more
aggressive therapy** and diagnostics. **Chronic vomiting** (2-3 weeks of regular
vomiting) with or without other systemic signs usually requires a systematic and
extensive diagnostic plan including a CBC, chemistry panel, heartworm test,
radiography, and endoscopy.

GI Disease

CATEGORY	DESCRIPTION	PLAN
Acute and Self-limiting Vomiting	• Onset of signs < 1 week • Patient looks and acts normal/acts healthy (no lethargy or inappetence)	• Check hydration if indicated (PCV, TP, BUN) • Fecal centrifugal float for intestinal parasites • May treat empirically
Serious and Life-Threatening Vomiting	History of • Toxic ingestion including drugs such as NSAIDS • Suspected foreign body ingestion (e.g. string in cats) • Kittens and puppies with no or incomplete vaccine history (PARVO, Panleukopenia) Clinical Signs & Physical Exam • Fever • Melena or hematemesis (perform a rectal and exam the feces obtained) • Lethargy or weakness • **Pain** on abdominal palpation • **Palpable abdominal mass** or abnormal organ size or shape • **Icteric mucous membranes** • Evidence of **dehydration**	• Perform CBC, chemistry panel (including T4 in cats), and urinalysis to rule out non GI causes of vomiting • Fecal centrifugal flotation • Dogs: SPEC cPL (Specific Canine Pancreatic Lipase) if pancreatitis is likely. Do not rely on amylase and lipase. • **Abdominal radiographs** and/or **ultrasound** are important to help rule out surgical cases (e.g. foreign body) from medical cases as well as for identifying GI and abdominal causes of vomiting (including neoplasia)
Chronic Vomiting	Chronic vomiting is defined as 2-3 weeks of regular vomiting with or without other signs of illness such as lethargy, depression, or anorexia. • Chronic vomiting rarely improves without work up and is often associated with serious life-threatening disease. • Common causes include IBD, hepatobiliary disease, hyperthyroidism (cats), chronic renal failure (cats), and GI malignancies.	Perform the same tests as for serious life-threatening vomiting. Also consider the following tests: • **Serum bile acids** • **TLI** for exocrine pancreatic insufficiency • **ACTH stimulation test** to rule out Addison's disease • **Gastroduodenoscopy** for ulcers, neoplasia, and biopsy • **Exploratory surgery** and full thickness biopsy

D. **INITIAL SUPPORTIVE TREATMENT:** If clinical signs are severe, stabilize the animal first and then perform the diagnostic work-up as soon as possible thereafter.
   1. **Fluids and electrolyte correction:** If the animal is dehydrated, initiate fluid therapy. Vomiting animals are usually hypokalemic and hyponatremic. Chemistry panel and CBC will help assess level of dehydration as well as electrolyte status.
   2. **Intractable vomiting:** In cases of severe, intractable vomiting where fluid therapy cannot keep up with the vomiting, anti-emetics are indicated. If vomiting is mild, you may elect to avoid anti-emetics as they can mask the signs of illness by which you are judging improvement.
   3. **In chronic cases,** conservative therapy may be initiated first. This includes:
      a. **Resting the GI tract by** withholding food **(NPO)** for several days or placing the animal on a **bland diet.**
      b. **Testing for food allergies or intolerances by** placing the animal on an homemade elimination diet (one novel protein and one novel carbohydrate), commercial prescription novel protein diet, or a hydrolyzed protein diet. Owners have difficulty maintaining the homemade diet. If vomiting is due to food intolerance, signs should improve within 2-3 weeks of being on such diets.
      c. Treatment with **pyrantel pamoate** (5mg/kg PO one time in dogs and cats) for *Physaloptera* will kill physaloptera, which is usually diagnosed on endoscopy or biopsy. The presence of as few as one organism may be

responsible for intractable vomiting. Pyrantel pamoate will also treat for ascarids but not whipworms (use fendendazole for whipworms).

d. **If ulcers are present**, treat with GI **protectants** and **hydrogen ion channel blockers**. This will not fix the underlying problem, but will improve the overall signs. When GI ulcers are present, etiology should be determined. Treatment include:

i. **H$_2$ blockers** such as famotidine (Pepcid®) and ranitidine (Xantac®). Avoid cimetidine; it is the least potent and has the most side effects because it inhibits the cytochrome P450 system, thus delaying metabolism of other drugs. Cimetidine is also QID, whereas famotidine (0.5-1.0 mg/kg PO SID-BID) and ranitidine (1-2mg/kg PO BID) can be taken less frequently. Ranitidine also works to promote gastric emptying.

ii. **H$^+$ pump blocker** such as omeprazol (Prilosec®) at 0.7-1.0 mg/kg PO SID in dogs and cats.

iii. **Prostoglandins** such as misoprostol (Cytotec®), 2-5 μg/kg TID-QID increase blood supply to the gastric epithelium and increase cell turnover.

iv. **Sucralfate** binds to and coats ulcers. It can cause constipation and inhibit absorption of other drugs. It can be used with other drugs but administration of other drugs should ideally be spaced by two hours; most gastroenterologists however, don't follow this practice due to lack of client compliance.

D. **DIAGNOSIS:** A minimum data base consisting of a complete blood count (CBC), urinalysis, and chemistry panel can rule out most non-GI causes of vomiting. It can also identify consequences of vomiting such as hypokalemia, dehydration, and acid-base imbalances (e.g. Dehydration plus poor perfusion leads to metabolic acidosis. Pyloric obstruction results in high acidity vomit, thus the patient is often alkalotic).

1. **History**

SIGNALMENT	Young unvaccinated animals: Consider PARVO, panleukopenia, distemper gastroenteritis
EXPOSURE/ TRAVEL	• Exposure to toxins or garbage (e.g. outdoor dog or cat) • Exposure to plants • Exposure to raw salmonid fish (salmon poisoning)
WHEN	**Immediately post-prandial (after eating)** • Overeating (engorging) • Excitement • Esophageal disorders (regurgitation) including hiatal hernias **Vomit > 8 hours later:** vomitus is undigested or partially digested. This indicates a distal motility disorder (pyloris) or obstruction. **Early morning vomiting before the first meal** may be due to bilious vomiting syndrome, which is a disorder involving delayed gastric emptying.
DESCRIPTION	• Blood or "coffee-grounds" (digested blood) • Undigested implies esophagus • Digested implied stomach or intestines • Bile implies vomiting (bile has been refluxed into the stomach)

GI Disease

2. Physical Examination

ORAL EXAM	• **Unusually bad breath:** Test for liver or renal disease (uremia) or diabetes mellitus (acetone). • **Icteric mucous membranes:** Rule out liver disease or hemolysis. • **Inflammatory pharyngitis** in cats: Look for an oral FB.
GENERAL	• **Generalized lymphadenopathy** indicates neoplasia (e.g. lymphosarcoma) or generalized inflammation as occurs with salmon poisoning. • **Fever** = inflammation
ABDOMINAL PALPATION	• Fluid distension of the intestines • Abnormally shaped or sized kidneys • Uterine distension (such as with pyometra) • Gaseous or fluid distension of the intestines • Pain • Enlarged mass
CNS	• **Vestibular disease**
RECTAL	• **Hematochezia** indicates the animal has colitis too • **Worms:** Exam may reveal hookworms or whipworms • A prominent **prostate** may indicate prostatitis or prostatic neoplasia.

3. Diagnostic Tests

CBC	**Eosinophilia** occurs with mast cell tumors, intestinal parasites, and Addison's disease **Leukocytosis** occurs with inflammation (e.g. pancreatitis or pyometra)
CHEMISTRY	• **Elevated bicarbonate** can occur with pyloric obstruction or upper duodenal obstruction due to loss of hydrogen ions from vomiting. • **Azotemia** and hyperphosphatemia suggest chronic **renal failure.** • **Hyperglycemia,** acidosis, glucosuria, & ketonuria indicate **diabetes mellitus** • **Hypernatremia** and hypokalemia indicate **Addison's disease.** • **Amylase and lipase** may be elevated with pancreatitis but are not specific or sensitive indicators of pancreatitis in dogs and are of no use in cats. • Elevated ALT, AST, and ALP point towards potential liver disease • **Hypercalcemia** can occur with **parathyroid tumors** or other neoplasia
FECAL CENTRIFUGAF LOTATION	• Roundworms • Whipworms
SURVEY RADIO- GRAPHS	Survey radiographs often don't give enough information to diagnose the disease (unless there is a radiodense foreign body), but they can give an indication as to which part of the GI system is affected and whether surgery is indicated. We may find the following clues: • Focal or diffuse abdominal contrast may indicate focal or diffuse peritonitis. If it's in the area of the pancreas, it may help indicate pancreatitis. • Gas or fluid-filled bowel loops indicate enteritis. If only the duodenum is affected and it's in the same position in all of the films, evaluate the animal further for pancreatitis or partial obstruction. • Markedly distended small intestines may indicate obstruction/neoplasia caudal to the distention. • Plicated intestines suggest the presence of a linear foreign body.

10.12

Diagnostic tests continued

CONTRAST RADIOGRAPHS (Barium Series)	Contrast Radiographs: When performing an upper GI series, be sure to use enough liquid barium (10 mg/kg in cats and 5 mg/kg in dogs) and take enough films (time 0, 15 min, 30 min, 45, min, 1 hour, 2 hours, etc). Contrast radiographs help us rule out: • **Radiolucent foreign bodies** • **Gastric outflow obstructions**: foreign bodies, antral hyperplasia, or neoplasia • **Intestinal obstructions**: foreign bodies, neoplasia, or intussusception • **Gastric masses** • **Thickened gut loops** indicating inflammation or infiltrative disease • **Delayed gastric emptying** (due to outflow obstruction or a functional problem such as inflammation): With delayed gastric emptying, liquid barium takes > 2-4 hours to pass the stomach and with kibble it takes over 8-12 hours to pass the stomach. So, if there is a large amount of liquid barium present after 4 hours or kibble-soaked barium after 8-12 hours, then the animal has delayed gastric emptying. Usually **ultrasound** is performed rather than a barium series.
ULTRASOUND	Ultrasound may also reveal thickened gut loops, enlarged mesenteric lymph nodes, and intestinal or other abdominal tumors. It's also a good diagnostic tool for pancreatitis, especially in cats (along with the fPL.
FLUORO-SCOPY	Fluoroscopy can be performed to look for a hiatal hernia or abnormal gastric or esophageal motility.
ENDOSCOPY	**Endoscopy** allows visualization of the gastrointestinal mucosa. It's more reliable than radiographs for the diagnosis of IBD, gastritis, ulcers, and neoplasia. The stomach and intestines should be biopsied.
EXPLORATORY SURGERY	During surgery, take full-thickness biopsies of the stomach, jejunum, and ileum, as well as pancreas and liver. The finding of pancreatitis, cholantitis/hepatitis, and duodenitis (IBD) are often associated with chronic vomiting and are diagnosed by biopsying all of these organs (**triaditis**). Biopsy via surgery is often preferred over biopsies obtained under endoscopy if lymphangiectasia or neoplasia is suspected because the surgical biopsy is a full-thickness biopsy whereas the endoscopic biopsy is just through the mucosa and submucosa. **Laparoscopy** can also be used to obtain a full-thickness biopsy.

GI Disease

TREATING SPECIFIC GI DISEASES

BILIOUS VOMITING SYNDROME	This is caused by gastric hypomotility and is characterized by early morning vomiting before meals. Treat by feeding the animal later at night and administering metoclopramide prior to meals as well as H2 receptor agonists such as famotidine at bedtime if needed.
ACUTE GASTRITIS e.g. Parvo, food intolerance etc.	**Correct the underlying cause** if possible. **Rest the stomach** by making the animal NPO (no food or water orally) for several days. Then place the animal on a bland diet using non-meat proteins such as tofu (non-meat proteins stimulate less acid secretion than meat proteins). Low fat and non-fat diets are better because they don't delay gastric emptying. **Control vomiting** (optional) Protect the gastric mucosa with H$^+$ blockers, sucralfate, etc. **Treat transient decreases in GI motility** with metoclopramide constant rate infusion.
CHRONIC GASTRITIS ± IBD	• **Chronic gastritis** can result from continued irritation by agents that cause acute gastritis. It is also often caused by food allergy. • **Place the animal on a controlled** diet of one carbohydrate source and one protein source (e.g. cottage cheese and rice or tofu and rice). The animal should start improving within days. After 2-3 weeks on the controlled diet (although some research recommends 12 weeks), gradually introduce one new antigen source at a time. If the controlled diet does not work, try corticosteroids. Steroids are indicated when the biopsy shows eosinophils (eosinophilic gastroenteritis) or lymphocytes and plasma cells (which suggest an immune-mediated pathologic response). Cats respond better to corticosteroids than dogs do. Don't use corticosteroids unless complete remission is not possible with a controlled diet. • **Surgical resection** may be indicated for areas of the stomach with granulomatous tissue (e.g. non-specific or eosinophilic gastroenteritis). Pyloromyotomy or resection may be indicated with mucosal hypertrophy or gastric outflow obstruction. • **Do not chronically inhibit gastric acid secretion** because it may lead to an increase in bacteria in the stomach (which is normally sterile). • Prostaglandins may be useful because they are cytoprotective. • Sucralfate is safe to use. It does not inhibit acid secretion.
GASTRIC ULCERS	**Gastric ulcers** are rarely primary. Find and treat the underlying cause and treat with GI protectants.
FOREIGN BODIES	In general, esophageal foreign bodies should be removed within 4-6 hours by endoscopy because they are highly painful and likely to cause neurologic damage to the esophagus as well as perforation. As a general rule, if the foreign body is causing obstruction or is likely to cause obstruction or perforation over time, remove it (surgically or endoscopically). After removing a foreign body, treat the animal as you would for acute gastritis. When removing the foreign body, also biopsy the stomach and intestines and save the samples in case the animal continues vomiting.
NEOPLASIA	**Neoplasia:** Tumors should be removed surgically if possible. Antral hyperplasia and gastric carcinoma look similar grossly. Biopsy is needed for a definitive diagnosis. The prognosis with tumors is poor unless they are caught early on and resected.
PYLORIC STENOSIS	**Pyloric stenosis:** Perform a pyloromyotomy and then treat for gastritis.

PANCREATITIS in DOGS

CLINICAL SIGNS	Clinical signs are non-specific and include the following (Hess, 1999): • Anorexia (91% of dogs) • Vomiting (90% of dogs) • Weakness or lethargy (79% of dogs) • Abdominal pain as exhibited by prayer position/abdominal guarding (58%). About 95% of humans with pancreatitis have marked abdominal pain. • Dehydration (46%) • Diarrhea (33%) is usually due to inflammation of the transverse colon • Fever (low grade)
RISK FACTORS	• **Overweight dogs** • Animals with a history of having eaten a **fatty meal**: Some dogs are more sensitive to fat than others and only need small amounts of fat in order to develop pancreatitis. • Small female spayed dogs that are middle-aged or old • Presence of conditions leading to **lipemic states**: diabetes mellitus, Cushing's disease, hypothyroidism, Schnauzer • **Hypercalcemia** • Exposure to **organophosphates** and some drugs such as KBr • Note: Glucocorticoids are no longer considered a risk factor
PATHO-PHYSIOLOGY	Pancreatitis occurs when pancreatic proenzymes are activated and released within the pancreas resulting in autodigestion. The pancreas makes a number of digestive enzymes which are stored in their inactive proenzyme forms in granules within the acinar cells of the pancreas. Normally, these proenzymes are released into ducts that converge into the pancreatic duct and empty into the duodenum. Once in the duodenum, **enterokinase** cleaves them to their active form. The pancreas also contains protease inhibitors that neutralize these enzymes in cases where small amounts are accidentally activated and released within the pancreas. Pancreatitis occurs when duodenal contents reflux back into the pancreas, proenzyme granules are released within the pancreas, or protease inhibitor levels are low. Signs associated with pancreatitis are caused by digestive enzymes acting on the pancreas and other organs. Trypsin and chymotrypsin cleave proteins. Lipase and phospholipases digest fats, leading to fat necrosis and membrane dissolution. Elastase digests elastin in blood vessels, resulting in hemorrhage. The severity of the disease depends on the level of cytokines and free radicals.
COMPLICATIONS	• **Ileus**: Pancreatitis may cause regional or diffuse ileus via several mechanisms. Peritonitis can cause a loss of motility due to inflammation extending into other organs such as the stomach or duodenum. Loss of potassium from extensive vomiting and diarrhea can also cause ileus. Stimulation of the sympathetic nervous system (shock) can cause loss of intestinal motility. • **Hepatic disease** occurs when pancreatic inflammation extends to the liver. Pancreatic inflammation may occlude the bile duct resulting in an **extrahepatic biliary obstruction**. • **Coagulopathies/DIC**: Pancreatic proteases activate and destroy clotting factors. • **Cardiomyopathy** (myocardial depressant factor) is the most likely cause of sudden death in animals with pancreatitis. If there's evidence for cardiac complications, monitor the animal using an EKG. • **Hypotension** due to vomiting and decreased water intake.
COMPLETE BLOOD COUNT (CBC)	The CBC shows non-specific changes. It may be normal or show a stress response. Toxic changes are usually absent because pancreatitis is a chemically-induced inflammation rather than a bacterial one. • **Thrombocytopenia**: These dogs often die from DIC due to massive inflammation. • **Neutrophilia** with a left shift • **Anemia**

The Small Animal Veterinary Nerdbook ™

GI Disease

PANCREATITIS in DOGS continued

CHEMISTRY PANEL	Most changes are non-specific: • ± increased **lipase** and **amylase**. Both of these enzymes are manufactured, stored, and secreted by the pancreas but are also present in other organs. Consequently, even pancreatectomized dogs can have circulating lipase and amylase. Serum lipase has only 54% or less sensitivity (levels 3X the reference range), and amylase has only 57% sensitivity and 62% specificity. Thus, there are many false negatives and false positives which make amylase and lipase poor tests for pancreatitis. • **Increased liver enzymes:** ALP (in 79% of dogs) and ALT (61% of dogs) are elevated due to cholestasis or inflammation extending to the liver. • **Bilirubinemia** (low grade): post-hepatic (up to the 20's) • **Hypoalbuminemia** due to vascular and peritoneal leakage • **Pre-renal azotemia** (in 59% of dogs): Check the urine specific gravity (concentrated vs. dilute urine) to be sure that it is pre-renal azotemia rather than acute renal failure due to vasoactive amine induced vasoconstriction or prolonged hypovolemia. • **Hyperglycemia** due to increased glucagon (39% of dogs) • **Hypoglycemia:** Glucose is used as energy during the massive inflammatory response. (30% of dogs) • **TLI** is not useful • **Decreased calcium** is caused by decreased albumin and by saponification of fat around the pancreas. • **Serum Spec cPL (pancreatic lipase)** is the test of choice with 81.8% sensitivity and 96% specificity, even in healthy dogs on prednisone, dogs with chronic renal failure, and those with gastritis.
RADIOGRAPH & ULTRASOUND	• **Radiographs:** Textbook changes include displacement of the duodenum to the right with a wide pyloroduodenal angle and dilated intestinal loops due to ileus as well as focal peritonitis which manifests itself as a ground glass appearance to the right cranial quadrant of the abdomen. On lateral, it shows up caudal to the liver and ventral to the stomach. The problem is that these findings are subjective and usually recognized better after pancreatitis is diagnosed. • **Ultrasound is much more useful than radiographs for diagnosing pancreatitis in dogs:** Findings include enlargement of the pancreas with fluid accumulation around it and increased echogenicity with fibrosis in chronic cases. The highest sensitivity of this test with an experienced examiner is 68%, so we still miss the diagnosis 32% of the time on ultrasound. • **Abdomenocentesis:** Results are consistent with a chemical peritonitis. We should see a non-septic exudate. Amylase and lipase levels in the fluid should be higher than serum levels. • **Biopsy:** Usually biopsies are only performed if the diagnosis is being made on surgery. Perform multiple deep biopsies even if the pancreas looks normal. Note that handling the pancreas does not cause pancreatitis.
MANAGE-MENT	Administer fluids to replace lost volume and to correct metabolic acidosis. Start off with crystalloids and monitor albumin. If albumin drops below 2.0, switch to colloids. Plasma is the best (but expensive) in this case because it also contains clotting factors, platelets, and circulating trypsin inhibitors. Remember that only half of the colloids stay in the vessels and half go into the interstitial space. Hetastarch is also a good colloid. Dextrans can cause coagulopathy because they stick to platelets. **Diet:** NPO if vomiting, but feed the patient as soon as it is willing to eat. Food may trigger CCK production by the duodenal cells. A nasogastric tube, esophagostomy tube, gastrostomy, or jejunostomy tube can be placed for feeding. Total Parenteral Nutrition (TPN) may be used if the animal has not eaten for > 3 days. Once the animal is eating, put it on a highly digestible fat-free or low-fat diet. It may need to be on a low-fat diet for the rest of its life. Some clinicians add pancreatic enzymes to the diet to try to decrease the pancreatic enzyme secretion in hopes of preventing recurrence of pancreatitis. There is no evidence that this practice has any beneficial effects.

PANCREATITIS in DOGS continued

MANAGEMENT continued	Anti-emetics such as chlorpromazine, metoclopramide (CRI), or dolasetron can be used to control vomiting. Cisapride (and metoclopramide) can be used for their prokinetic effects. (Refer to section p. 10.7 on anti-emetics). **Avoid anticholinergics.**
	Pain management: Opioid analgesics can be used (e.g. fentanyl 2-4 μg/kg IV followed by 1-4 μg/kg/hr CRI). Opioids can, however, exacerbate ileus, constipation, and vomiting. Lidocaine can be used at 20-30 μg/kg CRI. Ketamine at subanesthetic doses decreases pain build-up (2-5 μg/kg/min CRI).
	Dopamine (5 μg/kg/min) improves pancreatic perfusion.
	Antibiotics: Infection can occur due to translocation, secondary to GI compromise. Use an antibiotic with good gram negative and anaerobic coverage with severe disease or prolonged NPO periods. Pancreatic abscesses often follow acute pancreatitis and lead to a bad prognosis.
	Vitamin B complex supplementation should be instituted in patients with prolonged NPO or anorexia because they are not obtaining vitamin B from their diet.
	Monitor for arrhythmias because myocardial depressant factor (MDF; which is made in the pancreas) may be released in high amounts, thus predisposing the dog to premature ventricular contractions and ventricular tachycardia. Treat with lidocaine if the heart rate is greater than 200 bpm, if there are multiple foci, or if you see R on T phenomena.
	Corticosteroids: You may use 1-2 doses during the shock stage without harming the animal, but corticosteroids are not necessary. Use beyond this number of doses is controversial.
	Surgery may be indicated in cases of cysts, abscesses, and bile duct obstruction where medical management is not working.
	Monitor for impending DIC or shock.
	Identify and treat underlying etiologies such as diabetes mellitus.

PANCREATITIS in CATS

Pancreatitis is harder to diagnose in cats because the signs are more generic and the etiologies more varied. Consider pancreatitis as a rule-out for any unexplained disease in cats.

CLINICAL SIGNS	Lethargy, anorexia (97%), dehydration (92%), and jaundice (64%) are the most common signs. Vomiting (35%) and diarrhea (15%) are not commonly associated.
RISK FACTORS	• GI tract disease • Hepatobiliary infections • Trauma • Drugs (e.g. azathioprine; idiosyncratic reaction) and organophosphates • FIP • Idiopathic
DIAGNOSIS	Abdominal tenderness Amylase and lipase have no diagnostic value in the cat. fPLI (Feline pancreatic lipase immunoreactivity) is the test of choice (100% sensitivity and specificity). Ultrasound is a good diagnostic when the examiner is experienced (80% sensitivity in moderate to severe pancreatitis and 88% specificity in healthy cats). Pancreatic biopsy
TREATMENT	Treatment is similar to dogs with the following exceptions: • **Do not fast cats.** As obligate carnivores, fasting leads to fat mobilization which may exacerbate concurrent hepatic lipidosis. • **B-complex** is especially important in cats because they may have concurrent intestinal or liver disease which can compromise their ability to absorb dietary vitamin B12, putting them at even greater risk of B12 deficiency. (B-complex: 100 μg/kg SC q 4-6 weeks) • **Corticosteroid therapy** at anti-inflammatory doses. • **Pancreatic enzymes:** 1 tsp/feeding q 24 hours. It can be continued indefinitely as there is anecdotal evidence that doing so may decrease the incidence of recurrence.

GI Disease

LIVER DISEASE

LIVER FUNCTIONS	The liver has many functions which include the following: • To detoxify compounds by oxidizing and then conjugating them to make them more water soluble for excretion • To convert toxic ammonia (NH_3) waste products to urea (BUN) • To make albumin and cholesterol • To synthesize clotting factors and anticoagulants • To produce glucose, store glucose as glycogen, and release glucose • To break down gastrin (enzyme that stimulates gastric HCl secretion) When the liver is damaged, one or more of these functions can be impaired resulting in clinical signs and chemical changes in the blood.
ETIOLOGIES	**Cats** most commonly develop the following hepatic conditions: • **Toxic hepatopathy** (e.g. acetaminophen, aspirin, griseofulvin toxicosis) • **Hepatic lipidosis** • **Neutrophilic or lymphocytic cholangitis** which is often associated with IBD and pancreatitis • **Neoplasia:** primarily metastatic such as lymphoma or mast cell tumors • **Extrahepatic obstruction** due to conditions such as pancreatitis, neoplasia, cholelithiasis, inspissated bile duct plugs, parasite migration, abscess, or granuloma near the common bile duct • **Portosystemic shunts:** As in dogs, they can be congenital or acquired. **Dogs** most commonly develop drug-induced, neoplastic, or inflammatory non-infectious liver disease such as chronic active hepatitis.
CLINICAL SIGNS	• **Vomiting** ($\pm$ blood due to GI ulceration), **anorexia,** and **weight loss** • **Oral ulcers** are due to build-up of nitrogenous waste products lead to ptyalism in cats. • **Icterus** is due to elevated bilirubin. Examine the scleras, pinnae, soft palate, mucous membranes, and skin. • **Ascites** is due to hypoalbuminemia and congestion from elevated hepatic portal hypertension. Portal hypertension is most commonly caused by cirrhosis which leads to an increase in total portal blood flow or portal vessel resistance. Ascites is more common in dogs than cats. • **CNS signs** such as obtundation and head pressing are caused by toxic waste product build-up (ammonia, mercaptans, etc). • **Bleeding** is due to coagulopathies. • **PU/PD** is due to loss of BUN, which is needed for establishing the renal medullary concentration gradient.
CBC	Mild non-regenerative anemia is typical in cats with chronic liver disease; it is often secondary to blood loss from gastric ulceration caused by elevated waste products and gastrin. Thrombocytopenia due to DIC; Neutrophilia

CHEM PANEL	• **ALT: Alanine aminotransferase** is the most liver specific enzyme in dogs and cats. ALT is elevated with hepatocellular damage. Even in the absence of clinical signs, the animal likely has liver disease and further diagnostics should be performed if chemistries demonstrate any of the following:
	    • ALT $\geq$ AST
	    • ALT remains elevated 3-4 x normal for 2-3 weeks
	    • ALT remains moderately elevated for 6-8 weeks
	• **AST: Aspartate aminotransferase** is also elevated with hepatocellular damage, but can also increase due to muscle damage (so check CPK). If AST > ALT, look for muscle or RBC disorders.
	• **GGT: Gamma glutamyl transpeptidase** increases with biliary stasis and steroid hepatopathy.
	• **ALP: Alkaline phosphatase** is produced by the cells lining the bile canaliculi and is consequently elevated with biliary obstruction in both cats and dogs. However— the #1 cause of elevated ALP in dogs is **excess glucocorticoid levels (exogenous or endogenous).** Glucocorticoids induce an ALP isoenzyme with high activity. ALP can also be elevated due to non-hepatic sources. It is synthesized by bone, placenta, gut, and kidney, and is elevated in young growing animals.
	Note that in end-stage liver disease/fibrosis, liver enzymes are not elevated because the liver does not make enough enzymes. Also note that the magnitude of the elevation at one point in time does not indicate disease severity.

CHEMISTRY PANEL CONTINUED	**Elevated bilirubin:** Bilirubin, a breakdown product of heme, can be elevated due to **prehepatic** (RBC hemolysis), **hepatic** (the liver is unable to conjugate the bilirubin so it can be excreted), or **post-hepatic** (biliary obstruction or stasis) causes. To rule out prehepatic bilirubinemia, check for a low PCV. Also look for marked Heinz bodies, *Hemobartonella,* or spherocytes as an indicator of autoagglutination and reticulocytes as an indicator of a hemolytic event. If all are negative, then the elevation in bilirubin is due to hepatic or post-hepatic causes. If the PCV is borderline, recheck it in several days. Because the liver has a large reserve capacity for bilirubin (30 times the normal capacity), serum bilirubin concentration is an insensitive measure of hepatocyte function. Serum **hyperbilinemia** as well as bilirubin in the urine are **detectable at $\geq$ 0.6-0.8 mg/dL**; however, jaundice is not detectable until total bilirubin is $\geq$ 2-3 mg/dL. **BUN, albumin, and glucose can be depressed.** These values don't usually fall until the liver is severely impaired (70-80% loss of hepatic function). Note that glucose can be low with sepsis; albumin can be low due to GI , renal, or 3rd space losses; BUN can decrease with diuresis or anorexia. **Cholesterol** can be low late in disease. With some biliary diseases, it is elevated. Icterus plus cholesterolemia indicates biliary disease. **Increased total protein (TP) and PCV** due to dehydration: TP may be elevated due to high globulins in cases of cats with FIP.
URINE	**Decreased specific gravity** due to low BUN: BUN is required for establishing the renal medullary concentration gradient. **Bilirubinuria:** Dog have a low threshold for bilirubin excretion and their renal tubular cells can conjugate bilirubin. Consequently, small amounts of bilirubin in canine urine is normal. The presence of Bilirubinemia however, suggests hepatobiliary disease. Cats have a higher renal threshold for bilirubin; thus, any bilirubin in their urine is abnormal and indicates bilirubinemia.
SPECIFIC TESTS	**Serum Bile Acids (SBA) Tests** are used primarily to determine if the animal is likely to have a portosystemic shunt. It's not needed if the animal is icteric. This test is useful for cases where: 1) we suspect functional liver disease but there's no elevation in AST, ALT, or ALP 2) liver enzymes are elevated but clinical signs are mild or absent, or 3) it's difficult to distinguish pre-hepatic vs. hepatic disease {e.g. an icteric cat with moderate decrease in PCV (liver vs. hemolysis)}. The serum bile acids test is more sensitive and specific in cats than in dogs. **Ammonia Tolerance Tests** are useful in the same circumstances. Consider a **urine creatinine/bile acids** test.

1. SPECIFIC LIVER FUNCTION TESTS (Serum Bile Acids, Ammonia Tolerance Test)
   A. SERUM BILE ACIDS (one of the most useful).
      1. **Mechanism:** The gall bladder is important in fat digestion. When animals ingest a meal, the gall bladder contracts, releasing bile into the duodenum. Bacteria deconjugate the bile acids, which are then reabsorbed at the ileum and go into the circulatory system.
         a. In normal dogs, they are absorbed into the portal circulation and transported to the liver where they are cleared from circulation.
         b. In a portasystemic shunt dog, bile acids are absorbed from the ileum, enter the circulation (which bypasses the liver), and go directly to the systemic circulation without being cleared by the liver.

      2. **Running the test:** Fast the animal for 12 hours and then collect a pre-meal blood sample. Next, feed the dog a normal-sized meal high in fat and protein. Patients weighing $\leq$ 5 kg should eat at least 2 tsp of food whereas those $\geq$ 5 kg should eat at least 2 Tbsp of food. Two hours later, take another blood sample. In a normal dog, the bile acids should be cleared by the liver.

GI Disease

3. Interpreting the Test

	RESTING BILE ACIDS	POST-MEAL BILE ACIDS
Normal Dog	Normal	Normal (but higher than the resting bile acids)
Liver Shunt Dog	Normal or high	High
Cirrhotic Dog	High	High
Biliary Cirrhosis or Obstruction	High	High

a. **Normal dog:** The normal dog's liver clears the bile quickly.
b. **Liver shunt dog:** Bile acids are eventually cleared via the hepatic arterial circulation; therefore, fasting values can be normal or elevated.
c. **Cirrhotic dog:** The liver may be so small that it is only 1% of the dog's body weight. Resting values are elevated because the liver is so damaged that even with 12 hours to filter out bile acids, the hepatocytes can't completely clear the bile acids. Thus, the post-meal bile acid level is highly elevated.
d. **Biliary cirrhosis/obstruction:** Bile acids are made by the liver and are stored in the gall bladder. With a biliary tract obstruction, bile acids leak out into the circulation causing an elevation in resting and post-prandial bile acids.

4. Because bile acids are used and reused so efficiently through the enterohepatic circulation and because very little is needed, even the cirrhotic liver makes enough bile acids to cause elevated resting bile acids.

B. **AMMONIA TOLERANCE TEST:** Similar to the bile acid test, but in the bile acid test we use an endogenous substance, whereas in the ammonia tolerance test we administer a toxic substance.
1. **Performing the test:** Measure the resting ammonia. If it is elevated you don't need to proceed with the test. If the resting ammonia levels are normal, administer the ammonia via stomach tube or per rectum. The ammonia is absorbed by the gut and then it goes via the portal vein to the liver where it's incorporated into the urea cycle and made into urea.
2. **Advantages:** With this test the animal does not have to be eating because it can be stomach-tubed and the test only takes 30 minutes.
3. **Disadvantages:** This test is difficult to perform due to crucial sample handling factors which include keeping the samples on ice.
4. **Interpretation:** Animals with hepatic disease have elevated post-prandial ± elevated pre-prandial levels.

RADIOGRAPHS	Abdominal radiographs are used to evaluate for liver size. Hepatic lipidosis as well as steroid hepatopathy generally lead to hepatomegaly. Hepatic cirrhosis as well as portosystemic shunts are characterized by a small liver. Don't radiograph animals with ascites as the liver will be difficult to visualize. Perform ultrasound instead.
ULTRASOUND	Ultrasound should be performed as part of a diagnostic work-up if the bile acids test indicates hepatic dysfunction, or if the bile acids test is normal or equivocal but index of suspicion for hepatic disease is still high. Ultrasound allows evaluation of hepatic architecture as well as biliary tract and portal blood supply. **If the gall bladder is large and the bile ducts are dilated,** there's an extrahepatic bile duct obstruction. Look for extrahepatic plugs and for plugs in the common bile duct.
ASPIRATES	Biopsies/aspirates should be performed when ultrasound has ruled out post-hepatic obstruction. Aspirates are easy to perform and only require sedation; however, their sensitivity and specificity are low (approximately 50%). Consequently, if lesions are discovered on ultrasound, perform an aspirate (or a Tru-cut biopsy). If you find significant disease other than hepatic lipidosis in the cat, then the test was diagnostic. If you do not find significant disease, then perform a biopsy. Aspirates do not rule out disease. Additionally, finding fat cells can lead to a false diagnosis of hepatic lipidosis when an underlying disorder with patchy distribution exists. The gall bladder can be aspirated and cultured on ultrasound. Rupture is uncommon except in cases where the gall bladder is close to rupturing on its own.

BIOPSY	Biopsy is the only way to accurately diagnose the specific hepatic disease and consequently determine the appropriate treatment. Biopsy can be performed with ultrasound guidance (True-cut), laparoscopy, or via surgical exploratory laparotomy. The latter two cases are preferable as multiple wedge biopsies from different lobes can be taken. Tru-cut biopsies often do not yield adequate samples. Additionally, the gall bladder should be cultured. A biopsy is indicated for any case in which 1) the animal shows clinical signs and biochemical changes consistent with hepatic disease; 2) the patient has persistently abnormal serum hepatic enzyme activity (especially ALT) and other causes such as Cushing's disease have been ruled out; 3) the patient has microhepatica or persistent hepatomegaly even in the absence of biochemical or clinical signs, if other conditions are ruled out.
	Prior to biopsy, many clinicians perform a coagulation profile, but results do not correlate well with the incidence of post-biopsy bleeding. Additionally, clotting times are only prolonged when coagulation factors are decreased to 30% of normal. A more practical approach is to do a buccal mucosal bleeding time (BMBT) on all animals. If BMBT is prolonged, use cautery to control bleeding during the biopsy. Also use this method if the animal is thrombocytopenic or if it has prolonged bleeding on venipuncture. Vitamin K ± plasma transfusions can be given if BMBT is prolonged.
	Always warn clients that some patients with hepatic disease may acutely decompensate after hepatic biopsy even if they present with chronic, slowly progressive disease.

II. **APPROACH to NONSPECIFIC HEPATIC ENZYME ELEVATIONS:** We frequently find elevated liver enzymes on routine chemistry panels in addition to animals that present with clinical signs. It's important to determine whether elevations are associated with disease (rather than waiting for clinical signs of hepatic failure to present) because the ultimate goal is to diagnose the animal before it goes into hepatic failure. In dogs, by the time we see clinical signs, the prognosis is poor.

   A. **WHEN to PERFORM FURTHER DIAGNOSTICS BASED on ALT**

   ELEVATED ALT in the ABSENCE of CLINICAL SIGNS or other LABORATORY INDICATORS of HEPATIC DISEASE

   The following indicate the presence of hepatic disease and that further diagnostics (ultrasound and biopsy) should be performed to obtain a specific diagnosis:
   - ALT ≥ AST
   - ALT remains elevated 3-4 x normal for 2-3 weeks
   - ALT remains moderately elevated for 6-8 weeks, even in the absence of clinical signs. The animal likely has liver disease and further diagnostics should be performed.

   B. **STEPS to TAKE BASED on OTHER ELEVATED ENZYMES**

   ELEVATED ALP, GGT, and/or AST in the ABSENCE of CLINICAL SIGNS or other LABORATORY INDICATORS of HEPATIC DISEASE

   Elevations in ALP, GGT and AST can suggest presence of hepatic disease and indicate that further diagnostics (ultrasound and biopsy) should be performed to obtain a specific diagnosis:
   - Rule out other diseases associated with hepatic enzyme elevation such as Cushing's disease (ALP elevation due to isoenzyme induction) or diabetes mellitus, both of which can cause elevated ALP and ALT due to hepatocellular damage either related to lipid accumulation or glycogen storage. Both can also cause decreased BUN due to medullary washout from PU/PD.
   - Repeat a chemistry profile in 4-8 weeks. If hepatic enzymes are still elevated, run a bile acids test. If normal, repeat the hepatic function test and bile acids test 1-2 months later. If liver enzymes are still elevated and bile acids are equivocal, an ultrasound and biopsy may be warranted. Some clinicians opt for a trial on antibiotics prior to retesting.

III. **GENERAL MANAGEMENT** consists of supportive care. Specific treatments can be instituted once the specific disease is diagnosed via biopsy. Biopsy is encouraged so that specific therapies can be instituted.
   A. **Administer fluids to** patients that are dehydrated ± acidotic/hypokalemic:
      1. Supplement the fluids with 5-10% glucose if the animal is hypoglycemic, but not until dehydration is controlled.

GI Disease

2. **Plasma** can be given to replace albumin and clotting factors (fresh frozen plasma for clotting factors and frozen plasma for albumin). If the animal is severely anemic from gastric ulcers, it may need a blood transfusion.

B. **TREAT HEPATIC ENCEPHALOPATHY.** Hepatic encephalopathy is caused by a substance or combination of substances (including ammonia) produced by degradation of proteins by enteric bacteria. The goal of treatment is to decrease bacterial activity and decrease available protein substrates.

1. **Lactulose** (orally) promotes **osmotic diarrhea** and acidifies the colonic contents, thus trapping ammonia (NH_3) as ammonium ion (NH_4^+) in the intestinal lumen and providing a non-protein substrate for bacteria which decreases the production of ammonia.. The acidifiying quality also reduces bacterial numbers. Use just enough to make the feces soft. Good starting doses are 0.5 mg/kg PO BID or 3-10 mL PO TID in dogs (2-3 mL PO TID in cats). The goal is to have soft stools.

2. **Antibiotics** to decrease obligate anaerobe numbers.

C. **TREAT GASTRIC ULCERS** by administering sucralfate, H_2 blockers, or prostaglandins (misoprostol). Note that cimetidine must be metabolized by the liver cytochrome P_{450} system and consequently can alter the metabolism of other drugs (due to hepatic enzyme activation). For this reason, ranitidine and famotidine are the H_2 blockers usually used.

D. **PREVENT COAGULOPATHY** by administering **vitamin K_1** (3 mg/kg SC BID). For chronic disease, administer vitamin K at 1.5-5 mg/kg SC every 2-3 weeks.

E. **ANTIBIOTICS:**
1. Most **cats** have underlying infectious disease (bacterial related cholangitis) and require antibiotics.
2. **Dogs don't get bacterial hepatic infections** as frequently as cats, but may need antibiotics in order to decrease ammonia production if they are showing signs of hepatic encephalopathy.

F. **ANTIOXIDANTS:** Membrane damage due to oxidation exposes antigens which the body attacks. This leads to immune-mediated chronic hepatitis. Antioxidants work as a network at different regions of the metabolic pathway, thus multiple antioxidants should be used to prevent further oxidative damage.
1. **Vitamin E:** 15-20 mg/kg PO SID (100-200 units per small dog or cat and 400 units/ large dog). Use it with Vitamin B12 (100-500 μg/cat/day).
2. **S-Adenosylmethionine (SAMe):** 20-100 U/kg PO SID. SAMe is used to protect against acetaminophen toxicity because it replenishes the methyl groups needed in the conjugation phase of toxin handling by the liver.
3. **Silybum** (milk thistle) may protect against mushroom toxicity in dogs. The correct dose is not known, but 5-15 mg/kg is a good starting dose. Use the form that's complexed with phosphatidylcholine.

G. **URSODEOXYCHOLIC ACID (Actigal®)** at 10-15 mg/kg PO SID can be used to increase bile acid flow in cases of cholangitis once bile duct obstruction has been ruled out. Ursodeoxycholate neutralizes the detergent action of the hydrophobic bile salts which are toxic to hepatocytes.

H. **COLCHICINE** can be used to prevent fibrosis in chronic disease. It may cause vomiting/diarrhea.

I. **DIET:** Use a high quality, low protein (adequate levels) diet such as Hills k/d® or Royal Canin hepatic diet. Don't worry about branch-chain amino acids.

J. **ANTI-INFLAMMATORY DRUGS (IMMUNOMODULATORY DRUGS):**
1. **Corticosteroids** may be used in cases where histology reveals evidence of chronic immune-mediated hepatic disease (lymphocytic, plasmacytic cholangiohepatitis in cats or dogs) or where fibrosis is present. A dose of 1.0-2.0 mg/kg PO BID (SID in cats) prednisolone or prednisone can be used and then gradually tapered to 0.125-0.25 mg/kg q48 hours once the animal is improving. Although theoretically prednisolone should be used because it does not need to be converted by the liver, in practice, no difference has been shown between the two. Note that because glucocorticoids cause elevation in ALP and steroid hepatopathy (marked vacuolization and ballooning of hepatocytes), re-biopsy in 6 months to 1 year.
2. **Azothioprine (Imuran®) can be used in dogs** if prednisone alone is not effective. Some clinicians add azothioprine at a dose of 2 mg/kg/day and then taper to alternate day therapy. CBC/chemistry should be performed at 3- 6 weeks and every 2-4 months thereafter to monitor for myelosuppression.
3. **Chlorambucil (Leukeran®)**

IV. SELECTED HEPATIC DISEASE CONDITIONS

PORTOSYSTEMIC SHUNT

PATHO-PHYSIO-LOGY	Blood travels from the stomach, intestines, spleen, and pancreas via the portal vein to the hepatic veins where it delivers nutrients and tropic factors (e.g. insulin and glucagons) as well as toxins in need of detoxification (for excretion) to the hepatocytes. The blood then exits the liver into the systemic venous circulation. **Congenital shunts**: In the fetus, the importance of liver function is minimal; consequently, most of the blood is shunted from the portal vein directly to the systemic circulation. These vessels normally close after birth allowing the hepatic circulation to be established. In some animals, some shunts remain open and consequently the liver is not adequately perfused. This leads to liver atrophy due to lack of tropic factors and a decreased ability for the liver to perform detoxification and other functions. **Acquired shunts** are caused by chronic portal hypertension, which leads to opening of the fetal blood vessels that shunted blood from the portal system to the systemic circulation in the fetus. These extrahepatic shunts are multiple and tortuous shunts. The most common cause of portal hypertension is cirrhosis.
DESCRIP-TION	25% of congenital shunts are intra-hepatic (more common in large breed dogs) 50% are single extra-hepatic shunts (more common in small breed dogs)
CLINICAL SIGNS	Occurs primarily in animals < 1 year of age. Signs may be non-specific and may wax and wane throughout the day. • **Poor doer:** weight loss or slow growth, depression • **GI signs:** vomiting, diarrhea, anorexia • **Neurologic:** Approximately 90% of animals exhibit neurologic signs related to hepatoencephalopathy (depression, seizures, incoordination, aggression, etc). PU/PD Portosystemic shunts should be considered in any young animal where these signs persist. **Cats** with neurologic signs plus **salivation** should also be evaluated.
LAB FINDINGS	**Normal AST and ALT** is common because this condition does not lead to hepatocellular necrosis or leaking of enzymes. Rather, it's a condition of hepatic atrophy. • 50% have mild **hyperalbuminemia** • 70% exhibit low **BUN** • Serum **bilirubin** is usually normal • **Bile acids** are usually **elevated** • Approximately 30% have **ammonium biurate** crystals in the urine. They have elevated ammonia levels leading to increased formation of urea, yet the urea cannot be efficiently converted to allantoin by hepatocytes. These animal may also develop **ammonium biurate renal calculi**.
IMAGING	**Survey radiographs** usually reveal microhepatica. Contrast **radiographs** (portogram or splenic artery catheterization) **and nuclear scintigraphy are the most reliable methods for diagnosing portosystemic shunts.** • **Nuclear scintigraphy** (or contrast radiography) is the method of choice for a definitive diagnosis as well as identifying the shunt locations.
BIOPSY	Biopsy is not required for diagnosis but should be collected upon surgical correction. It reveals diffuse hepatic atrophy.
TREATMENT	Treatment of choice for single portosystemic shunts is surgical ligation. Animals must be stabilized medically first. Ligation leads to temporary portal hypertension which usually resolves after several weeks. The prognosis for single portosystemic shunts is excellent in dogs (unless severe portal hypertension exists) and favorable in 50-60% of cats. Prognosis for intrahepatic shunts is guarded due to the difficulty of identifying and ligating the shunts during surgery and the likelihood of severe portal hypertension.

GI Disease

TOXIC EXPOSURE

PATHO-PHYSIO	Up to 80% of blood entering the liver comes directly from the GI tract and spleen. Consequently, the liver is subjected to many toxins. Additionally, during the first step of detoxification by the liver (oxidation by the Cytochrome P450 system) some neutral foreign compounds are converted to more toxic metabolites. For instance, acetaminophen is not toxic but is oxidized to a toxic compound. As a result, some compounds can cause hepatic damage even after they are discontinued.
DIAGNOSIS	• **History** of exposure to chemicals or of being on medications +/- having stopped medications within the last several weeks. Drugs that are metabolized into toxins may continue to cause hepatic damage after they've been discontinued. Signs of toxicity may be acute or chronic. • **Discontinue the drugs.** If the only indication of liver disease is elevation of liver enzymes, then retest in 2 weeks. If the animal is sick, then pursue additional diagnostics immediately. Theoretically, animals that recover with drug removal alone should be rechallenged in order to diagnose drug reaction; this however, is usually not done. • **Biopsy:** Some toxins cause acute hepatic necrosis. Others such as those causing steroid hepatopathy cause marked vacuolization of hepatocytes.
SOME EXAMPLES	Some drugs and chemicals are **intrinsically toxic**. Their toxicity is dose dependent and reliably causes disease at these doses (e.g. acetaminophen, anticonvulsants, anabolic steroids, aflatoxins, etc). Other drugs such as carprofen (causes signs in 1.4/10,000 dogs), diazepam, and sulfa-antibiotics can cause **idiosyncratic toxicities** that are not dose dependent and difficult to reproduce experimentally. • **Anticonvulsants** such as primidone and phenobarbital often cause elevated liver enzymes. ALP may be elevated due to induction of the liver specific isoenzyme; however, elevated ALT probably represents low grade hepatocellular damage. Most patients are asymptomatic and have normal hepatic function tests. Some patients however, are sensitive to "safe" doses and develop hepatobiliary disease. By the time clinical signs are seen, disease is advanced. Consequently, chemistry panels should be evaluated every 6 months when animals are maintained on anticonvulsants. Follow the protocol for evaluation of hepatic enzymes to determine whether a biopsy should be performed. An estimated 6-15% of dogs on long-term anticonvulsants (especially primidone) develop hepatic disease. KBr does not have the same adverse effects. • **Steroid hepatopathy:** ALP can be greatly elevated due to induction of a liver-associated isoenzyme. Elevation in ALP is usually indicative of hepatopathy due to glycogen accumulation. Histopathology reveals marked vacuolization and ballooning of hepatocytes. Changes are reversible upon removal of excess glucocorticoids.

HEPATIC LIPIDOSIS in CATS

ETIOLOGY	Unknown. The classic presentation is an obese cat that has been anorexic, but it occurs in fit cats too. In some cases a known stressful event or illness has caused the anorexia. Disease can be attributed to the peculiarities of being a strict carnivore. Etiology is most likely related to low protein intake during starvation. Providing small amounts of high quality protein to obese cats during fasting states reduces hepatic lipid accumulation, reduces ALP elevation, and eliminates negative nitrogen balance. Providing lipids or carbohydrates to such cats does not have the same metabolic effects.
FINDINGS	• ALP >> GGT • **Ultrasound:** Areas of liver hyperechogenicity indicate presence of fat. **Cytology:** Hepatocytes look vacuolated because the vacuoles are fat-filled. Cytology can't rule out the presence of concurrent disease, so a diagnosis should be made on biopsy. • **Histopathology:** On gross examination, the liver looks yellow, is enlarged with rounded margins, and is friable. Histopathology reveals vacuolated hepatocytes.
TREATMENT	An estimated 80-95% of cats will recover with adequate nutrition. While cyproheptadine (5-HT$_2$ agonist) can stimulate appetite, nutritional support is most easily accomplished by placing a PEG tube or gastrostomy tube and giving antiemetics to control vomiting. The tube can be removed once the cat can eat on its own for 1-2 weeks.

CHOLANGITIS IN CATS

This disease was formerly referred to as cholangiohepatitis; however, in cats it primarily involves the bile ducts and is consequently called cholangitis.

PATHO-PHYSIOLOGY	Cholangitis arises from infections that ascend from the intestinal tract, through the common bile duct, into the bile ducts.
	Cholangitis is often associated with IBD and acute pancreatitis. The combination of the three conditions is referred to as triaditis. Cats with IBD are at increased risk for cholangitis because the chronic vomiting causes material high in bacteria (10^9 in cats compared to 10^4 in dogs) to reflux into the common bile duct which splits into the pancreatic duct and the bile duct. Thus with IBD in cats, efforts should be made to quickly control vomiting and clinical associated signs.
DESCRIPTION	In the past, cholangitis in cats has been classified as cholangiohepatitis; however in cats, bile duct inflammation is the predominant change and hepatic inflammation is a relatively insignificant factor. The **WSAVA International Liver Standardization Group** (2002) has devised the following classifications for liver disease in cats: • **Neutrophilic (acute) cholangitis** is characterized by neutrophilic infiltration of the bile ducts. • **Lymphocytic (chronic) cholangitis** is characterized by a mixed inflammatory response (lymphocytes, plasma cells, and neutrophils) primarily involving the bile ducts. Acute cholangitis progresses to chronic cholangitis. Inflammation may lead to bile duct hyperplasia or fibrosis of the ducts. Disease can progress to biliary cirrhosis and death. In severe cases, aspirates can yield an incorrect diagnosis of lymphosarcoma. Consequently, diagnosis should be confirmed on biopsy. • **Lymphocytic portal hepatitis** is a histologic finding where neutrophils and plasma cells are seen in patchy distribution through the portal tract. It's a normal histologic finding that probably does not correlate with disease. The bile ducts are not hyperplastic, there is no inflammation of the bile duct walls, and findings are not correlated with the presence of inflammatory bowel disease (IBD).
TREATMENT	In addition to fluids, antioxidants, and other supportive care, the following specific therapies can be instituted: • **Antibiotics:** Whether disease is acute or chronic, 66% of cats with cholangitis have a positive bacterial culture. Common bacteria include *E. coli*, Enterobacter, Streptococcus, Clostridium, and Pseudomonas. Prior to culture results, start with a broad spectrum antibiotic combination such as Clavamox (11 mg/kg PO BID) plus enrofloxacin 50 mg/kg PO BID. Metronidazole can be used instead of enrofloxacin for obligate anaerobes (10-25 mg/kg PO SID). • If biopsy reveals acute cholangitis, treat with antibiotics for 3-4 weeks. If it's chronic cholangitis, treat for 3-4 months. Some animals have to be on antibiotics life-long. • **Dietary modification:** Treat for IBD if the cat has associated IBD. • **Modulation of inflammation:** Inflammatory modulators such as corticosteroids can be used once bacterial infection is being treated if the other therapies alone are not effective as a treatment for IBD. • Colchicine or d-penicillamine can be used to help decrease fibrosis, however they may not be well tolerated (vomiting/diarrhea). • In severe cases, treatment includes surgical removal of the gall bladder.

GI Disease

DIARRHEA
Acute Diarrhea
Chronic Diarrhea
Symptomatic Treatment
General Work-Up & Specific Diseases

Diarrhea is defined as a change in the consistency, frequency, or volume of feces and is the primary sign of an intestinal problem. Healthy dogs with diarrhea should be examined if they've had 3 to 4 days of stool the consistency of soft-serve ice cream or looser. Cats are adapted for dry conditions and tend to conserve water, leading to very firm feces. Any loose stools in a cat are abnormal and diagnostics should be performed if such stools persist.

I. ACUTE vs. CHRONIC DIARRHEA
  A. **ACUTE DIARRHEA is often SELF-LIMITING but MAY ALSO BE LIFE-THREATENING.** Acute diarrhea such as that associated with diet change often improves with conservative therapy (bland diet) or empirical therapy such as fluids or a controlled diet. Such cases often require minimal work-up including fecal centrifugal flotation ($\pm$ Giardia SNAP test) and diagnostics to check for hydration status and rule out early indication of more serious problems. **Signs of fever, lethargy, anorexia, or dehydration indicate a more serious problem requiring more aggressive therapy** and diagnostics.
  B. **CHRONIC DIARRHEA** (2-4 weeks of regular diarrhea) with or without other systemic signs usually requires a systematic and extensive diagnostic work-up including CBC, chemistry panel, fecal, food trials, radiographs, and endoscopy.

II. ACUTE DIARRHEA
  A. ETIOLOGY of ACUTE DIARRHEA

CATEGORIES	DESCRIPTION
INFECTIOUS	• Parvovirus, Panleukopenia, FELV or FIV associated • Salmon poisoning • Giardia • Salmonella • *Clostridium perfringens* or *Clostridium difficile*
DIETARY INDUCED	• **Dietary intolerance:** Enzymes from the brush border increase or decrease in response to nutrients in the diet (e.g. dissacharides). When the diet is changed abruptly, the brush border enzymes don't have time to adapt. Thus, food is not digested and consequently not absorbed adequately. Furthermore, intestinal bacteria can then use the carbohydrate substrates. They proliferate and can cause gas. Some animal may never develop the ability to digest certain nutrients well (such as lactose) and therefore poorly digested nutrients should be avoided in these individuals. • **Garbage can:** Spoiled food may cause illness due to **enterotoxins** produced by bacteria. Some dogs can also develop **pancreatitis**, particularly after a high-fat meal.
OBSTRUCTION	• Intussusception, mesenteric torsion, and linear or non-linear foreign bodies can cause both vomiting and diarrhea.

  B. **WORK-UP for ACUTE DIARRHEA** can be conservative if the animal is not acting sick. If the animal is depressed, anorexic, or has blood in the stool, more aggressive diagnostics should be performed.

IF EATING and OTHERWISE ACTING HEALTHY:
• Bland diet for several days, then gradually switch back to regular diet
• Fecal for parasites (e.g. hookworms, whipworms, roundworms, coccidia—See Ch.17)
• PARVO test in puppies; FeLV and FIV test in kittens (See Ch. 11: Infectious Diseases)
• Giardia, *Tritrichomonas*
IF SICK or with AN APPROPRIATE HISTORY ADD:
• Fecal for salmon poisoning if there's a history of potential exposure to eating raw salmonid fish (trout, salmon)
• CBC, Chem to monitor for dehydration, electrolyte status, and signs of sepsis
• cPL for canine pancreatitis if there's a history of dietary indiscretion
• Radiographs or ultrasound to rule out obstruction or foreign body (surgical vs. medical)
• Enteric fecal culture for Salmonella, especially with a history of being on a raw food diet. Perform a fecal smear for Campylobacter.
• Antibiotic trial for *Clostridium perfringens* (dogs)

III. CHRONIC DIARRHEA
   A. SMALL BOWEL and LARGE BOWEL DIARRHEA
      1. **Small Bowel:** The small intestine is responsible for digestion of complex molecules and absorption of the resulting small molecules. The digestive enzymes are synthesized and secreted into the duodenum by the pancreas. Any problem leading to poor digestion or poor absorption (e.g. malassimilation problems) can lead to small bowel diarrhea.
         a. **Maldigestion** is the inability to digest complex food particles to constituents that can be absorbed by the small intestine. The usual cause of maldigestion is **pancreatic exocrine insufficiency** since the pancreas makes enzymes that degrade food particles into building blocks.
         b. **Malabsorption** is the inability to absorb digested food particles. It is usually caused by disease of the small intestinal mucosal cells.

      2. **Large Bowel:** The large intestine is responsible for water absorption.

      3. **Distinguishing between small and large bowel diarrhea:** The most consistent difference between the two is that the animals with small bowel diarrhea tend to **lose weight** because they have problems absorbing nutrients. The consistency and frequency of the stool may also help determine whether the problem is in the large or small intestines, but they are not very reliable indicators. Animals with severe colonic disease such as histiocytic colitis may also lose weight.

General Differences

	SMALL BOWEL	LARGE BOWEL
Blood	Digested	Fresh
Mucus	No	Yes
Weight loss	Yes*	No

* Weight loss may be seen prior to the appearance of diarrhea if the large bowel compensates by absorbing the excess water.

   B. ETIOLOGY of CHRONIC DIARRHEA

Chronic Small Bowel Disease	Chronic Large Bowel Disease
Maldigestion • Exocrine pancreatic insufficiency *Malabsorption* • Protein-losing enteropathy such as lymphangiectasia • Parasites: Giardia, roundworms, tapeworms, hookworms • Diet: Food allergy or non-allergic food intolerance • Antibiotic responsive enteropathy (*e.g. Clostridia*, Strep, Staph, etc.) • Neoplasia • Partial obstruction: Foreign body or intussusception • Inflammatory bowel disease	• Parasites: Whipworms, *Tritrichomonas*, Cryptosporidia • Diet: Food allergy or non-allergic food intolerance • Bacterial or antibiotic-responsive colitis (*e.g. Clostridia*, Salmonella, *Campylobacter*) • Neoplasia • Intussusception: Especially the ileocolic valve region • Fungal: *Histoplasmosis* • Inflammatory Bowel Diseases (this is a diagnosis of exclusion) • Fiber responsive inflammatory bowel disease. • Histiocytic colitis (Responsive to enrofloxacin and metronidazole) • Lymphocytic plasmacytic enteritis (cats)

IV. **SYMPTOMATIC TREATMENT** of CHRONIC or ACUTE DIARRHEA: Often the animal recovers whether or not it is treated. The goals of symptomatic treatment include: 1) Rest the GI tract 2) Maintain fluid balance 3) Prevent septicemia.

GI Disease

SYMPTOMATIC TREATMENT OF DIARRHEA

FLUIDS	This is the most important consideration in the diarrhea patient. Keep the animal hydrated and correct acid-base and electrolyte imbalances.
ANTIBIOTICS	**Use antibiotics when** there's evidence that bacteria have invaded the intestinal mucosa. Such evidence includes the following: • Hemorrhagic diarrhea (not just the occasional presence of streaks of fresh blood) • Fever • Depression • Marked left shift • Positive blood cultures **Choosing an antibiotic:** Don't use non-absorbable antibiotics orally (use them parenterally) because while they kill bacteria in the gut lumen, they don't kill bacteria in the gut mucosa where the invading bacteria are located. Use a drug that circulates in the blood stream. In addition, if the mucosa is disrupted, non-absorbable antibiotics (e.g. aminoglycosides) may be absorbed into the bloodstream in a non-regulated manner and may easily induce toxicity. **Use antibiotics effective against obligate anaerobes and enterics.** Penicillin can be used for anaerobes because it doesn't alter normal flora. **How long to treat?** For acute diarrhea, treatment for 1-2 days is sufficient. Usually we don't treat for more than 5 days. In Parvovirus cases, keep the dog on antibiotics for a longer period of time after it has recovered.
MOTILITY MODIFIERS	**Motility modifiers:** The goals are to increase resistance by increasing rhythmic segmentation and to decrease peristalsis so the gut contents are not rapidly propelled aborally. The second goal is difficult to attain, but we can achieve the first goal by using **opioids** (e.g. morphine, meperidine, **loperamide**) which increase rhythmic segmentation and decrease propulsive contractions; thus, opioids decrease the flow through the intestines. Opioids are only an adjunct therapy; they do not address the primary problem. Opioids may also delay gastric emptying time. • **Loperamide** (Imodium®) is a safe drug. It does not cause a narcotic analgesic effect and is available over-the-counter. • **Diphenoxylate** (Lomotil®) has a very potent narcotic analgesic effect, thus it can cause a "high." In order to prevent abuse, it is sold as a narcotic in combination with an anticholinergic. The anticholinergic produces side effects before the narcotic can produce a "high" effect. While anticholinergics are indicated in human patients with diarrhea, they are not indicated in animals with diarrhea.
LOCALLY ACTIVE PROTECTIVE AGENTS	Most of the so-called "protective drugs" (e.g. Kaopectate®) that are supposed to adhere to and protect the surface of the intestinal mucosa are not able to coat and protect the intestines well. If the clients want to use them, they can. • Bismuth salicylate (Pepto-Bismol®): 10-30 mL q 4-6 hours. Only for use in dogs as it contains salicylate. • Kaopectate® 1-2 mL/kg PO q 4-6 hours in dogs and cats.
DIETARY MANAGEMENT	**Dietary management:** Rest the GI tract by keeping the patient NPO for at least 12 hours. During GI inflammation, food has an abrasive action which results in loss of mucosal cells. By not feeding the animal, we give the GI epithelium time to regenerate, minimize changes in the bacterial microflora, and decrease the amount of dietary antigens. **Reintroducing food:** Intestinal cells get their nutrients from the intestinal contents, so it is important to provide food enterally as soon as possible but in frequent, small feedings to prevent osmotic overload. Put the animal on a controlled bland diet of one carbohydrate and one protein source and then wean it back to its normal diet over 3-5 days (unless you suspect food allergy as the cause of the diarrhea—in which case you will leave it on the diet for a longer period of time).

III. **GENERAL CHRONIC DIARRHEA WORK-UP:** The work-up for chronic diarrhea is often more extensive than that for acute diarrhea.
   A. **Take a detailed history and then perform a physical exam including a rectal exam.** Polyps, malignant tumors, and thickenings due to fungal infections

often present near the rectum and can be palpated. If the history (e.g. streaks of blood in the feces) suggests a rectal problem, palpate until you find the lesion.

B. **Determine** whether the animal has small bowel or large bowel diarrhea. If it's small bowel (weight loss with normal appetite), then rule out the following:

1. **Perform a fecal centrifugal flotation for parasites** and deworm if appropriate. Although parasites may not be the primary cause, they contribute to the overall health of the GI tract and thus affect the severity of disease.

   a. **Large Bowel:** Look for whipworms and Cryptosporidia. **Whipworms** are difficult to find on fecal float due to transient shedding and because they are dense and don't float well. Fecal centrifugal float or direct fecal exam should be repeated daily for several days in a row and/or the animal can be treated for whipworms without a diagnosis. Cryptosporidia are difficult to find due to their small size but DIF and ELISA's are available.

   b. **Small Bowel:** Rule out roundworms, hookworms, tapeworms, and coccidia.

2. **Multiple direct fecal exams** should be performed for both **Giardia (small bowel)** and *T. foetus (large bowel).* Giardia swim in a "falling leaf" pattern; *T. foetus* has an undulating membrane. Giardia shed intermittently and both parasites may be difficult to visualize. Thus, further tests should be performed if the results are negative.

   a. ELISA (Giardia fecal SNAP test) can be performed for Giardia. Sensitivity is good but specificity is unknown and false positives may occur. Some labs also perform DIF which has good specificity and sensitivity. Giardia can be treated with fenbendazole (50mg/kg PO x 3 days) or albendazole (25mg/kg PO for 2 days in the dog and 5 days in the cat).

   b. InPouch™ TF Culture (Biomed Diagnostics, White City, Oregon) should be performed if *T. foetus* is expected. *T foetus* can be treated effectively with Ronidazole (30-50 mg/kg PO BID for 2 weeks). Ronidazole can be obtained from some compounding pharmacies.

   c. *T. foetus* is common in purebred cats. At one international cat show, 31% of cats tested positive. 12% of cat show and cattery cats are co-infected with both Giardia and *T. foetus.*

3. **CBC, Chemistry, and Urinalysis:** If the diarrhea is **small bowel**, rule out **protein-losing enteropathy** by looking for hypoproteinemia. If it is hypoproteinemic, rule out glomerulonephropathy (proteinuria) and hepatic disease (bile acids, abdominal ultrasound, liver biopsy, elevated liver enzymes, BUN, etc). Hepatic disease and glomerulonephropathy are generally characterized by hypoalbuminemia whereas protein-losing enteropathies exhibit panhypoproteinemia. If the animal has low calcium and low cholesterol in addition to panhypoproteinemia, then **lymphangiectasia** is high on the differential list. Definitive diagnosis is based on full-thickness biopsies.

4. **Specialized blood tests for small bowel disorders:**

   a. Perform a **Trypsin-like immunoreactivity** test for **exocrine pancreatic insufficiency** (EPI) in dogs. Trypsin is normally secreted by the pancreas into the duodenum and some leaks back into the blood stream. If less trypsin is made, less will leak back into the blood (< 2.5 μg/L indicates EPI).

   b. **Measure serum specific pancreatic lipase (cPL)** in dogs if pancreatitis is suspected. This is usually an acute disease.

5. If the animal's condition is deteriorating at a fairly rapid rate, then perform further diagnostics such as ultrasound, endoscopy, and biopsy to rule out neoplasia and fungal infection (e.g. histoplasmosis). Radiographs rarely provide diagnostic information in cases of chronic diarrhea but they do help identify partial obstructions. Look for dilations cranial to the obstruction or plications indicating a linear foreign body. **Ceco-colic intussusception** can sometimes be diagnosed by barium enema if colonic endoscopy or ultrasound can't be performed.

   a. Aspirate (ultrasound-guided) or biopsy any enlarged lymph nodes as well as focal intestinal lesions (indicative of tumors or IBD).

GI Disease

6. If the animal is stable and can tolerate a delay of 4-8 weeks on diagnostics, then try a **therapeutic antibiotic trial** to rule in or out antibiotic responsive enteropathy or colitis.

    a. **Small intestinal bacterial overgrowth** (now referred to as **antibiotic responsive enteropathy**) is an interaction between GI bacteria and the host's immune system. It is a common disease but difficult to diagnose. In the past, **lymphangiectasia** was diagnosed by measuring levels of cobalamine (a nutrient absorbed in the ileum). Low levels of cobalamine plus high levels of folate were used as an indicator of bacterial overgrowth. These tests are specific but not sensitive so they do not rule out overgrowth. The cobalamine test may be useful in determining whether the animal (primarily cats) should receive vitamin B12 supplementation. The best way to diagnose is with antibiotic trials. The goal is to lower the bacterial levels until the GI tract can repair itself. The problem with an antibiotic therapeutic trial is that a response may be due to something else or the animal may have a second underlying GI disease.

        i.   Try a therapeutic trial with tetracycline and/ or tylosin or metronidazole and enrofloxacin for 2 weeks and evaluate response. If the response is good, continue for a total of 6-8 weeks. If the animal is still doing well at 6-8 weeks, we can say it is antibiotic responsive.

        ii. If upon discontinuation the diarrhea recurs, then repeat antibiotics. A different antibiotic may be necessary because the bacteria involved can change from week to week. This time, slowly wean the animal to SID or every other day and then to every 3rd day. Because this is a problem with the animal's immune system, antibiotic therapy may be life-long.

    b. **Large bowel bacterial disturbances: Trial therapy for Clostridia** (in dogs): *C. perfringens* and *C. difficile* are common pathogens and zoonotics of the large intestines. They are difficult to diagnose but are usually responsive to antibiotics within 3-7 days. For *C. perfringens*, try tylosin, ampicillin, or amoxicillin. Ampicillin is less available than amoxicillin but is retained in the bowel. Some animals have to be on low dose antibiotics for life (e.g. once every 1-3 days). For *C. difficile*, try metronidazole (10-15 mg/kg PO BID for < 10 days) or vancomycin. If the culture is negative for *C. difficile,* you can be fairly certain *C. difficile* is not present.

        DOSE of TYLOSIN (USE the POULTRY PREPARATION)

PATIENT SIZE	TYLOSIN DOSE
Small Dogs and cats	1/16 tsp BID to TID for 2 weeks
Dogs 7-15kg	1/8 tsp BID to TID for 2 weeks
Dogs > 15kg	1/4 tsp BID to TID for 2 weeks

        * Equivalent to about 10-40 mg/kg
        **The powder has a bad taste, so mix it with food or put it into capsules.

    c. **Other large bowel bacterial pathogens** can be found on fecal smears or bacterial cultures

        i.   **Campylobacter:** Fecal smear shows small, gram negative curved rods (like seagulls). Many are non-pathogenic. If you see a smear with a pure culture of these, treat with **xythromycin (7-15 mg/kg BID for 7-10 days)** or erythromycin (which however is noxious to the gut). Enrofloxacin is usually reserved as a second choice due to potential development of resistance.

        ii. **Enteric panel** (*E. coli* and Salmonella): It is unknown whether *E. coli* is an important cause of disease in dogs and cats because both healthy and sick cats and dogs carry *E. coli.* Salmonella causes severe diarrhea. Treat with enrofloxacin while waiting for enteric culture results. **Enteric panels should be performed:** 1) When there's an outbreak of diarrhea among pets on a **raw food diet** (One study found that 80% of raw meat diets contain Salmonella and 30% of dogs on raw meat diets culture positive for Salmonella), 2) When diarrhea appears in a dog after attending a dog show or after spending time in a boarding kennel, 3) Whenever there's an acute onset with evidence of sepsis (test for Clostridium too), 4) The patient has a fever and/or leukocytosis with left shift, or there are large numbers of neutrophils on fecal smear, or 5) When the client is immunocompromised

7. **Dietary trials** can be performed **in conjunction with or separate from antibiotic trials.** Diet and antibiotics work synergistically. If both are used together and the patient responds, you can stop one or the other to determine which was responsible for the difference. Diet trials should be performed early-on if the dog or cat has concurrent dermatologic conditions such as otitis externa (which raises the index of suspicion for food allergy). Dietary intolerance or allergy is a common cause for chronic diarrhea in dogs and cats and is under-diagnosed. Most of these pets respond to appropriate diets in 2-3 weeks, but a therapeutic trial should be carried out for 4-8 weeks before ruling a particular diet out. The trial should be carried out in such a way that it yields useful diagnostic information even if it fails. Two other dietary approaches include trying a highly digestible diet and trying a high fiber diet.

   a. Use an **elimination diet (a.k.a. novel protein diet)** made up of one novel protein and one novel carbohydrate. When performing a dietary trial, it is essential to obtain a thorough history to know which novel protein to use. Carefully explain to the client that: 1) No other foods or treats can be fed, and 2) Reserve a portion of the diet to be given as treats if the pet routinely gets treats. The gold standard is a one protein, one carbohydrate **home-made diet:** 1 part protein (boiled chicken) to 2 parts CHO (rice or cooked potato is best) + 1 multivitamin 2 days a week (non-flavored). Each diet should be strictly adhered to for 3-4 weeks and if the diarrhea resolves, the diet should be continued for another 3-4 weeks prior to switching over to a similar commercial diet.

      i. **Commercial** novel protein or **hydrolyzed protein diets:** Owners often have difficulty complying with home-made diets, thus commercial diets are a good option. There are many commercial prescription hypoallergenic diets available as well as several hydrolized protein diets. Be sure to get a thorough history so that you can make a logical choice. If one does not work, then try another. Frequently 2-3 diets may be required before an appropriate one is found, but an estimated 90% of dogs and cats are controlled within three trial diets.

      ii. **Trials with different commercial brands:** Sometimes the problem is a dietary intolerance rather than allergy, and random use of a commercial brand (where this is the only source of food for 2-8 weeks) solves the problem.

   b. **Highly digestible diet:** Some dogs and cats require a low residue, highly digestible diet.

   c. **Fiber supplementation:** Insoluble fiber works by soaking up excess water (thereby making the stool firmer) and by providing bulk which improves colonic motility. It can be used in conjunction with other therapies. Individual animals respond differently to differently types of fiber. Some animals do better on soluble fibers and others do better on insoluble fibers. Try one tablespoon of Metamucil or coarse wheat bran and adjust the levels as needed. Usually 2 weeks is enough to see improvement.

8. **Once parasite infection, antibiotic responsive disease and diet are ruled out** (note that frequently, the right diet has just not been found or the owner does not strictly adhered to the diet), the remaining rule outs are **tumors, fungal infections,** and **inflammatory bowel disease.** Ultrasound, endoscopy, and biopsies are used to rule out tumors and fungal infection. IBD is a diagnosis of exclusion and with the advent of good elimination diets, has been shown to be fairly uncommon in dogs. It does occur rather commonly in cats.

   a. **Lymphangiectasia:** If diagnostics indicate protein-losing gastroenteropathy, the next step is a biopsy to look for conditions such as lymphangiectasia. Each villus of **the small intestine is supplied with a lacteal through which** fatty acids and other fat soluble compounds are absorbed. With dilation, the lymph within the lacteals (high in protein,

10.31

GI Disease

lymphocytes, fatty acids, cholesterol, and vitamin D) leaks back into the gut. A full thickness biopsy is required because it's important to evaluate the crypts. Affected pets are treated with a low fat, highly digestible diet. Immunomodulatory drugs may be used too. Prognosis is poor.

b. **Histiocytic ulcerative colitis (Boxer colitis)** is a severe colitis characterized by severe diarrhea with hematochezia and mucous. Even though this is a large bowel disease, it can be associated with protein loss and subsequent weight loss. Early in the course of the disease, biopsies may reveal focal acute inflammation and epithelial cell degeneration at the luminal surface of the colon. Later, well-circumscribed ulcers appear. Histology reveals histiocytic infiltration of the mucosa. All potential histiocytic colitis biopsies should be stained with PAS because occasionally the histiocytes don't look characteristic (in the early stages of disease). In the past, this disease was usually fatal, however it's been found to respond well to antibiotics. Enrofloxacin is a good first-choice.

c. **IBD in dogs is not that common.** Many cases diagnosed as IBD do not respond well to immunomodulatory drugs because they are actually dietary intolerance or food allergy, requiring trial therapy until an appropriate diet is found. Cats however, clearly have an immune-responsive IBD called lymphocytic **plasmacytic enteritis** which is responsive to immunomodulatory drugs. In any case, it's best to combine immunomodulatory therapy with dietary therapy.

DRUG DOSAGES in CATS and DOGS for IBD

Osalazine (Dipentam®) is a dimer of 5-aminosalicylic acid molecules (an NSAID). Once in the colon, osalazine is cleaved by bacteria into two molecules of 5-aminosalicylic acid. Dosage in dogs is **10-20 mg/kg PO BID**. Don't try this until you're tried diet therapy first, because it can cause keratoconjunctivitis sicca (KCS).

Azulfidine: In cats: 125 mg/cat PO TID for at least 10-14 days. Monitor for adverse effects of NSAIDS in cats. Dogs: 50-60 mg/kg PO divided TID. Max = 3g/24 hours.

Metronidazole (10 –15 mg/kg PO SID-TID) has an immunomodulatory effect in some animals.

Corticosteroids are much more effective in cats than in dogs.
• **Prednisone** 1-2 mg/kg BID in cats. After 2 weeks remission, decrease to 0.5-1.0 mg/kg BID for a month and taper down. **Methylprednisolone** (Medrol®) may be more effective and can be given at 1/5 the dose.
• **Dexamethasone** 0.2 mg/kg PO **SID to BID** may be better in refractory cases.
• **Methylprednisolone acetate** (Depo-Medrol®) can be given (20 mg IM or SC q 2-4 weeks and then discontinue after 8-12 weeks of remission).

Azathioprine in dogs: 2 mg/kg SID to q 48 hours or start SID and taper to every other day in 2-4 weeks. Use for at least 2 weeks. It may take 4-6 weeks.

Chlorambucil is safer in cats: 1-2 mg q 3-4 days in cats < 7 pounds. 2 mg twice weekly for cats > 7 pounds. Use for at least 2 weeks. It may take 4-6 weeks.

SOME COMMON DRUGS
Other less commonly used drugs are listed within the chapter.

	CATS	DOGS
Butorphanol (1, 5, 10 mg tabs)		**Cough Suppressant:** 0.05 - 0.12 mg/kg PO BID-TID
Dextromethorphan (Robitussen® OTC)		**Cough Suppressant:** 1-2 mg/kg PO TID-QID. Use the pediatric formulation (no antihistamines).
Doxycycline	For Hemobartonella: 2.5-5.0 mg/kg PO BID for at least 21 days	**Salmon Poisoning:** 10 mg/kg PO BID for 7 days **Lyme Disease:** 10 mg/kg PO SID for 21-28 days **Ehrlichia:** 10 mg/kg PO BID
Hydrocodone bitartrate (Hycodan®) 1.5, 5 mg tablets, 0.3 mg/mL syrup		**Cough suppressant:** 0.22 mg/kg PO BID-QID (controlled substance)
Tetracycline	For Hemobartonella: 22 mg/kg PO TID for at least 21 days	**Lyme Disease:** 22 mg/kg PO BID for 21-28 days

Infectious Dx

FADING PUPPY SYNDROME RULE OUTS
Herpes Virus
Infectious Canine Hepatitis
Naval III (Septicemia-not included in these notes)

Within the first few weeks of life, puppies can become infected with a number of agents that cause peracute illness and sudden death.

CANINE HERPESVIRUS (CHV)

TRANSMISSION	Canine herpesvirus is shed in oral and nasal secretions. Consequently, the virus is transmitted by casual contact (i.e. mucosal contact). It is also spread by fomites but does not survive long in the environment. It is not usually spread venereally.
SIGNALMENT	Up to 80% of dogs in high density environments such as breeding kennels are infected, but the virus causes only a mild respiratory infection. Infection can cause problems in two populations of dogs: • Pregnant bitches that have never been exposed to herpesvirus (these bitches are described as **"naive"**) • Puppies of a naive bitch up to 3 weeks of age
PATHOGENESIS	The virus enters via the mucous membranes (MM) and replicates locally at cooler temperatures, destroying MM cells and leading to mucosal erosions. Immunity takes over and the virus hides in ganglions where it remains latent and doesn't replicate. Later, when the animal is stressed (sick, parturition), the genome reactivates and the virus travels up the nerve to re-infect the mucous membranes again. Virus particles are shed. These particles may be shed without recurrence of signs or lesions (i.e. asymptomatic shedders).

CLINICAL SIGNS	**Adults on their first exposure** can be asymptomatic or may exhibit a mild respiratory infection with serous oculonasal discharge. On rare occasion, they can also develop genital lesions with or without preputial or vaginal discharge. Most dogs that develop clinical signs are young and have not been previously exposed to herpes.
	
	Naive bitch and her puppies: The naive bitch does not have immunity to herpes, so infection during pregnancy is significant because her puppies do not receive protective antibodies against the virus. As the bitch matures and develops better immunity, her subsequent litters are unlikely to develop herpes infection.
	• **The young, naive bitch may have a spontaneous abortion or still birth.** If infected during gestation, one of three courses can occur:
	  ▪ If exposure occurs early in gestation, she could mount a quick, strong immune response in which case neither she nor her puppies develop significant disease.
	  ▪ She could develop a viremia in which case her puppies are infected *in utero*, leading to abortion or death of the puppies within 24-48 hours after birth. Usually 100% of the puppies die.
	  ▪ She could develop genital shedding and infect her puppies as they pass through the birth canal. In this case, the puppies can develop disease shortly after birth, but typically not as many die as compared with *in utero* infection.
	
	• **Puppies < 3 weeks old: Neonatal death.** These puppies are susceptible to infection because they don't receive antibodies against herpesvirus in the colostrum. Clinical signs include signs of failure to thrive (poor nursing, poor weight gain). Death may occur within 48 hours. Whole litters can be affected over 5-7 days with up to 100% mortality.
	
	• **Puppies > 3 weeks old: Mild respiratory signs.** At this age the puppies are usually able to mount a good immune response.

CANINE HERPESVIRUS continued

DIAGNOSIS	A diagnosis must be confirmed since other more common causes of fading puppy syndrome look similar clinically and histopathologically. • **PCR is now the gold standard.** • **Necropsy** of the dead pups specifically identifying herpes inclusion bodies in infected cells. • **Antibody titers:** Titers are often negative in affected animals (prepatent infection), but an increasing titer indicates infection with herpesvirus. • **Virus isolation, IFA** on nasal or genital discharge reveals which animals are shedding virus. It won't detect early infection though.
TREATMENT	Once puppies are showing signs, it's usually too late to save them. • **Provide supportive care** (IV fluids, keep them warm, ± antibiotics). • **Separate the healthy puppies** from the bitch and from the sick puppies and tube feed them with milk replacer. Keep them warm. At the first sign of herpes infection, provide supportive care. **Treat the entire litter as if they've been exposed/infected using anti-viral medications (acyclovir).**
PREVENTION	The best prevention is for the bitch to develop immunity. Exposing her to older dogs who've previously been infected with canine herpesvirus (80% of kennel dogs are infected) will help her establish immunity. **Husbandry:** From late gestation (3 weeks prior to whelping) to three weeks after whelping, keep the bitch and her puppies away from other dogs that may be carrying herpesvirus. People handling the puppies should wash their hands so they don't inadvertently spread herpes from infected dogs to the litter.

INFECTIOUS CANINE HEPATITIS

ETIOLOGY	Canine Adenovirus - type I (CAV type II causes respiratory disease)
SIGNALMENT	Dogs in kennels, shelters, pet stores. It's uncommon but can affect whole litters.
CLINICAL SIGNS	• Can cause **peracute death in puppies.** The puppy looks healthy one minute and very sick and shocky the next. The puppy can die within hours of onset, making the disease **look like a case of poisoning.** • Puppies can develop diarrhea (± hemorrhage), vomiting, fever, tonsilitis, oculonasal discharge, and depression. After the initial fever, the temperature may decline to subnormal temperatures. • **CNS signs include seizures and coma** • Hepatic signs: icterus • Following recovery, the dog may develop **blue eye (anterior uveitis and corneal edema)**
TRANSMISSION	Virus is shed in feces and urine. Infected individuals shed the virus in their urine for up to one year. Virus enters the new host via the oronasal route.
PATHOGENESIS	The virus enters the oronasal cavity and replicates in the tonsils and lymph nodes. Virus particles are released from infected cells resulting in viremia. They then infect hepatic parenchymal cells and endothelial cells where they replicate and cause cellular damage. This cellular damage leads to vasculitis and hepatitis, which both contribute to DIC and death.
DIAGNOSIS	• Increased liver enzymes (ALT) and DIC • Virus isolation from oropharyngeal secretions, feces, and urine (early in the disease) • Rising paired antibody titers (A 4-fold increase in titers taken 2-4 weeks apart indicates infection.) • Intranuclear inclusion bodies in hepatic parenchymal cells on necropsy
PREVENTION	Vaccinate with CAV-II. CAV II gives good cross-immunity with CAV I but doesn't cause blue eye (which CAV I vaccine can cause). Use the parenteral MLV vaccine, not the killed. The MLV vaccine provides a more effective immune response.
TREATMENT	Supportive.

Infectious Dx

SICK PUPPY/ DIARRHEA in PUPPIES
Parvovirus
Coronavirus
Distemper

Parvovirus is the most common cause of severe diarrhea in puppies. Coronavirus is an enteric virus that occasionally causes clinical disease in dogs (and cats). Distemper is a systemic disease that can cause diarrhea/vomiting but can also cause neurologic and upper respiratory disease.

CANINE PARVOVIRUS

SIGNALMENT	• Dogs in kennels, pet stores, and animal shelters are most likely to develop "Parvo". Even vaccinated animals (especially between puppy vaccinations) can get the disease. Some vaccines may cause disease in debilitated or stressed puppies. • Infection is most severe between 6-14 weeks of age (up to 60% mortality in some populations). • Certain factors such as viral load, concurrent GI parasites, and genetic factors predispose dogs to developing parvovirus infection. Rottweilers, Doberman pinschers, and pitbulls are more susceptible to parvovirus infection.
PATHOGENESIS	Parvovirus is spread by fecal-oral transmission. Since the virus is stable in the environment for years and is resistant to many disinfectants, the disease is **highly contagious** and does not require direct dog-to-dog contact. Once virus is ingested, it infects **crypt cells** of the **small intestines**, leading to destruction of intestinal villi. As a result, water, electrolytes, and nutrients aren't absorbed well and the animal develops diarrhea. Infection can be subclinical, , or the dog may present with mild to severe disease. Virus is shed in feces for 13-30 days after recovery.
CLINICAL SIGNS	Signs range from mild to severe and may be peracute. They begin 4-14 days after infection. • **Vomiting** and **diarrhea** are the primary clinical signs.Puppies typically present with fever, depression, anorexia, vomiting, and severe (often bloody), diarrhea. The diarrhea may smell bad due to increased protein in the feces. Dehydration, shock, and death can result if not treated promptly and appropriately.
DIAGNOSIS	• CBC/Chemistry: Leukopenia (often profound), blood loss anemia, hypoproteinemia • **Fecal ELISA for antigen**: Antigen is present for the first several days. Later it may be blocked by the animal's own antibodies, resulting in false negatives. False positives can occur shortly after vaccination with a modified live virus vaccine. An animals that tests negative but is highly suspicious for Parvo should be treated as a Parvo case and retested in 48 hours, or should undergo a serum IFA test if exposure occurred greater than 8 days earlier. • **Abdominal radiographs** or **palpation** sometimes reveal intussusception, a consequence of diarrhea. • **Necropsy/histology:** Positive IFA on the small intestinal crypt cells and widespread damage to the crypt cells.
TREATMENT (Continued on next page)	• Treatment consists primarily of supportive care. • **Keep the dog NPO** (no food or water) **until vomiting stops.** • **Give fluids with potassium and vitamin B1 supplementation** to compensate for losses from vomiting, diarrhea and decreased intake. • **Plasma transfusion or colloid (hetastarch) administration** is indicated when the albumin falls below 1.5 g/dL or if total protein falls below 3.5 g/dL. Use whole blood if the dog is also anemic from GI blood loss. • **Broad spectrum parenteral antibiotics** combat secondary infection caused by anaerobes and gram negative enterics passing from the severely damaged intestines into the circulation. Bacterial infection is also likely because the marked leukopenia results in impaired immunity. For severe cases, enrofloxacin* (5 mg/kg BID IV)/ampicillin (22 mg/kg TID IV), or gentamicin (2.2 mg/kg TID IV)/amoxicillin (15 mg/kg BID IV) are good combinations. For milder cases, ampicillin (20 mg/kg TID IV), or cefazolin (10 mg/kg TID IV) are good choices. *Caution in puppies (per label). Advise client of risks.

PARVOVIRUS in Dogs continued

TREATMENT (continued)	• **Anti-emetics** such as metoclopramide, chlorpromazine, or ondansetron (Zofran®) may reduce vomiting (For more info refer to pp. 10.7 and 10.11) • **Glucose:** Toy-breed puppies are prone to developing hypoglycemia if they are anorexic and may need glucose supplementation. • Treat for concurrent **GI parasites.** • **Recombinant granulocyte colony-stimulating factor (rG-CSF)** also known as Neupogen® (Amgen, Inc.) can be used when WBCs are markedly depressed and the dog is not responding well to supportive care (5-10 µg/kg/day) but there is no evidence that it improves outcome.
PREVENTION	**Husbandry:** The owner should clean the house and yard where the dog lives with bleach diluted 1:30. Owners must be diligent about picking up after the dog for at least one month following recovery so that the dog doesn't contaminate the environment. Make sure any new dog in the home is over 16 weeks old and fully vaccinated. **Vaccination:** Use a **modified live parvovirus vaccine.** Puppies should be vaccinated every 3-4 weeks starting at 6-8 weeks of age with the last vaccination occurring between 14-16 weeks (24 weeks if it's a breed that's more susceptible to developing parvovirus infection e.g. Rottweilers, Doberman pinscher, pitbulls). Revaccinate every 3 years.
VACCINES	The vaccine can back-pass to virulence, so **don't vaccinate sick** or wormy **animals.** The vaccine must get to the lymphatics before it can cause an immune response. The MLV high-titer, low-passage vaccine gives the strongest immune response.

CORONAVIRUS in DOGS

ETIOLOGY	RNA virus (has ray-like surface projections on the envelope). Each species of animal has its own disease-causing, species-specific coronavirus.
SIGNALMENT	• **Puppies** around 4-14 weeks old that are from kennels, animal shelters, and pet stores are more susceptible. • **Elderly dogs** going to shows may be more susceptible to infection with coronavirus too (debatable).
PATHOGENESIS	Virus particles are ingested and within 12-24 hours they invade the **mature columnar epithelium** of the **lower small intestines** (distal duodenum to terminal ileum). Intestinal crypts remain intact so villi regenerate faster than with parvovirus. Clinical signs appear within 96 hours (5 days after infection) and may last 3-20 days. It may be followed by **prolonged virus shedding.**
CLINICAL SIGNS	**Corona virus is usually not a serious disease in dogs.** It can cause mild vomiting and diarrhea.
CANINE CORONAVIRUS	**Prevention:** Coronavirus should not be part of a routine puppy/kitten vaccination program because disease is rare and mild and the vaccine efficacy is questionable. A MLV vaccine can be used in high risk dogs (e.g. show dogs). Some boarding kennels require vaccination.
DIAGNOSIS	**Biopsy/necropsy:** Small intestinal villous atrophy. **Feces:** Virus isolation, serum IFA.

Infectious Dx

CANINE DISTEMPER VIRUS (CDV)

Canine distemper is a disease that affects both young and old dogs. It is characterized by a variety of **neurologic, respiratory,** and/or GI signs. Anytime a dog has multifocal **neurologic disease, distemper should be on the rule out list.**

SIGNALMENT	Distemper occurs most commonly in young, unvaccinated puppies raised in stressful environments (e.g. puppy mills, poor neighborhoods, animal shelters). Dogs that are stressed or immunosuppressed can develop distemper regardless of vaccine history and can occasionally develop distemper from the modified-live vaccine.
TRANSMISSION	CDV is shed in the secretions of subclinical, sick, and recovering dogs (and wildlife hosts such as raccoons and coyotes). Recovered dogs may shed for 10-60 days. The virus usually enters the new host via aerosol route but does not persist long in the environment.
PATHOGENESIS	Virus is inhaled and replicates in lymphoid tissue. In 10-14 days, it invades the CNS and various epithelial tissues (e.g. pulmonary, GI, footpads). Animals can respond to infection in several ways: • Rapid immune response leading to quick recovery with few or no signs • Weak, slow immune response leading to rapidly progressive systemic and/or neurologic signs • Delayed or intermediate response leading to progressive neurologic disease
CLINICAL SIGNS	Most dogs have subclinical infections or only show signs of mild respiratory or mild GI infection. Young, unvaccinated dogs are more likely to develop severe generalized disease which they may or may not recover from, followed 1-3 weeks later with neurologic signs. Older dogs often develop only a chronic, progressive neurologic disease characterized by tetraparesis. • **Respiratory signs** include oculonasal discharge and sneezing which can progress to pneumonia. • **GI signs:** Diarrhea • **Foodpads and nasal planum** may exhibit hyperkeratosis (e.g. hardpad disease) • **Neurologic signs** vary depending on the distribution of virus within the CNS and the location of the lesions. Signs include: ataxia, vestibular signs, seizures (including chewing gum seizures due to polioencephalomalacia of the temporal lobes), myoclonus of the muscles of the head and limbs (due to encephalomyelitis), hyperesthesia, tetraparesis, and blindness.
DIAGNOSIS	**History:** Diagnosis based on history is difficult to make when you don't get the classic systemic signs followed by development of neurologic signs. Additionally, neurologic signs vary widely. **Any time you see multifocal neurologic disease, rule out distemper and other infectious diseases.** **Retinal exam** may reveal: • Optic neuritis • Ill-defined pink densities in the tapetal or non-tapetal retina • Well-delineated hyperreflective areas (chronic inactive disease) **Enamel hypoplasia** indicates past infection. **CBC** may show a persistent **lymphopenia.** The worse the lymphopenia, the worse the prognosis. Occasionally inclusion bodies are found. **Cytology** of conjunctival or respiratory epithelium: CDV antibodies are present on IFA early in the infection. **CSF tap** can be normal or may show elevated protein and an increase of mononucleated cells, indicative of viral encephalitis. **Biopsy and PCR or IFA** for viral antigen on the skin, footpads, CNS.
TREATMENT	Supportive and non-specific. The prognosis for dogs with neurologic signs is poor. Seizures are very hard to treat.
PREVENTION	Vaccinate with the MLV vaccine or recombinant Canine Distemper Virus Vaccine (rCDV) every 3-4 weeks starting at 6-8 weeks of age continuing through 12-14 weeks of age. In adults, one dose of MLV is considered protective. Two doses of rCDV are needed. Then revaccinate every 3 years. MLV can backpass to virulence so avoid its use in shelter and other stressed/immunosuppressed animals.

KENNEL COUGH (INFECTIOUS TRACHEOBRONCHITIS)

ETIOLOGY	Most commonly caused by *Bordetella bronchiseptica* and/or canine parainfluenza or canine hepatitis (CAV-2). Also rule out distemper based on vaccine history, and if signs are systemic and severe, consider submitting serology for canine influenza.
SIGNALMENT	Dogs that are kenneled with many other dogs and are stressed are most likely to develop kennel cough. The immunity following infection is short-lived. The agent is shed for prolonged periods.
PREDISPOSING FACTORS	In the respiratory tract, the mucocilliary apparatus, IgA, phagocytes, and bactericidal compounds in the mucus help keep the numbers of pathogenic bacteria down. Anything that impairs this defense system allows increased replication of viruses and bacteria. Many of the respiratory viruses, especially parainfluenza virus, cause a rapid and sometimes complete denudation of the villous processes of the respiratory mucosal cells. This severely limits the animal's ability to clear irritants from the respiratory tract and allows resident bacteria and Mycoplasma to descend into distal areas of the respiratory tree.
PATHOGENESIS	Clinically ill as well as asymptomatic carriers shed organisms. Sick animals shed more. The aerosolized organisms are inhaled by other animals and cause acute tracheobronchitis for 4-6 days. Animals may spontaneously recover or may develop a secondary bacterial/viral infection. Clinical signs occur 3-10 days following exposure.
CLINICAL SIGNS Outbreaks of either respiratory or systemic forms can occur in kennels and shelters.	• **Productive** or **non-productive cough**: Dry, hacking cough usually ends in the production of some amount of foam. A cough is often easily elicited on tracheal palpation. The animal is usually alert and active, and is normal on thoracic auscultation. • **Systemic signs** can occur in some dogs and can be fatal in puppies if untreated. Signs include anorexia, fever, oculonasal discharge, or respiratory distress. Dogs can also develop secondary pneumonia. Such signs can also be caused by canine influenza.
DIAGNOSIS	• **History** of being in a kennel situation or being exposed to another dog with kennel cough plus appropriate clinical findings. • All lab tests are essentially normal. If the disease is non-responsive to treatment, then perform a tracheal wash and culture the sample. • Rule out other causes of cough (e.g. pneumonia, cardiomegaly, etc.)
TREATMENT	Kennel cough is usually self-limiting. Isolation from other dogs and rest for 2 weeks if often adequate. If the dog has signs of 2° infection such as purulent nasal or ocular discharge, then antibiotics are justified. **Antibiotics:** Doxycycline (5-10 mg/kg PO SID for ≥ 2 weeks) works against Bordetella, Mycoplasma, and most of the 2° bacterial invaders. Since Bordetella can live in the respiratory tract for several months, longer treatment (e.g. 1 month) is warranted in some cases (such as multidog households with multiple dogs affected). Doxycycline should be given with food as it often causes GI upset. Clavamox (14 mg/kg PO BID) can be used as an alternative to Doxycyline. **Cough suppressant:** Break the cough–tracheal irritation cycle. Treat with cough suppressants for 3-5 days: • **Dextromethorphan** (Robitussin®): 1-2 mg/kg PO TID-QID. When using Robitussin®, use the pediatric formula since it does not contain other drugs such as antihistamines. • **Butorphanol:** 0.05-0.12 mg/kg PO BID-TID (1, 5, 10mg tabs) • **Hydrocodone bitartrate** (Hycodan®): 0.22 mg/kg PO BID-QID (1.5 and 5 mg tabs; 0.3 mg/mL syrup) • **Glucocorticoids** (prednisolone: 0.25-0.5 mg/kg) can be used short-term (≤ 5 days) in conjunction with antibiotics to decrease inflammation leading to coughing. Continue antibiotics 7 days beyond completion of glucocorticoids. **Avoid antitussives in animals with productive coughs.** **Nebulization** and **coupage** can be used if secretions are excessive (6-10 mL sterile saline over 15-20 minutes SID-QID). **Bronchodilators** (e.g. aminophylline, albuterol, or terbutaline) may help in some cases.
PREVENTION	**Vaccination:** Keep the pet current on distemper and CAV-2 vaccines. Vaccinate dogs 5 days prior to exposure (kenneling). Immunity lasts ≤ 6 months. Intranasal vaccination has a quicker onset of immunity.

Infectious Dx

SALMON POISONING

Salmon poisoning is a fatal rickettsial disease affecting dogs but not cats. It is one of the few causes of severe generalized lymphadenopathy (besides lymphoma, severe generalized skin disease, and other tick-borne diseases) in dogs.

ETIOLOGY	*Neorickettsia helminthoeca* (a rickettsia) is the causative agent. The fluke *Nanophyetus salmincola* harbors the agent, and the snail *Oxytrema silicula* is the intermediate host. Disease occurs in the Pacific Northwest (California to Washington) where the intermediate host lives. There are foci of infection in the north coast and Lake Tahoe area.
TRANSMISSION	Dogs get salmon poisoning when they ingest raw Salmonidae fish (salmon and trout) that are infected with the fluke *Nanophyetus salmincola* which in turn is harboring *Neorickettsia helminthoeca*, the causative agent of salmon poisoning. *N. salmincola* harbors the rickettsial organism throughout its life cycle from the egg stage to the adult. Dogs can also get salmon poisoning from ingesting the fluke eggs or the snail intermediate host when the snail is harboring the rickettsia-carrying fluke.
PATHOGENESIS	Life cycle: Fluke eggs are passed in feces and hatch in an aquatic environment. The resulting miracidia penetrate the snail host (*Oxytrema silicula*) which lives in fast-moving streams. The fluke exits the snail and infects salmonid fish. The dog eats the fish. On ingestion, the flukes mature and attach to the dog's intestinal lumen. Then, 8-12 days later, rickettsial organisms can be found in monocytes and macrophages. The organisms multiply in lymph nodes and other lymphoid tissue and have a special trophism for intestinal tissue.
CLINICAL SIGNS	Signs usually appear 5-7 days after ingestion of raw fish, but occasionally take up to 30 days to appear. • **Fever**, lethargy, and depression • **Lymphadenopathy** • Signs of **severe intestinal infection** such as vomiting, diarrhea (± blood), and anorexia. Rule out infection with parvovirus, distemper, or canine adenovirus.
DIAGNOSIS	You must have an index of suspicion in order to make the diagnosis (e.g. a vomiting dog that's recently been exposed to salmon or trout from the target area). • Diagnosis is most commonly based on finding trematode (**fluke**) **eggs** in the feces of dogs with the appropriate history, clinical signs, and physical exam findings. (Eggs are about 90μm x 45μm in dogs.) A negative fecal sedimentation does not rule out salmon poisoning because the fecal may have been taken during the prepatent period. Fluke eggs appear before clinical signs or as clinical signs appear. • **CBC** reveals activated monocytes • **Lymph node cytology** may reveal rickettsial organisms within macrophages • **Serology** is not done due to time constraints.
TREATMENT	• **Emetics** can be given immediately after the animal has ingested raw fish • **Doxycycline** (10 mg/kg IV BID for 7 days) is administered parenterally because the patient is usually vomiting. Tetracycline, oxytetracycline, and chloramphenicol are also good drug choices. Dogs rapidly improve over the first 24 hours. Continue treatment for 7-14 days orally. • **Praziquantel** to treat for the fluke which can contribute to enteritis. This treatment is optional. • **Supportive therapy:** Administer fluids to correct the acid-base balance. Monitor the animal for anemia due to bloody diarrhea and vomiting.
PROGNOSIS	Prognosis is good if animals are treated early in the disease. 90% of untreated dogs die. Recovery provides good immunity.

LYME DISEASE

Borrelia burgdorferi (a spirochete) is the agent associated with Lyme disease. It is transmitted by *Ixodes dammini* (the Deer Tick) or, on the West Coast, *Ixodes pacificus,* the Western Black Legged Tick.

SIGNALMENT	Dogs: Many dogs exposed to Lyme never exhibit clinical signs of disease. 50-80% of dogs in endemic areas are seropositive, but only 5% of this population develop clinical signs attributable to the disease.
PATHOGENESIS	The adult ticks jump off rodents and wait on brush for deer. They inject spirochetes into the skin on the lower limbs of people and animals. The spirochetes replicate locally at the site of infection for a period of several weeks or more. At this time the animal develops a spirochetemia. Dogs develop antibodies 2-3 weeks after exposure and these antibody levels remain high for approximately 18 months.
CLINICAL SIGNS	**Humans** develop a rash where they were bitten followed by flu-like signs. Weeks later they may develop arthritis ± neurologic and cardiac signs. Doxycycline cures the disease, however some people appear to have a chronic immune-mediated form that persists after the organism has been cleared with antibiotics. **In dogs, acute signs** include lameness due to one or more inflamed joints (**polyarthritis**), anorexia, lethargy, fever, ± lymphadenopathy. They do not get the initial skin rash. Some dogs develop an immune-related nephropathy.

DIAGNOSIS	A sick dog with positive Lyme titers doesn't necessarily have **Lyme disease.** In order to arrive at a diagnosis of Lyme disease, the dog must: 1. Have a history of exposure to the *Ixodes* tick in a Lyme disease endemic region (www.cdc.gov/ncidod/dvbid/lyme/index.htm) 2. Exhibit appropriate clinical signs 3. Have positive serology 4. Respond rapidly to appropriate antibiotic therapy (within several days), and finally, the clinician must rule out other causes of the dog's clinical signs (e.g. neutrophilic inflammation of joints can also be due to *Ehrlichia*, immune mediated disease, etc).
	 • **Perform a joint tap:** 43-85% neutrophils. The rest of the cells are primarily monocytes with a few lymphocytes. Culture the fluid.
	 • **CBC/Chem** may be normal but will help rule out other diseases. CPK may be elevated.
	 • **Radiograph ≥ one joint** to help rule out osteoarthritis, panosteitis, HOD, and HO. Chest radiographs and abdominal ultrasound may be needed to rule out underlying neoplasia.
	 • **Test for antibodies or disease agent.** Serology proves past exposure but not present disease.
	     • **ELISA Serology:** Detection of Lyme disease antibodies via ELISA test indicates the presence of Lyme disease. **Dogs that have been vaccinated with the Lyme bacterin may be positive on ELISA.** The antibody levels should be elevated if the animal's signs are due to Lyme disease. They may be elevated in asymptomatic animals too. This test should only be run by labs that properly validate the test and that correct for cross-reacting antibodies (such as antibodies to leptospirosis).
	     • **IFA Serology** works on the same principal as the ELISA but is more subjective and variable.
	     • **Western Blot test** and the newer SNAP 3Dx® ELISA test can differentiate natural infection from vaccine-induced antibodies.
	     • **PCR** on joint fluid, serum, and CSF
	     • Spirochete isolation is difficult.
	 • **Perform titers to rule out leptospirosis, toxoplasma, neospora, rickettsias, etc.**
	 • **Check for proteinuria** since dogs can develop "Lyme nephropathy."

TREATMENT	Dogs: Doxycycline (10 mg/kg PO SID or BID x 1 month) may be used if the disease is diagnosed. If there's no response in 1-2 days, consider other differentials. If the dog has no clinical signs, do not treat, but do monitor for proteinuria ("Lyme nephropathy") and treat accordingly.
PREVENTION	Prevent tick bites by removing ticks from pets within 24-48 hours of attachment. Frontline® or Amitraz (Preventic®) collars (or both together) work well. Because only 5% of dogs in endemic areas develop clinical signs, disease is easy to treat, and because the vaccine is variably effective, vaccination is generally not recommended.

Infectious Dx

RICKETTSIAL DISEASES IN DOGS

Ehrlichia and *Rickettsia rickettsii* (Rocky Mountain Spotted Fever, RMSF) are intracellular blood parasites (bacteria) transmitted by ticks to dogs. Both diseases can cause subclinical to severe disease with varying, non-specific signs. They are both found worldwide. *E. canis* is transmitted by the brown dog tick (*Rhipicephalus sanguineus*) and RMSF is transmitted by *Dermacentor* ticks. RMSF signs and treatment are similar to that of *E. Canis* which is decribed below.

EHRLICHIOSIS

PATHOGENESIS	Signs may be acute, sub-clinical, or chronic. Upon infection, the organisms invade mononuclear cells and reproduce. They form **morulae** within these cells (colonies surrounded by vacuolar membranes). During this early stage at 1-3 weeks of infection, the dog may develop mild, vague signs. The most common changes are thrombocytopenia due to vasculitis. **Subclinical stage**: Most dogs clear this stage completely or become subclinical. In this asymptomatic stage, dogs harbor organisms in splenic mononuclear cells. They may be thrombocytopenic and have elevated globulins. **Chronic stage**: This is the ehrlichiosis stage, the stage where dogs present with clinical signs.
CLINICAL SIGNS	Signs are nonspecific and include fever, depression, anorexia, and lymphadenopathy. • **Signs associated with bleeding** occur in 25-60% of dogs. They include hyphema, ecchymosis, melena, epistaxis, and retinal hemorrhage. • **Neurologic manifestations** can occur. They include ataxia, paraparesis, decreased proprioception, and head tilt, among others. • **Glomerulonephropathy/ nephrotic syndrome** can occur due to the marked humoral response leading to increased globulins. • **Pancytopenia** can lead to secondary infections as well as anemia due to bleeding.
DIAGNOSIS	The diagnosis is difficult to make because no one test is definitive. Diagnosis is based on a combination of clinical and lab findings as well as response to treatment. • Ehrlichia should be on the differential list whenever a dog comes in with **acute polyarthropathy** and/or **bleeding** that leads to a non-regenerative anemia with thrombocytopenia and increased globulins. • Finding morulae on a blood smear or within cells on a CSF tap is diagnostic but not common. • **Serology**: Positive titers indicate past or present infection. Negative titers don't completely rule out disease because the animal may not have mounted an antibody response yet. Paired negative titers (at 4-6 weeks apart) rule out disease. The test of choice is the IFA for antibody. There's currently an in-house SNAP 3Dx® ELISA test that's both sensitive (71%) as well as specific (100%). It also tests for heartworm and Lyme disease. It correlates with an IFA of 1:500. • **PCR**: Identifies the Ehrlichia.
TREATMENT	**Tetracycline** (22 mg/kg TID for 14-21 days) or **Doxycycline** (10 mg/kg PO SID-BID for 1 month). In the acute case, dogs should improve in several days. In the more chronic case, it may take 1-2 weeks to see significant change. **Chloramphenicol** (15-20 mg/kg PO, IM, or IV TID for 14-21 days) **Imidocarb dipropionate** (5mg/kg IM BID on day 1 and day 14) Therapy may need to be extended up to 2-3 months. **Corticosteroid therapy may be added** in cases of severe thrombocytopenia, if the animal has polyarthritis or vasculitis, or if the animal is not improving as quickly as expected. **Re-evaluate for signs of improvement in 1-2 weeks**. It's difficult to evaluate progress by measuring titers since they decline at different rates in different animals and don't correlate consistently with clinical signs. PCR can be used to monitor for organisms.
PREVENTION	Use tick control such as Frontline Plus®, Advantage®, or Preventic® collars (see Lyme disease for more information).

LEPTOSPIROSIS IN DOGS

Leptospirosis is a zoonotic disease caused by infection with the *Leptospira* spirochete (a spiral-shaped filamentous bacteria). The organism has a propensity for renal tubules and can cause **hepatic** and **renal disease. Whenever a dog has either hepatic or renal disease, consider leptospirosis as a rule out.**

AGENT	There are at least 8 serovars in dogs including: *L. canicola, L. icterohaemorrhagia, L. pomona, L. grippotyphosa,* and *L. bratislava.* Each serovar has a different reservoir host in nature. The organism lives in the host kidney and is shed in the urine but does not cause disease in the reservoir host.
TRANSMISSION	Leptospirosis is transmitted primarily through urine but can also be transmitted transplacentally, venereally, through bite wounds, and through ingestion of infected meat. It can be indirectly transmitted through infected water, soil, and vegetation. It survives best in warm, wet environments such as stagnant or slow-moving water.
PATHOGENESIS	The organisms are ingested or they penetrate the mucous membranes and then get into the blood stream where they multiply. They colonize many tissues including renal tubular epithelium, hepatic cells, vascular endothelium, the CNS, and spleen. Antibodies clear *Leptospira* from most tissues but organisms usually persist in the kidney, leading to persistent renal shedding. The organisms cause renal disease, liver disease, and vasculitis within various organs, which can lead to DIC.
CLINICAL SIGNS	Clinical signs can be peracute, acute, or chronic. Signs of illness are due to bacteremia, vasculitis, renal failure, and hepatic failure. • **Peracute infections:** Animals may die suddenly in the absence of clinical signs due to overwhelming bacteremia. • **Acute infections:** Early signs of fever, myalgia, and shivering may be followed by vomiting, dehydration, and shock. Vasculitis can lead to bleeding (epistaxis, petechiae, melena, etc.). Animals with acute infection often die before they develop liver or renal disease. • **Chronic infections may be the most common presentation:** These dogs develop smoldering inflammation of the kidneys and their clinical signs are vague (lethargy, vomiting, anorexia). Diagnostic findings are the same as with renal disease. These dogs often develop low grade hepatic disease too.
DIAGNOSIS	• **Lab findings indicate liver or kidney disease:** Refer to sections on liver and renal disease (pp. 10.18 and 21.20) • **Identify the organisms in urine:** It's difficult to identify organisms in urine because urine is leptocidal. • **Microscopic Agglutination Test (MAT):** A 4 fold increase in MAT titers (based on the serovar with the highest titer) between the first test and 2-4 weeks later indicates active infection. A single titer of > 1:800 with classic signs of renal disease in an animal who has never been vaccinated also indicates infection. Titers can also be used to monitor treatment. • PCR is available.
TREATMENT	Treatment is usually based on a presumptive diagnosis rather than waiting for titer results. Use penicillins (PO or SC) to decrease bacteremia early in the disease. Then after at least 1 week of therapy, follow up with a second antibiotic to clear the organism from the kidneys. Tetracyclines such as doxycycline (10 mg/kg PO SID) and the newer macrolides work well. Fluoroquinolones do not work well.
PREVENTION	• *Leptospira* bacterin protects only against serovars included in the vaccine, so use either a multivalent vaccine or one that contains serovars appropriate for the geographic region. • Older bacterins were relatively allergenic because they were produced from inactivated whole cultures. The newer subunit vaccines released in 2000 contain purified proteins from the bacteria's outer envelope. • Give 2-3 vaccinations 3 weeks apart to dogs in rural areas. Start vaccinations after 9 weeks of age and booster annually in dogs at risk. • **Eliminate carriers:** Get rid of rodents. Isolate infected dogs.

Infectious Dx

FUNGAL DISEASES

AGENT	GENERAL INFO	PATHOGENESIS	CLINICAL SIGNS	DIAGNOSIS/TREATMENT
COCCIDIOMYCOSIS *Coccidioides immitis*	**Signalment:** Most common in dogs, especially outdoor dogs in endemic areas. **Location:** A soil fungus native to the San Joaquin Valley in California **Route of infection:** Inhalation or direct inoculation. With direct inoculation, the disease usually remains localized and recovery is common but slow. **Public health:** Culturing this organism is dangerous. Vegetative arthrospores are infective. Spherules (tissue phase) are not. For fistulous lesions, change the bandage often in order to prevent arthroconidia.	Vegetative *C. immitis* hyphae in the environment fracture and release infectious arthroconidia. The spores are inhaled into the lungs and small airways and are ingested by phagocytic cells. The spores proliferate as spherules which enlarge until they burst, disseminating hundreds of endospores (which go on to become spherules). The result is a peribronchial granuloma. Organisms can spread to hilar lymph nodes and disseminate into the blood stream. Spores can also be introduced into skin and soft tissue via trauma or wounds. Incubation period is 1-3 weeks.	Flu-like signs: Chronic, low grade fever, malaise, myalgia, arthralgia, and anorexia 1° respiratory signs such as coughing: The cough may be soft if it's caused mainly by pneumonia or may be harsh and dry if it's caused by the hilar lymph nodes compressing the trachea. Pets may have joint pain. Disease may become disseminated leading to signs of specific organ involvement (bone-HOD, lung lesions, skin, etc.).	**Diagnosis:** Nonspecific anemia of chronic disease, hypergammaglobulinemia, hyperfibrinogenemia, neutrophilia. Radiograph the affected areas. **Cytology or histology:** Organisms are present. **Serology:** If organisms aren't found on cytology/histology but signs coincide with possible infection, serology can be used. IgM antibodies appear shortly after infection and disappear a short time after recovery. Increased IgM indicates current or recent infection. IgM ≥ 1:32 indicates active infection. **Treatment:** Fluconazole, itraconazole, or amphotericin B. Consider voriconazole in refractory life threatening cases. Monitor progress with serology.
HISTOPLASMOSIS *Histoplasma capsulatum*	**Location:** A soil fungus most commonly found in Mississippi, Missouri, and the Ohio River Valleys. Organisms reach high concentrations in chicken, bat, and wild bird feces. Histoplasma is easily cultured from soil in endemicareas. **Public health:** It is not considered a public health hazard.	Similar to coccidioidomycosis except that histoplasmosis is usually self-limiting and dissemination beyond the lung and its regional lymph nodes is uncommon. Dissemination can involve the GI tract, spleen, and liver. With lung dissemination, radiographs reveal a miliary pattern. Note: Corticosteroid use can lead to dissemination. Incubation period is 2 weeks.	Transient or subclinical signs include fever, malaise, and a cough lasting several weeks. Chronic, localized form: Interstitial pneumonia with hilar lymphadenopathy. Recovery can occur spontaneously in 1-2 months. Dissemination with GI signs is the most common presentation, leading to upper or lower bowel signs.	**Diagnosis:** Serology is not very useful. Cytology or biopsy is required for a diagnosis. **Biopsy:** Organisms are present. **Treatment:** This disease is more amenable to treatment than coccidioidmycosis. Amphotericin B (0.44 mg/kg IV in dextrose solution every 48 hours for 12 treatments) Other drug choices: fluconazole, itraconazole

			Dog/Cat	Diagnosis/Treatment
BLASTOMYCOSIS *Blastomyces dermatitidis*	**Location:** Found in the soil around the great river valleys and tributaries in North America and Canada (e.g. Mississippi, Missouri, and the Ohio River Valleys.)	Hyphae produce conidiophores which are inhaled into the lungs causing microgranulomas. Yeast rapidly form and divide within macrophages and disseminate to lymph nodes. Infected individuals more frequently develop severe or progressive disease than with histoplasmosis or coccidiomycosis. Dissemination from the lungs to the skin is common.	**Dog:** Pulmonary (cough, dyspnea), bone (osteolysis and periosteal proliferation), ocular (uveitis, chorioretinitis, retinal detachment), and skin (papule, nodule, draining tract) forms are most common. The CNS can also be involved. **Cat:** Same as dogs but CNS involvement is more common.	**Diagnosis: Cytology** of draining tracts is the best method (many organisms are found). **Serology** can be helpful. It tests for A-antigen. Agar diffusion has a 60-90% sensitivity and 96% specificity. You can get false negatives due to production of antibodies though. **Treatment:** Itraconazole at 5 mg/kg PO BID for 5 days and then SID for 3 days past resolution of signs is the therapy of choice. (Cats stay on BID treatment). 70-75% of cats and dogs do well with treatment. Fluconazole or amphotericin B can also be used.
CRYPTOCOCCOSIS *Cryptococcus neoformans*	**Location:** Pigeons and doves are vectors. **Public health:** Any fungus is hazardous to AIDS patients, though AIDS patients that get cryptococcosis are most likely experiencing recrudescence of infection that they had had prior to developing AIDS. **Prognosis** is guarded. Treatment is prolonged and relapses frequently occur. Prognosis is better when there's no evidence of systemic spread and blood antigen levels are low.	Organisms are in dust or dried pigeon manure. They are inhaled into the lungs where they cause mild, often inapparent pulmonary infections. The animal either recovers or organisms disseminate to the CNS, uveal tract, bone, nasal passages, etc.	More common in cats than in dogs. Cats with FIV or FeLV have a worse prognosis. Corticosteroid therapy in dogs or cats can exacerbate infections. **Upper respiratory infections** are common. Signs include sneezing, facial or nasal deformity, and nasal discharge. Many cats have skin lesions (nodule, mass, draining tract). Ocular and CNS signs can also occur (retinal detachment or chorioretinitis; vestibular disease). **Lower respiratory tract signs are uncommon.**	**Diagnosis:** CSF tap (organisms may be present in large numbers) or cytology of exudates. Stain the exudate (wet exudate) with india ink or methylene blue. CSF can also be cultured. **Serology:** Latex particle agglutination test. This serologic test is used more for monitoring treatment than for diagnosing the disease. **Treatment:** Itraconazole, fluconazole, amphotericin B. Prognosis is good for cats if infection does not involve the CNS. Prognosis is worse in dogs. Serology can be used to monitor progress.

Infectious Dx

RABIES IN SMALL ANIMALS

RESERVOIRS	America: wild carnivores (e.g. skunk, raccoon, fox, bat, coyote, etc.)
INCIDENCE	While the incidence of rabies is relatively low (60,000 people worldwide die from rabies annually), the number of suspected exposures in humans resulting in expensive post-exposure prophylaxis is high. Cats contract rabies 3x more than dogs and more than any domesticated species.
TRANSMISSION	Infected animals shed for about five days and then die. Virus is transmitted via: saliva/bites, urine, eating infected animals, and through an infected mother's milk.
PATHOGENESIS	When an infected animal bites another animal or a person, rabies virus is inoculated into the bite wound where it proliferates locally for a variable period of time and then attaches to nerve endings. (Note: If you cleanse a bite wound thoroughly, you can prevent the infection from taking). The virus travels up the peripheral nerve for 12-180 days towards the CNS. At the same time it reaches the CNS, it also reaches other organs and is shed in the saliva, milk, urine, etc. Within one week of reaching the CNS, the animal develops progressive neurologic signs. The animal dies within 4-5 days of onset of signs.
CLINICAL SIGNS	Rabies infection should be considered in any unvaccinated animal with rapidly progressive neurologic signs. • Prodromal/paradoxical behavior stage: A normally aloof animal becomes very friendly, etc. • Aggressive/furious stage: Affected animals may roam, snap, hypersalivate, and exhibit no fear. The expression in dogs connotes fear. Affected animals may have a "far-away" staring expression. • Paralytic/dumb stage: Characterized by local muscle incoordination, convulsions, and loss of brainstem function. Pharyngeal and masseter paralysis is common. The animal can't swallow, so it drools more. Paralysis of the diaphragm leads to death.
RABIES TREATMENT IN HUMANS	• Wash the wound well. • Within 48 hours of exposure, inoculate with **human rabies immune globulin (HRIG)**. This treatment is used only in people who have not previously been vaccinated for rabies. • Initiate the immune series (human diploid cell rabies vaccine) immediately at 3, 7, 14, and 28 days after the first dose. People previously vaccinated receive a booster on day 0 and day 3.
DIAGNOSIS	Perform the **fluorescent rabies antibody (FRA)** test on the brain of the rabies suspect. This test is fast (overnight) and reliable. A rabid animal will demonstrate rabies in the brain by the FRA test whether or not it has Negri bodies.
PREVENTION	Prevent overpopulation, vaccinate all dogs and cats that spend time outdoors (even occasionally), and keep pets away from wildlife. All dogs and cats should be vaccinated against rabies using a killed vaccine with a 3-year duration (or annually with a non-adjuvanted vaccine). It takes about one month for peak rabies titers to be reached, so animals are not considered immunized until 30 days after vaccination. The first rabies vaccine can be given as early as 3 months of age in dogs and cats (4 months of age in dogs in California). All animals should receive their second vaccination one year after their first vaccination and then every 3 years for the best control program. For cats, the non-adjuvanted, recombinant, or transdermal vaccines decrease the likelihood of sarcoma.
MANAGING ANIMALS THAT BITE HUMANS	• Wild or stray animal: Euthanize the animal and submit the head refrigerated to the state health department. • Healthy vaccinated animal: Quarantine for 10 days. • Healthy unvaccinated animal: In endemic areas, the animal may be euthanized and the brain submitted for testing, or it may be quarantined for 10 days. • Any animal that develops signs of rabies during the 10 days of quarantine should be euthanized.
MANAGING ANIMALS BITTEN BY ANIMALS	Animals bitten by wildlife or by animals with unknown vaccine history should be regarded as having been exposed to rabies. • If the animal is unvaccinated, it should be euthanized or isolated for 6 months and vaccinated 1 month prior to release. • If it's vaccinated, revaccinate immediately.

FELINE PANLEUKOPENIA (Feline Distemper)

Panleukopenia virus is a parvovirus that affects rapidly dividing cells (e.g. lymphoid, GI, bone marrow) causing diarrhea, vomiting, and bone marrow suppression.

SIGNALMENT	Most common in animal shelters and rural and feral cat populations (large populations of unvaccinated kittens in close contact with older unvaccinated cats). It is the most common infectious cause of sudden death in such populations. • **Young, unvaccinated kittens** ($\leq$ 5 months): Up to 75% of these kittens die. • **Older kittens and adults** develop subclinical or milder disease with a better chance of recovery. • **Chronic carriers** are rare. • **Neonates:** Transplacental infection may result in cerebellar and vestibular disease in neonatal kittens.
PATHOGENESIS	Virus is shed in feces and is ingested by another cat. It replicates in the tonsils and lymph nodes and then spreads via the blood (viremia) to rapidly dividing cells such as bone marrow and GI crypt epithelium causing vomiting, diarrhea, and bone marrow suppression. Infected animals shed large numbers of virus particles into the environment. The virus can survive for months to years in the environment.
CLINICAL SIGNS OF PERACUTE DISEASE	Clinical signs are worst in young, unvaccinated kittens. Infection can be subclinical, acute, or peracute. • Sudden hypovolemia and death in a kitten that seemed healthy a few hours ago (often mistaken for poisoning). • Fever, vomiting, anorexia, painful abdomen • Diarrhea usually occurs later on in disease. It may become a chronic problem. The bowel may become fibrotic and unable to regenerate its epithelium. Return to normal stool may take weeks. • Ataxia and hypermetria are caused by **cerebellar hypoplasia**, which can occur if the queen is infected in the last trimester of gestation. The virus can selectively infect fetuses and knock out the cerebellar Purkinje cells. The signs of cerebellar hypoplasia are noticeable at 2-3 weeks of age when the kittens first ambulate. Some kittens can learn to compensate and lead a normal life. The queen is typically asymptomatic. • **Vision problems** are due to optic nerve and retinal damage that occurs with in-utero infection. Retinal degeneration appears as gray foci and retinal folds.
DIAGNOSIS	• **CBC** reveals **leukopenia** (50-300 cells/μL) during the fever stage. The severity of leukopenia parallels the severity of the disease. With chronicity, cats may develop leukocytosis. • **Fecal EM for virus particles** (20 nm). Suspend feces and react it with RBCs. **Hemagglutinins** on the virus will bind to RBCs. • **Fecal ELISA** for antigen (using the canine kit). • **Necropsy** reveals hemorrhagic, fluid-filled **bowel loops** with fibrinous exudate and liquid **bone marrow**. Submit lung, kidney, and CNS tissue for virus isolation or PCR.
TREATMENT	• Antiemetics • NPO while the animal is vomiting plus **parenteral fluids**: Fluids can be given subcutaneously unless the animal is hypovolemic. • **Antibiotics** combat secondary bacterial infection from intestinal bacteria. Use bactericidal antibiotics with good efficacy against anaerobes and enterics. Ampicillin/gentamicin is a good combination. • **Vitamin B1** since the cat is not eating much. • **Plasma or blood transfusion:** Perform these if the cat is severely anemic or hypoproteinemic (TP < 4g/dL or WBC < 2000 cells/μL). • Some clinicians report good success with GM-CSF (granulocyte macrophage- colony stimulating factor). • Monitor for DIC.
PREVENTION	Vaccinate with a MLV vaccine or adjuvanted killed virus (KV) vaccine. Start at 6-8 weeks of age and vaccinate every 3-4 weeks until the kitten is $\geq$ 12 weeks old. For older cats, administer 2 doses 3-4 weeks apart. Revaccinate every 3 years (may provide protection for 5-6 years though). Avoid MLV vaccines in pregnant queens and kittens < 4 weeks old but ensure that the queen is vaccinated (KV is safe during pregnancy).

Infectious Dx

FELINE UPPER RESPIRATORY TRACT INFECTIONS

Herpesvirus and Calicivirus are the two most common causes of upper respiratory tract infections in cats. In terms of treatment, it's not vital that infection with herpes be distinguished from calicivirus infection (unless you are considering using anti-herpetic drugs) because both infections are treated similarly. Herpes tends to be more severe and is associated with herpetic corneal ulcers. Calici infection often involves oral ulcers, stomatitis, and lameness. Mycoplasma and Chlamydia can also cause upper respiratory infections, but are frequently limited to causing conjunctivitis. Upper respiratory infections may progress to pulmonary infections. With most of these diseases, recovered animals can become persistent carriers and can shed pathogenic organisms into the environment continuously or intermittently. Veterinarians routinely vaccinate for these diseases, but in general, immunity is short-lived and not particularly high.

DISEASE	PATHOGENESIS	CLINICAL SIGNS	DIAGNOSIS	TREATMENT/PREVENTION
FELINE HERPESVIRUS 1 (FHV-1) Rhinotracheitis	**Signalment:** All cats. Herpes is one of the most important diseases in catteries. The herpes virus remains in the trigeminal ganglion until an animal is stressed then the virus is activated, travels down into the nerve, and reinfects the mucosal cells (conjunctival and respiratory epithelium) where it replicates and is shed. Infected animals become latent carriers. 1° infection lasts weeks while recurrence lasts 3-10 days.	**Ocular signs:** Bilateral keratoconjunctivitis, nasal discharge, and blepharospasm. Painful dendritic or herpetic ulcers may occur, especially in lagophthalmic breeds (those with incomplete closure of the eye). **Systemic signs:** • **Rhinitis:** characterized by sneezing, watery nasal discharge, ulceration of the mucosa, plus 2° bacterial infection and crusted nose. Some cats develop a chronic rhinitis/sinusitis due to permanent turbinate damage (e.g. Siamese cats). • **Pneumonia** in young kittens (death)	**Culture** nasal, ocular, or oropharyngeal exudates using a viral culturette. **Conjunctival scraping** reveals intranuclear inclusion bodies.	**Treatment:** Antiviral drugs are the best treatment but they're expensive, must be given frequently, and are only palliative. • Idoxuridine 1% drops (Herplex®) q 4-6 hrs. • Vidarabine 3% ointment (Vira-A®) • Trifluridine drops (Viroptic®) q 6-8 hrs. **Antibiotics** to prevent 2° infection Keep the nasal passages clear **Fluid therapy** if indicated **Steroids are contraindicated** as they reactivate infection Vaccination
CALICIVIRUS	**Victims:** Kittens. 20%-30% of all cats shed this virus. It's shed from the oropharynx into the saliva. **The virulent systemic form** can affect any cat regardless of vaccination history. Outbreaks can lead to sudden death (within 1-2 days). Virus is transmitted by fomites and can survive in the environment for ≥ 4 weeks. Recovered animals continue to shed for up to several years.	Clinical signs include fever, rhinitis, conjunctivitis, oral ulcers, and chronic stomatitis. Affected individuals can also show lameness or skin ulcerations, or may develop pneumonia. **Any time you see a limping kitten, look for oral lesions and take its temperature.** If signs of calici are present, keep the cat isolated; clean the area with bleach, wash hands, and change scrub tops since any cat could have the virulent systemic form that was first diagnosed in 1998 (These cats may also have ulcerative facial dermatitis and cutaneous edema).	**Swab the lesion** (virus isolation). If negative, the cat probably does not have calici. A positive result doesn't mean calici is responsible for clinical signs however. Diagnose based on history of being around other cats (kennel, shelter) prior to onset, plus history of disease spread in a population (house or vet hospital). **Necropsy**	**Treatment:** Broad spectrum antibiotics for 2° infection. **Vaccine:** Over 100 strains exist and only a few are contained in the vaccines. In an outbreak, use the MLV intranasal for healthy cats. Killed vaccine requires a booster. **Virulent systemic form:** Clean and then bleach the area. Isolate affected cats. Contact owners of all cats seen and all vet clinics, shelters, kennels in the area. Don't admit cats to affected hospitals for 2 weeks after the last the affected cat is gone.

11.16

CHLAMYDIA PSITTACI	**Signalment:** Cattery cats. It primarily affects kittens around weaning when they have decreased maternal antibody. They are usually infected by adults or older kittens. Shed in nasal discharge and feces. Recovered animals may become carriers and often don't develop good immunity. Recurrent infections can occur but decrease in incidence as the immune system matures.	**Ocular:** Unilateral conjunctivitis, Ophthalmia neonatorum (conjunctivitis contracted by newborns as they pass through the vaginal canal). **Systemic:** Infection is usually limited to ocular signs. Occasionally, young (2-4 weeks) kittens develop pneumonia leading to death. These kittens often don't exhibit respiratory signs— they just die. Possible abortion.	**Conjunctival scraping** reveals elementary or inclusion bodies in the epithelial cells in the first two weeks. The scraping shows primarily neutrophils with some lymphocytes and plasma cells. You can send the sample to a livestock lab for IFA (cross reacts with cat chlamydia). **PCR.** Inclusion Body	**Treatment:** Tetracycline BID to TID for 2 weeks after resolution of signs. **Prevention:** vaccination and clean environment. **Vaccine:** The modified live virus (MLV) vaccine has marginal activity and provides short-lived immunity (even shorter than that in recovered animals). Possible zoonosis.
MYCOPLASMA M. gatae M. felis	**Signalment:** Cattery cats. Recovered animals can become carriers. Shed in nasal exudates.	**Ocular:** Unilateral or bilateral conjunctivitis. Not very painful. Cats can get concurrent chlamydial infection. **Systemic:** Pneumonia has been described in 3-4 week old kittens. Possible abortion.	**Conjunctival scraping:** See intracellular or extracellular coccobacilli Intra and extracellular Coccobacilli Some mycoplasmas can be grown on special agar plates	**No vaccine.** **Treatment:** Tetracycline BID to TID for 2 weeks. Tetracycline is bacteriostatic, thus the cat's own immunity must kick in. Consequently, you should treat as described and hope the cat's immune system kicks in rather than treating for > 2 weeks.

Infectious Dx

FIV and FeLV

Feline Immunodeficiency Virus (FIV) and Feline Leukemia Virus (FeLV) are two of the most common infectious diseases of cats. Cats can be infected with FIV at any age. The virus is transmitted through bites from infected animals. FeLV infection occurs through casual contact— but it primarily infects kittens. Both FIV and FeLV cause immune deficiency; consequently, death is commonly a result of secondary infectious diseases (or leukemia).

FELINE IMMUNODEFICIENCY VIRUS (FIV)

GENERAL INFO	Approximately 5% of cats have both FIV and FeLV. The incidence of cancer increases 6x with FIV, 60x with FeLV, and 80X with both. Despite these numbers, FIV positive cats can go many years before developing clinical signs of disease, so the prognosis for FIV cats is good.
TRANSMISSION	• **Bites**: This is the most common mode of transmission; consequently, FIV is most common in outdoor, intact male cats. • *In utero* infection is rare but kittens of infected queens have circulating FIV antibody due to passive transfer. • **FIV transmission does not occur through casual contact.** Infection is characterized by a transient viremia but the levels quickly drop and the virus is rapidly destroyed by enzymes in the mouth, just as HIV is in humans.
CLINICAL SIGNS	• Clinical signs can start as soon as 6-8 weeks after infection. Usually there are no clinical signs this soon however. • Fever and leukopenia • Ocular disease • Neurologic signs— especially those indicating cerebral lesions (behavioral changes, ataxia, seizures). • Clinical signs are associated with neoplastic disease (lymphoma), or more commonly **infectious diseases** since FIV infected cats are immunosuppressed. Cats can be asymptomatic for years. During this time they can infect other cats. Any sick cat should be tested for FIV (as well as FeLV).
PATHOGENESIS	Pathogenesis involves immunodeficiency, cancer (especially lymphoma and myeloproliferative disorders), and neurologic disease. Upon infection, cats experience a transient viremia. Kittens and geriatric cats may exhibit clinical signs of illness such as lymphadenopathy, fever, or neutropenia. These signs can last days to months. After the initial infection, the virus goes into a long phase of clinical latency where the cat is asymptomatic. During this period the number of T helper cells (CD4+) decreases gradually. This phase may last 4-8 years. Eventually the cat may develop generalized signs of disease such as fever, lymphadenopathy, or stomatitis. In the last stage, when the immune system is depleted, the cat starts to develop secondary infections.
DIAGNOSIS	Since antigen levels are low with FIV infection, we measure antibody to FIV. This measurement is fairly accurate because most cats infected with FIV become lifetime carriers. Due to the low incidence of FIV in many populations, tests may frequently lead to false positives. Consequently, positive ELISA tests should be confirmed with Western blot. • **ELISA**: using serum or whole blood (more accurate on serum) is the initial test of choice. • **Western blot**: All positive FIV results should be confirmed with Western blot.
PREVENTION	**Prevent exposure** to infected cats by keeping them indoors so they are not at risk of being bitten by FIV positive cats. Avoid adopting FIV positive cats who might fight with FIV negative cats in the household. Since casual transmission is rare and indoor cats rarely bite each other, FIV positive cats don't need to be separated from their housemates.
	Only 5% of cats in multiple-cat households develop FIV from an FIV positive housemate. FIV positive cats should be kept indoors and away from neighborhood cats since fights are common among non-housemates. **Vaccination** is generally not recommended because it causes antibody production, so the ELISA can no longer be used to diagnose infection. Additionally, while it is effective against two strains of FIV, we don't know its efficacy against other strains. Thus, the FIV vaccine should be used only in high risk cats.

FIV Prevention continued

PREVENTION / WHO to TEST	Exposure can best be prevented by testing cats and preventing FIV cats from infecting other cats. Who to test: • All **cats and kittens should be tested** on their first veterinary visit regardless of age because a negative result is very reliable. Kittens may test positive due to maternal antibody; thus, those who test positive should be retested after 6 months of age. **Note:** Cats should be tested even if being introduced into a household with no other indoor cats for several reasons: 1) they may occasionally escape and infect other cats, 2) other cats may join the household in the future, and 3) positive status may affect their future healthcare. • Cats with **possible recent exposure** to FIV positive cats (e.g. whenever a cat's been in a cat fight): Antibodies usually appear within 2-4 weeks after exposure, but some cats don't produce antibodies for up to one year. The AAFP recommends testing 2 months after exposure. • **Any sick cat:** especially those with stomatitis, neurologic disease, or bone marrow dyscrasias. • **Cats at risk** for contracting disease (e.g. outdoor cats, cats with abscesses, cats recently mated to cats with unknown FIV status, cats living with FIV positive cats) should be **retested yearly**.

FELINE LEUKEMIA VIRUS (FeLV)

GENERAL INFO	FeLV causes or contributes to many different disease states including lymphoma, anemia, and secondary infections.
TRANSMISSION	FeLV is shed in the **saliva** (richest source), milk, urine, and feces. As a result, it's transmitted through: • **Bites** (virus is inoculated into the tissues) • **Intimate contact** such as mutual grooming, shared water bowls, etc. • **Transplacentally** from queens to their kittens. Most of these kittens are aborted or are born sick and die. Some survive and become carriers and shedders.
PATHOGENESIS	Upon infection, virus particles inject their RNA into lymphoid cells. This RNA is converted to cDNA, which is integrated in varying locations throughout the cat's DNA. Where it integrates in a given cell determines what will happen. For instance the virus may just replicate itself, or if it integrates in a way that activates the latent onc gene, it can lead to the production of a solid tumor. Thus, FeLV can transform normal cells in different parts of the body into cancerous cells. In the early stages, FeLV replicates in oropharyngeal lymphoid tissue. If the infection is not eliminated by the immune system, then it can disseminate through the circulatory system to other lymphoid tissues. During this early transient phase of infection (usually 2-6 weeks), if the immune system fights off infection, the cat develops a **regressive infection**—one in which it has no signs of illness and either clears the virus completely or the virus goes into a latent phase. Most infected cats (97% in single cat households and 72% in multiple-cat households) develop regressive infection. If the virus is not neutralized, the cat develops **progressive** infection. That is, the virus invades bone marrow and infects monocytes, granulocytes, and platelets which are then released into the circulation. Cats with progressive infection as well as those in the transient phase shed virus and test positive for FeLV. Some cats in the transient phase show signs of illness (e.g. lethargy, fever, lymphadenopathy). Cats that go into the progressive phase tend to develop FeLV-related illnesses and the majority die within 3 years, although they can live longer. Cats with latent infection can convert to progressive infection later on. They are more likely to do so if they live in multiple-cat households or are under greater stress. The likelihood of converting decreases over time, and is much less likely one year after infection with the virus.

Infectious Dx

CLINICAL SIGNS	During the 3-6 week transient phase, kittens may experience malaise, fever, or lymphadenopathy. During progressive infection, clinical signs depend on the organ system involved. • **Anemia** is one of the most common sequelae. • **Thombocytopenia and leukopenia:** FeLV is the most common cause of thrombocytopenia and leukopenia in cats. • **Lymphosarcoma** • Signs are often non-specific and related to general immunodeficiency (e.g. fever, infections, etc.). • Any sick cat is a candidate for FeLV.
DIAGNOSIS	Unlike FIV, FeLV is characterized by an extremely high antigen load. As a result, the diagnostic tests screen for FeLV antigen (p27, a core protein). Since both ELISA and IFA test for antigen rather than antibody, we don't have to worry about maternal antibody causing false positives in kittens. Testing can start at any age. Vaccination does not interfere with test results either. • **ELISA** is the standard test. It tests for FeLV core antigen in free circulating virus. This test is more accurate on serum than on whole blood. • **IFA test** detects FeLV core antigen located intracellularly within lymphocytes and monocytes. A positive test result indicates the cat is in the progressive phase, the stage where bone marrow is affected. These cats are less likely to develop the antibodies needed to clear infection (seroconversion). Consequently, these cats tend to remain FeLV positive and develop signs of FeLV-related disease. • In areas with low FeLV incidence, false positives may occur. A positive ELISA should be confirmed with IFA. If tests results are discordant, repeat both tests in 2 months to see if the cat has overcome the infection and is no longer a carrier. Repeat annually until both tests agree.

FELINE LEUKEMIA VIRUS (FeLV) continued

INTERPRETING the FeLV TEST	Because IFA detects FeLV antigen during a more specific stage of infection than ELISA, the two tests may be discordant. The ELISA is a more sensitive test but IFA may be more specific. • A negative test means the cat is negative for FeLV or has latent infection (no circulating antigen in either case; not infectious to other cats). • A positive test may be a false positive, or may mean the cat is in the transient phase of viremia and may still fight off infection. Kittens that test positive should be retested in 1-3 months since the transient phase can last up to 3 months. • A healthy FeLV positive cat should be rechecked using IFA. If the results are discordant, repeat testing in a month until the 2 tests agree. • Cats that test positive for > 16 weeks and those that test positive by IFA (which indicates bone marrow involvement) are less likely to seroconvert. They are in the progressive phase and will remain positive.
WHO to TEST	Who to test: • **Any cat being introduced to a new household** even if there are no other cats in the house: Positive cats can infect other cats and, if in the progressive phase, will require more frequent and prompt medical attention than FeLV negative cats. • **Any cat with unknown FeLV status:** The presence of FeLV will affect the intensity and duration of treatment for related diseases in the future. • **Sick cats**— regardless of age, FeLV vaccination status, and previous negative FeLV tests: Previous FeLV tests may have occurred during the latent phase. • **Cats who will be receiving the FeLV vaccine:** Because the vaccine does not prevent infection in cats already infected, test before giving the FeLV vaccine. • **Cats with recent exposure:** Cats that go outdoors unsupervised should be rechecked even though adult cats are relatively resistant. Test cats after 28 days and retest at 90 days since some cats take much longer to develop viremia. Alternatively, just test at 60 days.

PREVENTION	Keep FeLV out of the household by keeping cats indoors and keeping FeLV positive cats out of the household.
	Vaccination: The FeLV vaccines are effective. Avoid adjuvanted vaccines due to their association with sarcomas. The intradermal recombinant vaccine is a good choice as it is non-adjuvanted. Two vaccinations should be given 2-4 weeks apart. Restart the series if they are spaced further than 4 weeks apart. Booster annually. Kittens can be vaccinated starting at 9 weeks of age.
	Who to vaccinate:
	• **Kittens < 4 months** of age. They are at greatest risk of infection.
	• **Outdoor cats** are more likely to be bitten and have a high risk of exposure.
	• **Households with > 2 cats,** especially where cats are regularly introduced.
LIVING with a POSITIVE CAT	Cats that seroconvert may still have latent infections, but if they are FeLV negative, they do not have circulating virus and are not infectious. Later in life, however, they can convert to progressive infection and become infective. At that time their FeLV test will be positive. Converting to the progressive phase is not that likely, but the owner may opt for annual testing in a multi-cat household or before adding FeLV negative cats to the household.
	If one cat in a household is positive and the rest of the cats are adults, and because primarily kittens are infected, the likelihood that the adult cats will get FeLV from the positive cat is low.

MANAGING FeLV/ FIV POSITIVE CATS

- **Confine infected** cats indoors to prevent exposure to parasitic and infectious diseases and to prevent spread of disease. Separate FeLV cats from unaffected ones. If the owner can't do this, have the owner vaccinate the unaffected cats and test them yearly.
- **Nutrition:** Cats should be on a balanced cat food and should avoid raw meat, eggs, and unpasteurized milk due to food-born bacterial and parasitic diseases.
- **Deworming:** These cats should be routinely tested for GI and ectoparasites and possibly for heartworm. Perform fecals on those with exposure to intestinal parasites or a history of GI disease.
- **Semi-annual wellness check:** Look closely at the oral cavity, lymph nodes, ocular lesions, and skin lesions. Stress dental care since it is the number one problem in aging cats.
- **Body weight:** Check for weight loss.
- **Complete Blood Count:** Perform a CBC yearly for FIV cats and 2x a year for FeLV cats.
- **Chemistry and Urinalysis:** Perform these tests yearly.
- **FVRCP Vaccine:** Stay current using either a killed or MLV vaccine.
- **Neuter** to decrease the stress associated with estrus and mating behavior.
- **Immune modulators:** There is no evidence of beneficial effects. AZT antiviral therapy may be beneficial in cats with stomatitis and seizure disorders.
- **Promptly identify** secondary diseases as longer treatment may be required for FIV/FeLV positive cats. Avoid immunosuppressive drugs except when they're clearly indicated. Avoid griseofulvin in FIV cats since it can cause bone marrow suppression.
- **Avoid corticosteroids and immunosuppressive drugs** unless required for treatment of a specific disease. Also avoid them in the FeLV negative cat in a house with FeLV positive cats, because the FeLV negative cat can have latent infection which may convert to progressive infection.

Reference:
Association of Feline Practitioners: *Report of the American Association of Feline Practitioners and Academy of Feline Medicine Advisory Panel and Feline Retrovirus Testing and Management.* 2000.

FELINE INFECTIOUS PERITONITIS (FIP)

FIP is a disease affecting primarily **young cats** (3 months to 3 years of age) from large **multi-cat environments** (shelter, pet store, cattery). It is caused by an enteric coronavirus (FECV) that mutates and gains the ability to infect macrophages (FIPV).

EPIDEMIOLOGY	FECV is endemic in most large multiple-cat environments with 75-100% of cattery cats affected vs. 25% of cats from single cat households. Mutation of the virus to the FIP virus results in FIP outbreaks in high risk populations. Mutations usually result in single sporadic cases. Epidemics are rare and cause is unknown since most cats with FIP do not shed FIP. Outbreaks of disease usually occur in spurts where a few cats develop disease within a several month period and then no more cats are affected for several years.
TRANSMISSION	FECV is transmitted via the **fecal-oral route**. Once ingested, the virus replicates on epithelial cells of the small intestines causing subclinical or mild signs of intestinal disease. Humoral immunity (IgA) is important in combating FECV infection. FIP occurs when FECV mutates and gains the ability to replicate in macrophages making it a systemic, intracellular pathogen. Cell mediated immunity is the most important factor in fighting FIP.
CLINICAL PRESENTATION	General signs: • Intermittent fever that doesn't respond to antibiotics consistently. FIP is immunosuppressive and fever may respond if it's due to secondary infection. • Anorexia and weight loss • Stunted growth in kittens, general poor-doers **Wet or effusive form:** 50-75% of cats have the wet form which is characterized by ascites or pleural effusion. The fluid is a yellow modified transudate (< 20,000 cells/μl) and is rich in globulins. The albumin:globulin ratio is < 0.41. Many fibrin tags may be present in the fluid. **Dry or non-effusive form** is harder to diagnose because it's characterized by diffuse granulomas. Signs may be vague (e.g. fever, lethargy). Affected cats may present with the following: • **Granulomas** in the peritoneal cavity. • **Enlarged lymph nodes**, especially the mesenteric lymph nodes. • **CNS involvement** is common because in this case the immune system is doing a fair job of controlling the disease in the body core, but can't get to the CNS to combat the virus. (Conversely, wet FIP animals have very little cell-mediated immunity, thus other organs collapse before the virus has a chance to significantly invade the CNS.) The most common CNS lesion is **spinal cord** damage, but the virus can also affect other portions of the CNS causing paralysis, seizures, and polyneuropathies. In young cats with neurologic disease, always consider FIP as a rule out. • **Anterior uveitis with keratic precipitates** and a dark, discolored pupil. • Cats usually start with an episode of the wet form (may be transient or unnoticed) and then go into the dry form where the disease smolders. The cat either contains the virus or the virus starts taking over and the disease gets worse.

DIAGNOSIS	Diagnosis is based on the appropriate history and clinical signs plus biopsy/histopathology with immunohistochemical stains. PCR for FECV can be performed on the feces. Few other organisms cause a similar overall picture.
	Peritoneal effusion: The fluid is a yellow, thick, high protein, pyogranulomatous exudate. It may be bloody.
	CSF tap may reveal elevated neutrophils and total protein, and it may be positive for FeCV (Titer $\geq$ 1:25).
	Serology does not differentiate between FECV and FIP. FECV Titers are elevated in FIP cats but can also be as low as 1:25 in end-stage disease. Titers are of less value in cats from catteries because catteries are usually positive for FECV. More cats are killed from FIP serology (misdiagnosis) than from FIP. Do not use serology alone to diagnose FIP. High FIP titers in the presence of appropriate clinical signs indicate FIP infection.
	Necropsy: • **Wet FIP**: Histopathology reveals diffuse inflammation of serous membranes (of the thoracic and abdominal organs) with small pyogranulomatous lesions. • **Dry FIP**: Granulomatous lesions occur primarily in the abdomen and most commonly affect the kidneys, mesenteric lymph nodes, and liver. Histopathology reveals macrophages surrounded by plasma cells and lymphocytes, indicating an active process.
PROGNOSIS	Cats that mount a rapid, strong cell-mediated immunity can contain the disease and recover. These cats often have no clinical signs of disease. Cats that develop clinical signs of wet of dry FIP have a poor prognosis (99% mortality rate).
PREVENTION	In order to prevent FIP infection, you must prevent FECV infection. Since FECV is transmitted in feces, good husbandry may decrease FECV infection, but even catteries with excellent husbandry have FECV. The best recommendation is to keep the cat population low ($\leq$ 4 cats). **Cattery situation:** • Isolate pregnant queens in a pathogen-free area so they and their kittens are not exposed to high levels of FECV. • If the queen has an FIP titer of > 1:100, she may be shedding FECV. Her kittens should be weaned at < 6 weeks of age. Up until this time, the queens maternal antibodies protect the kittens from FECV infection. • Raise kittens in isolation until they are 12-16 weeks old, then do an FIP test. If this test is negative, they are free of FECV. This is very hard to do and requires premature weaning which puts kittens at risk for developing other diseases since they stop receiving maternal immunity via the milk. It also may affect their behavioral development.
	FIP Vaccine: The FIP modified live virus vaccine made by Primucell-FIP has low efficacy. That means that in the cattery situation, the queen and kittens must still be isolated as described above. The vaccine can be used in cats from single cat or small cat households of 2-3 cats because these cats are likely seronegative for FECV/FIP. These cats are not at high risk for developing FIP anyway.
	MANAGING FIP POSITVE CATS (cats with clinical signs and a positive titer): • **Cattery**: Remove the infected cats. • **Single or small cat household**: If the other cats are adults, the infected cat does not have to be isolated. Adult cats rarely develop FIP (unless they contracted it when they were young and the disease recrudesces as described in the pathogenesis section).

Infectious Dx

MYCOPLASMA HEMOFELIS (HEMOBARTONELLA) IN CATS

M. hemofelis is an agent that parasitizes feline red blood cells causing potentially fatal hemolytic anemia. Many cats infected with the organism are asymptomatic carriers.

SIGNALMENT	Infection in cats can occur at any age. Clinical signs are more likely to occur in cats with concurrent inflammatory, infectious, immunosuppressive, or neoplastic disease (e.g. FeLV, FIV, FIP, lymphosarcoma).
OTHER RULE OUTS for HEMOLYSIS in CATS	• Other RBC **parasites** such as *Babesia spp* (originated in Africa) and *Cytauxzoonosis felis*. • **Oxidative damage** (e.g. onion toxicity, acetaminophen toxicity) leading to Heinz body formation. Cats normally have some Heinz bodies, but they don't develop anemia unless they have very large or excessive numbers of Heinz bodies. • **Immune-mediated disease** is often a component of hemolysis involving RBC parasites and Heinz bodies. • DIC
TRANSMISSION	Spread by carrier cats via blood transfusion and other unknown modalities (possibly fleas). Once infected, the cat can act as a carrier for several years to the rest of its life.
PATHOGENESIS	*M. hemofelis* is transmitted from the blood of an asymptomatic carrier cat to another cat. The new cat may develop peracute or acute anemia, which can lead to death. *M. hemofelis* causes red blood cell hemolysis and anemia through several different mechanisms: • When the organisms attach to the red blood cell surface, they expose membrane antigens to the immune system. The immune system responds by producing auto-antibodies that attack the red blood cells and activate complement-associated hemolysis (intravascular hemolysis). Thus, the cat develops an **immune-mediated anemia.** • Damaged RBCs are also phagocytized by cells of the mononuclear-phagocytic system (MPS) primarily in the spleen and liver (**extravascular hemolysis**). • Macrophages of the MPS can strip parasites out of the RBCs (pitting) and then release the RBCs back into the circulation. Each time parasites are stripped out, the RBC is damaged making it less deformable; consequently, its lifespan decreases. Note that parasitism with *M. hemofelis* causes an **immune-mediated hemolytic anemia**. The parasites themselves do not create extensive RBC damage. Diseases that depress blood elements (infectious, inflammation, neoplasia, renal disease, etc.) can activate latent Hemobartonella infection and can depress the bone marrow erythroid response to Hemobartonella-induced anemia.
CLINICAL PRESENTATION	Many cats are **asymptomatic** with no hemogram changes. The **most common presentation** is the cat with low grade anemia and a moderate regenerative response. The **classic presentation** (uncommon) is characterized by fever, lethargy, icterus, anemia, and autoagglutination.

MYCOPLASMA HEMOFELIS (HEMOBARTONELLA) continued

| DIAGNOSIS | Diagnosis is based on finding a regenerative anemia with evidence of *M. hemofelis* organisms in the RBCs. These organisms are sometimes difficult to find and a presumptive diagnosis is often based on finding an anemia responsive to tetracycline antibiotics.

CBC indicates a **regenerative anemia** if blood is taken 3-5 days following the onset of the hemolytic event. With severe anemias, nucleated red blood cells are often present as part of the regenerative response. The anemia may not be adequately regenerative if:
• The animal has an underlying immunosuppressive, infectious, inflammatory, or myelosuppressive disease (e.g. FeLV, neoplasia, FIV, abscess, etc.).
• Iron is sequestered in the spleen and liver.

Blood cytology: Finding *M. hemofelis* in blood smears is diagnostic. Less than 25% of blood smears in infected cats reveal organisms however. To increase the probability of finding organisms, submit fresh blood smears (organisms are more difficult to find in EDTA samples) on multiple days.

Autoagglutination indicates an immune component to the disease.

Direct Coombs' test detects RBC fragility. It is neither sensitive nor specific for hemobartonellosis.
Chemistry/Urinalysis: occasionally bilirubinemia and bilirubinuria are seen.
PCR test |
|---|---|
| TREATMENT | Always determine if the Hemobartonella infection is associated with FIV, FeLV, FIP, abscess, neoplasia, etc.

Tetracycline (25 mg/kg PO BID) or doxycycline (2.5-5.0 mg/kg PO BID) for a minimum of 21 days. Doxycycline is tolerated better in cats. Cats may vomit when on tetracycline.

Corticosteroids should be used if the anemia is acute and severe or if the disease relapses despite appropriate therapy for an adequate time period. Corticosteroids suppress antibody production.
• Prednisone 2 mg/kg PO BID
• Dexamethasone 0.15 mg/kg PO BID

Whole blood transfusions should be reserved for severely anemic cats since cats infected with Hemobartonella are at risk for transfusion reactions. Perform a cross-match prior to transfusing.

Cats may be chronically infected from their first infection and go into remission with therapy. Treatment won't abolish the carrier state. You still need an immune response to the organism (in addition to antibiotics) in order to get rid of the clinical disease. |
| PROGNOSIS | Some cats present with severe clinical signs due to strains that cause severe anemia in otherwise healthy cats. Other cats have underlying disease. Those with underlying disease (e.g. FIV, FeLV) have a guarded prognosis because they are likely to have recurrent bouts. |

Infectious Dx

VACCINATIONS

For decades, pets have benefited from vaccines. In recent years, however, vaccines have been increasingly implicated in adverse events in both dogs and cats. In 1985, two adjuvanted vaccines—one for rabies and one for FeLV—were introduced onto the U.S. market and shortly thereafter veterinarians began to recognize fibrosarcomas in cats. A number of studies have demonstrated an association between vaccines and fibrosarcoma; particularly with regard to these two adjuvanted vaccines. Additionally, anaphylactic reactions are known to occur in some dogs, and immune-mediated diseases have anecdotally been reported. Because there is no national vaccine adverse event reporting agency for pets, the process of validating such anecdotes is slow.

In the U.S., up to 19% of pet owners purchase and administer vaccines themselves because they are unaware of the complex issues involved with vaccinating. Virtually all patients receive vaccines and there are many more vaccines on the market now than 10-15 years ago. All of these factors make it imperative for veterinarians understand when to vaccinate, whom to vaccinate, and which vaccines to use. Veterinarians should devise individualized vaccine programs for their patients.

I.   **IMPORTANCE OF VACCINATING:** Despite recent findings, vaccines are generally safe and effective and are very important in controlling infectious diseases. Without vaccines, the U.S. would experience outbreaks similar to those seen in developing countries. For instance, 60,000 people worldwide die from rabies annually and domestic dogs are the principal vector. In the U.S., where dogs and cats are routinely vaccinated, only several hundred cases occur annually and dogs are rarely the vector.

II. **TYPES of VACCINES:** There are three general types of vaccines on the market:
   A.   **KILLED:** Killed vaccines are usually adjuvanted because without adjuvant they do not elicit a strong enough immune response to be protective.
   B.   **MODIFIED LIVE VIRUS** vaccines generally elicit a stronger response than killed vaccines and do not use adjuvant, but some back-pass to virulence.
   C.   **RECOMBINANT VACCINES:** Recombinant vaccines all involve recombination of genes. There are three types of recombinant vaccines. The current recombinant vaccines for dogs and cats do not require adjuvant.
   1.   **Subunit vaccines:** For the subunit vaccine, recombinant refers to how the product is manufactured. The gene encoding the outer-surface protein is isolated and placed into *E. coli* and then expressed such that the pure protein product can be collected and used in the vaccine. Currently there are several recombinant Lyme vaccines. One contains adjuvant and the other does not.
   2.   **Gene deletion vaccines** contain the pathogenic organism but the genes responsible for pathogenicity have been deleted. These vaccines can be used during an outbreak because we can distinguish between vaccinated animals and infected animals. Those infected have a larger array of antibodies since they do not have the gene deletions.
   3.   **Virus vectored vaccine:** Virus vectored vaccines are somewhat different. Here, the genes that express the immunoprotective proteins are separated from the pathogenic virus and are subsequently recombined with the DNA of a virus vector, such as the canarypox virus. Upon vaccination, the canarypox virus vector transports the selected genes into the patient. Antigen presenting cells (APC) then capture the vaccine virus and rapidly present the immunoprotective proteins to the lymphocytes. Because the canarypox virus will not replicate in mammalian cells, antibody against the vector virus is not produced. Studies performed at the University of Wisconsin have demonstrated that the recombinant canine distemper is capable of immunizing puppies (based on challenge studies) despite the presence of maternal antibody. This is a unique advantage when trying to protect puppies in a high risk environment.

III. **RECOMMENATIONS**
   A.   Use non-adjuvanted vaccines in order to avoid the inflammation that contributes to problems in susceptible animals.
   B.   Where appropriate, vaccinate every 3 years instead of annually.
   C.   Administer only those vaccines for diseases which the animal is reasonably likely to encounter.
   1.   **Recommentations in cats:**
      a.   **Core vaccinations:** Panleukopenia, herpes, calicivirus, and rabies
      b.   **FeLV:** All kittens should receive FeLV vaccine since they have the greatest risk (compared to adults). After one year of age, outdoor cats and those living with FeLV positive cats are most at risk.
      c.   **FIV and FIP** vaccines are not generally recommended.
   2.   **Recommendations in dogs:**
      a.   **Core vaccinations:** Distemper, hepatitis, parvovirus, and rabies

11.26

COMMON DRUGS in NEUROLOGY

DRUG	DOSAGE
Dexamethasone	Cerebral edema: 0.1 mg/kg PO SID
Diazepam (Valium®) 2, 5, 10 mg tablets 5mg/mL for injection	Status epilepticus: dogs and cats: 0.5-1.0 mg/kg IV (5-20 mg IV). For constant rate infusion, use 0.5 mg/kg per hour. 1 mg/kg per rectum (PR). If receiving phenobarbital, give 2 mg/kg PR Seizure control in cats (maintenance): 0.25 to 0.5 mg/kg PO BID-TID. Fatal hepatic necrosis reported in cats
Edrophonium (Tensilon®) 10mg/mL solution	0.1 mg/kg IV
Methylprednisolone Sodium Succinate 40 mg/ml, 62.5 mg/mL (40, 500, 1000mg/vial)	Not recommended for treatment of spinal cord trauma.
Pentobarbital 50mg/mL	2-4 mg/kg (up to 15 mg/kg) IV bolus 0.5-4 mg/kg per hour constant rate infusion.
Potassium Bromide	With or without phenobarbital, give 35-45 mg/kg PO q 24 h. Loading dose if needed: 400-600 mg/kg PO over 24 h. stop if excessive sedation occurs.
Phenobarbital 8, 16, 32, 65, 100 mg tablets 4mg/mL elixir	Dogs 2.0-5.0 mg/kg PO BID Cats 1.5-2.5 mg/kg PO BID
Prednisone or prednisolone 1, 5, 20 mg tablets	**Immunosuppressive dose** Dogs and cats: 2-4 mg/kg daily **Degenerative Disk:** Give 0.5 mg/kg PO BID (controversial)plus strict cage rest. Other options include NSAIDS and other analgesics. Don't use NSAIDS and corticosteroids together.
Pyridostigmine (Mestinon®) 60mg or 180 mg tablets 12 mg/mL elixer, 5 mg/mL injectable solution	**Dogs:** 0.2 - 2.0 mg/kg PO BID-TID. Start at the low end and gradually increase the dose (for myasthenia gravis). Cats: Use with caution. 0.1-0.25 (PO) mg/kg q 24 hours.
Thiamine (Vitamin B1) 25, 50,100, 250, 500 mg tablets OTC 100, 200, 500mg/mL liquid	50-100mg PO SID 20 mg IM SID

Neurology

THE NEUROLOGIC EXAMINATION
History
Physical Exam
Neurologic Exam
Specific Lesion Localization
Differential Diagnoses

The purpose of the neurologic examination is to first determine whether the animal has neurologic disease and then to localize the lesion. A good history is important in establishing the presence or absence of neurologic disease (e.g., seizure vs. syncope), especially when the animal is functionally normal on examination (e.g., animals with seizure disorders). Once neurologic disease is ascertained, localize the lesion, and try to explain the neurologic signs with as few lesions as possible. Localizing the lesion to the brain, spinal cord, or peripheral nerve/muscles helps us list possible causes and then decide what diagnostic tests need to be performed. It doesn't, however, tell us the cause of the lesion (e.g., a myelopathy may be caused by a tumor, disc herniation, foxtail, etc.).

I.   **HISTORY:** The history can be vital in determining the disease affecting the patient. A good history includes the signalment of the patient, onset and progression of signs, possibility of exposures to toxins and infectious diseases, and presence of pain or of systemic signs such as vomiting.

   A.   **SIGNALMENT** (age and breed): Young animals are more likely to have congenital or hereditary diseases, develop infectious diseases, and be exposed to toxins.

AGE	YOUNG	OLD
	• Anomalous (congenital or hereditary) • Infectious disease • Toxic exposure	• Degenerative • Neoplastic
BREED	Some breeds are at greater risk of developing certain neurologic diseases. Examples include: **Pug:** hemivertebra **Dachshund:** disc disease **Dalmatian:** deafness	

   B.   **ONSET of SIGNS** (acute vs. chronic)

ONSET	DEFINITION/RULE-OUTS
PERACUTE	Rapid onset of signs that reach their maximal intensity within minutes or hours. • **Toxic:** Signs are often progressive or improve on their own. • **Trauma** (e.g., hit by car, head trauma, spinal trauma, etc.) • **Vascular disorders** (e.g., infarction or hemorrhage)
SUBACUTE	Signs progress over days or weeks. They usually get worse, not better. • **Inflammatory/infectious diseases** (e.g., FIP) • **Neoplasia:** Some tumors (e.g., lymphosarcoma) and metastases develop rapidly.
CHRONIC	Clinical signs may be insidious and progress slowly. Some animals with chronic diseases present with an acute onset of signs due to sudden worsening of the chronic condition (e.g., a tumor that hemorrhages).

   C.   **PROGRESSION of SIGNS**

PROGRESSIVE	• Degenerative (e.g., degenerative disc disease) • Anomalous (congenital) • Metabolic (e.g., portosystemic shunt) • Nutritional (e.g., thiamine deficiency) • Neoplastic • Inflammatory (e.g., granulomatous meningoencephalitis, or GME) • Infectious • Toxic
NON-PROGRESSIVE or IMPROVING	• Anomalous (congenital) • Vascular disorders

D. **EXPOSURE to TOXINS and INFECTIOUS DISEASES**

RULE OUTS	
EXPOSURE to INFECTIOUS DISEASES Vaccine history History of illness	Determine whether the animal is indoors or outdoors and if it's at risk for developing certain infectious diseases. Is there a history of illness or presence of signs consistent with infection? **Rule-out the following** • Distemper (p. 11.7; myoclonus, seizures, etc.) • Rabies • Panleukopenia (causing cerebellar hypoplasia) • FeLV, FIV, and FIP
EXPOSURES to TOXINS	• History of chewing and ingesting objects • Use of rat, ant, mouse poisons, or other toxic pest controls • Use of yard and lawn sprays • History of bath or dip in flea products • Presence of household chemicals • Presence of toxic plants/moldy walnuts • Presence of other sick animals or people in the house. • Presence of human or pet medications in the house • Presence of lead products (paint, car batteries, stained glass windows, areas undergoing renovation).

E. **SIGNS of PAIN:** Indications of pain include stiff or stilted gait, aggression or hiding, reluctance to jump or go up stairs, and licking the painful area. Pain may indicate an orthopedic problem as well as a neurologic problem.

F. **SYSTEMIC SIGNS:** Look for systemic signs of disease such as fever, weight loss, anterior uveitis, joint pain, heart murmur, or vomiting.

II. **PHYSICAL EXAM:** Remember to perform a thorough physical examination so that you don't miss problems such as an **orthopedic issue** or a mass in the abdomen that's metastasized to the central nervous system.

III. **NEUROLOGIC EXAMINATION:** Perform the examination in a quiet environment to alleviate distractions and patient anxiety. Be complete and consistent. Have an assistant other than the owner help you. Test pain perception last (if you need to) so that you don't make the patient overly anxious.

SEVEN FACTORS in the NEUROLOGIC EXAMINATION
1) **Mentation/behavior**

2) **Gait and posture**
   • Walk normally (without ataxia or circling)
   • Stand with normal posture (no head tilt)
   • Coordination

3) **Cranial nerves**
4) **Postural reactions:** conscious proprioception in all four limbs
5) **Muscle size**

6) **Spinal reflexes:** UMN vs. LMN signs
   • **Thoracic limb:** biceps and triceps tendon reflexes, withdrawal reflex
   • **Pelvic limb:** patellar and gastrocnemius tendon reflexes, withdrawal reflex
   • **Perineal and panniculus reflexes**

7) **Palpation/pain evaluation:** spine, neck flexion, muscle tone

Neurology

A. **MENTATION/BEHAVIOR:** Before even touching the animal, observe its behavior and gait as it wanders around the room.

1. **Mentation: level of consciousness.** Decreased consciousness indicates abnormal function of the reticular activating system (RAS), located in the brainstem. The RAS sends projections to the cerebral cortex. This functional problem may be due to a lesion in the cerebral cortex or brainstem, or it may be secondary to an extracranial condition such as toxicity or metabolic diseases (e.g., hypoglycemia). Animals may also exhibit decreased consciousness due to generalized illness or weakness.

MENTATION: LEVEL of CONSCIOUSNESS	
NORMAL	Alert
OBTUNDED	Lethargic, dull, less responsive to normal stimuli
STUPOROUS	Asleep, but may be aroused by strong stimulation; only aroused when stimulated
COMATOSE	Unconscious; no cerebral response to noxious stimuli
DEMENTED	Inappropriate response to normal stimuli

2. Animals may also be alert with normal consciousness but exhibit **abnormal behavior** such as episodes of aggression, fly biting, or tail chasing.

B. **GAIT and POSTURE**

1. **Can the animal walk normally** or is it **ataxic, paretic, weak, or nonambulatory?**
   a. **Ataxia** is incoordination due to **vestibular or sensory deficits.**
   b. **Paresis** (mono-, para-, hemi-, tetra-) is a **decrease** in voluntary movement. **Paralysis is** the absence of voluntary movement.
      i. Monoparesis: paresis in one leg
      ii. Paraparesis: paresis in pelvic limbs
      iii. Hemiparesis: paresis of a thoracic and pelvic limb on the same side
      iv. Tetraparesis: paresis of all four limbs
   c. **Weakness** reflects a lack of strength and a problem of the motor unit (peripheral nerve, neuromuscular junction, or muscle fiber).

2. **Does the animal exhibit involuntary movement?**
   a. **Tremors** are involuntary muscle tremblings. They can occur at rest or only when the animal is moving. Intention tremors (those associated with movement) indicate cerebellar disease. Tremors also occur due to disorders of myelin.
   b. **Myoclonus** is the repetitive contraction of a group of muscles. For instance, the biceps may contract repetitively causing the elbow to bend repeatedly. Myoclonus is noted in some dogs with distemper virus infection.
   c. **Muscle fasciculations** are small, local, involuntary muscle contractions visible under the skin. They represent spontaneous discharge of fibers innervated by a single motor nerve.

3. **Posture/attitude:** Does the animal have a normal stance and head position?
   a. **A head tilt** is named in terms of which ear is pointing downward. An animal with its left ear pointing downward has a head tilt to the left. A head tilt indicates central or peripheral vestibular disease or a foreign body in the ear.
   b. **Decerebrate rigidity:** The animal is comatose and all four limbs are extended. It is caused by a lesion in the rostral brainstem (midbrain or pons).
   c. **Decerebellate rigidity:** The animal is **not** comatose and can move its limbs, but the thoracic limbs are extended when the animal is in lateral recumbency. Decerebellate rigidity is associated with an acute lesion of the cerebellum. If the rostral lobe of the cerebellum is affected, then the head and neck may be extended dorsally (**opisthotonus**). If the entire cerebellum is involved, then all four limbs are extended. If the caudal vermis is spared, the pelvic limbs may be flexed.
   d. **Opisthotonus** is the rigid extension of the head and neck. It can occur with decerebrate or decerebellate rigidity.
   e. **Schiff-Sherrington syndrome** occurs in animals that are paraplegic. The forelegs function normally (no neurologic deficits) but are excessively

hypertonic so that they are extended when the animal is in lateral recumbency. This syndrome indicates severe spinal cord damage anywhere along T3-L7. Depending on the site of the lesion, the animal may have UMN or LMN deficits and usually has no deep pain perception. Signs may resolve and the animal may recover, but generally the prognosis is guarded.

C. **CRANIAL NERVES** (Refer to the chart on the next page.)
1. **Check for muscle atrophy** of the temporalis muscle (CN V).
2. **Check for strabismus.** Presence of strabismus indicates a lesion of CN III, CN IV, or CN VI; abnormal vestibular input; or damage to the ocular muscles.
3. **Look for physiologic nystagmus** by moving the head from side to side. Also look for spontaneous nystagmus, which indicates vestibular disease. Spontaneous nystagmus may only present in some head positions. Look at the eyes with the animal on the right and left sides, as well as in dorsal recumbency.
4. **Stimulate the lateral and medial canthus of each eye** and watch for a **blink reflex.** This tests the ophthalmic and maxillary branches of CN V (sensory) and the facial nerve (CN VII). Presence of **ptosis** may be indicative of a problem with the sympathetic nerve or with CN III.
5. **Check the menace response.** This tests CN II, the cerebral cortex, and CN VII. Approach laterally so that you're testing the visual field of the retina and the contralateral cerebral cortex. Be sure you don't hit the animal's whiskers when performing the test. Also, remember that the menace response is learned, so young puppies and kittens may not respond. Other vision tests include the visual placing test and tossing a cotton ball for the animal to visually track.
6. Hold the eyelids open and **touch the cornea** with a moist Q-tip. Watch for the eyeball to reflexively retract. This tests the ophthalmic branch of CN V (sensory) as well as CN VI (motor).
7. **Stimulate the inner ear** in the area where you fold the pinna, and watch for an ear twitch or eye blink (CN VII—both sensory and motor).
8. **Stimulate the maxillary whiskers** or skin and watch for a **reflex blink.** This tests the maxillary branch of CN V (sensory) and CN VII (motor).
9. **Pinch the skin of the mandible** lateral to the canine tooth and look for blinking and **conscious withdrawal.** This response involves the mandibular branch of CN V, CN VII, and the cerebral cortex.
10. **Tilt the head up** and look at the ventral mandible to check the commissures of the mouth for asymmetry **(CN VII).**
11. **Check the tongue for symmetry (CN XII)** by opening up the mouth and looking at the tongue.
12. **Check the gag reflex (CN IX, CN X)** by gently putting your finger into the back of the animal's mouth (as if you were going to give them a pill or gently squeeze the larynx). The animal should swallow.
13. **Check the brachiocephalicus** and **trapezius** muscles for atrophy **(CN XI).**
14. In the dark, check for **anisocoria** (the oculomotor nerve, CN III, provides parasympathetic innervation to the eye; sympathetic nerves travel with CN V to innervate the eye).
15. **Check the pupillary light responses** to evaluate the retina, optic nerve, and sympathetic and parasympathetic nerves (direct and consensual). If the direct PLRs are normal in both eyes, there's no need to test the consensual PLRs.
    a. Lack of direct and consensual responses suggests a lesion in the afferents to that eye. That is, if a light is shone in the right eye, and neither the right pupil (direct response) nor left pupil (consensual response) constricts, the animal has a lesion in the retina or optic nerve of the right eye. (A right consensual response means that the light was shone in the right eye.)
    b. If the animal lacks a direct response in one eye, but that eye responds when light is shone in the other eye, it has a lesion in either CN II or the retina.
    c. **Swinging flashlight test:** Normally light causes a less marked constriction in the opposite eye. If you quickly swing the light to the opposite eye, the eye should constrict further. If the eye dilates instead, this confirms an afferent deficit to that eye.

Neurology

THE CRANIAL NERVES

CRANIAL NERVES	FUNCTION	SIGNS of LOST FUNCTION
I-OLFACTORY	Smell	Loss of ability to smell
II-OPTIC	Sight	Loss of vision Dilated pupil Loss of PLR (direct and consensual when light is shone in the affected eye)
III-OCULOMOTOR	Motor to dorsal, medial, ventral rectus; ventral oblique; levator of the eyeball	CN III carries parasympathetic fibers to the iris and controls iris constriction. Dilated pupil Loss of PLR on the affected side (regardless of which eye light is shone into) Ventrolateral strabismus
IV-TROCHLEAR	Motor to the dorsal oblique	Slight dorsomedial eye rotation (most visible in cats)
V-TRIGEMINAL	Sensory to skin of the face (mandibular, ophthalmic, maxillary branches) Motor to the muscles of mastication (mandibular branch)	Analgesia of innervated areas (face, eyelids, cornea, nasal mucosa) Atrophy of temporalis, masseter muscles; loss of jaw tone and strength Dropped jaw (if bilateral)
VI-ABDUCENT	Motor to the lateral rectus ± retractor bulbi	Medial strabismus Impaired lateral gaze Poor retraction of the globe
VII-FACIAL	Motor to the muscles of the face for facial expression Sensory to the inner surface of the pinna Taste	Lip, eyelid, ear droop Inability to blink Inability to retract lips ± tear production
VIII-VESTIBULO-COCHLEAR	Hearing and balance	Ataxia Head tilt Nystagmus Deafness
IX-GLOSSO-PHARYNGEAL	Motor to the palatopharyngeal Muscles, some salivary glands Sensory to the caudal tongue (taste)	Loss of gag reflex Dysphagia
X-VAGUS	Cervical, thoracic, abdominal viscera	Loss of gag reflex Laryngeal paralysis Dysphagia
XI-ACCESSORY	Motor to the trapezius, sternocephalicus, brachiocephalicus	Atrophy of trapezius, sternocephalicus, and brachiocephalicus muscles
XII-HYPOGLOSSAL	Motor to the tongue	Loss of tongue strength (causes relaxation of the ipsilateral side; tongue hangs to the contralateral side) Chronic damage: the damaged side contracts; tongue points to the ipsilateral side

D. **POSTURAL REACTIONS** are responses that allow the animal to remain upright and in a normal position. Conscious proprioceptive (CP) placing should be tested in all animals. The other tests can be performed if the CP or hopping responses are abnormal.

1. **Proprioceptive placing** tests **conscious proprioception (CP).** That is, it tests the animal's conscious knowledge (sensorimotor cortex of the cerebrum) of where its limb is. For this test, place the animal on a non-slip surface. Support the animal's front or hind end, and then flex a foot so that the dorsal surface is on the floor. The animal should reposition its foot. The signal for CP travels from the sensory nerves of the skin through the spinal cord to the brain stem, and then to the sensory cortex of the cerebrum. The signal continues via motor pathways to the LMN of the limb. A CP deficit can be caused by a lesion anywhere along this pathway (including the cerebral cortex). If the animal has a **cortical** lesion, it will have **contralateral** deficits. A **brainstem** lesion will result in **ipsilateral** deficits. Conscious proprioception is an early indicator of spinal cord damage because the fibers for CP are large in diameter; thus, they are sensitive to compression. CP deficits are the earliest indicator of compressive spinal cord disease and the last deficits to reverse in animals recovering from spinal cord compression.

2. **Hopping** tests the animal's ability to hop on individual legs as well as the ability to hop sideways when we hold two legs on the same side. A hopping abnormality indicates that the animal has either a proprioceptive deficit, a motor deficit (weakness), or a cerebellar disorder.

3. **Visual placing** tests vision and motor function. Pick the animal up and carry it towards the table at a level at which it can place its paw on the table. As the animal nears the table, it should raise its paw and place it on the table.

4. **Tactile placing** is similar to visual placing except that the animal's eyes are covered. The animal is carried towards the table and the dorsum of a paw is touched to the edge of the table. The animal should place its paw on the table. As with proprioceptive placing, the signal travels from sensory nerves on the skin through the spinal cord to the brain stem, and then to the sensorimotor cortex of the cerebrum. The signal continues down motor pathways to lower motor neurons of the limb. A deficit anywhere in the pathway (including the sensorimotor cortex) can cause a diminished tactile placing response. A lesion in the **cerebral cortex** results in **contralateral** deficits. If a lesion is in the **brainstem, ipsilateral** deficits will appear. If the animal has normal visual placing but lacks tactile placing, then it has a sensory deficit.

5. **Wheelbarrowing:** Elevate the hind end and walk the animal forward quickly. This tests proprioception and strength in the thoracic limbs.

6. **Extensor postural thrust:** Support the animal by its torso and lower it to the ground at an angle so that one leg touches the floor first at an angle. Then walk the animal backwards. The animal should put the leg down at an appropriate angle to bear weight and then move it backward in a caudal walking motion. If the leg is placed in an abnormal fashion or the animal is unable to step backwards symmetrically, it may have a vestibular deficit or a CP deficit.

7. **Cat jump test:** Place the cat on a chair or other slightly elevated surface and gently tilt the surface until the cat jumps off. Evaluate for weakness, ataxia, and proprioceptive deficits.

E. **MUSCLE SIZE:** Evaluate muscle size (atrophy, normal, hypertrophy) and tone (flaccid, normal, or hypertonic). Muscle tone can give a clue to the location of the lesion. Upper motor neuron disease causes increased tone and hyperreflexia, while lower motor neuron disease causes decreased tone and hyporeflexia.

Neurology

F. **SPINAL REFLEXES:** Place the animal in lateral recumbency to check the limb reflexes.

SPINAL REFLEXES
(Refer to the section on myelopathies on p. 12.21 for more information.)

REFLEX	STIMULUS	RESPONSE	SPINAL CORD SEGMENT
THORACIC LIMB WITHDRAWAL	Pinch the interdigital skin of the forelimb.	The limb withdraws.	C6, C7, C8, T1, T2
TRICEPS	Bend the elbow, abduct the elbow, and strike the triceps muscle proximal to the elbow.	The elbow extends, and the triceps muscle contracts.	C7, C8, T1
BICEPS	With the elbow in extension, palpate the biceps tendon with your finger. Strike your finger while it is overlying the biceps tendon.	The elbow flexes slightly, and the biceps muscle contracts.	C6, C7, C8
PATELLAR	Strike the patellar ligament.	The stifle extends.	L4, L5, L6, femoral nerve
GASTROC-NEMIUS	With the stifle in extension and the hock in flexion, strike the tendon of the gastrocnemius muscle just above the tibial tarsal bone.	The hock extends. The semimembranosus and semitendinosus muscles contract.	L6, L7, S1, S2
PELVIC LIMB WITHDRAWAL	Pinch the foot of the pelvic limb.	The limb withdraws.	L6, L7, S1, sciatic nerve
PERINEAL (bulbo-cavernosus reflex)	Stimulate the perineum of the penis or vulva.	The anal sphincter contracts.	S1, S2, S3, pudendal nerve
PANNICULUS	Stimulate the skin over the dorsum just lateral to the vertebral column starting at the iliac crest and moving cranially.	The cutaneous trunci twitches unilaterally or bilaterally, depending on the strength of the stimulus.	Lateral thoracic nerve. Response is absent or reduced caudal to a spinal cord lesion. Segmental sensory input travels up the spinal cord and then at C8-T1, it enters the lateral thoracic nerve (motor) and travels to the cutaneous trunci. This response is used primarily to localize lesions between T3 and L3. It may also be helpful with polyneuropathies since it's a long nerve and is often affected first.

1. Grading tendon reflexes is difficult due to individual variation. It's easier to state that reflexes are present, clonic, or absent.

UPPER MOTOR NEURON vs. LOWER MOTOR NEURON DAMAGE

	UPPER MOTOR NEURON (UMN)	LOWER MOTOR NEURON (LMN)
MUSCLE TONE	Hypertonic	Hypotonic or atonic
SPINAL REFLEXES	Hyperreflexic, clonic, or normal	Hyporeflexic or areflexic
MOTOR FUNCTION	Spastic paresis or paralysis	Flaccid paresis or paralysis

2. Withdrawal reflex and crossed extension: Crossed extension is an abnormal withdrawal reflex. Normally, a walking animal flexes one leg and extends the opposite. If the animal is lying down, it should not have this response. Consequently, if you test the withdrawal reflex on a laterally recumbent dog by pinching between the toes on a hind leg, the dog should withdraw that leg, but it shouldn't extend the opposite leg. Crossed extension is a sign of an upper motor neuron dysfunction.

G. PALPATION/PAIN EVALUATION: Some diseases—such as traumatic type I disc extrusions—are painful, whereas others—such as fibrocartilaginous emboli—are usually not.
   1. Evaluate for neck pain by carefully flexing and extending the neck in different directions.
   2. Palpate each vertebra.
   3. Palpate the muscles of the head, and open the mouth.
   4. Check for limb and joint pain, as they may indicate orthopedic disease.
   5. Check for hyperesthesia.

IV. SPECIFIC LESION LOCALIZATION: By now the lesion should be localized to the brain, spinal cord, or peripheral nerves/muscles. We should know whether the disease is unifocal (our initial assumption) or multifocal, and if it is diffuse/generalized, symmetric, or asymmetric. We may also have localized the lesion more specifically within the primary category.

A. ABOVE or BELOW the FORAMEN MAGNUM

SIGNS INDICATING a LESION ABOVE the FORAMEN MAGNUM
Seizures
Mentation changes
Cranial nerve deficits
Head tilt
Postural deficits on the contralateral side (decreased conscious proprioception)

B. SECONDARY NEUROANATOMIC LOCALIZATION (localization within a major subdivision)

BRAIN	SPINAL CORD SEGMENT	PERIPHERAL NERVE/MUSCLE
• Cerebral cortex (visual system, limbic system, olfactory) • Diencephalon (hypothalamus, thalamus) • Midbrain • Pons, medulla, vestibular system • Cerebellum	• C1-C5 • C6-T2 • T3-L3 • L4-S3	• Peripheral nerve, dorsal roots and ganglia, ventral roots • Neuromuscular junction • Muscle

Neurology

V.   DIFFERENTIAL DIAGNOSES
     A. USE the DAMN IT-V SYSTEM.

DIFFERENTIALS		
DEGENERATIVE	• Degenerative myelopathy	• IV disc degeneration
ANOMALOUS (congenital)	• Hydrocephalus • Deafness • Storage diseases	• Spina bifida • Hemivertebra • Atlanto-axial luxation
METABOLIC	• Hypo- or hyperglycemia • Hypo- or hypercalcemia • Hypo- or hyperkalemia • Hypo/ hyperadrenocorticism • Hypo- or hyperthyroidism	• Uremic encephalopathy • Hepatic encephalopathy • Hypoxia • Acid-base disturbance • Osmolality disturbance
NUTRITIONAL	• Hypervitaminosis A	• Thiamine deficiency
NEOPLASTIC	• **Primary tumors, including** lymphosarcoma, oligodendroglioma, meningioma, astrocytoma • **Secondary metastatic tumors**	
INFLAMMATORY & IMMUNE	• Myasthenia gravis • Polymyositis • Polyradiculoneuritis	• Granulomatous meningoencephalitis • Necrotizing encephalitis
INFECTIOUS	• **Viral:** distemper, panleukopenia, rabies, FIP • **Bacterial:** meningitis, discospondylitis • **Fungal:** blastomycoses, cryptococcosis, histoplasmosis, aspergillosis • **Protozoal:** toxoplasmosis, neosporosis • **Rickettsial:** *Ehrlichia*, Rocky Mountain spotted fever • **Parasites:** heartworm disease	
IDIOPATHIC	• Idiopathic vestibular syndrome	• Idiopathic epilepsy • Facial paralysis
TRAUMATIC	• Head or spinal cord injury • IV disk herniation	• Peripheral nerve injury
TOXIC	•Lead • Organophosphates • Ivermectin • Piperazine • Hexachlorophene • Botulism and tick paralysis	• Ethylene glycol • Aminoglycoside antibiotics • Chlorinated hydrocarbons • Chocolate • Strychnine • Tetanus
VASCULAR	• Infarct or fibrocartilaginous embolic myelopathy • Vasculitis or hemorrhage	

B.   DEVISE a DIAGNOSTIC PLAN
   1. **A minimum data base** should include a CBC, chemistry, and urinalysis to help rule out metabolic causes, systemic infection, and inflammation.
   2. **A clotting profile** rules out coagulation problems.
   3. **Radiography:** Thoracic radiographs rule out metastasis and infection. Survey spine or skull radiographs help rule out degenerative, anomalous, and infectious problems (e.g., discospondylitis). A myelogram assists in identifying spinal cord compression or intramedullary disease.
   4. **CSF analysis** helps rule out infection, neoplasia, and inflammation.
   5. **A CT scan and MRI** provide advanced imaging to further define the disease.
   6. **Electrodiagnostics** localize the lesion and in some cases diagnose the disease.
      a. **Electromyography** (EMG): Abnormal muscles have electrical activity (fibrillation potentials and positive sharp waves) at rest, whereas normal muscles do not. Activity at rest indicates myopathy or neuropathy.
      b. **Nerve conduction studies** measure the velocity of the electrical signals along the nerves. If the EMG is abnormal and the nerve conduction velocities are normal, the animal likely has a myopathy rather than a neuropathy.
      c. **Brainstem auditory evoked potential (BAEP or BAER)** records potentials generated by different regions in the brainstem in response to a click stimulus in the external ear. With this test, we can evaluate both the peripheral auditory system and brain function.
      d. **Electroencephalography (EEG)** demonstrates the electrical activity on the surface of the cortex. Diffuse increase in activity suggests encephalitis. We may localize an area of abnormality consistent with signs of an epileptic focus.
   7. **A biopsy** of a muscle, nerve, spinal cord mass, etc. may be helpful.

I.   BRAIN ANATOMY

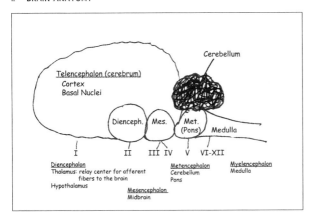

A.   General info
  1.   Ascending and descending motor tracts traveling in the brain stem cross over in the midbrain to the cortex. Thus motor lesions in the cortex manifest on the contralateral side. Lesions caudal to the midbrain manifest on the ipsilateral side.

  2.   The reticular activating system involves the brainstem and cerebrum. Thus lesions in the brainstem or brain can cause decreased mentation.

II. PUPIL SIZE and PLRs in BRAIN INJURY: The **sympathetic innervation** to the eye travels via the **ophthalmic nerve** (branch of the trigeminal nerve V). The **parasympathetic innervation** travels via the **oculomotor nerve** (cranial nerve III). They are both susceptible to midbrain swelling. In general, dilated, unresponsive pupils carry a worse prognosis than miotic pupils, although prognosis is often guarded with miotic pupils too. Pupillary abnormalities following intracranial trauma do not always reflect destruction of the parasympathetic or sympathetic neurons to the eye.

FINDING	PUPIL SIZE	SIGNIFICANCE	PROGNOSIS
Equal and responsive	◉ ◉	Normal	Good
Unilateral constriction	⊙ ◉	Retrobulbar damage to the dilated side (damage to the ophthalmic nerve), or unilateral brain swelling.	Good
Unilaterally dilated, unresponsive pupils	● ◉	Ipsilateral oculomotor compression (to the axons or the cell bodies located in the midbrain) or ipsilateral tentorial herniation with impending irreversible damage. Consider hernia.	Guarded
Bilateral pinpoint pupils	⊙ ⊙	Acute, extensive brain damage (pathophysiology unknown)	Guarded but signs are reversible
Bilateral dilated and fixed pupils	● ●	Damage to the midbrain most often due to hemorrhage or compression (associated with brain swelling).	Grave

Neurology

SEIZURES
Etiologies
Treatment

A seizure is an episode of abnormal electrical activity in the brain most commonly characterized by loss or altered consciousness, altered muscle tone (usually tonic-clonic contractions), and involuntary urination or defecation. **Epilepsy** is the condition in which an animal has recurring seizures from an intracranial cause.

Seizures may be preceded by a period of unusual behavior called the **preictal phase** (may last minutes to hours), and most seizures are also followed by a **postictal phase** during which the animal is disoriented and possibly ataxic or blind (cortical blindness). Most seizures in dogs and cats are generalized tonic-clonic seizures where the animal first becomes stiff and then goes into repetitive muscle contractions usually followed by paddling of the feet. In **generalized seizures**, the animal also loses consciousness. Animals can also have **partial seizures**, which can be localized to a specific part of the brain based on presentation. For instance, psychomotor seizures arising from the limbic system can cause transient behavior changes such as sudden aggression, screaming, or aimless running. Fly-biting, tail-chasing, and flank sucking can sometimes be attributed to partial seizures.

I. **Seizure vs other causes for collapse:** It's important to distinguish seizures from other episodic conditions such as narcolepsy, syncopal episodes and episodic muscle weakness.

SIGNS ASSOCIATED WITH COLLAPSE	MOST LIKELY CONDITION
Flaccid muscles + loss of consciousness	**Narcolepsy:** Recurring, sudden attack of sleep **Syncope:** Transient loss of consciousness due to ischemia to the brain. Most frequently due to cardiac or pulmonary disease
Flaccid muscles + no loss of consciousness	**Weakness** due to **neuromuscular disorder** **Weakness** due to **metabolic dysfunction** **Syncope** can also occur without loss of consciousness.
Tonic-clonic muscles + loss of consciousness	Generalized seizure (often with involuntary urination and defecation)

II. **INTRACRANIAL vs. EXTRACRANIAL ETIOLOGIES of SEIZURES:** Seizures can be classified as having intracranial or extracranial causes. Intracranial etiologies are caused by primary CNS disease, whereas extracranial etiologies are caused by metabolic diseases and toxins that have secondary effects on the CNS.

  A. **Rule out EXTRACRANIAL causes of seizures first** by taking a thorough history (including questions about exposure to toxins as well as questions about diet, and relationship of seizures to time of day, exercise, and meals), and a minimum database including a CBC, chemistry, fasting blood glucose, and urinalysis. Run a fecal centrifugal flotation for parasites, and perform serum lead levels and thoracic or abdominal radiographs if indicated by physical exam, history and signalment.

EXTRACRANIAL CAUSES of SEIZURES

ETIOLOGY	DIAGNOSIS
Metabolic disease • Hypoglycemia • Hepatic disease, portocaval shunt • Renal disease • Electrolyte disturbance: hypoCa^{2+}	Serum electrolytes, CBC, chemistry panel, T4 levels and urinalysis can rule out most metabolic diseases. Note: Seizures in renal and hepatic disease are due to high levels of nitrogenous waste products. **Hypocalcemia** leads to instability of the neural membranes leading to increased firing and seizures. If a lactating bitch presents with seizures treat for **eclampsia** (Refer to repro p. 19.13) and then evaluate serum calcium levels. Also check for hypoglycemia. **Hypoglycemia:** Sudden drops in glucose lead to muscle weakness due to low energy. Fasting in these dogs can lead to seizure due to decreased glycolysis and thus decreased ATP needed for depolarization of the nerve. Take a 12-hour fasting blood glucose to check for hypoglycemia. Extend to 12-24 hours if normal and you still suspect hypoglycemia.

EXTRACRANIAL CAUSES of SEIZURES cont.

ETIOLOGY	DIAGNOSIS
Nutritional • Thiamine deficiency in cats (fish diet) • Thiamine deficiency in dogs (cooked meat diet)	Diagnosis is based on a history of all-fish diet in cats (fish contains thiaminase which degrades thiamine resulting in thiamine deficiency) and cooked meat diet in dogs plus response to a therapeutic trial of vitamin B1 given IV (50-100mg per day) on day one and then IM thereafter. Animals should rapidly improve within 1-2 days.
Toxins • Strychnine • Metaldehyde • Organophosphates, carbamates • Chlorinated hydrocarbons • Lead • Moldy walnuts • Metronidazole (esp. cats) • Human medications or supplements such as 5-HT, a human dietary supplement that is a precursor to serotonin	History of exposure to toxins or acute onset of severe progressive seizures, plus presence of clinical signs characteristic for the specific toxins CBC: Basophilic stippling, microcytic, hypochromic anemia, and nucleated RBCs indicate lead toxicity. Measure whole blood lead levels for a diagnosis. Cholinesterase activity: Reduced activity indicates exposure (Refer to toxicology section page 20.9 and 20.10 for more information).

B. Rule out INTRACRANIAL CAUSES once you've ruled out extracranial causes. Diagnostic tests include—MRI or CT of the brain, CSF tap, and EEG, Owners may opt to forego diagnostic imaging and treat without a diagnosis; however, if the affected animal is a dog < 1 year or > 5 years of age or is a cat, an intracranial diagnosis should be sought since the seizures are likely due to a specific diagnosable cause and the specific etiology may change the prognosis and ease or difficulty of treatment. In older animals, perform thoracic radiographs and abdominal ultrasound to screen for neoplasia. If a specific diagnosis is not obtained and the seizures are difficult to treat, intracranial diagnostics should then be performed. If a diagnosis is obtained, the animal treated, and the seizures are difficult to manage, diagnostics should be repeated.

C. INTRACRANIAL CAUSES of SEIZURES

ETIOLOGY	DIAGNOSIS
DEGENERATIVE Degenerative storage disease in the CNS	Signs develop in young animals and are progressive and severe. In these storage diseases, the lysosomes of the CNS cells lack certain enzymes. Undigestible material builds up within the affected lysosomes resulting in death of the cell.
ANOMALOUS (Congenital) Hydrocephalus	Breed Predispositions: Pugs, Chihuahua, Maltese, English Bulldog, Pomeranian Congenital defect: These dogs are slow learners and may seem dull. Presence of an open fontanelle (predisposed breeds may have open fontanelles and mild hydrocephalus without signs of disease though). Exam: ± tetraparesis, slow postural reactions, decreased proprioception, hyperactive reflexes, and bilateral divergent strabismus. Diagnosis: • Ultrasound of the brain and lateral ventricles through an open fontanelle • Skull radiographs in animals with closed fontanelles may show thinning of the calvarium. • CT or MRI Hydrocephalus can also occur secondary to CNS neoplasia, granulomas, and inflammation.
Arachnoid Cysts	

Neurology

INTRACRANIAL CAUSES of SEIZURES continued

ETIOLOGY	DIAGNOSIS
NEOPLASTIC **Primary** (meningioma, oligodendroglioma, astrocytoma) **Secondary** or **metastatic** neoplasia (prostatic carcinomas, mammary carcinomas, hemangiosarcomas, and melanomas all metastasize to the brain)	Signalment: Usually occurs in older animals, although lymphoma can affect an animal of any age. History: Gradual onset of slowly progressive neurologic signs, although onset may be acute if there's hemorrhage, edema, or build up of CSF fluid (acquired hydrocephalus) associated with the tumor. Examination: These animals may be normal or they may have deficits dictated by the portion of the brain that's involved. They may also show peripheral evidence of neoplasia (enlarged lymph nodes, splenic or hepatic involvement, etc.). Some animals with cerebral neoplasia have altered mentation. CBC, chemistry panel: Look for evidence of metabolic disorders that can be caused by neoplasia (i.e. elevated liver enzymes due to lymphoma in the liver). CSF Analysis: Look for neoplastic cells and for increased protein with normal cell counts. Neoplastic cells are rarely seen in cats and dogs with intracranial brain tumors unless the tumors are lymphosarcoma in which we see a high number of abnormal lymphocytes in the CSF fluid. Skull radiographs: Occasionally, we see a calcified brain tumor (usually a meningioma) or a tumor rupturing through the cribriform plate. Thoracic Radiographs: Check for evidence of metastasis. MRI or CT: MRI is better for evaluating soft tissue. CT is best for evaluating bone. Electroencephalogram (EEG) can help further characterize the seizures. At this point in time, it is mostly done for academic purposes, and usually does not help individual animals. It may be helpful to confirm that an animal is having a seizure, although if the EEG is normal, it does not rule it out.
INFECTIOUS • Bacterial (abscess) • Fungal • Viral (distemper, rabies, FIP) • Protozoal (*Toxoplasmosis*) • Parasitic (larval migrans)	History of exposure to animals that can transmit the diseases, of travel to areas where the disease is endemic, or an incomplete vaccine history Signalment: More common in young animals Physical exam: Evidence of systemic illness CBC: Look for evidence of infection such as neutrophilia with toxicity, left shift, monocytosis, and elevated fibrinogen. CSF Analysis: Look for elevated protein and elevated cell counts.
INFLAMMATORY (non-infectious) Granulomatous meningoencephalitis or Necrotizing encephalopathy (Refer p.12.20)	Signalment: Young adult dogs of small breeds (e.g. poodle, terrier). CSF: Increased protein and mononuclear cells Presumptive diagnosis is based on inflammatory, non-infectious CSF, ruling out of other intracranial etiologies and somewhat on pattern of CT, MR. Definitive diagnosis is made via biopsy or necropsy.
IDIOPATHIC Idiopathic "True" Epilepsy	Signalment: Usually occurs in animals 1 to 5 years of age and is due to a single neuron or group of neurons in the cerebrum discharging autonomously. It's a functional disorder of the brain and no changes are seen on MRI or CT but changes can be seen on EEG Diagnosis is based on ruling other causes out.
TRAUMATIC Traumatic Epilepsy	History of head trauma resulting in unconsciousness. Seizures usually start within 2 years after the trauma. EEG may be abnormal.
Vascular Accident	Signalment: More common in older dogs with renal failure or hypothyroidism and cats with hyperthyroidism. History of acute, non-progressive onset of seizures or other neurologic signs. CSF may be xanthochromic Many animals spontaneously improve dramatically over 3-10 days following onset of signs.

III. **TREATMENT:** The most common anti-seizure drugs work by enhancing the effects of gamma-amino butyric acid (GABA), the inhibitory neurotransmitter of the central nervous system. GABA causes the chloride channels to open so that chloride ions flow into the cell resulting in hyperpolarization of the cell membrane. This hyperpolarization makes the cell membrane less likely to fire. Phenobarbital, valium and potassium bromide (KBr) enhance the membrane chloride ion channels though GABA. Other antiepileptics work by reducing effects of glutamate, the excitatory neurotransmitter, by blocking its receptor, the n-methyl-D-aspartate receptor (NMDA).

A. **FIRST MAKE A DIAGNOSIS:** It is important to make a diagnosis prior to treatment, especially in cats and in dogs < 1 year of age or > 5 years of age.
   1. **Young dogs** frequently have underlying metabolic problems such as liver disease or inflammatory conditions of the brain. In addition to MRI they should have a CSF tap to look for inflammation.
   2. **Older dogs:** Many dogs over 5 years of age have a specific intracranial problem leading to their seizures. MRI should be encouraged. Additionally, prognosis in cases of tumors is often good because meningiomas, which can be surgically removed, are the most frequent brain tumor.

B. **START TREATMENT EARLY:** Epilepsy is a disease that should be treated proactively rather than reactively by waiting for seizures to become frequent. Approximately 80-90% of dogs that have one seizure have recurrent seizures. Additionally, the more seizure activity the brain undergoes, the more epileptic foci develop and the lower the threshold for future seizures. Starting earlier leads to a potentially better outcome for treatment of seizures.

CRITERIA for TREATMENT with ANTICONVULSANTS
• The etiology of the seizure is an identified structural brain lesion.
• The animal is in status epilepticus.
• The animal has ≥ 3 seizures within 24 hours.
• The animal has ≥ 2 cluster seizure events within one year.
• The animal has ≥ 2 isolated seizures within 6 months.
• The pet has a seizure within a week of head trauma.
• The pet has a preictal period lasting > 5 minutes.
• The pet has a prolonged, severe, or unusual postictal period.

C. **LONG TERM TREATMENT with PHENOBARBITAL:** Phenobarbital is the drug of choice for controlling seizures in dogs and cats.
   1. **Treatment:**
      a. **Start with 3-5mg/kg PO BID in dogs and 1.5 to 2.5 mg/kg PO SID in cats.** Start with a lower dose if the dog is on medications that inhibit liver enzymes, such as chloramphenicol or cimetidine. Since the half-life of phenobarbital is 45-90 hours, and it take 5 half-lives to reach a steady state, it takes 10-20 days for the animal to reach steady-state levels of phenobarbital. As a result, wait at least 2 weeks before testing the phenobarbital levels. Repeat testing at 45, 90, 180 and 360 days following start of treatment and then every 6 months thereafter. Also repeat phenobarbital levels if the dog has ≥ 2 seizures between testings and two weeks after every dose change.
      b. **Measuring and Interpreting Phenobarbital levels:** Take the blood sample right before giving the normal dose of phenobarbital (**trough value**). An effective **therapeutic range** in dogs is **15-35 mg/mL** but dosing should also be based on clinical signs. Phenobarbital levels can be useful in determining whether the owner is giving medications appropriately and whether phenobarbital is the appropriate medication—if the blood levels are low yet the dog or cat continues to show adverse effects, then phenobarbital may not be the right choice.
      c. Phenobarbital has a number of **side effects**; consequently, chemistry panel should be performed every 6 months. Side effects include:
         i. Polyuria, polydipsia and polyphagia
         ii. Sedation: Animals may be sedated for up to two weeks after starting phenobarbital or after increasing the dose.
         iii. Hyperexcitability: Animals may become hyperexcitable at low doses..
         iv. Hepatotoxicity (elevated liver enzymes).

       d. **If Phenobarbital is discontinued, don't stop suddenly.** Even normal dogs on phenobarbital will seizure if taken off suddenly. When discontinuing phenobarbital use, decrease the dose 25% every 4-8 weeks.

D. **LONG TERM TREATMENT with DIAZEPAM (Cats)** An alternative to phenobarbital in cats is valium at a dose of 0.25-0.5 mg/kg PO BID-TID. There have been a few reports of hepatic failure following several days of treatment with diazepam. These are probably idiosyncratic reactions, so some clinicians elect to avoid valium even if a chemistry panel (and possibly a bile acids) reveals no indication of liver disease.

D. **LONG TERM TREATMENT with POTASSIUM BROMIDE (KBr):** Chemical grade KBr can be compounded by a compounding pharmacist into capsules or dissolved in water (100-250 mg/mL) and used for seizures in dogs. It can be used instead of or in conjunction with Phenobarbital. Bromide is associated with asthma in cats, and therefore should be used with caution in this species.

    1. **Dose** is 35-45 mg/kg PO BID whether on phenobarbital already or just starting with KBr.
       a. **Oral loading Dose:** To reach serum levels quickly when needed and for animals not already on phenobarbital, give 400-600mg/kg PO with food divided q 12h for 5 days and then measure serum levels on day 6 to check for a goal level of 1-1.5 mg/mL.
    2. **Monitoring:** Test the serum levels at 2 months and then again at 4 months. Due to the 25-day half-life, it takes about 4 months to reach steady-state levels. Then recheck every 6-12 months. If the animal is geriatric, has renal problems, or is on a varying diet (varying chloride intake as with urolith dissolving diets) then recheck more frequently.

    3. **Adverse effects** include polyuria, polydypsia, polyphagia, sedation, incoordination, anorexia and constipation. If animal vomits due to gastric irritation, divide treatment into 2-4 equal doses to be given with food.

F. **TREATING STATUS EPILEPTICUS:** Number one priority is to stop the seizures and then keep the animal seizure free for 12-24 hours.
    1. **Start with valium at 0.5-1.0 mg/kg IV which comes to 0.1 –0.2 ml/kg if valium is 5 mg/mL.** Total amount is usually a 5-20 mg IV bolus depending on the size of the animal. Give 1-2 mg/kg rectally if there's no IV access. If uncontrolled, repeat every 5 minutes for up to 3 doses (Give 2 mg/kg PR if receiving Phenobarbital).

STARTING VALIUM DOSE (5 mg/mL solution)
• **Intravenous:** 0.1-0.2 mL/kg (usually 5-20 mg IV bolus)
• **Rectal administration:** 0.4 mL/kg

    2. **Pentobarbital:** If uncontrolled on valium, bolus 2-4 mg/kg pentobarbital or phenobarbital IV every 30 minutes. In the case of pentobarbital, if ineffective, give 10-15 mg/kg boluses. Redose as needed or put the animal on a pentobarbital continuous infusion at a rate of 0.5-4 mg/kg per hour depending on how sedate you want the animal. The difficulty is determining whether seizures are controlled. EEG can reveal seizure activity even in immobile dogs. In human medicine, patients are treated until EEG reveals flat brainwaves. Dogs frequently need to be kept at a deep level of anesthesia. In the meantime, perform basic diagnostics for seizures (PCV, glucose, BUN, electrolytes, etc) and provide supportive care. Appropriate body temperature and blood pressure should be maintained in order to maintain good cerebral perfusion.

    3. **Vitamin B Complex** can be administered in dogs since thiamin and pyridoxine are important for brain metabolism of nutrients.

    4. If the animal was already on phenobarbital prior to status epilepticus, continue to administer phenobarbital treatments on time.

Horner's Syndrome

Pupil size is controlled by parasympathetic and sympathetic innervation. The
parasympathetic innervation responds to light and causes **pupillary constriction**
(via the oculomotor nerve; CN III) whereas the **sympathetic innervation** responds to
factors such as fear and anger that cause excitement and leads to **pupillary dilation**
(via the trigeminal nerve; CN V). At rest, both systems are active and balance each
other. Horner's syndrome is caused by damage to the sympathetic innervation to the
eye.

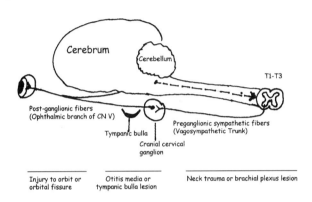

CLINICAL SIGNS	Miosis Ptosis Enophthalmus Protruding nictitans *Corneal ulcers produce similar sign, so be sure to stain the eye with fluorescein dye.
PATHO-PHYSIOLOGY	Horner's syndrome is caused by **damage to the sympathetic innervation to the eye.** • **Preganglionic sympathetic fibers** originate from the T1-T3 spinal cord. The nerve fibers travel up the cervical region within the vagosympathetic trunk and synapse in the **cranial cervical ganglion.** • Then the **postganglionic nerve** passes near the tympanic bulla and enters the **ophthalmic nerve** (ophthalmic branch of the **trigeminal nerve**) which enters the orbit via the orbital fissure. • Fibers from the ophthalmic nerve distribute to the smooth muscles of the orbit, the ciliary muscle (pupillary dilation), the nictitans, and the upper eyelid. Thus, damage to the sympathetics causes enophthalmus, pupillary constriction, protruding nictitans, and ptosis
ETIOLOGIES	Injury to any of these areas can lead to Horner's syndrome. Thus, etiologies include: • Injury to the T1-T3 spinal cord • Avulsion of the brachial plexus (nerve roots are in the C6-T2 region of the spinal cord) • Neck injury or trauma • Otitis media • Retrobulbar injury • Peripheral neuropathy • Idiopathic (often resolves spontaneously)

Neurology

VESTIBULAR DISEASE
Clinical Signs
Diagnostic Work-up
Etiologies and Treatment

I.   **DIAGNOSING VESTIBULAR DISEASE:** The vestibular system regulates balance and
     equilibrium. It is comprised of receptors in the inner ear which send signals up the
     vestibulocochlear nerve (CN VIII) which synapses in the medulla. Lesions causing
     vestibular disease can either be **central** (due to a lesion of the brain stem or the
     cerebellum) or **peripheral** (inner ear receptors and vestibulocochlear nerve). Both central
     and peripheral lesions cause ataxia, head tilt, circling, falling or rolling, spontaneous
     nystagmus (nystagmus that present when the animal's head is stationary), and vomiting.

Clinical Signs of Vestibular Disease

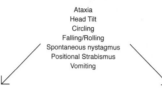

Ataxia
Head Tilt
Circling
Falling/Rolling
Spontaneous nystagmus
Positional Strabismus
Vomiting

Central Vestibular Disease

Spontaneous nystagmus (vertical nystagmus
   or positional–where direction changes with
   position–point to central disease)

Altered mental state (e.g. obtunded or stuporous)

Cranial nerve deficits (CN VII and/or
   sympathetics to the eye)

Decreased proprioceptive placing or motor nerve
   deficits (ipsilateral)

Peripheral Vestibular Disease

Spontaneous nystagmus

Horner's Disease

Facial nerve paralysis (CV VII)

Normal CPs and postural responses

A.   CLINICAL SIGNS ASSOCIATED WITH VESTIBULAR DISEASE

SIGNS	COMMENT	Towards or away from the lesion
Head tilt	Head tilt may occur with peripheral or central vestibular disease but can also sometimes occur with external ear infections. **Note:** in paradoxical vestibular syndrome the head tilt is opposite the major signs (proprioceptive deficits, etc.)	Towards Except with **paradoxical (central) vestibular.**
Circling	Tight circles	Towards
Falling or rolling		Towards
Nystagmus	Spontaneous nystagmus occurs when the head is stationary. May occur only in some body positions. Look at the eyes in different head positions	Away (Named in the direction of the fast phase)
Positional strabismus	Ventrolateral strabismus may occur. It usually occurs when the head is tilted up. This positional strabismus is unique to vestibular disease.	Towards
Postural reaction deficits	Occur with central disease	Towards
Vomiting	Signals reach the vomit center in the brain (medulla).	NA

B. CLINICAL SIGNS ASSOCIATED with CENTRAL and PERIPHERAL VESTIBULAR SYNDROME: Once we've determined that the animal has vestibular syndrome we should try to determine whether it has central or peripheral disease. Often we can make this determination based on clinical signs.

CENTRAL vs. PERIPHERAL VESTIBULAR DISEASE

SIGNS	CENTRAL	PERIPHERAL
Nystagmus	Vertical or with direction changing with change in body position	Spontaneous and direction (phase) doesn't change with body position
Altered mental state	+ Reticular activating system is in the brain stem	-
Horner's syndrome	± Not usually	± The sympathetic fibers to the eye pass through the middle ear.
Facial nerve paralysis (CN VII)	± The facial nerve exits the brain stem at the level of the medulla with CN VIII.	±
Other cranial nerve deficits	± Brainstem disease may affect other CN nuclei	No (only Horner's syndrome & VII)
Conscious proprioception	Absent or decreased Ipsilateral	Normal
Paresis	+ May have hemiparesis.	Normal

C. PARADOXICAL VESTIBULAR DISEASE is a form of central vestibular disease in which one or more of the vestibular signs (usually head tilt or nystagmus) is in the direction opposite the other localizing signs (paresis and CP deficits are usually ipsilateral). It's generally caused by lesions of the flocculonodular lobes or the caudal cerebellar peduncles.

II. DIAGNOSTIC Work-Up: At this point, we may or may not have localized the disease as central or peripheral. Diagnostics consist of trying to rule out peripheral disease first.

A. RULE OUT PERIPHERAL DISEASE
   1. **Check for otitis externa**, the most common cause of peripheral vestibular disease because it often extends to the middle ear and inner ear.
   2. Check for **submandibular lymphadenopathy** on the affected side. Lymphadenopathy can indicate infection, neoplasia, inflammation.
   3. **Chemistry profile/CBC:** Check for hypothyroidism which can cause peripheral vestibular disease and check for signs of systemic infection or neoplasia that could also cause a vestibular lesion.
   4. **Check for otitis media:** Animals can have otitis media and interna without having otitis externa, thus additional diagnostics may be needed.
      a. Examine the eardrum under deep sedation or anesthesia to see if it's intact and if there's fluid beneath it (causing an opaque, bulging appearance). If the eardrum is ruptured, collect and culture the fluid. If it's intact and abnormal, perform myringotomy to collect fluid. A spinal needle can be used. Lack of abnormalities on exam does not rule out otitis media.
   5. **Skull radiographs** often don't yield much information and **MR and CT scan** may be needed. Look for evidence of fractures, fluid or bony changes of the osseous bulla. Bony changes may indicate a tumor or osteomyelitis from chronic disease. Also look for evidence of nasopharyngeal polyps and exudate in the middle ear. If there's evidence of either in the tympanic bullae, you should surgically explore the area and drain it (e.g. bulla ostectomy) or remove the polyp. Negative findings on radiographs do not rule out peripheral vestibular disease or otitis media.
   6. **BAER** can help localize the lesion to central vs. peripheral.
B. CHECK for BRAIN INVOLVEMENT:
   1. **MRI and CT:** Look at the middle ear and to look for masses in the brain.
   2. **CSF Analysis** to rule out inflammation, infection, neoplasia: Advanced imaging should be performed first.

III. ETIOLOGIES and TREATMENT of VESTIBULAR DISEASE

DIFFERENTIAL	CENTRAL	PERIPHERAL
Metabolic	**Hypothyroidism** Test for hypothyroidism. Signs should resolve with supplementation.	
Nutritional	**Thiamine Deficiency** (cats on all–fish diets) causes bilateral central vestibular deficits and cerebellar deficits.	
Neoplastic	**Primary neoplasia of the nervous tissue** Metastatic tumors	

Infectious	Animals may show systemic signs too.
	Distemper
	FIP
	Rabies
	Toxoplasma, neospora
	Fungal: *Histoplasmosis Coccidiomycosis, Blastomycosis, Cryptococcus*
	
	Bacterial infections are not common. Bacterial otitis media-interna may extend to involve the brainstem
		Bacterial and fungal otitis is common: Prognosis is good unless there's osteomyelitis. Facial nerve paralysis/Horner's syndrome and KCS (VII) may be permanent.
		   Treat **otitis externa** topically. If the eardrum is ruptured, use oral antibiotics ± topical medications that are water soluble or safe for aural use. Avoid oil-based, irritating topical medications as they can cause peripheral vestibular disease.
		   For **otitis media,** treat with oral antibiotics for a minimum of 6-8 weeks. **The goal is to prevent central vestibular infection!**

Inflammatory	**Granulomatous meningo-encephalitis (GME)** occurs primarily in small dogs. Presumptive diagnosis is based on inflammatory, non-infectious CSF, rule out of other intracranial etiologies and somewhat on pattern of CT,MRI. Definitive diagnosis is made via biopsy or necropsy.	**Corticosteroids:** Dexamethasone IV (0.25 mg/kg) and then prednisone 1-2 mg/kg PO BID (immunosuppressive dose). Taper the prednisone if possible based on clinical response and CSF. Cytosar is often used concurrently with prednisone.
Idiopathic		**Old Dog Vestibular Syndrome** **Feline idiopathic vestibular syndrome:** Both diseases have acute onset with marked improvement over 72 hours. Signs resolve completely within 1-3 weeks (except for the head tilt).
Toxic	**Metronidazole** (systemic) can cause ataxia and nystagmus as well as seizures, opisthotonus and coma in some animals. Mildly affected animals recover within a few weeks. Severely affected animals may not recover.	**Aminoglycosides** (systemic or topical) can cause irreversible deafness and vestibular signs (may be reversible). Signs may be unilateral or bilateral. They usually occur only after prolonged use of the drug.
Traumatic	**Head injury/fracture** **Radiograph** for evidence of fractures to the skull (i.e. the tympanic bullae). **Observe** for 48 hours with repeat neurologic exams. Prognosis is good with peripheral disease. These animals usually improve rapidly. Animal may have a permanent head tilt. Prognosis is poor with central disease.	
Vascular	**Infarct or hemorrhage** Provide supportive care. Signs should improve over 5-7 days. Diagnosis is based on MRI.	

MYELOPATHIES
Clinical Signs
Localizing the Lesion
Diagnosis
Diseases Causing Transverse Myelopathies
Intervertebral Disk Disease

I. CLINICAL SIGNS

CLINICAL SIGNS
• Pain - holds neck out or hunches back
• Stiff gait
• Paresis or paralysis
• Stumbling gait, knuckling
• Lameness

II. **LOCALIZING THE LESION:** The neurologic examination localizes the lesion to a specific spinal cord segment or segments.

A. **SPINAL REFLEXES** (also refer to neurologic exam p. 12.8)

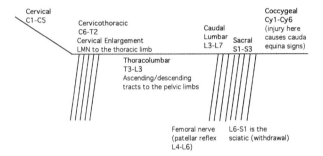

Signs Based on Lesion Location (Spinal Cord Segments)

C1-C5	C6-T2	T3-L3	L4-S3	Coccygeal
UMN signs to all four limbs	LMN signs to thoracic limbs UMN signs to pelvic limbs	UMN signs to pelvic limbs Severe damage causes temporary or permanent Schiff-Sherrington posture (T3-L3 damage)	L4-L6: LMN signs with patellar reflex and UMN signs with sciatic. L7-S3: LMN signs to sciatic.	LMN signs to bladder and anus LMN signs to pelvic limbs

B. **SIGNS to the ANUS and BLADDER:** (These signs are not always consistent): Animals may be incontinent (Refer to incontinence 21.13).

	BLADDER	ANUS
UMN Signs	The bladder is hyperreflexic. That is, it fills then reflexly contracts. It may not contract completely, and you can't predict what the bladder pressure is when it contracts. The danger with UMN disease to the bladder is that urine pooling may predispose the animal to urinary tract infections and may stretch the detrusor muscle causing temporary or permanent damage. UMN bladders are difficult to express.	The anus is hyperreflexic
LMN Signs	The bladder is hypotonic, thus it's always dribbling. It's easy to express (Lesions in S1-S3 or cauda equina lesions cause lower motor neuron signs to the bladder).	The anus is atonic and areflexic.

* Usually these animals don't have problems with fecal incontinence

Neurology

C. **SPINAL vs VERTEBRAL SEGMENTS**: In dogs and cats, the spinal cord segments are shorter than the vertebral column segments. As a result, in the dog, the spinal cord ends at the L6 vertebral area and spinal roots extend caudally down the rest of the vertebral canal. The collection of spinal roots occupying the vertebral canal caudal to the end of the spinal cord is called **the cauda equina**. Lesions of the coccygeal spinal cord segments and the cauda equina cause LMN signs to the bladder, anus and tail.

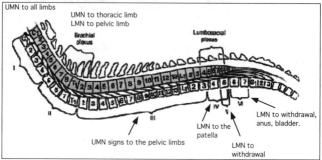

From Oliver and Lorenz: Handbook of Veterinary Neurology. 2nd edition. Philadelphia, WB Saunders, 1993. (Used with permission - figure 2-2.)

The importance of the difference in length between the spinal cord and vertebral segments is that on further diagnostics, (e.g. radiographs), you must be sure to correlate the clinical signs with a lesion in the appropriate spot. For example, LMN signs to the patella (L4-L6 spinal segments) correlate with a lesion at L3, L4 disk space.

D. **Pain**: Once you've narrowed the lesion down to specific region of the spinal cord, palpate the vertebra and gently flex and extend the neck to localize areas of pain.

III. DIAGNOSTIC TESTS
A. DIFFERENT TESTS

DIAGNOSTIC TEST	PURPOSE
Survey spinal radiographs	Helps find or rule out the following: • Fractures • Vertebral malformations • Traumatic luxations, subluxations • Vertebral neoplasia • Discospondylitis • Spondylosis • Narrowing of disc spaces, compatible with disc disease
CSF analysis	Can help rule out inflammation, infection, neoplasia
Myelogram is needed to get a better view of the spinal cord	Best used for extradural lesions. Myelograms identify **compressive** (IV disk herniation and spinal cord tumors/masses) and **expansive** (intramedullary spinal cord masses) **lesions**.
MRI can also be used to get a multiplanar picture of the spinal cord.	Less invasive than a myelogram
Surgical exploration	May be needed for specific diagnosis

B. MYELOGRAMS: Contrast is injected into the subarachnoid space.

LOCATION OF THE SPINAL CORD MASSES BASED ON MYELOGRAMS

MASS LOCATION	CROSS SECTION	VD	LATERAL
Extradural (e.g. disk protrusion)		or **	
Intradural, extramedullary			
Intramedullary			

** If the mass (e.g. disk material) is ventrolateral, the spinal cord will be pushed to the side as well as being pushed dorsally.

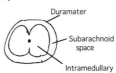

Duramater

Subarachnoid space

Intramedullary

Neurology

IV. DISEASES CAUSING TRANSVERSE MYELOPATHIES

RULE OUT	DIAGNOSIS
DEGENERATIVE Chronic, progressive disease	**Degenerative myelopathy** is a degeneration of the white matter. It occurs primarily in German Shepherd dogs and is a chronic, progressive, asymmetric, non-painful disease with a grave prognosis. **Type II disk disease** (Refer to disk disease p. 12.25). **Spondylosis** indicates a degenerative change between two vertebral bodies. It is usually not associated with any clinical problems.
ANOMALOUS (congenital) Chronic, progressive or non-progressive disease	**Spina bifida** is incomplete fusion of the dorsal vertebral arches. It occurs most often in the lumbosacral area and results in signs of cauda equina syndrome (fecal and urinary incontinence, rear limb ataxia, rear limb paresis). When the meninges and spinal cord protrude through the defect, it's called **myelomeningocoele**. Spina bifida occurs in Manx cats and in screw-tailed dogs (pug, bulldog etc). **Lumbosacral stenosis** results in signs of cauda equina syndrome. **Hemivertebrae** are sometimes associated with spinal cord compression. **Cervical vertebral instability** occurs most often in Dobermans.
NEOPLASTIC Chronic progressive disease	Primary spinal or bone tumor Metastatic tumor Bone tumors can be diagnosed based on survey radiographs. Myelogram is often needed to specifically localize the lesion. Prior to a myelogram, you should check for thoracic metastasis, and perform blood panel, If these are negative, then myelogram, CSF tap are indicated. Chemotherapy is not very useful for tumors involving the spinal cord. Surgery can be performed for extradural and intradural/extramedually masses. Tumors are usually slowly progressive except for lymphosarcoma and acute hemorrhage of metastatic masses.
INFECTIOUS	**Discospondylitis** is most often caused by *Staphylococcus*, *Streptococcus* or *Brucella*. Disk aspirate and culture is the best method for determining etiology. Blood culture is the next best method. In the mean time, treat for *Staphylococcus and Streptotoccus* and run *Brucella* titers. If positive for *Brucella*, then neuter the animal too. The animal may require surgical decompression and stabilization.
INFLAMMATORY (non-infectious) Subacute, progressive	**Granulomatous meningoencephalitis:** Use CSF anaylsis to rule out infection. Long term prognosis is poor.
TRAUMATIC Acute, progressive or non-progressive	**Fracture, luxation, subluxation** Stabilization and decompression first choice for treatment. Steroids are not indicated. **Type I disk** (signs are acute and non-progressive): Perform decompressive surgery if there are any neurologic deficits. (Refer to the following page for additional information).
VASCULAR Acute, non-progressive	**Fibrocartilagenous emboli** (acute/non-painful): Animals may improve immediately or over 6 weeks. Those that don't improve within the first 7-10 days and those with LMN signs have a worse prognosis. About 50% of animals will recover. Corticosteroids have not been shown to affect outcome.

V. **DEGENERATIVE INTERVERTEBRAL DISK DISEASE in DOGS:** Disk herniation is one of the most common causes of myelopathy in dogs.
  A. **THE TWO TYPES OF DISK DISEASE—EXTRUSIONS and PROTRUSIONS**

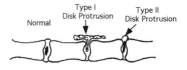

TWO TYPES OF DISK DISEASE

	TYPE I (EXTRUSION)	TYPE II (PROTRUSION)
PATHOGENESIS	Occurs primarily in chondrodystrophic dogs such as Dachshunds, Pekingeses, Pugs, and Basset Hounds. It's characterized by calcification and degeneration of the nucleus and anulus of the disk. Ultimately, nuclear material is **extruded.**	Occurs primarily in big dogs such as Labrador Retrievers (cervical), and German Shepherds (lumbosacral junction). It's characterized by bulging of the annulus.
CLINICAL SIGNS	Rapid onset (over 1-2 days) of back pain and reluctance to move due to meningitis and nerve root irritation. The dog may stand with its back arched or it may have a stiff neck. Paralysis or paresis may ensue within a few hours to a few days after the onset of pain. Some of the signs may be due to edema, inflammation, or hemorrhage around the spinal cord.	The signs are usually chronic and slowly progressive (the annulus is smooth and does not irritate the spinal cord as much as the nuclear material in type I protrusion). These animals are usually non-painful or only have mild pain.
TREATMENT	For **pain with no deficits,** restrict activity to cage rest x 3 weeks followed by 3 weeks of leash walks only. Treatment with 0.5 mg/kg prednisone BID (is controversial) for 3 days hasn't been shown to change her outcome. NSAIDS and other analgesics are an option. Don't use NSAIDs and corticosteroids together. For **repeat episodes** or cases of neurologic deficits, do surgery. If signs are **acute** and the animal is **non-ambulatory,** as with acute spinal cord trauma and perform surgical decompression immediately.	These animals often don't present until they have significant myelopathy. Surgical decompression is indicated.

  A. **DIAGNOSIS:**
    1. **History and Clinical Signs**
    2. **Localize the lesion** during your neurologic examination of the animal.
    3. **Survey radiographs:** May reveal collapse of a disc space or calcification of nuclear material. If the calcification is located within the intervertebral disk space, you cannot determine that the calcification is the cause of the signs. If the calcification is located within the spinal canal, it is much more likely to be the cause of the signs. Always correlate the lesions seen with the clinical signs.
    4. **CSF analysis:** Before injecting the contrast material for the myelogram, CSF fluid should be obtained and submitted. Perform a lumbar tap for spinal cord disease and a cisternal tap for brain disease.
    5. **Myelogram:** May reveal elevation of the ventral contrast column in the area of the ruptured disk plus thinning of the dorsal contrast column in the same area. VD views reveal thinning of the contrast column in the same area on one or both sides of the cord. Disk herniation may cause significant cord edema, inflammation or hemorrhage. So while a dog may have only one disk protrusion, the lesion may span several disk spaces.

B. **TREATMENT CONSIDERATIONS:**

1. In mild neuropathies and myelopathies, if you have ruled out contraindications for steroids (Check for other infections such as an infection caused by foxtails- typically the neurologic signs are of a T_2, L_3 myelopathy), **corticosteroids** may be used, **(0.5 mg/kg BID) for several days** but this is controversial. It hasn't been shown to help and may mask signs allowing the animal to exercise and exacerbate the condition. The most important component of treatment is strict cage rest for at least three weeks ($\pm$ physical therapy) followed by gradual increase in activity. Corticosteroids theoretically work by decreasing the inflammation and giving the spinal cord time to adapt to the insult. They don't decrease the spinal cord compression though. The cord is less able to adapt to additional insult and the healing process slows down. Finally, any extruded disk material will be much more difficult to remove in several months than it is presently. Advise the owner that any time the dog has neurologic signs, a neurologic work-up should be performed. Warn the above owner that the animal should be worked up if the signs get worse or don't improve, and that the dog needs strict cage rest.

2. Animals that only have CP deficits and/or pain on their first episode may be treated medically. If they have repeated painful episodes, the pain is not resolving, or they develop neurologic deficits, they should undergo surgical treatment.

C. **PROGNOSIS for RECOVERY from MYELOPATHIES:**

1. **Order of Progression of Neurologic Signs:** The normal progression of signs when an animal has a compressive transverse myelopathy is as follows: First the animal loses conscious proprioception to its limbs while retaining the ability to ambulate normally. Then it develops paresis or paralysis. Lastly, superficial, and then deep pain is lost.

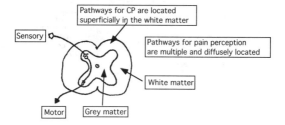

2. **Prognostic indicators**

a. **Presence of deep pain sensation:** The absence of deep pain lends a poor prognosis. When eliciting deep pain, make sure that the animal is consciously reacting to the stimulus rather than just reflexly reacting. That is, when you clamp the dog's toes, the dog should cry out or move his head to look at you. The animal may lack deep pain but retain normal spinal reflexes.

b. **Upper motor neuron signs vs lower motor neuron signs:** Animals with transverse myelopathies that have lower motor neuron signs have a worse prognosis than those with upper motor neuron signs because the pathways for lower motor neuron tracts are in the gray matter.

NEUROMUSCULAR DISORDERS
Clinical Signs
Classifications
Specific Diseases

Neuromuscular diseases are disorders affecting the motor unit. A **motor unit** is comprised of an individual peripheral neuron and all the muscle fibers it innervates. Neuromuscular disorders can affect any component of the motor unit—the **peripheral nerve, neuromuscular junction, or muscle fibers.**

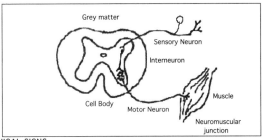

I. CLINICAL SIGNS
    A. CLINICAL SIGNS of NEUROMUSCULAR DISEASE: Neuromuscular disease is characterized by **lower motor neuron signs** (flaccid paresis or paralysis and muscle atrophy).

CLINICAL SIGNS of NEUROMUSCULAR DISEASE
• Episodic weakness or paralysis (In cats, weakness of the extensors of the neck is characterized by ventral neck flexion). • Stiff gait, stumbling, knuckling • Muscle atrophy • Dysphonia (change in voice character) • Regurgitation (due to megaesophagus) • Decreased spinal reflexes (may be normal too) • Normal or decreased CPs

1. **Fatigue**, weakness exacerbated by exercise, can occur with any neuromuscular disorder.
2. **Conscious proprioception** is often normal in animals with neuromuscular disease. With spinal cord damage, CP deficits occur early in the disease process (precedes weakness) because the CP deficits are due to damage to the ascending CP pathways which are located superficially within the spinal cord. These CP deficits occur because the animal does not sense where its paws are. With neuromuscular disease, the sensory pathways may be intact and CP deficits occur due to motor dysfunction. That is, the animal knows where its paws are but it can't move them into the correct position. So in neuromuscular disease CP deficits won't occur until the motor deficits are bad enough to prevent the animal from moving its legs into position at the normal rate unless the sensory nerves are involved in the disease process. In short, a hallmark of neuromuscular disease is weakness with intact CPs whereas with spinal cord disease, CP deficits precede ataxia and weakness.

> If the animal is paretic but has normal CPs, think neuromuscular disease.

B. **CLASSIFICATION:** We can classify neuromuscular diseases based on the region (peripheral nerve, neuromuscular junction, muscle fibers) of the motor unit that's involved.

1. **Polyneuropathy** consists of diseases affecting multiple peripheral nerves.
2. **Neuromuscular junction** disorders are caused by problems with acetylcholine (ACH) release at the neuromuscular junction or uptake of ACH at the postsynaptic membrane of the neuromuscular junction.
3. **Myopathyies** consist of diseases of the muscle fibers such as **myositis** (inflammation of the muscle) and **muscular dystrophy.**

CLASSIFICATION of NEUROMUSCULAR DISEASES

	POLYNEUROPATHY	NEUROMUSCULAR JUNCTION	MYOPATHY
Rule Outs	• Diabetes Mellitus (plantigrade stance in cats) • Hypothyroidism • Insulinoma (paraneoplastic syndrome) • Thiamine Deficiency • Tumor (paraneoplastic syndrome) • SLE (systemic lupus erythematosus) • Coonhound paralysis (polyradiculoneuritis) • Organophosphate toxicity	• Tick paralysis • Botulism • Myasthenia Gravis (Rule out thymoma and other tumors as an underlying cause) • Aminoglycoside toxicity	• Idiopathic polymyositis • Hypokalemia • Excess glucocorticoids • Tumor (e.g. thymoma) • Infectious-*Toxoplasma* or *Neospora*
Electro-diagnostics	• EMG shows spontaneous activity. • Nerve conduction is decreased.	• Normal EMG	• EMG shows spontaneous activity, normal nerve conduction.

C. **DIAGNOSTIC STEPS**
1. History:
   a. Is the cat on a fish-only diet. Fish diets contain thiaminase, which degrades thiamine leading to thiamine deficiency (vitamin B1). Perform a trial therapy of 20 mg thiamine IM per day (or 50-100 mg PO). Signs should rapidly improve in 24 hours.
   b. Are other dogs in the household affected? Have any of the pets had diarrhea within the last week (botulism)?
   c. Are the animals in a tick area or have they been treated for ticks or fleas? Check for ticks (tick paralysis).
   d. Travel history?
   e. History of a voice change?
2. Physical exam and neurologic exam
3. Blood count, chemistry panel, thyroid levels and urinalysis will rule out most metabolic causes of neuromuscular disease. ANA, biopsy of any suspicious skin lesions, examination of urine for elevated protein: creatinine, and joint taps can help rule out SLE.
4. Screen for tumors
   a. **Thoracic radiographs** will rule out thymomas and may reveal metastasis. They will also identify **megaesophagus** and **aspiration pneumonia.**
   b. **Abdominal ultrasound**
   c. **Lymph node aspirate, bone marrow sample and abdominal ultrasound** can be used to help identify multicentric lymphosarcoma.
5. Nerve Conduction/ EMG
6. Muscle or nerve **biopsy** and antibodies to acetylcholine receptors.
7. **Tensilon® Test:** is based on keeping ACH available in the neuromuscular junction for a longer period of time by blocking its degredation with an anticholinesteras such as edrophonium (**tensilon** 0.1mg IV). Induce weakness by exercising the animal and then administer edrophonium (**tensilon 0.1 mg IV**). If affected, the dog should show rapid improvement within 30-60 seconds.

II. **SPECIFIC DISEASES**
A. **DISEASES THAT PRESENT ACUTELY vs CHRONICALLY**
1. **Acute onset of progressive neurologic signs: Coonhound Paralysis, Tick Paralysis, and Botulism** are all characterized by acute onset of

progressive neurologic signs. Animals typically develop an ascending paralysis. They can also develop megaesophagus, dysphonia, and respiratory paralysis which may lead to death. Signs often do not progress to this severe an extent though and prognosis is often good unless the animals have megaesophagus which predisposes them to developing aspiration pneumonia

2. **Chronic, progressive neuromuscular diseases: Myasthenia Gravis and idiopathic polymyopathy** are both characterized by weakness exacerbated by exercise. They are often associated with megaesophagus and dysphonia. Most of the metabolic polyneuropathies are also chronic and progressive.

B. POLYNEUROPATHY
  1. **Coonhound Paralysis (polyradiculoneuritis):**
      a. **Etiology:** unknown. It most commonly affects hunting dogs that have been exposed to raccoons.
      b. **Clinical Signs:** Usually cranial nerves are not involved. Animals often develop hyperesthesia. Signs develop about 7-9 days after exposure and can lead to paralysis within 12 hours to one week. Prognosis is good with supportive care for an average of 3-6 weeks.
      c. **EMG:** Evidence of denervation or slow nerve conduction.

C. NEUROMUSCULAR DISORDERS (Go to www.nerdbook.com/extras for the handout *Overview of the Neurologic System* for additional information.):
  1. **Tick paralysis:**
      a. **Etiology:** Caused by *Dermacentor* ticks that secrete a **neurotoxin**. The neurotoxin blocks ACH release at the neuromuscular junction. Diagnosis is made based on presence of ticks on the animal and rapid recovery once ticks are removed. Animals in the U.S. improve rapidly with removal of the ticks. Treat with a dip that kills ticks. Be sure to remove the tick heads as leaving the heads can lead to worsening signs. Also, check the ears and digits for ticks too. Failure to treat leads to rapid death within a week. Signs occur about 1 week after exposure to ticks and can progress to complete paralysis within 12-24 hours. Note that since this is a neuromuscular disorder, nerve conductions are normal.

  2. **Botulism:** This disease is rare in dogs and cats.
      a. **Etiology:** It occurs due to ingestion of food contaminated with *Clostridium botulinum* which releases a toxin that blocks the release of ACH at the neuromuscular junction. Signs develop within 6 days of exposure.
      b. **Diagnosis** is supported by a history of multiple animals affected. The toxin can be identified in the vomitus, food, or feces.
      c. **Treatment** involves supportive care including antibiotics to decrease the amount of *Clostridia* in the GI tract and enemas or laxatives to help decrease GI toxins. Recovery is good with mild signs. If the signs are rapidly progressive, the prognosis is poor.

  3. **Myesthenia Gravis:** Signs are due to deficiency in ACH receptors at the post-synaptic membrane of the neuromuscular junction. The congenital form is rare. The acquired form is due to antibodies against the ACH receptors at the neuromuscular junction. Administration of an anticholinesterase such as tensilon® (edrophonium) or neostigmine leads to marked improvement in muscle strength.

      a. **Treatment:** Give an anticholinesterase such as Mestinon® (pyridostigmine bromide) at a dose of 0.2 to 2 mg/kg PO BID to TID in dogs and 2.5 mg PO BID in cats (elixir). Be careful with this medication, particularly in cats. The goal is to improve muscle strength without causing increased regurgitation in animals with megaesophagus. Consequently, most animals don't achieve normal muscle strength. **Prednisone** is not usually used in dogs, but is usually used in cats. Once the disease is controlled, decrease and possibly discontinue the Mestinon® and taper the prednisone. Some of these animals go into remission and can be taken off prednisone too. It's also important to manage the megaesophagus by placing a PEG tube if needed and to treat aspiration pneumonia with antibiotics.

Neurology

D. **MYOSITIS:**
1. **Etiologies:** Rule out SLE and thymoma as an underlying cause. Also, rule out hypokalemia and thiamine deficiency in cats because they have a similar presentation.
2. **Diagnosis:**
   a. Elevated creatine kinase (over 15,000)
   b. EMG: positive sharp waves and fibrillation potentials.
   c. Biopsy

3. **Treatment:** For dogs, give 2 mg/kg **prednisone** per day for at least two weeks and then taper slowly once signs are controlled. The animal will be on prednisone for at least one month. For cats give 2-6 mg/kg prednisone daily and taper over two months.

E. **THYMOMAS** are commonly associated with neuromuscular disease. Thymus cells are isolated from the body's immune system. As a result, the body does not recognize them as self. When a thymoma develops, the cell antigens are exposed to the immune system and antibodies against them are made. Because thymoma cell antigens resemble ACH receptor antigens and myocyte membrane antigens, these new antibodies bind to ACH receptors at the neuromuscular junction and to muscle cells. In cases where animal show weakness with exercise, rule out thymoma.

NOTE: Animals with concurrent megaesophagus are much more difficult to manage since they are predisposed to developing aspiration pneumonia. Placing a PEG tube early on is helpful. When treating for aspiration pneumonia, avoid using **aminoglycosides** because they may cause neuromuscular blockade.

Suggested Reading

Pibot P, Biourge V, Elliott D (Eds). Encyclopedia of Canine Clinical Nutrition. Italy: Diffo Print Italia, 2006.

Hand MS, Thatcher CD, Rimillard RL, Roudebush R (Eds.). Small Animal Clinical Nutrition, 4th Edition. Marceline, Missouri: Walsworth Publishing, 2000.

Nutrition

PET FOODS
Understanding Pet Food Labels
Feed Additives and Supplementation
Feeding Recommendations

I. **UNDERSTANDING PET FOOD LABELS:** Pet food labeling is regulated at the federal and state levels. The FDA establishes standards that apply to animal feeds, and the American Association of Feed Control Officers (AAFCO) provides additional standards. AAFCO is an advisory panel with representatives from all 50 states, Canada, and Puerto Rico. Pet food labels must provide information in a standardized format. The information is divided into two groups: the display panel and the information panel.

A. **THE PRINCIPLE DISPLAY PANEL** must include the following:
- Product name
- Net weight/quantity
- The words "Dog Food" or "Cat Food" and "Snack" or "Treat," if applicable

1. **Product names are regulated based on the ingredients.** Manufacturers design product names to be catchy and descriptive, sometimes causing confusion about the ingredients. Regulations on the usage of ingredient names in the product name help avoid misrepresentation.

PRODUCT NAME EXAMPLE	INTERPRETATION
100% Chicken	The ingredient list contains only chicken as its main ingredient. The product can also contain preservatives, minerals, vitamins, etc.
Chicken for Cats	Chicken makes up 95% or more of the product, not counting water. If water is counted, then chicken must still make up $\geq$ 75% of the product. If two products of animal origin are listed in the name (e.g., "Chicken 'n' Liver Cat Food"), together the two products must comprise 95% or more of the food, and the first ingredient must be present in higher amounts than the second. This rule applies only to products of animal origin. So, if the product name says "Lamb and Rice Dog Food," lamb must comprise $\geq$ 95% of the product.
Chicken Dinner (or Supper, Nuggets, Entrée, Formula) for Cats	Chicken constitutes $\geq$ 25% and less than 95% (not including water for processing) of the product. Chicken is probably listed third or fourth on the ingredient list. If two ingredients are in the product name, then both—regardless of whether they are of animal origin—must total $\geq$ 25%. So, "Lamb and Rice Dinner" must have $\geq$ 25% lamb and rice combined.
Chicken Flavored	The flavor source for the food is chicken in sufficient amounts to be detected by animals. This can be tested using animals trained to prefer specific flavors. Flavors are often obtained from digests (materials that are treated with heat and enzymes and/or acids).
Cat Food With Chicken	The food contains at least 3% chicken.
Light, Lean, or Reduced	Dog food: • 1409 kcal/pound and < 9% fat (dry foods) • 1136 kcal/pound and $\leq$ 7% fat (semimoist foods • 409 kcal/pound and $\leq$ 4% fat (canned foods) Cat food: • 1477 kcal/pound and $\leq$ 10% fat (dry foods) • 1205 kcal/pound and $\leq$ 8% fat (semimoist foods) • 432 kcal/pound and $\leq$ 5% fat (canned foods)
New and Improved (brand name) Cat Food	The words "new and improved" can only be used for 6 months following the initial release of the newly revised product.
Contains no additives or preservatives	Such claims must be true and substantiated.

B. **THE INFORMATION PANEL** yields nutrient information including the guaranteed analysis, ingredient statement, nutritional adequacy statement, and FDA required information for health claims. It also contains the name and address of the manufacturer and the feeding instructions.

1. **The guaranteed analysis** includes the minimum levels of crude protein and fat and the maximum levels of moisture and fiber. It does not include the exact amounts of these components or information about the digestibility or quality of the nutrients. Furthermore, the nutrient levels are displayed on an "as fed" (AF)

basis rather than a metabolizable energy (ME) basis. To compare products, you must first convert to a metabolizable energy basis. Converting removes diet moisture, fiber, and ash content variables. This allows you to accurately compare different types of foods (i.e., dry vs. canned foods).

a.   **Step 1:** To calculate % ME, first calculate the carbohydrate content of the food by subtracting the following from 100: % protein AF, % fat AF, % fiber AF, % moisture AF, and % ash AF. As an example, look at the guaranteed analysis below.

Guaranteed Analysis	% (AF)
Protein	10%
Fat	5%
Fiber content	3%
Moisture	75%

Based on these amounts, the carbohydrate (CHO) content equals 7. [100% - (10% + 5% + 3% + 75%)] = 7% = carbohydrate

b.   **Step 2:** Convert % protein AF, % fat AF, and % carbohydrate AF to a ME basis using the modified Atwater values (3.5 kcals/g of protein, 8.5 kcals/g of fat, and 3.5 kcals/g of carbohydrate). Remember that 1% is equivalent to 1 g/100 g of food. This also calculates the total kcals in 100 g of food.

Guaranteed analysis (% AF) (g of nutrient/100 g food)		Multiply by kcal/g of nutrient		Total kcal from that nutrient/100 g food
10 g protein/100 g food	x	3.5 kcal/g protein	=	35 kcals from protein
5 g fat/100 g food		8.5 kcal/g fat		42.5 kcals from fat
x		=		
7 g CHO/100 g food	x	3.5 kcal/g CHO	=	24.5 kcals from CHO

Add these kcals (35 + 42.5 + 24.5) to get **102 kcals total/100 g** of food.

c.   Finally, divide the kcals from protein, fat, and carbohydrates by the total kcals calculated from step 2 to get the percentages on a ME basis.

Guaranteed analysis (% AF) kcal/100 g of food		Divide by total kcal/100 g food		% metabolizable energy (% of nutrient in food)
35 kcals from protein/100 g	÷	102 kcals total/100 g	=	34.3% protein
42.5 kcals from fat/100 g	÷	102 kcals total/100 g	=	41.7% fat
24.5 kcals from carb/100 g	÷	102 kcals total/100 g	=	24.0% carb

2.   **Ingredients:** The ingredients are arranged in decreasing order based on weight.
   a.   Manufacturers improve the appearance of their ingredient list for marketing purposes by:
      i.   Separating different forms of similar ingredients so that they can place the ingredients further down on the list. For example, wheat may be broken into **ground wheat and wheat fiber** when the only difference between the two is that one is more finely ground. Wheat may be the #1 ingredient in the food, but by separating the ingredients, the manufacturer may be able to list chicken as the #1 ingredient while listing the wheat forms as the #3 and #5 ingredients.
      ii.   Contents are listed in order based on an "as fed" weight rather than on a dry matter basis. Manufacturers may add high quality ingredients, such as meat, in the high moisture content form and add low quality ingredients, such as wheat, in the dry matter form. This allows the meat, which may be present in significantly smaller quantities than the wheat, to be listed higher in the ingredient list. This is not a problem with dry foods, but it can be a problem with canned foods, which contain products of vastly differing moisture content.

   b.   **Variable and fixed formula diets**
      i.   **Variable formula diets:** Most generic and many name brands contain ingredients that vary from batch to batch depending on market price.
      ii.   **Fixed formula diets:** Most premium brands contain fixed ingredients in a fixed order, which is one reason why they are more expensive. Contact the company to determine if their formula is fixed.
3.   **Nutritional adequacy statement:** All pet foods in interstate commerce (not including treats or snacks) must contain a statement of nutritional adequacy.

Nutrition

The nutritional adequacy statement indicates that the product meets or exceeds the AAFCO nutritional requirements for one or more of the following life cycle stages: gestation/lactation, growth, maintenance, or all stages.

a. Life cycle stage:
   i. Foods that are labeled as "100% complete and balanced" for adult maintenance must be adequate for adults but may not be adequate for growth or gestation/lactation.
   ii. Foods labeled for all stages must support growth, gestation/lactation, and maintenance.
   iii. Foods labeled for puppies will *in theory* also support gestation/lactation needs and maintenance needs; however, they may not have been tested via feeding trials on lactating or pregnant females. Contact the company to see if gestation/lactation trials were performed.

b. The claim of nutritional adequacy is based either on AAFCO-sanctioned feeding trials or on AAFCO-sanctioned laboratory analysis. **Feeding trials are far superior** because they account for the differences in digestibility, bioavailability, and dietary interactions. Diets tested in feeding trials have a statement that says *"Animal feeding tests using AAFCO procedures show that (brand) provides complete and balanced nutrition for (life stages)."*

4. **Daily feeding instructions:** The package should contain instructions on the amount to feed. This value is usually a calculated average maintenance energy requirement and can vary as much as 50% from the animal's true requirement. Therefore, owners should be instructed to monitor the pet's body weight and feed to maintain an ideal body weight.

II. FEED ADDITIVES and SUPPLEMENTATION

A. **SUPPLEMENTATION:** Modest supplementation with table foods (< 10% of the daily caloric requirement) or multi-vitamin/mineral supplements designed to be given with commercial pet foods is neither detrimental nor beneficial. Vitamins and minerals designed for human consumption or home-cooked diets, however, may result in nutritional imbalances, deficiencies, or toxicities if added to a commercial diet. Adding more than 10% table foods can lead to serious digestive disturbances and an imbalanced diet.

B. **ANTIOXIDANTS and FOOD ADDITIVES**
   1. **Ethoxyquin:** Research involving ethoxyquin has not substantiated claims of reproductive failure and poor condition. Some hemoglobin-related pigments have been shown to accumulate in the liver but only at doses higher than those used in pet foods. The clinical significance of these changes is unknown.
   2. Many manufacturers use **vitamin E, C, or beta carotene** as natural antioxidants. They are less potent and less stable then ethoxyquin.
   3. Canned diets don't require preservatives. Semimoist diets often use **BHA** or **BHT** to preserve the fat in the diet. Propylene glycol is no longer used to preserve semimoist cat foods as it causes Heinz bodies in cat RBCs. It may still be found in semimoist dog foods.
   4. **Additives:** Food intolerances are most commonly due to dietary proteins rather than additives.

III. FEEDING RECOMMENDATIONS

A. **NO ONE FOOD is BEST** for all dogs or all cats.
   1. In general, foods that have been tested via feeding trials are better than foods that haven't.
   2. Premium brands may be better than supermarket and generic brands because they are specifically formulated to meet the animal's needs, use better quality ingredients, and have better quality control. Generic brands and popular brands are formulated to be palatable. They may use ingredients with lower bioavailabilities and have poorer quality control leading to less consistency among batches.

B. **DIETARY CHANGES**
   1. With dogs, it is best to stick to one food rather than constantly changing diets unless you change gradually. Sudden diet changes can lead to digestive upset.
   2. With healthy cats, it's safer to vary brands to guard against dietary deficiencies not yet discovered.
   3. Dry food is more energy dense. Wet food is more palatable and provides increased water intake.

OBESITY and WEIGHT REDUCTION

Obesity is the most common nutritional disorder in cats and dogs. Up to 44% of pets in North America are obese (overweight by 15-20%). This condition can seriously affect a pet's quality of life. On average, dogs that are in athletic body condition (approximately 4-5 out of 9 BCS) live several years longer and tend to develop orthopedic problems several years later than those that are slightly overweight (approximately 6-7 out of 9 BCS).

ETIOLOGY	Obesity occurs when an animal consumes more energy than it needs. The excess energy is stored as fat. During the growth stage of life, the number of fat cells an animal has is determined. The more energy the growing animal consumes, the more fat cells it develops. Once fat cells are formed, they are permanent; weight loss occurs through reduction of fat cell size rather than fat cell number. Because fat cells must retain some triglyceride stores, they never become devoid of fat. The result is that animals with more fat cells have a greater minimum fat content than animals with fewer fat cells. In other words, pets that become fat during the growth phase and form many adipocytes have more trouble losing weight than pets that become obese in adulthood. Consequently, preventing obesity in growing animals is important. Adult animals that consume more energy than used gain weight by increasing the size of their fat cells (hypertrophy). Over time, they can also develop higher numbers of fat cells (hyperplasia).
PRE-DISPOSING FACTORS	• Old age • Neutering: Neutering decreases the energy requirement and tends to increase food intake or **appetite.** • Being female • Overweight owners, sedentary lifestyle (e.g., indoor cats) • Free-feeding (especially dogs) • More than one pet in the household (competition for food) • **Genetics** (e.g., Labrador Retrievers, Beagles, Dachshunds, Shelties) • Obesity as puppies or kittens
ADVERSE EFFECTS of OBESITY	• Dermatoses • Hypertension and possible heart failure • Immune suppression • Diabetes mellitus • Hepatic lipidosis in cats • Orthopedic and locomotor dysfunction • Increased risk in surgery and under anesthesia • Respiratory difficulties
BENEFITS of WEIGHT REDUCTION	• Decreased stress on joints • Easier for veterinarians to examine and perform surgery • Better cardiovascular function • Increased athleticism • Reduction or elimination of medications (e.g., insulin in diabetic cats)
CANINE and FELINE BODY CONDITION SCORING (BCS)	**Determining whether an animal is fit or fat:** Body condition should be scored on a scale of 1 to 9 at each visit (See a video on body condition scoring at www.drsophiayin.com/resources/videos.) Very thin (BCS 1-3) • The ribs, lumbar vertebrae, pelvic bones, and $\pm$ other bony prominences are visible. • The pet has a severe waist and abdominal tuck. • The pet may have decreased muscle mass. Ideal weight (BCS 4-5) • The ribs are easily palpable (without applying pressure). • The abdomen is tucked up when viewed from the side, and the last rib is visible. • When viewed from the top, a waist is visible behind the ribs. Obese (BCS 7-9) • A layer of fat is palpable over the ribs; that is, you must apply pressure to feel the ribs. • No abdominal tuck is seen. The abdomen may even be distended. • The pet may have fat deposits over the lumbar area, base of the tail, or inguinal area. The skin feels thick around the neck and shoulders.

I. ACHIEVING WEIGHT LOSS: The goal is to lose fat while retaining lean muscle mass. Prior to starting a weight loss program, evaluate the pet for other problems that may need treatment (e.g., pregnancy, Cushing's disease, hypothyroidism).

Nutrition

A. **DETERMINE the ANIMAL'S CURRENT CALORIC INTAKE,** and decrease the daily total kcals fed by 20%. If the current caloric intake cannot be accurately calculated, determine the pet's **ideal weight** and then calculate the metabolic energy requirement (MER) for a normal pet of that weight.

$$\text{Cat MER} = 1.2 \, [70 \times (\text{kg BW})^{3/4}]$$

$$\text{Dog MER} = 1.6 \, [70 \times (\text{kg BW})^{3/4}]$$

As a guideline, feed dogs 60% of their ideal MER and cats 70% of ideal MER. Dogs can safely lose 1-2% of their body weight per week, and cats about 1%, until they are at their desired weight. Initially, the pet should be reweighed every two weeks and appropriate adjustments made in the amount of food fed to achieve the desired rate of weight loss. Once a desired rate of weight loss is achieved, the pet should be rechecked at least monthly.

B. **CHOOSE a FOOD** that is designed for active weight loss. Veterinary therapeutic weight loss foods are higher in protein, vitamins, and minerals, helping ensure that a protein or nutrient deficiency does not develop during caloric restriction. Feeding multiple small meals per day will help increase metabolism and satiety. Avoid table scraps and situations where table scraps are likely to be given. Scraps or treats should be $\leq$ 10% of the animal's daily caloric intake.

C. **EXERCISE** the pet for at least 15 minutes BID to increase its metabolic rate and retain lean body mass.

FELINE MER CHART

WEIGHT (lbs)	WEIGHT (kg)	MER (kcal)	70% x MER (kcal)	WEIGHT (lbs)	WEIGHT (kg)	MER (kcal)	70% x MER (kcal)
1	0.5	47	33	9	4.1	242	169
2	0.9	78	55	10	4.5	261	183
3	1.4	106	74	11	5.0	281	197
4	1.8	132	92	12	5.5	300	210
5	2.3	155	109	13	5.9	318	223
6	2.7	178	125	14	6.4	337	236
7	3.2	200	140	15	6.8	354	248
8	3.6	221	155				

CANINE MER CHART

WEIGHT (lbs)	WEIGHT (kg)	MER (kcal)	60% x MER (kcal)	WEIGHT (lbs)	WEIGHT (kg)	MER (kcal)	60% x MER (kcal)
7	3.2	267	160	50	22.7	1166	699
9	4.1	322	193	55	25.0	1252	751
11	5.0	374	225	60	27.3	1337	802
13	5.9	424	255	65	29.5	1419	852
15	6.8	473	284	70	31.8	1500	900
17	7.7	519	311	75	34.1	1580	948
19	8.6	564	339	80	36.4	1659	995
21	9.5	608	365	85	38.6	1736	1041
25	11.4	693	416	90	40.9	1812	1087
29	13.2	775	465	95	43.2	1887	1132
33	15.0	854	512	100	45.5	1961	1176
37	16.8	930	558	105	47.7	2034	1220
41	18.6	1005	603	110	50.0	2106	1264
45	20.5	1077	646	115	52.3	2177	1306

FOOD COMPARISON CHARTS

FELINE DIET	kcal	CANINE DIET	kcal
Eukanuba RC can	34/oz	Eukanuba RC can	32/oz
Eukanuba RC dry	277/cup	Eukanuba RC dry	238/cup
Hill's r/d can	21.1/oz	Hill's r/d can	22.9/oz
Hill's r/d dry	263/cup	Hill's r/d dry	205/cup
Purina OM can	27.3/oz	Purina OM can	15.1/oz
Purina OM dry	326/cup	Purina OM dry	276/cup
Waltham Calorie Control dry	208/cup	Waltham Calorie Control dry	226/cup

DIETS of CHOICE

ALLERGIES	Animals can develop food allergies (an immune-mediated disorder) or food intolerances (e.g., food poisoning, sensitivity to histamine in the food, etc.) at any age. If you suspect a food allergy/intolerance, place the animal on a commercial veterinary uncommon allergen diet or homemade diet consisting of one novel protein source and one novel carbohydrate source. (Cats need only a novel protein source, no carbohydrate required.) Animals with GI signs should show improvement within 2-3 weeks. Those with dermatologic signs may not show improvement for up to 10 weeks. If the owner elects to continue with a home-cooked diet, a veterinary nutritionist must review and balance it for long-term feeding. If the animal is on an elimination diet, once it has improved, gradually add in suspect agents individually to determine the inciting factor (and to confirm the diagnosis of food allergy/intolerance). Or place the pet on a commercial low-allergen food containing the same protein and carbohydrate used in the homemade diet. **Beef, dairy products, wheat, and soy** are the most commonly reported food allergens, possibly because they are common in many commercial pet foods.
ASCITES, EDEMA, EFFUSION	Determine the etiology and correct the problem if possible. If indicated (e.g., ascites due to congestive heart failure), use a diet low in sodium. This will decrease the amount of water retained in the intravascular space, and thus decrease the hydrostatic pressure causing fluid leakage into the abdomen and other body cavities. If the effusion is due to hypoproteinemia, the animal's diet should contain adequate protein (many of the low sodium diets are also protein-restricted diets).
DIABETES MELLITUS	The goal of dietary therapy is to correct obesity and control hyperglycemia. Place **dogs** on a diet of low carbohydrates and moderate to high fiber. Be sure the dog will eat it and experience few side effects (such as flatulence, constipation, or diarrhea). Avoid semimoist foods since they are high in simple sugars. It's better for glycemic control to feed diabetic dogs small, frequent meals rather than one large meal. However, it is important to have a consistent feeding schedule from day to day to best coordinate insulin injections. **Cats** should be on a low carbohydrate (< 15% on a ME basis), high protein diet such as Hill's m/d or Purina DM. They may also benefit from a restricted calorie diet since most diabetic cats are obese. Because cats are carnivores and get glucose through gluconeogenesis, feeding in meals vs. free-feeding does not drastically affect their glycemic control.
CONSTIPATION	Use bulk-forming laxatives such as psyllium fiber (Metamucil®, 1-6 tsp mixed with each meal) or bran (1-2 tbsp per 400 g canned food). Lubricant laxatives such as Laxatone® or osmotic laxatives such as lactulose may be useful, too.
HYPERLIPIDEMIA and LYMPHANGECTASIA	Feed a diet with reduced fat and adequate protein. Usually a homemade diet works best because many of the commercial low fat diets are also low in calories; thus, they may not provide adequate calories for the patient's needs. Examples of appropriate homemade diets include cottage cheese and rice, tuna (in water) and rice, or turkey and rice.
PANCREATIC DISEASE	**Pancreatitis:** Keep the animal NPO if it's vomiting, but feed it as soon as it is willing or able to eat (nasogastric tube, gastrostomy tube, etc.). Use a highly digestible low fat diet. There is no evidence that supplementing with pancreatic enzymes is beneficial; however some clinicians recommending supplementing. **Exocrine pancreatic insufficiency:** Feed a highly digestible diet and avoid high fiber because it impairs pancreatic enzyme activity. Supplement with a non-enteric-coated pancreatic enzyme at a dose of 1 tsp/10 kg body weight. Do not use enteric-coated enzymes or enzyme capsules (unless they are crushed) because they have unreliable activity. Pre-incubation of enzyme with food does not improve the enzyme's effectiveness.

Nutrition

DIETS of CHOICE (continued)

LIVER DISEASE	Do not restrict protein unless the animal is showing evidence of protein intolerance. Animals with liver disease need a diet containing highly digestible, high quality protein and adequate carbohydrate and fat calories to prevent protein catabolism. **Hepatic lipidosis in cats:** These cats usually do well if kept on long-term (3-8 weeks) feeding via a gastrostomy or nasogastric tube. Force-feeding and the use of appetite stimulants usually fail to provide the cat with enough calories. These cats need 60-80 kcal energy/kg daily and about 3.3 g protein/kg daily (20-24% protein). Some appropriate diets include Clinicare® Feline, Hill's Prescription a/d®, and Hill's Prescription Feline i/d®. Food should be warmed to room temperature and pureed so that it can be fed through the nasogastric or gastrostomy tube. Animals should be fed 3-4 times per day. Initially, cats should receive 20-50 mL per feeding. Within a week they should be getting closer to 100 mL per feeding. These cats should not receive any food orally for at least 10 days. **Dogs with liver disease:** Dogs need about 2.0-2.2 g/kg protein and 5-8 g/kg fat and carbohydrate daily to prevent protein catabolism. **Animals with signs of protein intolerance:** If the animal is hyperammonemic and showing signs of hepatic encephalopathy, place it on a reduced protein diet and increase the non-protein calories. The goal is to reduce the amount of nitrogenous wastes. A prescription diet is indicated.
RENAL FAILURE	Provide adequate nutrition and high quality protein or the body will use its own protein for energy, which results in elevated BUN. Place an esophagostomy or gastrostomy tube if needed, rather than trying to force-feed. Feed in frequent, small meals. **In the azotemic animal** with signs of renal insufficiency, feed a diet reduced in protein and phosphorus and high in vitamin B and omega-3 fatty acids. This may help reduce inflammation, hypertension, and clotting seen with DIC. Although protein restriction does not appear to prevent the progression of renal disease, it can aid in making the patient feel better by decreasing uremia. Phosphorus restriction is the most important dietary modification for delaying the progression of renal disease. Some patients also require phosphate binders. Sodium restriction is recommended to help prevent systemic and renal hypertension. Cats often need to receive potassium supplements.
UROLITH - CALCIUM OXALATE	**Calcium oxalate uroliths can't be dissolved** with dietary management, but they may be prevented with the right diet. A canned food low in oxalate-containing ingredients is recommended. Increase the amount of water consumed by adding water to the food, and aim for a urine specific gravity of less than 1.020. Some commercial foods use high sodium to drive thirst and increase water intake.
UROLITH- STRUVITE	**Struvite uroliths can sometimes be dissolved** with dietary management, especially in cats, because the entire urolith is usually comprised of struvite (whereas in the dog, the inner layer may be made of a different compound). The most important step in dissolving or preventing struvite uroliths is keeping the urine pH between 6.0-6.5 by placing the animal on an acidifying diet. Most feline commercial diets are acidifying. Do not use urinary acidifiers (such as DL-methionine) on top of an acidifying diet because the urine pH may become too acidic. Diets that avoid excess magnesium and phosphorus may also help prevent the formation of struvite crystals and uroliths but are not as important as diets that acidify the urine. Free-feeding or providing frequent, small meals helps avoid an alkaline tide. Encourage water drinking by always providing fresh water and possibly by adding water to dry food or feeding canned food.

Suggested Reading

Withrow, S.J., Vail, D.M. *Withrow and MacEwen's Small Animal Clinical Oncology, 4th edition.* New York: WB Saunders, 2006.

Oncology

ONCOLOGY WORK-UP

I   **DIAGNOSIS:** Any mass that's prominent or persistent should be examined for neoplasia.
   A. **NOT ALL MASSES ARE NEOPLASMS**

RULE OUTS for MASSES
Abscess
Cyst
Granuloma
Hematoma
Tumor

   B. **EXAMINE THE MASS:** Note the size, location, consistency, fixation to surrounding
       tissues and skin, and ulceration of the skin. These factors help us determine tumor
       type. Also examine the lymph nodes draining the area. When describing the mass in
       the medical record, it helps to pretend that you are describing the mass over the
       telephone to a colleague.

RULE OUTS for SOLITARY DERMAL MASSES in the DOG	
• Mast Cell Tumor	• Adnexal Gland Adenocarcinoma (sweat
• Melanoma	gland/sebaceous gland tumor)
• Squamous Cell Carcinoma	• Sebaceous Adenoma
• Histiocytoma	• Lipoma
• Plasmacytoma	• Kerion (dermatophytosis)
• Viral Papilloma	• Mycosis fungoides (rare)*

       *(Typically a widely disseminated disease that's slowly progressive)

   C. **CYTOLOGY:** Although biopsy is usually required for a definitive diagnosis of
       neoplasia, aspiration cytology is often performed first because it's easy, inexpensive,
       and can yield a definitive diagnosis. The disadvantages of aspiration cytology are
       that the sample may not be representative of the entire process in the mass, and
       that the architecture of the mass can't be evaluated.
       1. Fine needle aspiration is a common screening step for distinguishing
           inflammatory from **neoplastic** lesions. Cytological examination of the mass
           may also differentiate **epithelial tumors from discrete cell tumors.**
           Discrete cell tumors can be round cell tumors or mesenchymal tumors.
           Mesenchymal tumors usually do not exfoliate easily. Consequently, a **negative
           aspirate does not rule out neoplasia.**

ROUND CELL TUMORS
Histiocytoma
Mast Cell Tumor
Melanoma
Lymphoma
Transmissible Venereal Tumor (TVT)
Plasmacytoma

       2. **Aspiration Technique:** The mass can be aspirated using a 22 or 25 gauge
           needle. Insert the needle and then apply suction using a syringe. Redirect the
           needle several times. Aspirates can also be performed without a syringe by just
           inserting a needle and redirecting several times. Material collects in the needle
           even without suction. This method is good for avoiding blood contamination
           with vascular tumors. With sarcomas and other tumors where the cells do not
           exfoliate well, it's best to use a large gauge needle and a syringe.
       3. **Scrape/shave biopsy technique:** Scrape the tissue gently with a surgical
           blade and smear the contents across a slide. This technique works well for
           suspected squamous cell carcinomas in cats. Shave biopsies are performed as if
           you are peeling a potato.
   D. **BIOPSY** is the definitive diagnostic technique for neoplasia. It can reveal the tumor
       type and grade (e.g. well-differentiated vs. undifferentiated).
       1. **Biopsies should be performed prior to definitive therapy in the
           following cases:**
           a. If it will **alter the type of therapy used** (e.g. surgical vs. chemotherapy
               or aggressive vs. conservative surgical resection, especially if the tumor is
               in an area that will require extensive reconstruction).
           b. When the **results will influence how the owner decides to treat
               the animal:** For example, the owner may decide to have a tumor surgically
               removed if it's malignant, but not if it's benign.
       2. **When to wait until after surgical excision to perform histopathology:**

a. When the prognosis **won't affect the treatment** (e.g. small skin mass on the back: just perform a wide surgical excision)
b. If the biopsy procedure is as **dangerous** as the surgical excision procedure (e.g. brain tumor)
c. When excision is just as easy as biopsy (e.g. splenectomy for splenic masses or small mast cell tumors)
3. **Rules for taking a biopsy:**
   a. **Biopsy at the margin** of the normal and abnormal tissue. An exception for this rule is for suspected osteosarcoma, where the biopsy should be obtained from the center of the lesion. Biopsying at the margins allows the histopathologist to determine the invasiveness of the mass. Avoid biopsying necrotic or ulcerated tissue.
   b. Get the **largest sample** possible because it's more likely to yield an accurate diagnosis.
   c. **Don't use electrocautery, and be careful not to crush** the tissue as it damages tumor architecture.
   d. Make the biopsy incision **following the lines of skin tension** (e.g. on the tail, the incision should be longitudinal, not transverse).
   e. When collecting an aspirate or biopsy, **be careful not to seed healthy tissue.** That is, perform the procedures in a manner so that if the mass is later removed, removal can include the biopsy tract.
   f. **Fix the tissue in 10% formalin** for 24-48 hours. If the tissue is greater than 1 cm wide, place incomplete slices through it (like a loaf of bread). Any samples that will be submitted for culture should not be placed in formalin. Large tumors may be placed in saline in the refrigerator until your pathology service comes to collect the sample. This will allow the pathologist to evaluate the tumor *in situ* and orient her/himself when collecting margins.
   g. **Mark the margins** of interest by dipping them in india ink or with special tissue stains. When the ink has dried, place the sample in formalin. You can use different colored ink to denote different margins (so you know which side needs the wider excision in the case where you do not have clean margins). Suture and/or staples can also be used to identify margins.
   h. Submit the sample to a **skilled veterinary pathologist** along with a **detailed history.** If the results are not what you expected, do not be afraid to call your pathologist and discuss both the case and the results.
4. **Types of biopsies:** Where local anesthesia is used, be careful not to distort the tissues being biopsied with the lidocaine.

TYPES of BIOPSIES

TECHNIQUE	ANESTHETIC	TISSUE	OTHER
Punch Biopsy	Local anesthetic or brief general	Dermis only	Include the junction of normal and abnormal tissues.
Core Needle Biopsy	Local or brief general	Dermal, epidermal, or subcutaneous tissues	(Tru-cut®, BiopT) The small tissue sample may not be diagnostic. Use a blade to make a stab incision in the skin, then insert the biopsy needle. Take 3-5 samples.
Incisional Biopsy (wedge resection)	General or local anesthetic	Dermal, epidermal, or subcutaneous tissues	Provides a larger tissue sample than the first two methods. Be sure to include the junction of normal and abnormal tissue. Remember that subsequent excisional surgery must remove the entire tumor and past surgery sites. Use incisional biopsies on the distal limbs where you want to get a big sample but don't want to remove the whole mass (reconstructive surgery required).
Excisional Biopsy	General anesthesia	Any mass	Use this when the tissue is small enough that wide surgical excision can be easily performed. Cytology should be performed first to determine whether conservative or wide excision is needed (cyst vs. tumor) even if the mass is small. Sometimes small tumors appear easily excisable but have tendrils that extend much farther into normal tissue than expected.

Oncology

II. **ADDITIONAL WORK-UP:** Once diagnosis is confirmed and before initiating treatment, evaluate the general health of the animal, identify paraneoplastic syndromes, and determine the anatomic extent of the disease or stage of the disease.
  A. **BLOODWORK:** Perform a complete CBC, chemistry panel, and urinalysis to rule out complications of disease such as infection from immunosuppression, and to rule out the presence of liver or renal failure, which would make chemotherapy more dangerous.

  B. **LYMPH NODE BIOPSY or CYTOLOGY:** Biopsy or aspirate any suspicious lymph nodes.

  C. **IMAGING—Radiographs, ultrasound, CT scan, or MRI:** Take radiographs (Always include thoracic radiographs), and/or perform an ultrasound, CT scan, or MRI to detect metastatic disease, determine the extent of the primary disease, and help plan the best surgical approach. For example, abdominal ultrasound is commonly performed for diseases such as lymphosarcoma to look for abdominal lymph node, splenic, or hepatic involvement (i.e. imaging is used to help stage the disease).

  D. **BONE MARROW ASPIRATE or BIOPSY** should be collected in cases of hematopoietic neoplasms or unexplained cytopenias. They are commonly performed to stage lymphosarcomas.

III. **TREATMENT:** Three treatment modalities are commonly used in oncology.
  A. **SURGERY** can be used for solitary tumors that have not metastasized.
  B. **RADIATION THERAPY** is indicated in cases of microscopic disease following incomplete surgical excision, as a primary treatment of specific tumors, and as palliative therapy for non-resectable tumors.
  C. **CHEMOTHERAPY** is indicated with systemic neoplasms, for adjuvant treatment of incompletely excised or metastatic tumors, and for palliation of non-resectable tumors.
  D. **COMBINATIONS of the three.**

  Immunotherapy and hyperthermia are also used, but their discussion is beyond the scope of this book.

CANINE MAMMARY TUMORS

Mammary tumors are the most common tumors affecting intact female dogs. Over 50% of all tumors in female dogs are mammary tumors, and dogs are three times more likely than humans to get mammary tumors.

PREDILECTIONS	• Toy and miniature poodles, English springer spaniels, pointers, and German shepherds are some of the breeds predisposed to mammary tumors.
	• Occurs most commonly in older adult bitches (9-11 years) that are intact or have been spayed after their second heat.
	• Dogs spayed before their third heat are less likely to develop mammary tumors.
	  • Spay before 1st estrus = 0.5% risk
	  • Spay after 1st estrus = 8% risk
	  • Spay after 2nd estrus = 26% risk
	• Obesity at 1 year of age and high red-meat diets are linked to increased incidence of mammary tumors.

NATURE	50% are malignant carcinomas, adenocarcinomas, or sarcomas. 50% are benign tumors.
CLINICAL PRESENTATION	• These tumors present as single or multiple mammary masses. The masses may be associated with the nipple or with the glandular tissue. A majority of tumors affect the 4th and 5th glands because these glands contain more mammary tissue. • Those that present acutely and are more aggressive may carry a worse prognosis than those that grow slowly over several months. Benign tumors are often small, well-circumscribed, and freely movable. Malignant tumors are often attached to the underlying tissue. • Some tumors present as hot swollen glands (looks like mastitis).
DIAGNOSIS	**Cytology** is often not useful in differentiating between benign or malignant epithelial malignancy. It's better to do an incisional or excisional biopsy. One case where cytology may be helpful is in distinguishing between mastitis and inflammatory carcinoma. **Biopsy:** Incisional or excisional biopsy is diagnostic. Core needle biopsy can also be performed, but it is not as reliable as the other two methods. Prior to excisional biopsy, take **thoracic radiographs** to evaluate the lungs and sternal lymph node for metastasis. If the caudal mammary glands are affected, perform a rectal exam to check the internal iliac nodes. Sublumbar lymph nodes can be examined using radiographs or ultrasound. Aspirate enlarged lymph nodes. If cytology is positive or questionable, you may elect to excise the affected lymph node. **Complete blood count, chemistry** panel and **urinalysis** should be performed to check overall health prior to anesthesia.
TREATMENT	**Surgical excision is the treatment of choice.** • **Lumpectomy:** If the mass is < 5 mm in size, firm, superficial, and well circumscribed, just remove the mass. It's most likely benign. • **Mammectomy** (a.k.a. mastectomy): If the mass is greater than 1 cm or is associated with glandular tissue, remove the entire gland. If it involves the 4th or 5th gland, then remove both glands because these glands are associated. • **Radical mastectomy** has not been proven more effective. • **Lymph node removal:** Remove the inguinal node when it's enlarged and positive for cancer and whenever gland 5 is removed (they are intimately associated). Don't remove it prophylactically. The use of chemotherapy and radiation therapy in the management of this disease has not been adequately evaluated in the canine patient.
PROGNOSIS	**Tumor size and type** are the most important prognostic indicators. Mammary **adenocarcinomas** that are small (< 3 cm), non-ulcerated, and freely movable yield a better prognosis because they are probably benign. If the regional lymph nodes are affected, the prognosis is worse. Tumors that are less differentiated yield a worse prognosis. Sarcomas and inflammatory carcinomas yield a poor prognosis. Two year survival time is 25-40% (however this number does not differentiate between tumors size or clinical stage).

Oncology

CANINE MAST CELL TUMORS (MCT)

MCTs are the most common cutaneous tumors in the dog, accounting for up to 20% of all cutaneous canine tumors. They are usually easy to diagnose on cytology.

PREDILECTION	Can occur in any age or breed of dog but are usually found in older dogs (mean = 8-9 years). They occur more commonly in brachycephalic breeds (boxers, bulldogs, Boston terriers, pugs), Labrador retrievers, and sharpeis. MCTs in boxers are usually well-differentiated, low grade tumors. Those in shar-peis tend to be aggressive.
PATHO-PHYSIOLOGY	Upon activation, mast cells degranulate, releasing vasoactive amines such as histamine and heparin, as well as cytokines and other inflammatory mediators. These products cause local hypersensitivity (wheal), or worse, systemic hypersensitivity (anaphylactic shock).
CLINICAL PRESENTATION	SKIN: MCTs can look like anything. They may present as solitary dermal or subcutaneous masses, but can also present as multiple skin tumors (frequently very small). MCTs are often alopecic, erythematous, and may be ulcerated. They can also mimic many other skin lesions such as lipomas, papules, crusts, nodules, and tumors. MCTs can be slow growing (> 6 months) or can be recognized acutely, especially when manipulation leads to degranulation and consequently wheal formation (Darier's sign). These masses can have a history of growing and then shrinking within a short time period (24 hours) such that it mimics a bug bite or bee sting. This is most common with high grade MCTs. SYSTEMIC SIGNS: • **35% of dogs with MCTs have GI ulcers** (due to histamine release which induces H_2 receptors in the parietal cells, subsequently leading to increased gastric acid production). Systemic signs include **vomiting, anorexia, melena**, and subsequent **hematochezia**. • **Heparin** release can result in signs associated with **coagulation abnormalities**.
DIAGNOSIS	Diagnosis can often be made on aspiration cytology: Cytology reveals a monomorphic population of round cells with basophilic granules. Eosinophils may be present due to their attraction to histamine. A small percentage of high grade MCTs (less differentiated) have granules that don't stain well. In these cases, the diagnosis is based on histopathology. Due to the need for larger surgical margins, all skin masses should be aspirated for evidence of MCTs prior to excision. A negative aspirate does not rule out MCT though. A biopsy is needed for grading.
GRADE	Histological grade is based on biopsy. If the tumor can be surgically excised with wide margins and the animal has no systemic signs or evidence of lymph node metastasis on physical exam (no LN enlargement and aspirate is negative), remove the mass and submit it for histopathological grading and margin analysis. Then stage it if it's a grade II or III tumor. If you're unable to remove the mass due to size, location, etc., perform a punch biopsy. Tumors that are more differentiated are less likely to spread systemically, thus they have a better prognosis. • **Grade I MCTs are well-differentiated** and stay within the dermis. These tumors have a low metastatic potential (< 10-25% metastasis). • **Grade II MCTs are moderately differentiated** and invade into surrounding tissues. They have a moderately low metastatic rate (15-40% metastasis). • **Grade III MCTs are poorly differentiated** and invade into the surrounding tissues. Grade III MCTs have a high metastatic rate (50-95%). Special stains may be required to identify the intracytoplasmic granules in these MCTs.

Canine Mast Cell Tumors (MCT) continued

WORK-UP (CLINICAL STAGING)	Regional lymph nodes should be routinely aspirated and if results are equivocal, they should be removed. Further staging is indicated in cases where:
	1) The animal shows signs of systemic illness or has lymphadenopathy
	2) The tumor requires extensive, aggressive surgery for removal
	3) The tumor requires expensive radiotherapy or the tumor is grade III and likely to metastasize
	4) The patient has had a MCT before, has multiple MCTs, or has regional lymph node involvement (regardless of grade).
	Because metastasis is rare with grade I tumors, clinical staging is not mandatory like it is for grade II and III tumors.
	The goals of further work-up are to **look for systemic spread** and screen the animal for concurrent disease that would make it a poor candidate for extensive treatment.
	• **Aspirate** the regional lymph nodes regardless of size but especially enlarged **lymph nodes.**
	• **Abdominal radiographs and ultrasound:** Look for hepatomegaly or splenomegaly and evidence of metastasis to these organs or abdominal lymph nodes. Aspirate abnormal looking organs.
	• **Thoracic radiographs:** If the MCT is on the cranial half of the body take thoracic radiographs to look for intrathoracic lymphadenopathy.
	• **CBC:** Look for eosinophilia, basophilia, and mast cells, all of which may indicate systemic mast cell spread (rare). Anemia may occur due to GI bleeding from histamine release.
	• **Bone marrow aspirates and buffy coat smears** are not needed. Only about 2% of patients have positive buffy coats.
	• Occult blood in stool indicates GI ulceration.
TREATMENT	• **Surgically excise** solitary tumors that are amenable to wide surgical margins and that have no lymph node or systemic involvement (3 cm margins on all sides and one fascial plane below is the standard in surgical oncology. Some recent studies indicate that 2 cm margins or margins that are equal to the width of the MCT may be adequate). Surgical excision is **curative in that spot** if the margins are wide and there is no metastasis. If histopathology reveals incomplete surgical margins, consult an oncologist. Incomplete margins are associated with recurrence in some cases.
	• **Radiation therapy** when combined with surgery offers an excellent prognosis for local control (> 80% for grade I and II MCTs).
	• **Chemotherapy** is indicated in cases of grade III disease, metastatic disease, grade II tumors in locations where they are likely to metastasize (e.g. prepuce, oral), and any MCT with lymph node metastasis. The prognosis is poor and treatment is palliative; however, in cases with complete resection and no metastasis, chemotherapy may markedly prolong life span. Drugs used include prednisone, vinblastine, cyclophosphamide, chlorambucil, and lomustine, among others.
	Treat with diphenhydramine (2-4 mg/kg PO BID) prior to surgery and use GI protectants if needed (Refer to GI section p. 10.11).
PROGNOSIS	**Tumor grade and clinical staging are the best predictors of prognosis.** Dogs with higher grade tumors, with lymph node involvement, or those that are systemically ill have a worse prognosis.
	• Well differentiated tumors: 80-90% long term survival
	• Intermediate differentiated: 50-85% long term survival if completely excised
	• Undifferentiated: Most patients die within 6 months due to metastasis or local recurrence
	Tumor location: Tumors located on the extremities have a better prognosis. Tumors on the prepuce, perineum, muzzle, or in the oral cavity tend to have a poorer prognosis because they are usually less differentiated and have metastasized by the time of diagnosis.
	Growth rate: Tumors that grow quickly and are ulcerated have a poorer prognosis.
	Systemic signs: Dogs with systemic signs have a worse prognosis.

Oncology

SELECT TUMORS
Hemangiosarcoma
Melanoma
Lymphoma
Canine Oral Tumors

HEMANGIOSARCOMA (HSA) IN DOGS
Hemangiosarcomas are malignant endothelial cell tumors (tumors of the blood vessels).

COMMON SITES	Spleen and right atrium are the most common locations. Solar-induced cutaneous HSA occurs in areas lacking fur or coloration.
BIOLOGIC BEHAVIOR	This tumor is very aggressive with infiltration and metastasis occurring early in the course of the disease (except in the cutaneous form). The cutaneous form has decreased metastatic potential but the subcutaneous form can be aggressive.
CLINICAL SIGNS	Signs range from lethargy to acute collapse and death from hemorrhage (tumor rupture or coagulopathy). Animals are frequently **anemic** due to intracavitary bleeding or microangiopathic hemolysis. DIC can occur. **Splenic HSA** may lead to abdominal distention (due to size or bleeding). **Cardiac HSA** can cause arrhythmias and/or right congestive heart failure (pericardial tamponade or obstruction of the caudal vena cava). **Cutaneous HSA** may appear as a mass or nodule.
DIAGNOSTIC FINDINGS	• **Anemia** that is strongly regenerative: Bleeding is internal so iron is conserved and reused which allows a robust regenerative response. • **Thrombocytopenia** is consistent with DIC (about 90,000 cells/μL rather than being really low as with ITP). • **Left shift** and monocytosis: Blood loss causes release of cells from the marginal pool. • **Schistocytes** and acanthocytosis occur because the blood vessels are abnormal and have fibrin strands in them (which shear the RBCs). • **Elevated nRBCs:** The bone marrow releases immature RBCs in response to anemia. Usually the spleen pulls out nuclei from nRBCs, but with splenic HSA the spleen can't perform this function. On further evaluation using **ultrasound** (and sometimes **radiographs**), look for a primary or metastatic mass that can be biopsied for a definitive diagnosis of hemangiosarcoma. Always perform an echocardiogram to look for signs of HSA affecting the heart. **Histopathology** is the definitive way to diagnose hemangiosarcoma. Unfortunately, cytology of effusions most commonly contains only blood. Therefore, surgical removal of the affected organ will allow a diagnosis and stop the life-threatening hemorrhage. Since 50-60% of splenic masses in dogs are non-neoplastic, surgery can cure the bleeding in some dogs.
PROGNOSIS/ TREATMENT	Disease has metastasized in 80% of HSA dogs by the time they present. Most dogs die from metastatic disease within 2-4 months. Adjuvant chemotherapy may increase survival in a subgroup of dogs.

MELANOMA

SITES	**Dogs:** Cutaneous, sublingual, or oral (most common canine oral tumor). **Cats:** Usually ocular (most common feline ocular tumor) or oral; cutaneous is less common.
CLINICAL PRESENTATION	**Dogs:** Usually a solitary mass. It can be a black macule or it can be a dark brown or amelanotic mass. Malignant tumors are frequently ulcerated with secondary infection. They often invade bone. Metastases are common but may be slow-growing. Dogs may not develop signs from metastasis for months to years. **Cats:** Buphthalmos, change in iris color (iridal melanoma), glaucoma.
TREATMENT	• Wide surgical excision of any melanoma. • Early enucleation in cats with ocular melanoma.
PROGNOSIS	**Dogs:** Ungual melanomas metastasize in 30-50% of patients. Most patients with oral or mucocutaneous melanomas die from distant metastases. The one-year survival in dogs with oral melanoma is 40%. If these tumors are < 2 cm the dog may survive 18 months. These tumors often metastasize to the lymph nodes and lungs. **Cats:** Ocular melanomas are often malignant, although metastasis may not be apparent for years. Prognosis for cutaneous melanomas is good. In both dogs and cats, benign melanomas carry a good prognosis with surgical excision.

LYMPHOMA

Lymphoma is a malignant tumor of the lymphocytes that originates in lymphocytes of solid organs (peripheral lymph nodes, Peyer's patches of the GI tract, etc). It's the most commonly treated systemic cancer in veterinary medicine and is highly treatable.

CLINICAL SIGNS	Palpate firm, markedly to severely enlarged peripheral lymph nodes. Lymphoma that originates in the GI tract may cause vomiting, diarrhea, lethargy, anorexia, and weight loss.
DIAGNOSIS	Cytology and biopsy of an affected lymph node reveals high numbers of immature or undifferentiated lymphocytes with multiple nucleoli and mitotic figures. Biopsy is occasionally required for a definitive diagnosis. Perform cytology or histopathology on any unexplained enlarged lymph node. If you suspect a tumor, it's best to take an excisional biopsy because this preserves the lymph node architecture and includes the lymph node capsule, which the pathologist evaluates for cell invasion. When possible, avoid obtaining the sample from the submandibular lymph nodes since these nodes are usually reactive because they drain the oral cavity.
STAGING	Stage I: Neoplasm is limited to one lymphoid tissue or organ (e.g. one lymph node is involved). Stage II: A chain of lymph nodes is involved (e.g. a chain of nodes in the submandibular area may be involved). Stage III: Generalized lymph node involvement (e.g. all peripheral lymph nodes are involved). Stage IV: The spleen or liver is involved. Stage V: Bone marrow is involved. B-cell lymphoma is bad, but T-cell lymphoma is terrible (worse prognosis).
PROGNOSIS	Without therapy, animals survive an average of 2-6 weeks. With chemotherapy, 75% go into clinical remission. The average length of survival ranges from about 7 months (cats) to 12-14 months (dogs). 30% may survive 2 years.

CANINE OROPHARYNGEAL TUMORS

All of these tumors should be biopsied and oral radiographs or CT scan should be taken to determine the type and extent of bony involvement prior to devising a treatment plan.

	DESCRIPTION	TREATMENT
Malignant Melanoma	The mass may be pigmented or non-pigmented. This tumor is aggressive. Bone invasion and metastasis are common. Animals usually die from metastasis or recurrence.	Radical surgical excision ± radiation
Fibrosarcoma	Pink, sessile, fleshy, firm mass on the gingiva or palate. Fibrosarcomas deeply infiltrate soft tissue and bone.	Radical surgical excision ± radiation
Squamous Cell Carcinoma	Sessile, fleshy, friable mass or progressive, ulcerative, and infiltrative lesion (usually invading bone). The behavior is location dependent. More rostral masses are locally invasive with low metastatic potential. They may travel down the marrow cavity though. More caudal masses (tonsils, tongue base, pharynx, etc.) are very infiltrative and metastatic.	Radical surgical excision ± radiation
Epulides	Fleshy tumors of the gingiva. They are sessile and deeply invasive, usually located in the rostral or pre-maxillary gingiva. Fibromatous or ossifying epulides are benign and easily cured with surgery. Acanthomatous epulides invade bone and can cause severe facial distortion and mechanical interference with mastication.	Wide *en bloc* excision is indicated for acanthomatous epulides. Radiation is an option if excision is incomplete or impossible.

For all malignant oral tumors and acanthomatous epulides, biopsy is required for a diagnosis. Radiographs should be performed to evaluate bone involvement, however a CT provides a much better assessment of the extent of disease. Because aggressive surgery is needed to remove the tumor, gathering together an oncology team is the best approach to the management of these diseases.

Oncology

CHEMOTHERAPEUTICS / ANTINEOPLASTIC DRUGS

DRUG	MECHANISM OF ACTION	USE	TOXICITY
ANTIMETABOLITE 5-fluorouracil Azothioprine Methotrexate Cytosine arabinoside Gemcitabine	Inhibit enzymes of the purine and/or pyrimidine biosynthesis	**5-Fluorouracil (5-FU):** Carcinomas of glandular structures such as: • Mammary glands • GI carcinomas • Thyroid carcinoma • Squamous Cell Carcinoma **Azothioprine (Imuran):** • Autoimmune disease **Cytosine arabinoside (Cytosar):** • Lymphoma • Myeloproliferative diseases • CNS lymphoma **Methotrexate:** • Lymphoma • (Osteosarcoma and CNS neoplasia)	• Neurotoxicity: cerebellar signs • Contraindicated in cats! • Mild myelosuppression • GI: moderate signs • Crosses the BBB • Myelosuppression • Moderate myelosuppression, thrombophlebitis (Crosses the BBB) • GI: vomiting, diarrhea • Bone marrow depressant • Renal tubular necrosis is a side effect of excretion
ALKYLATING AGENTS Cyclophosphamide Chlorambucil Lomustine	Covalently bind to DNA causing crosslinking and miscoding	**Cyclophosphamide (Cytoxan):** • Lymphoma or Leukemia • (Some solid tumors) • Autoimmune disorders **Chlorambucil (Leukeran):** • Lymphoma or Leukemia (CLL)	• Myelosuppression in 7-14 days • Chemical cystitis, especially with > 9 weeks of continuous use • GI: vomiting, diarrhea (rescue with Mucomyst) • Mild leukopenia • Cummulative hepatotoxicity
ANTITUMOR ANTIBIOTICS Doxorubicin Bleomycin Mitoxantrone	Form stable complexes with DNA, inhibiting DNA replication or mRNA transcription	**Doxorubicin (Adriamycin):** • Lymphoma • Myeloproliferative diseases • (Sarcomas or Carcinomas) **Mitoxantrone:** Squamous cell carcinoma, transitional cell carcinoma, and sarcomas	• Moderate to severe myelosuppression in 10-12 days, irreversible dilated cardiomyopathy (DCM) in dogs • Alopecia, hyperpigmentation • GI: anorexia, vomiting, and diarrhea, especially in cats • Nephrotoxicity occurs more commonly in cats Anaphylaxis, vesicant (e.g. causes blistering) • Myelosuppression • Rare GI signs

14.10

PLANT ALKALOIDS Vincristine Vinblastine	Interfere with microtubule formation, preventing formation of the mitotic spindle. Resistance to one drug does not imply resistance to the other drugs.	**Vincristine (Oncovin):** • Lymphoma • Transmissible venereal tumors • (Sarcomas or carcinomas) • (Mast cell tumors) **Vinblastine (Velban):** same as vincristine	• Peripheral neuropathy • GI: pancreatitis, constipation, ileus • Rare myelosuppression • Myelosuppressive in 4-7 days • Peripheral neuropathy • GI: pancreatitis, constipation, ileus
HORMONAL AGENTS Glucocorticoids Estrogens Androgens	Lympholytic Suppresses antibody function Suppresses RES function	**Glucocorticoids:** • Lymphoma • Lymphoproliferative diseases • Myeloproliferative diseases • Mast cell tumors • Immune mediated diseases	• GI: stomach ulcers, pancreatitis • Metabolic: Cushings; PU/PD, panting
Miscellaneous Carboplatin Cisplatin (Platinol®)	Inhibits DNA synthesis by cross-linking complimentary strands of DNA	• Osteosarcoma • Transitional cell carcinomas (TCC) • Squamous cell carcinomas (SCC) • (Primary bronchiogenic carcinomas)	• Nephrotoxicity (acute tubular necrosis) • Primary pulmonary toxicity • **Contraindicated in cats** (carboplatin is used in cats) • Mild leukopenia and thrombocytopenia in an unpredictable fashion. Vomiting is common during administration.
Miscellaneous L-asparaginase (Elspar®)	Destroys extracellular stores of L-asparagine, leading to death of cancer cells lacking the enzymatic ability to synthesize this amino acid.	• Lymphoma • Lymphoproliferative disorders • (Mast cell tumors)	• Myelosuppression (rare alone) • Anaphylaxis • Pancreatitis • Peritonitis

* For diseases in parentheses, treatment has not been proven to increase survival, thus use of the given drug for the specific tumor is controversial.

CONVERTING BODY WEIGHT TO m^2

Table for Converting Body Weight in Kg to Body Surface Area in Meters Squared for the DOG			
Kg	Square mm	Kg	Square mm
0.5	0.06	25	0.85
1	0.10	26	0.88
2	0.15	27	0.90
3	0.20	28	0.92
4	0.25	29	0.94
5	0.29	30	0.96
6	0.33	31	0.99
7	0.36	32	1.01
8	0.40	33	1.03
9	0.43	34	1.05
10	0.46	35	1.07
11	0.49	36	1.09
12	0.52	37	1.11
13	0.55	38	1.13
14	0.58	39	1.15
15	0.60	40	1.17
16	0.63	41	1.19
17	0.66	42	1.21
18	0.69	43	1.23
19	0.71	44	1.25
20	0.74	45	1.26
21	0.76	46	1.28
22	0.78	47	1.30
23	0.81	48	1.32
24	0.83	49	1.34
		50	1.36

Conversion From Pounds of Body Weight to Body Surface Area (m^2) for the CAT		
Weight (pounds)	Weight (Kg)	BSA (m^2)
5	2.3	0.165
6	2.8	0.187
7	3.2	0.207
8	3.6	0.222
9	4.1	0.244
10	4.6	0.261
11	5.1	0.278
12	5.5	0.294
13	6.0	0.311
14	6.4	0.326
15	6.9	0.342
16	7.4	0.356
17	7.8	0.371
18	8.2	0.385
19	8.7	0.399
20	9.2	0.413

$$\frac{\text{Weight (grams)}^{2/3} \times \text{K (constant)}}{10^4} = \text{m}^2\text{BSA} \qquad \begin{array}{l} \text{K (cat)} = 10 \\ \text{K (dog)} = \end{array}$$
10.1

COMMON OPHTHALMIC DRUGS and DOSAGES

DRUG	DOG DOSE	CAT DOSE
Aspirin 65, 81, 325, 500 mg	Anterior uveitis 20-30 mg/kg PO TID	
Atropine ophthalmic ointment	Treat affected eye q 6-12 hours initially and then decrease the dose to the minimum effective dose.	
Azathioprine (Imuran®) 50 mg tablets Monitor CBC for leukopenia.	1 mg/kg PO SID for 1-2 weeks, then every other day to every 4-7 days for maintenance.	
Clindamycin 25 mg/mL in 20 mL bottle 25, 75, 150 mg capsules		For cats with suspect toxoplasmosis: 12.5 mg/kg PO BID for 21 days or 30 mg/cat divided BID-TID.
Cyclosporine (Optimmune®)	SID or BID	
Dexamethasone 1% (Maxidex® or Maxitrol®)	q 2-6 hours	q 2-6 hours
Dichlorphenamide (Daranide®): a carbonic anhydrase inhibitor 50 mg tablets	2-5 mg/kg PO TID	1 mg/kg PO BID-TID
Diclofenac sodium 0.1% (Voltaren®): a topical NSAID Caution: Can elevate IOP	1 drop BID. Caution: Should be used with discretion in patients prone to secondary glaucoma.	
Dipivefrin HCL 0.1% (Propine®): an epinephrine prodrug	1 drop BID	1 drop BID
Dorzolamide HCL 2% (Trusopt®): a carbonic anhydrase inhibitor	1 drop BID to TID	
Flubiprofen 0.03% (Ocufen®)	1 drop q 2-6 hours	1 drop q 2-6 hours
Glycerine (90%)	1-2 mg/kg PO	
Idoxuridine (0.1% solution or 0.5% ointment), compounded		1 drop q 4-6 hours until signs of herpes infection resolve. Then BID for 1-2 weeks.
Latanoprost (Xalatan®)	1 drop SID-TID	1 drop SID-TID
Mannitol 20% solution	5-7.5 mL/kg over 15-20 minutes (1-1.5 g/kg) IV. Withhold water for 3-4 hours post IV mannitol. Contraindicated in azotemic or dehydrated patient. Administer using an in-line IV filter (0.22 μm) with solutions this concentrated.*	
Methazolamide (Neptazane®): a carbonic anhydrase inhibitor	1-2 mg/kg PO BID-TID	1-2 mg/kg PO BID-TID
Prednisolone acetate (1% Pred Forte®)	q 4-6 hours or more frequently	q 4-6 hours or more frequently
Prednisone (oral) 5, 20 mg	Anterior uveitis 0.5-1.0 mg/kg PO BID for at least one week and then taper.	
Timolol 0.5% (Timoptic®) and 0.25% (dogs < 10 kg) 2.5, 5, 10, 15 mL bottles	1 drop BID. Caution: May cause bradycardia, particularly in animals less than 10 kg. Use with caution in cardiac patients.	
Trifluridine (Viroptic®)	TID-QID. Can be topically irritating.	

*http://www.utmb.edu/rxhome/Operations/Filtrations.htm

THE OPHTHALMOLOGY EXAMINATION

The ophthalmology exam must be methodical and complete. If you don't perform all of the steps and specifically look for problems, you won't find them.

OVERVIEW: STEPS in the OPHTHALMOLOGY EXAM

- **At a distance,** assess vision and symmetry (including strabismus, which assesses cranial nerves III, IV, VI).
- **Blink and menace responses** assess cranial nerves II, V, VII.
- **Adnexa:** Assess the eyelids, nictitans, conjunctiva, and eyelashes.

Turn the light out and use an ophthalmoscope. Check the pupillary light responses (PLR), and then examine the cornea and anterior chamber on each side.
- **Pupillary light responses**
- **Cornea:** Vessels, pigment, edema, lipid/calcium deposits, scar, ulcer
- **Anterior chamber:** Check the anterior chamber for content and size abnormalities. Then examine the iris. Remember to check for aqueous flare.

Dilate the pupils, and then examine the lens and fundus. Perform a Schirmer's tear test first if indicated. Do so prior to instilling any type of drops in the eye. Do not dilate the pupils if the animal has glaucoma or signs of lens luxation (aphakic crescent or vitreous in the anterior chamber). If you suspect glaucoma, then measure the intraocular pressure. In general, if the eye is nonpainful and the PLRs are intact, then it's okay to dilate the pupils.
- **Other tests:** While waiting for the pupils to dilate, other tests such as fluorescein stain, cytology, culture, lacrimal cannulation, and performance in an obstacle course can be conducted.
- **Fundic reflection:** Check for opacifications. Then do a retinal exam.

I. STEPS in the OPHTHALMOLOGY EXAM
   A. **EXAM FROM A DISTANCE:** From a distance, evaluate orbital symmetry, vision, and cranial nerves II, III, IV, VI.
      1. **Evaluate vision at a distance** (cranial nerve II and cerebral cortex): Can the animal maneuver around the room, or does it walk tentatively and bump into things? Does it look at objects that it hears? Vision can be further evaluated later in the exam.
      2. **Symmetry of the palpebral fissures and of eye placement within the sockets**
         a. Are the palpebral fissures symmetric or is one side too large or small?

ABNORMAL FINDINGS	RULE-OUTS	DIFFERENTIATING FEATURES
Palpebral fissure too large on one side	Buphthalmos (large globe)	• Look down from the top. The exophthalmic eye often protrudes more than the buphthalmic eye. • Compare cornea size. The buphthalmic cornea is larger than the cornea of the normal eye.
	Exophthalmos (protruding globe)	• Retropulse the globes. The exophthalmic eye does not retropulse well since it's often malplaced due to retrobulbar hemorrhage, abscess, or mass. • Open the mouth. With retrobulbar abscesses, the animal may show pain on opening its mouth, or you may see evidence of an abscess in the pharyngeal area on the side of the affected eye.
Palpebral fissure too small on one side	Blepharospasm (spasm due to pain)	• If the cornea size is decreased, the eye is microphthalmic. • Check for evidence of **pain. Blepharospasm** and **enophthalmus** can be caused by pain. Blepharospasm should disappear with topical anesthetic or iridocycloplegics.
	Enophthalmos (retracted globe)	
	Ptosis (droopy upper eyelid)	• **Miosis** can occur with pain but can also occur with sympathetic nerve damage (e.g., Horner's syndrome - miosis, ptosis, and enophthalmos). • Check for **neurologic deficits** on the same side as the affected eye (e.g., facial paralysis, lameness, etc.).
	Microphthalmos (small globe)	• Check for evidence of corneal ulceration (corneal ulcers are painful).

   b. Are the eyes symmetrically placed within the sockets or is
       strabismus present? Do the eyes move symmetrically (conjugate
       motion) when they are following an object? If there is no strabismus
       and the eyes move symmetrically, then cranial nerves III, IV, VI are intact.

The rest of the ophthalmology exam is done "hands-on" at eye level.

B   CRANIAL NERVES (VISION and BLINK)
   1. **Test for the blink response** (cranial nerves V and VII): Touch the lateral or
       medial canthus and watch for a blink response. Is the blink response complete
       and symmetric? This tests cranial nerves V (sensory to the face) and VII (motor
       to the face and ears). If the blink is not complete, the animal has
       lagophthalmos. Look for exposure keratitis in the central or ventromedial
       portion of the cornea.

   2. **Menace response** only works if the animal has learned to respond (it tests
       cranial nerves II and VII and the cerebral cortex). If you're unsure about the
       animal's vision, then go to the cotton ball test.

   3. **Cotton ball test:** Drop a cotton ball in front of the animal and see if it
       watches the cotton drop. Test different visual fields by tossing the cotton ball
       from behind the animal into different visual fields. If the animal is uninterested in
       the cotton ball, find a toy or treat that it shows interest in, and move the object
       in and out of its visual field to see if it tracks the toy or treat. Alternatively toss
       increasingly smaller treats and see if the animal can track and find them easily
       by sight. If needed, you can test for night and day vision with an obstacle
       course at the end of the examination.

C. **ADNEXAL EXAMINATION:** The adnexa consist of the eyelids, conjunctiva, nictitans,
    lacrimal ducts, etc. Look for:
   1. **Discharge:**
       a. Ocular discharge, both serous and purulent, indicates irritation (e.g., viral,
           bacterial, trauma, etc.). It can also be caused by blocked lacrimal ducts.
           Note: Purulent discharge is not pathognomonic for bacteria. Any
           chemotactic stimulation of neutrophils can cause a purulent discharge.
       b. Mucoid discharge may indicate keratoconjunctivitis sicca (KCS).
   2. **Chemosis:** Chemosis and conjunctival edema indicates acute irritation due to a
       chemical irritant, foreign body, trauma, etc. Cats with *Chlamydophila* often
       develop chemosis, too.
   3. **Nictitans:** Look for protrusion of the nictitans, erythema, and follicles.
       Lymphoid follicles located on the external surface of the nictitans indicate
       chronic antigenic stimulation or chronic irritation.
   4. **Eyelid disorders:**
       a. **Eyelid agenesis:** Lack of a complete eyelid.
       b. **Entropion** or **ectropion:** Note any asymmetry in the length or position of
           the eyelid margins and the globes. Be careful to differentiate entropion
           from spastic blepharospasm due to pain. You can do so by applying topical
           anesthetic and an iridocycloplegic to the eye. **Blepharospasm** will
           disappear.
       c. **Lagophthalmos:** Poor closure of the upper eyelid.
       d. **Chalazion** is an eyelid mass or pustule caused by inflammation of the
           Meibomian gland and inspissated secretory material within the gland. It's
           painless and can be viewed from the palpebral conjunctiva as a yellow mass.
       e. **Stye (or hordeolum)** is a bacterial infection of the Meibomian gland. It
           should be treated with hotpacks and systemic or local antibiotics. Surgical
           incision/drainage may be required.
       f. **Eyelid tumors**

   5. **Eyelash disorders:** Use some form of magnification to see eyelash disorders.
       a. **Distichiasis** is the presence of abnormally placed eyelashes that arise from
           the Meibomian gland opening (lid margin).
       b. **Trichiasis** is the presence of normally located hairs directed abnormally so
           that they contact the globe (e.g., nasal folds). When you see pigmentation

in the medial canthus of brachycephalic dogs with prominent nasal folds, don't assume the pigment is due to trichiasis; it may be caused by lagophthalmos.

c. **Ectopic cilia** are eyelashes that arise from the Meibomian gland and emerge through the palpebral conjunctiva. Evert the eyelid slightly or palpate the palpebral conjunctiva to find ectopic cilia. They most commonly occur at 12 o'clock on the upper eyelid, but lower eyelids can also be affected.

Use an ophthalmoscope or transilluminator for the rest of the examination. Check the PLRs here.

D. CHECK the PUPILLARY LIGHT RESPONSE. (Refer to neurology p.12.5 for more information.)

E. **CORNEA:** The corneal surface should appear smooth with a bright luster. Using a transilluminator, evaluate the cornea for evidence of blood vessels, pigment, and other opacities.

1. **Vessels** are a nonspecific indicator of disease.
   a. **Superficial vessels** are long and thin, and branch like a tree. They indicate superficial disease.
   b. **Deep vessels** are short and nonbranching. They indicate deep ocular disease (e.g., glaucoma, scleritis, anterior uveitis).
2. **Pigmentation** indicates irritation to the cornea. The location tells us where the irritation is coming from. Pigmentation is a secondary disease. Look for the underlying cause.
3. **Lipid/calcium deposits** in the corneal stroma indicate corneal dystrophy. Steroids can make the problem worse. You must distinguish it from a scar.
4. **Edema** causes corneal opacity.
5. **Scar**
6. **Ulceration:** For better evaluation of corneal ulcers, stain the eye with fluorescein (described later on p. 15.6).

F. **THE ANTERIOR CHAMBER** is the area bounded by the cornea, iris, and anterior lens capsule. The anterior chamber and lens should be translucent. When examining the anterior chamber, first transilluminate the chamber from the front. Then get a side view to look for synechia, masses pushing on the iris, and aqueous flare.

1. **Content abnormalities:** e.g., aqueous flare, hemorrhage (hyphema), hypopyon, lipids, masses, parasites.
   a. **Aqueous flare:** The anterior chamber normally contains very little protein. With breakdown of the blood-aqueous barrier, such as with anterior uveitis or iritis, protein escapes from the uveal vessels into the aqueous. When an abnormally large amount of protein is in the aqueous, light is partially scattered so that if you shine a narrow beam of light into the eye, you can see the beam passing through the anterior chamber. This phenomenon is called aqueous flare, and it indicates **anterior uveitis.** To see aqueous flare, put the ophthalmoscope on the slit setting and hold it less than 1 cm away from the eye with the lights turned out. Then look at the anterior chamber from the side. In the normal eye, you see a beam at the cornea and through the lens but none through the aqueous. With aqueous flare, the beam extends through the aqueous.
   b. **Hypopyon** is the accumulation of purulent material or white blood cells in the anterior chamber. Neutrophils accumulate with any chemotactic stimulus and usually are not due to infection. In cases where there's a deep corneal ulcer, the neutrophils migrated from the iris chamber, not from the cornea.
   c. **Hyphema** is blood in the anterior chamber.
   d. **Keratic precipitates** are accumulations of cells adhered to the corneal endothelium. They can be very small and diffusely located, or large and isolated masses called **mutton fat precipitates.**

2. **Size and shape abnormalities:** Lens luxation, hypermature cataracts, synechia
3. **Iris abnormalities:** Look for iris discoloration, swelling, vessels, persistent pupillary membranes, anterior synechiae (adhesions between iris and cornea), dyscoria, or cysts/tumors. Cysts can be distinguished from tumors because cysts transilluminate.

Dilate the pupils for the rest of the examination.
If the animal needs a Schirmer's tear test (STT), do the STT first. Do not dilate the pupils if the animal has glaucoma or a lens luxation. In general, if the eyes are comfortable and the PLRs are normal, the animal doesn't have glaucoma. When in doubt, measure the IOP first!

Dilate the pupils by placing 1-2 drops (make sure you place the same number of drops in each eye) of **1% tropicamide** onto the dorsal bulbar conjunctiva/cornea of each eye. Normally, maximal dilation of the pupils will take **15-20 minutes**. While waiting for the pupils to dilate, perform ancillary tests such as fluorescein stain, cytology, and culture.

G. **FUNDIC REFLECTION:** With the transilluminator approximately an arm's distance away from the animal and the lights off, shine the light into the animal's eyes and look for the tapetal reflection. This is the most sensitive way to look for an aphakic crescent and abnormal intraocular translucencies (e.g., incipient cataracts). It is also the best way to distinguish nuclear sclerosis from cataracts.
   1. **Lens examination:** If an opacity moves in the same direction as the eye, it is located in the anterior lens. If it moves in the opposite direction of the vision, it is in the posterior lens. If it does not move, it is in the lens.

H. **RETINAL EXAM:** Indirect ophthalmoscopy gives a wider field of view and is the best method for screening patients for fundic abnormalities.
   1. **Optic disk:** Evaluate the color for signs of edema.
   2. **Vessels:** Are they abnormal in caliber? Spare vessels may indicate retinal degeneration.
   3. **Retina:** Is the retina in focus? If not, the animal may have retinal detachment. Also look for retinal hemorrhage. Retinal hemorrhage can be associated with hypertension (especially in cats).

II. **ANCILLARY TESTS:** Schirmer's tear test should be performed prior to any test requiring ophthalmic drops or irritating substances (e.g., fluorescein stain, IOP measurement, conjunctival scraping). The other tests can be performed in any order.

A. **SCHIRMER'S TEAR TEST (STT):** Perform a STT if the animal has a history of mucoid or purulent discharge from either eye, if the conjunctival surfaces appear red, or if there is corneal disease. These signs may indicate inadequate aqueous tear production, which is termed **keratoconjunctivitis sicca** (KCS). Prior to performing the STT, remove any mucoid or mucopurulent material from the conjunctival fornices. This test should be done prior to instilling any ophthalmic drops or irritants (e.g., fluorescein strip).

Normal STT for dogs $\geq$ 15 mm/minute
(for cats, the value is much lower)

B. **TONOMETRY for MEASURING INTRAOCULAR PRESSURE:** Although the equipment is relatively inexpensive, Schiotz tonometry is time consuming, inconvenient, and difficult to perform on many animals. The **Tono-Pen®** is a much better piece of equipment for measuring IOP. Normal pressure is 10-26 mmHg in dogs and 15-25 mmHg in cats.
   1. **Schiotz tonometry:** If your only option is Schiotz tonometry, then first anesthetize the cornea with several drops of **proparacaine**. Proparacaine takes effect in 10 seconds and lasts about 15 minutes when one drop is used and 25 minutes when 2 drops are used. Occasionally, if the eye is quite painful and the conjunctival vessels are congested, several applications 2-3 minutes apart may be necessary.
      a. **Zero the Schiotz tonometer.** The most accurate readings are obtained when a total of 7.5 g is used. To get this, snap the 7.5 g weight onto the plunger. (Actually, the plunger weighs 5.5 g and you are adding 2.0 g when you add the 7.5 g weight.) Grasp the tonometer by the finger plates and rest the corneal plate on the steel dome that is in the holding case. Slowly push down toward the dome until the needle begins to move. When the tonometer is working properly, it will record a value of zero when placed on the dome. If the needle does not register zero, the tonometer may need to

be adjusted. (The instrument must be sent to the manufacturer for proper adjustment. DO NOT BEND THE NEEDLE.)

b. **Take the readings:** Position the animal so that the eye is directly vertical. Place the tonometer on the center of the cornea. Take three readings that are relatively consistent and record the numbers over the total number of grams of weight (i.e., 8/7.5). The normal range for readings is $\pm$ **2.5 scale units** of the total number of grams of weight. For example, if 7.5 grams are being used, the normal range is between 5-10 scale units. Since this is an inverse scale:
   - A low scale reading indicates an elevated IOP (intraocular pressure), or glaucoma.
   - A high scale reading indicates a lowered IOP, which is commonly seen with anterior uveitis due to impaired aqueous production.
   - The human chart (Friedenwald) that comes with the tonometer is also appropriate for dogs and cats.

C. **FLUORESCEIN STAIN** tests the integrity of the corneal epithelium and the patency of the lacrimal ducts. Apply **topical sodium fluorescein dye** to the eye (using a strip). Remove excess dye by flushing the eye with saline. Then examine the eye using a UV light. Corneal uptake indicates a defect in the corneal epithelium (e.g., a corneal ulcer). Passage of fluorescein stain into the nares indicates patent nasolacrimal ducts. If there's no passage, perform a nasolacrimal flush to determine patency. Occasionally, the ducts may enter the oral cavity prior to exiting the nares; consequently, the stain may enter the mouth instead of the nares.

D. **CONJUNCTIVAL/CORNEAL SCRAPING for CYTOLOGY:** This procedure is **contraindicated** in eyes with **deep corneal lesions.**
   1. Place multiple drops of topical anesthetic onto the conjunctiva.
   2. Use a Kimera spatula or the **blunt end of a scalpel blade** to collect material from the conjunctival surface. Resting your hand on the patient's head, use your index finger to retropulse the globe by applying pressure on the upper lid. This causes the third eyelid to slide up over the cornea, protecting the globe and exposing more conjunctival surface for sampling. Scrape the anterior surface of the third eyelid firmly in one direction. Gently tap the cellular material onto a clean microscope slide and allow it to air dry.

E. **CONJUNCTIVAL/CORNEAL CULTURE**
   1. Topically anesthetize the eye (proparacaine) and then crush the protective casing of a **micro-tip culturette** and allow the transport media to wet the tip of the culturette wand. A wet tip will improve the microbial load. Remove the wand from the casing and, while steadying your hand on the lateral aspect of the animal's head, gently roll the tip over the affected region of the cornea. Any conjunctival area will do for a conjunctival culture. Avoid touching the eyelids or conjunctiva if you are doing a corneal culture, since the normal flora in these regions may contaminate your sample. After the tip has contacted the corneal lesion, replace it into the transport casing and submit it to the microbiology lab. Unlike with equines (where the sample should be evaluated for fungal and bacterial organisms), corneal cultures in small animals usually need only be evaluated for bacteria.

F. **LACRIMAL DUCT CANNULATION**
   1. **Indications:**
      a. Chronic epiphora
      b. Dacryocystitis
      c. Diagnosis and treatment of imperforate punctum, dacryocystorhinography
      d. Identification and preservation of punctum and canaliculi after traumatic eyelid laceration

G. **OBSTACLE COURSE/MAZE:** Put the animal through an obstacle course both in a lit room and a dark room. You can use a treat or toy to encourage the animal to approach you through the maze, or toss either in both a lit and dark environment and observe the animal's ability to find the item (if the pet's hungry or motivated to get the toy). If the animal shows signs of nyctalopia, it may be developing **progressive retinal atrophy**—an autosomal recessive trait characterized by increased tapetal hyper-reflectivity, retinal vessel attenuation, decreased nontapetal pigmentation, night blindness that progresses to day blindness, and cataract formation.

APPROACH to the "RED EYE"

First determine the source of the redness, then determine whether the animal has superficial or deep ocular disease.

I.   **SOURCE:** When a patient presents with a chief complaint of red eye, first determine the source of the redness.

SOURCES of the RED
• Conjunctival vessels
• Scleral vessels
• Cornea
• Anterior chamber
• Iris neovascularization

II. **SUPERFICIAL or DEEP OCULAR DISEASE:** Determine whether the redness indicates superficial or deep ocular disease. Deep ocular disease most often requires urgent treatment and may result in blindness if not treated appropriately.

SUPERFICIAL	DEEP
• Conjunctiva • Superficial corneal vessels	• Scleral vessels • Deep corneal vessels • Anterior chamber • Iris neovascularization

III. **ETIOLOGIES of "RED EYE"**

SOURCES of REDNESS

SOURCE of the REDNESS	ETIOLOGIES	DESCRIPTION
Conjunctival vessel prominence indicates superficial disease	Keratoconjunctivitis sicca (KCS) Distichiasis or trichiasis Primary corneal disease or irritation	These are thin and branching, and they move with the conjunctiva. You can distinguish conjunctival engorgement from prominent scleral vessels by placing a drop of phenylephrine or epinephrine into the affected eye. Conjunctival vessels will blanch within 15 seconds.
Scleral vessel engorgement indicates deep ocular disease and can be associated with blindness within 24-48 hours if the underlying disease isn't treated.	Anterior uveitis Glaucoma Scleritis Deep corneal disease	Scleral vessels are thick, straight, and nonbranching. They don't move with the conjunctiva, and they don't blanch when a vasoconstrictor is added.
Corneal vasculature can indicate superficial or deep disease depending on where the vessels are located.	**Superficial vessels** indicate nonspecific irritation (e.g., ulcer, foreign body, KCS). **Deep vessels** are nonspecific indicators of reaction to deep disease (scleritis, deep corneal disease).	**Superficial vessels** cross the limbus and are often long and branching. **Deep vessels** are short and straight with brush borders. You can't see them crossing the limbus because they are deep. They all grow out to the same intensity.
Anterior chamber - hyphema	Same etiologies and appearance as hemorrhage elsewhere in the body. These include: trauma, tumor, hypertension (especially in old cats with renal disease), uveitis, clotting problems, retinal detachment secondary to neovascularization (the retina releases agents that cause neovascularization; these new vessels may be leaky).	
Iris neovascularization	Chronic uveitis Lymphosarcoma (especially in cats with retinal detachment)	In cats with lightly pigmented irises, you normally see the major arterial circle.

CORNEAL ULCERS

CLINICAL SIGNS	• Signs of pain: blepharospasm, photophobia, epiphora • Hyperemic conjunctiva • Corneal edema • ± Corneal vascularization or pigmentation (if chronic)
DIAGNOSIS	• Stain the cornea with **fluorescein** dye. The ulcer takes up stain evenly. Presence of a clear spot in the center of a stained area indicates a descemetocele. Descemet's membrane does not retain stain. • Look for **underlying causes** such as KCS, entropion, distichiasis, ectopic cilia, foreign body. Be sure to fully inspect the eyelids and fornices for foreign bodies and irritants. Also assess blink function and perform a Schirmer tear test (STT). STT should be performed prior to fluorescein staining. • Perform a bacterial culture and/or corneal cytology if the ulcer is progressing rapidly or you suspect infection. This should be done before anything is put into the eye (except for topical anesthetics).
ANATOMY and PHYSIOLOGY of the CORNEA	The cornea is comprised of five layers: the precorneal tear film, the epithelium and its basement membrane, the stroma, Descemet's membrane, and the endothelium. • **Endothelial cells** remove fluid from the stroma into the aqueous. Intraocular pressure (IOP) forces fluid into the cornea. When the IOP is elevated, more fluid enters the cornea than is removed, resulting in corneal edema. • The **epithelium** also removes fluid. If the epithelium is damaged, fluid enters the cornea resulting in corneal edema.

NORMAL CORNEAL HEALING	**Epithelium:** When the epithelium is damaged, the epithelial cells surrounding the margins of the lesion slide in to cover the lesion. The whole cornea can be covered in 4-7 days.
	
	Stroma:
	• **Superficial defects** are filled with epithelial cells.
	• **Deeper defects** are covered by epithelium, but the stroma beneath undergoes further **avascular or vascular healing.**
	  ◦ In **avascular healing**, neutrophils from the tear film or from limbal conjunctival vessels migrate to the defect. Keratocytes in the area transform into fibrocytes and synthesize collagen and mucopolysaccharides, which fill the defect. The collagen fibers are laid down irregularly, resulting in an opaque scar. The density of the scar decreases over time but does not disappear.
	  ◦ In **vascular healing**, the area is invaded by blood vessels from the limbus, allowing inflammatory cells and melanocytes to enter the damaged area. Granulation tissue is laid down and forms a denser scar than that formed with avascular healing. The vessels will eventually collapse and become difficult to visualize. They can still be visualized with a slit lamp, though.

TREATMENT of UNCOMPLICATED ULCERS	Treatment for superficial and deep corneal ulcers is similar, but treatment is more frequent with deep ulcers or ones that are infected or complicated (e.g., treatment TID vs. hourly). • Determine the etiology and use specific therapy to eliminate it (e.g., correct the entropion or remove foreign bodies). • **Topical antibiotics** should be used either prophylactically (disruption of the corneal epithelium makes the eye susceptible to bacterial infection) or based on culture results if the eye is infected. Triple antibiotic ointment and oxytetracycline/polymyxin are good broad-spectrum antibiotics for prophylactic use. • **Atropine** should be used as needed as an iridocycloplegic. • **Oral NSAIDs** such as Rimadyl® or Metacam® can be used for pain in dogs. Metacam® can be used in cats. **Tramadol** (2 mg/kg PO BID in dogs and 1/4 of a 50 mg tablet PO BID in cats) can be used. Be sure to use the formulation that is acetaminophen-free. • **Note:** When administering multiple eye medications, wait 5 minutes between each medication and administer any ointments last. • Place an Elizabethan collar on the animal if it is likely to rub its eye.

CORNEAL ULCERS (continued)

TREATMENT of COMPLICATED ULCERS	**Indolent ulcers (or refractory ulcers)** are ulcers in which the corneal epithelium does not adhere well to the stroma; thus, the ulcers have redundant corneal epithelial edges. Suspect an indolent ulcer if a superficial ulcer persists for 7-10 days and no cause for persistence can be found. They occur in any breed of dog but are more common in Boxers. Treat with corneal debridement and grid keratotomy. Remove the loose epithelial edges using a sterile cotton-tip swab. Then with the dog sedated (if calm) or under general anesthesia (if the dog is energetic or difficult), use a 25-gauge needle. Make linear striations across the cornea in a cross-hatch pattern. These improve the epithelial attachment to the cornea. This may need to be repeated in 10-14 days. Herpesvirus: Cats with non-healing ulcers may have herpesvirus. Herpes can be identified on IFA or PCR, but diagnosis is often made based on response to empirical treatment with antiviral agents such as idoxuridine (q 4-6 hours until clinical signs are gone and then BID for 1-2 weeks) or trifluridine (Viroptic®). Cats often dislike receiving drops but can be quickly counter-conditioned to accept the treatments if owners feed a treat (including the cat's regular wet food, tuna, or cat treats) immediately before, during, and right after the treatment.
TREATMENT of DEEP CORNEAL ULCERS	• **Protease inhibitors** inhibit enzyme destruction. Acetylcysteine is commonly used; however, serum can be collected from the patient, placed in a sterile dropper bottle, and used as a protease inhibitor. With melting ulcers, use protease inhibitor treatment. It should be refrigerated. • **Surgery** (e.g., third eyelid flap, conjunctival flap, corneal graft, corneal suturing) may be needed to maintain corneal integrity and produce optimal healing conditions. Surgery should be performed if the corneal defect is half the thickness of the cornea or deeper. Such deep ulcers, as well as melting corneal ulcers and descemetoceles, are surgical emergencies and require conjunctival or corneal graft surgery.

KERATOCONJUNCTIVITIS SICCA (KCS): dry eye or xerosis

CLINICAL SIGNS	• **Red eye:** The red is due to conjunctival hyperemia. • **Blepharospasm,** accompanied by enophthalmos, is often the first sign. It results from pain and discomfort. • **Mucoid and mucopurulent discharge:** When the aqueous phase of the precorneal tear film (PTF) is absent or the lipid phase is abnormal, mucus accumulates and is not washed down the lacrimal system. The mucus is usually a ropey gray material but may become mucopurulent if the animal develops a secondary bacterial infection. Animals with red eyes and a mucoid or purulent discharge should be tested for KCS (Schirmer tear test). • **Dry, lusterless cornea** ± corneal ulceration • **Corneal vascularization and pigmentation:** In chronic cases, superficial and deep corneal vascularization and pigmentation occur. • **Dry ipsilateral nostril** can indicate neurogenic KCS.
ETIOLOGY	• **Drug-induced: Sulfur-containing drugs** such as sulfadiazine (e.g., trimethoprin/sulfadiazine) and sulfasalazine can cause KCS. EtoGesic® (NSAID) has also been implicated. • **Autoimmune:** 75% of idiopathic KCS cases may involve autoimmune destruction of the lacrimal gland. • **Surgically induced:** KCS can result clinically from removal of a prolapsed gland of the third eyelid. It often does not develop for months to several years after the gland is amputated. • **Orbital and supraorbital trauma** may result in direct damage to the lacrimal gland or to the nerves innervating the lacrimal gland (i.e., damage to the facial nerve can cause KCS). • **Canine distemper:** Canine distemper virus affects the lacrimal gland and gland of the third eyelid and may result in acute KCS with temporary or permanent dysfunction. • **Idiopathic:** Senile atrophy is sometimes attributed as idiopathic.
DIAGNOSIS	• **History:** KCS can be intermittent. • **Clinical signs** may be more frequent during hot, dry times of the year when tear evaporation is the greatest. • **Schirmer tear test:** ≥ 15 mm of tears/min is normal in dogs. STT times of ≤ 15 mm/min in dogs indicate KCS if accompanied by clinical signs (mucoid discharge, conjunctival hyperemia or keratitis). A qualitative tear film deficiency (abnormal lipid or mucous phases **with normal aqueous phase**) may also cause clinical signs of KCS.
TREATMENT	• If caused by drugs, stop medication with the inciting drugs. • **Topical cyclosporine BID is the first line of defense.** Animals with ≤ 2 mm/min of wetting on a STT have a 50% chance of responding to cyclosporine. Those with ≥ 2 mm/min wetting have an 80% chance of response. It's important to diagnose autoimmune KCS and begin early treatment before the lacrimal glands undergo atrophy secondary to chronic inflammation. Some normal aqueous tear gland tissue must be present for cyclosporine to be effective. It may take 8 weeks or longer for cyclosporine to clear the inflammation and allow the tear gland to function; therefore, intensive therapy with topical antibiotic ointments and artificial tears is necessary until tear production returns to normal. Topical antibiotic therapy is needed to treat and/or prevent secondary bacterial conjunctivitis. Dogs with KCS are also prone to developing corneal ulcers, which may easily become infected. It's impossible to overlubricate the eye, so owners should be encouraged to treat as often as possible (4-8 times daily). Surgical removal of the proptosed glands of the third eyelid is contraindicated (except with neoplasia) as it will predispose animals to developing KCS. Cyclosporine therapy must be continued indefinitely or else clinical symptoms (as well as increased destruction of the aqueous tear glands) will occur. Cyclosporine should initially be used BID to TID. After tear production returns to normal, the frequency may be decreased to SID to BID. • **Artificial tears** help replace the precorneal tear film. Preservative-free artificial tear preparations are less irritating to the eyes. Products with a methylcellulose base are more viscous and have a longer effect. • **Ointments:** Lanolin-based ointments (Lacri-Lube®) can be used. • **Parotid duct transposition:** Use this treatment in dogs that are non-responsive to cyclosporine and in cases where the owner can't give the medications frequently enough.

ANTERIOR UVEITIS

Uveitis occurs when blood vessels of the iris and ciliary body become inflamed, leading to leakage of proteins and even blood cells into the aqueous humor. Signs of uveitis are dramatic in dogs but subtle in cats.

CLINICAL SIGNS	**Red eyes:** The red is due to scleral vessel engorgement (including ciliary flushing where the episcleral vessels are hyperemic), indicating involvement of the deeper structures of the eye.
	Pain manifests as blepharospasm, epiphora, enophthalmos, and photophobia. Ocular pain is caused by **spasms of the ciliary muscles** (unlike with corneal ulcers, where pain is due to irritation of the free nerve endings of the trigeminal nerve). It can be alleviated with **iridocycloplegics (tropicamide** or **atropine**) but not with topical anesthetics (such as proparacaine). If you aren't sure whether the pain is due to anterior uveitis or corneal ulceration, apply topical anesthetics. Pain-induced corneal ulceration will cease within a minute of application. **Chronic anterior uveitis is less painful than acute uveitis.**
	Corneal edema occurs if the corneal endothelial cell layer is inflamed.
	Miosis may result in detectable **anisocoria**. In addition, **the affected eye will dilate more slowly with 1% tropicamide** than a normal eye will. **Horner's syndrome** may be confused with uveitis because both cause miosis, ptosis, and enophthalmos. Horner's syndrome isn't painful and doesn't have associated aqueous flare. Additionally, atropine does not eliminate the miosis, ptosis, or enophthalmos. Pharmacologic testing with 1 drop of 1:10 dilution of 10% **phenylephrine** alleviates the clinical signs of post-ganglionic Horner's syndrome. Clinical signs need to be present for at least 2 weeks before testing to allow the muscle receptors to become supersensitive to dilute phenylephrine. The normal eye should also be treated and acts as a control (no response).
	Iris inflammation is characterized by: • **Ragged pupillary borders** • **Neovascularization** of the iris, which can be localized or diffuse • **Multiple gray** or **pink nodules** scattered throughout the anterior surface of the iris stroma • **Darkening of the iris.** More visible in cats.
	Anterior or posterior synechia: The inflamed iris may adhere anteriorly to the cornea or posteriorly to the lens. Circumferential adherence to the lens is called **iris bombe.** Synechia with or without iris bombe can lead to secondary glaucoma.
	Aqueous flare is caused by increased protein in the aqueous. The protein leaks from the inflamed vessels of the iris and ciliary body.
	Hyphema, hypopyon, keratic precipitates • **Hyphema** occurs when blood from the inflamed iris and ciliary blood vessels leaks into the anterior chamber (may be free floating, clotted, or unclotted). It usually settles ventrally. Hyphema can be caused by any process that causes third-space compartment, including hypertension, coagulopathy, and neoplasms. • **Hypopyon** is the accumulation of purulent material or white blood cells in the anterior chamber. **It doesn't generally indicate infection, although it can be caused by infection.** In cases of corneal ulcerations caused by *Pseudomonas spp*, leukocytes migrate into the anterior chamber due to the leukotactic toxins produced by the bacteria. The hypopyon is still sterile. • **Keratic precipitates** are accumulations of inflammatory cells adhered to the corneal endothelium. They are usually found in the ventral central cornea but can also be found on the anterior lens capsule. They can be very small and diffusely located, or large and in isolated masses called **mutton fat precipitates.**

ANTERIOR UVEITIS (continued)

CLINICAL SIGNS continued	**Blindness:** When blindness occurs it is usually due to associated optic neuritis or retinitis and retinal detachment. Since disease involving the posterior segment can drastically change the prognosis for vision, the posterior segment of both eyes must be carefully evaluated in all cases of anterior uveitis. Any medication for the posterior segment must be administered systemically.
ETIOLOGIES	Uveitis can be a primary ocular disease or an ocular manifestation of a systemic disease. Any process that causes inflammation of vessels can lead to ocular manifestation of systemic disease. Primary ocular • **Trauma:** e.g., proptosis, keratitis with superficial or deep corneal ulcers, other globe trauma • **Hypermature cataracts:** Lens proteins may leak from the cortex of the lens through the anterior lens capsule into the aqueous, inciting an immune response. • **Primary intraocular tumors** include malignant melanomas, ciliary body adenomas and adenocarcinomas, and medulloepitheliomas. Anterior uveitis is often present early in tumor formation in a subtle form but is more often recognized as a late manifestation of primary intraocular tumors. The inflammation is usually associated with bleeding as the mass extends into the uveal tissue. With primary ocular neoplasms, we can often identify a mass lesion. Secondary to systemic disease • **Mycosis:** The most common ocular manifestations of systemic mycosis (e.g., blastomycosis, histoplasmosis, coccidioidomycosis) are anterior uveitis and chorioretinitis. • **Canine adenovirus vaccine:** Severe, usually unilateral anterior uveitis may develop 10-21 days after the first vaccine with modified live canine adenovirus-1 (CAV-1, the agent of infectious canine hepatitis). Corneal edema occurs because the virus attacks the endothelial cells of the cornea. Large protein precipitates are frequently found in the anterior chamber. • **Other infectious agents:** FIV, FeLV, *Coronavirus* (FIP), and *Toxoplasma gondii* (toxoplasmosis) are the four main infectious agents to consider in cats. Others that occur in cats and dogs include *Ehrlichia* bacteria (Ehrlichiosis), *Bartonella,* etc. • **Immune-mediated** anterior uveitis can be associated with drug reactions, lens-induced uveitis from resorbing cataracts, or traumatic lens-capsule rupture (termed "phacoclastic uveitis"). Vogt-Koyanagi Harada syndrome, or uveodermatologic syndrome, is an autoimmune disease of primarily arctic breeds (most commonly the Akita). The uveitis is caused by an immune reaction to pigmented uveal cells. The uveitis may result in posterior synechia, iris bombe, retinal detachment and secondary glaucoma. Immunosuppressive doses of prednisone and sometimes azathioprine therapy are necessary to control the disease. Dermatologic signs include poliosis (patch of white hair near the eye due to loss of pigment), vitiligo, and alopecia around the eyes and on the nasal planum. Neoplasm: • **Malignant lymphoma** is a common metastatic tumor of the dog and cat eye. • Any tumor has the capability of metastasizing to the eye. **Idiopathic:** Frequently, the cause of uveitis cannot be determined.

ANTERIOR UVEITIS (continued)

DIAGNOSIS	Clinical findings **Decreased intraocular pressure:** Active aqueous production is significantly reduced in cases of anterior uveitis, resulting in decreased intraocular pressure. If clinical findings indicate uveitis and pressures are normal, suspect **secondary glaucoma.** Once anterior uveitis is diagnosed, if it's nontraumatic in origin, a white blood cell count, chemistry panel, and urinalysis should be performed as an initial work-up to look for the underlying etiology. Other tests to run include: • FIV, FeLV, FIP titers in cats • Rickettsia titers • Toxoplasma IgM and IgG titers (Positive blood titers indicate past or present infection. Compare serum titers to aqueous humor titers. High relative aqueous humor titers indicate present infection.) • Lymph node aspirate, cytology of the aqueous or vitreous (perform if you suspect neoplasia), or ultrasound to look for intraocular tumors. • Enucleation and histopathology of the blind eye to look for neoplasia Although you often can't find a cause of anterior uveitis, it's important to look for an underlying cause because identifiable etiologies are usually serious systemic diseases.
SEQUELA	• **Glaucoma** can occur if the pupil fails to dilate and the iris adheres completely to the lens (**posterior synechia**). It can also occur with broad peripheral synechia or angle blockage with inflammatory cells. Secondary glaucoma may develop after treatment for anterior uveitis has been instituted, because the treatment improves the integrity of the ciliary processes so that aqueous production is increased toward the normal rate. If the outflow pathway is not open, the intraocular pressure starts to rise. If the blockage is due to posterior synechia, the iris begins to bulge toward the cornea, resulting in iris bombe and a shallow anterior chamber. • **Phthisis bulbi:** If the inflammatory reaction is severe, the ciliary processes may be destroyed resulting in little aqueous production and a small, soft globe. The animal becomes blind but usually is not painful (unless iritis or keratitis persist). • **Cataracts:** Anterior capsular and subcapsular opacities can develop following uveitis. Pigment deposits frequently occur on the anterior lens surface. Cataracts are also caused by posterior synechia. A complete cataract may develop if the lens damage is severe. • **Corneal scars and edema:** Anterior synechia may cause full-thickness corneal scars. If the damage to the endothelial layer of the cornea is severe, edema may persist. • **Iris atrophy:** The iris may become heavily pigmented or depigmented due to chronic inflammation, or it may become severely atrophied leaving strands of tissue or pigment on the lens capsule. • **Lens luxation:** Zonules become weakened with chronic uveitis and can break.
TREATMENT	**Treatment:** If a cause can be identified, treat the primary disease. Goals of treatment are to dilate the pupil, reduce ocular pain, reduce inflammation, and prevent and monitor complications. **Cycloplegics and mydriatics: Iridocycloplegics** paralyze the iris and ciliary body musculature, reducing pain associated with muscle spasm. **Mydriatics** dilate the pupil, which reduces the incidence of posterior synechia, secondary cataracts, and secondary glaucoma. The inflamed iris resists dilation, so the eye with anterior uveitis will take longer to dilate. • **Atropine** is both a mydriatic and iridocycloplegic. It also reduces vascular permeability, thus reducing aqueous flare. Use atropine topically q 6-12 hours initially and then decrease the dose to effect. Remember that one drop of 1% atropine contains 0.5 mg atropine. An animal can easily become systemically atropinized with this topical application.

ANTERIOR UVEITIS (continued)

| TREATMENT continued | **Corticosteroids** decrease the inflammation, inhibit fibroblastic proliferation, and improve vascular permeability. Dexamethasone 0.1% (Maxidex® or Maxitrol®) or prednisolone acetate (1% Pred Forte®) have good potency and penetrate through the intact epithelium well. Prednisolone penetrates even more effectively, though. Use every 2-6 hours or more frequently. If not due to an infectious disease, severe anterior uveitis and posterior uveitis may be treated systemically with 0.5 mg-2 mg/kg prednisone per os initially and then taper the dose. Topical and systemic therapy may be used in combination as long as there is no corneal ulceration. Topical corticosteroids are contraindicated in the presence of an ulcer. Dogs can be given subconjunctival injections (triamcinolone, betamethasone, dexamethasone).

Azathioprine (Imuran®) has been used successfully in cases of severe anterior uveitis. Perform a CBC first since azathioprine suppresses the bone marrow, causing leukopenia, thrombocytopenia, and anemia. Give the drug with a meal to reduce GI disturbance (1 mg/kg daily for 4-7 days, then decrease to every 2-7 days). Monitor the CBC every 2-3 weeks while azathioprine is being used.

NSAIDs reduce capillary permeability, stabilize lysosomal membranes, and suppress leukocytic migration via a mechanism different than that of corticosteroids.
• **Flurbiprofen** (0.03%: 1 drop q 2-6 hours)
• **Aspirin** 20-30 mg/kg TID in dogs. To prevent gastritis, you can use Ascriptin® and give it with a meal.
Be careful when using NSAIDs together with prednisone, as both can cause GI ulcers.

Antibiotics should be used if there's a deep corneal ulcer that may be infected or in cases of suspected toxoplasmosis (**clindamycin** 12.5 mg/kg PO q 12 hours for 21 days or 30 mg/cat per day divided BID-TID). In the case of toxoplasmosis, also use corticosteroids to suppress the immune component of the disease. Use antibiotics that penetrate into the eye (e.g., fluoroquinolones). |

COMPARING CORNEAL ULCERS, ANTERIOR UVEITIS, and GLAUCOMA

	CORNEAL ULCER	ANTERIOR UVEITIS	GLAUCOMA
Pain	Due to irritation of free nerve endings in the cornea. These nerves lead to the ciliary muscle, resulting in ciliary spasms, too.	Due to spasm of the ciliary muscles. Use iridocycloplegics such as tropicamide or atropine.	Painful due to increase in intraocular pressure
Injection	± Conjunctival injection	Engorged episcleral vessels ± engorged conjunctival vessels	Engorged episcleral vessels ± engorged conjunctival vessels
Corneal edema	Yes	Yes	Yes
Anterior chamber	Usually normal	Aqueous flare ± keratic precipitates ± hyphema, hypopyon	Normal ± aqueous flare
Pupil size	Normal or miotic	Often miotic	Often dilated
Iris changes	None	± Ragged edges ± neovascularization ± darkening of iris	May become dull in chronic cases
IOP	Normal	Decreased	Increased

GLAUCOMA

Glaucoma, an **elevation in intraocular pressure** (IOP), is one of the leading causes of irreversible blindness in dogs and cats. Because it can lead to blindness within 24-48 hours of onset, it is an emergency requiring aggressive medical treatment and immediate referral to a veterinary ophthalmologist. Glaucoma is easy to miss, especially in cats. All red eyes in which corneal ulcers and infectious or purulent processes have been ruled out, and red eyes in dogs with predilections for glaucoma should be checked for the disease.

PATHOGENESIS	Glaucoma is caused by impaired outflow of aqueous humor from the eye. Aqueous humor normally exits the eye through the iridocorneal drainage angle. Anything that blocks or narrows this angle can lead to glaucoma. Narrowing of the drainage angle can be **primary** (inherited problem) or **secondary** to intraocular neoplasia, lens luxation, inflammation (anterior uveitis), etc.
CLINICAL SIGNS	Most cases of glaucoma are not diagnosed in time to prevent vision loss, but once diagnosed, owners can monitor and manage the unaffected eye to delay development of disease. Suspect primary glaucoma in any Cocker Spaniel, Basset, or Samoyed with painful or red eyes, and secondary glaucoma in terriers, Border Collies, and Shar-Peis with painful eyes. • **Ocular pain** manifests as blepharospasm, **pawing at the eye,** and/or **lethargy.** The affected eye is usually very painful, especially in the early stages of acute glaucoma. Signs may be subtle to the owners, but the pet usually feels better once the IOP is decreased. • **Vision deficits:** Loss of vision can occur within 24-48 hours due to optic nerve damage and retinal atrophy. Higher IOPs, longer duration of elevation, and more acute onsets lead to quicker vision loss. • **Red eye:** The red is due to engorged episcleral vessels ± engorged conjunctival vessels. • **Corneal edema:** Elevated IOP impairs the corneal endothelium's ability to remove water from the corneal stroma. It also allows aqueous humor to get into the stroma, forcing collagen fibers apart, which leads to opacity. • **Buphthalmos and Descemet's streaks (also known as Haab's Striae):** Elevated IOP causes the cornea and sclera to stretch irreversibly (more common in young animals). Be careful to distinguish buphthalmia (increase in globe size; the corneal diameter is increased) from exophthalmia (protruding globe). Buphthalmic globes still retropulse into the orbit when pressure is applied to the lids. An exophthalmic eye has normal dimensions but will not retropulse normally due to space-occupying lesion in the orbit. **Descemet's streaks** are permanent linear ruptures in Descemet's membrane caused by stretching of the cornea. They indicate past glaucoma or glaucoma of some duration. • **Fixed, dilated pupil (mydriasis):** As IOP increases (> 50 mmHg), the pupillary constrictor muscle is paralyzed, leading to pupillary dilation. • **Lens luxation:** Luxation can cause glaucoma (anterior luxation) or result from glaucoma. In the latter case, lens zonules break as the globe enlarges, allowing the lens to fall out of position. Exam shows an aphakic crescent. Lens luxation is common in terriers, Border Collies, and Shar-Peis. • **Chronic anterior uveitis** can lead to glaucoma. A normal IOP (15-25 mmHg) in an animal with anterior uveitis indicates that either the animal has concurrent secondary glaucoma or is at risk of developing glaucoma. These animals should initially be treated for glaucoma (timolol or dipivefrin HCL) in addition to using corticosteroids. Avoid using atropine in these cases. If the pupil is miotic, use dipivefrin HCL. These cases are best referred to an ophthalmologist.
DIAGNOSIS	**Diagnosis is based on finding elevated intraocular pressure (IOP) plus appropriate clinical signs.** Measure IOP using an applanation tonometer (e.g., Tono-Pen® or TonoVet®) or a Schiotz tonometer. Normal pressures are below 10-26 mmHg in dogs, 15-25 mmHg in cats. Take into consideration clinical signs, breed, and whether the pet was struggling or had pressure on its neck when the IOP pressure was measured. It's best to take the measurement when the animal is holding its eyelids open voluntarily.

GLAUCOMA (continued)

OTHER DIAGNOSTIC CONSIDERATIONS	Once glaucoma is diagnosed, the next step is to determine whether it is primary or secondary to something that needs to be treated. • Look for signs of underlying causes such as anterior uveitis or lens luxation. • Check IOP in the unaffected eye. Elevation (as well as breed predilection) supports a diagnosis of primary glaucoma. • **Gonioscopy** can reveal whether the iridocorneal angle is blocked or malformed. **Determine whether the animal is visual.** If the animal is still visual or just recently blind, then institute aggressive therapy.
TREATMENT	**Treat glaucoma as an emergency, and then refer** the patient to an ophthalmologist. The goal of treatment is to reduce intraocular pressure (IOP). This can be accomplished by decreasing aqueous pressure or increasing aqueous drainage. **Decrease aqueous production** • **Carbonic anhydrase inhibitors:** dichlorphenamide (Daranide or methazolamide systemically; brinzolamide (Azopt) or dorsolamide (Trusopt®) topically. • **Adrenergic agents:** dipivefrine (Propine®, an epinephrine dimer), timolol (Timoptic®), a ß adrenergic agent). We don't know why both the adrenergic agonist and antagonists work. • **Cyclocryotherapy** (ophthalmologist) • **Increase aqueous drainage** • **Topical prostaglandins are the most potent and effective drugs** for canines: latanoprost (Xalatan®) and bimatoprost (Lumigan®). • **Cholinergic:** topical pilocarpine (minimally effective, rarely used), demacarium bromide (used more commonly, longer acting). • **Osmotic diuretic:** mannitol or glycerin • **Surgical** (ophthalmologist) • **Paracentesis** can be performed by an ophthalmologist.
EMERGENCY TREATMENT	• **Mannitol or glycerin:** Glycerin dose is 1-2 mg/kg PO of 90% glycerin. Withhold water for 3-4 hours. This treatment is easy and inexpensive. Mannitol dose: 2.0 g/kg IV or 10 mL/kg of 20% solution over 15-20 minutes can reduce IOP profoundly within an hour. Use with an in-line IV filter (22 μm). • **Timolol 0.25%, 0.5%** decreases aqueous production. Use 1 drop BID of 0.5% solution. It may cause bradycardia. • **Carbonic anhydrase inhibitor: methazolamide** (Neptazane®) 1-2 mg/kg PO TID in dogs and cats. Side effects include metabolic acidosis, vomiting, and panting. **Dorsolamide 2% (Trusopt®) and brinzolamide** are topical carbonic anhydrase inhibitors. Dose is 1 drop BID-TID. • **Topical prostaglandin:** latanoprost (Xalatan®) SID-BID. • **Topical corticosteroids** can be used with anterior uveitis. **ATROPINE is CONTRAINDICATED.**
LONG-TERM MANAGEMENT	Medical management is usually temporary until surgery can be performed. Glaucoma is difficult to control medically. In cases of primary glaucoma, the other eye can be treated with **timolol (Timoptic®).** Owner should examine the eye BID for signs of glaucoma (redness, pain). **Surgical options:** Surgery should be performed even in the blind pet because glaucoma is a painful condition. • **Cyclodestructive procedures:** Cyclocryotherapy or cyclophotocoagulation (laser) procedures, in conjunction with a drainage device and medications, may be useful in prolonging vision in a visual eye. Estimated success: 50-60% of patients are visual at 1 year. • **Enucleation** is for blind and/or painful eyes. A second option is an **intraocular prosthesis** (used for cosmetic purposes). Because pressure around the neck can increase IOP, these dogs should be trained using positive reinforcement to walk on leash without pulling. Choke chains and pinch collars should be avoided. Head halters or harnesses where the leash attaches to the front (e.g., SENSE-ation® or Gentle Leader® Easy Walk™ harnesses) can be used.

CATARACTS

Cataracts are lens opacities of varying etiologies. They may be located in the capsular, cortical, or nuclear region of the lens. Cataracts can be focal or diffuse, progressive or non-progressive, and should be distinguished from nuclear sclerosis on fundic examination. With nuclear sclerosis, the fundus can easily be seen, but it cannot be visualized through a cataract. Animals with cataracts usually present with visual difficulties only after the cataract has progressed to a mature stage and usually only if the cataract is bilateral, unless they have marked nuclear sclerosis in the nonaffected eye.

ETIOLOGY	• **Trauma** • **Nutritional:** Esbilac and KMR are low in arginine and can lead to cataracts in young kittens and puppies. • **Metabolic: Diabetes mellitus** is the most common metabolic cause. These cataracts develop rapidly. • **Toxins:** PRA leads to the release of compounds that affect the lens. The tapetum is hyperreflective due to the retinal atrophy. • **Radiation therapy** profoundly affects the eye. • **Congenital** • **Hereditary:** Cataracts are often hereditary in purebred dogs. • **Uveitis**
CLASSIFICATION by STAGE	**Incipient:** The opacities are localized and vision is not affected. **Immature:** The opacity is more marked and generalized, and the fundus may be partially obscured on fundic exam. In bilaterally affected dogs, vision may be decreased. This is the ideal time to refer the animal to an ophthalmologist since the fundic evaluation can still be performed. **Mature:** The lens is totally opaque and the fundus is obscured on exam. The animal has severe visual deficits. This may be the ideal time for lens removal. **Hypermature:** The lens begins to liquefy and resorb, and some vision may return. Surgery should be performed prior to this stage because lens resorption may result in leakage of protein out of the lens into the anterior chamber. This causes anterior uveitis, glaucoma, and retinal detachment, all of which reduce surgical success. In cases where the nucleus liquefies and sinks to the bottom of the lens, the cataract is called a **Morgagnian cataract.**
DIAGNOSIS	• **Dilate the pupils** and examine the lens with indirect ophthalmoscopy or a slit lamp. Cataracts obscure the tapetal reflection. • Note that **nuclear sclerosis** (which occurs because new fibers on the periphery are constantly being laid down and are thus compressing the older fibers at the center of the lens) begins at about 5 years of age in dogs and 8-9 years of age in cats. These lenses appear almost pearlescent. Tapetal reflection can be seen. • **Retinal detachment** may obscure the tapetal reflection, thus appearing like a mature cataract.
TREATMENT/ MANAGEMENT	Clients interested in cataract surgery should be referred as early as possible to an ophthalmologist. This allows the ophthalmologist to evaluate the fundus for signs of PRA or retinal detachments. Many cataracts, especially juvenile onset (1-5 years of age) and diabetic cataracts, may begin to resorb and cause a lens-induced uveitis (LIU). The LIU needs to be treated promptly, to prevent secondary glaucoma and ensure that the eye will be a good surgical candidate. Because most cataracts are now removed by phacoemulsification, surgery is best performed in the early stages of cataract formation before visual impairment becomes severe. Surgical treatment also involves medical follow-up and regular monitoring of the eye with biannual ophthalmology exams. Success rate of surgery is 90-95% short term and 70-75% long term. The most common complication is glaucoma.

OCULAR EMERGENCIES

An ocular emergency is any condition that will cause loss of vision or loss of the globe if left untreated. They are most commonly traumatic in origin.

CONDITION	ASSESSMENT/CLINICAL SIGNS	TREATMENT/PROGNOSIS	SEQUELAE if UNTREATED
ACUTE BLINDNESS	• **History:** Usually the animal was visual and then blindness seemed to occur overnight. • Maze test the animal to see if it's blind. • PLR present or absent? • Fundic examination normal or abnormal? Etiologies include: • Retinal separation or detachment • Sudden acquired retinal degeneration (SARD) • Optic neuritis • Brain tumors • Patients with progressive retinal degeneration (PRD) may appear to the owner to suddenly go blind, especially if their environment has changed. Diagnose through ophthalmic, physical, and neurologic examination, and then ERG if indicated.	Treatment depends on the cause. • **Optic neuritis:** Oral corticosteroids reduce inflammation. If the animal has neuritis, you should evaluate it systemically to rule out fungal causes. • **SARD:** There is no treatment. • **Retinal detachment:** Small retinal tears may be treated with laser photocoagulation. Diffuse subretinal edema secondary to posterior uveitis may respond to systemic prednisone. (Be sure to diagnose and treat underlying infectious causes first, before using systemic steroids.) Detachments due to systemic hypertension may improve after treatment for the hypertension, but prognosis for vision is poor. • **Brain tumor:** CT scan followed by surgery. • With no improvement in 2 weeks, an animal has a poor prognosis for recovery.	• Permanent blindness • Retinal degeneration
ANTERIOR UVEITIS	Refer to section on anterior uveitis, p. 15.11.		
CHEMICAL INJURY/ KERATITIS	• **History:** The animal may have been seen around fertilizer, drain cleaner, acids, mace. • Determine if the cornea is edematous or if there's an ulcer. With alkaline products, usually less pain is present. A blanched or gray conjunctiva yields a bad prognosis.	**Acid burns** are usually self-limiting due to precipitation of corneal stromal proteins. Lavage the eye with 2-3 liters of LRS. Then treat with topical antibiotics and cycloplegics (atropine) QID. Recheck the eye in 1-3 days. If the cornea looks intact at 3 days, re-evaluate in another 3 days and at 3-day intervals until the cornea no longer stains with fluorescein. **Alkaline burns** cause melting of the cornea, but not immediately. Changes may occur in 7-10 days. Lavage the eye with 2-3 liters of LRS. Then apply an anticollagenase (such as EDTA, Mucomyst™, or serum), antibiotics QID, and cycloplegics. Re-evaluate every 3 days until the cornea heals (may take 3-5 weeks). You may want to consult with an ophthalmologist due to the chronicity, aftercare, and possible sequelae.	• Corneal perforation

OCULAR EMERGENCIES (continued)

CONDITION	ASSESSMENT/CLINICAL SIGNS	TREATMENT /PROGNOSIS	SEQUELAE if UNTREATED
CORNEAL LACERATION or DEEP ULCER For more information, refer to corneal ulcer section on p. 15.8.	**ALL CASES are URGENT** • **Perforation:** With perforation, iridal tissue and fibrin protrudes from the lesion. If you aren't sure whether there's a perforation, stain with a sterile fluorescein strip. The anterior chamber will fluoresce or the fluorescein stain will flow away from the lesion (Seidel sign) if the cornea is perforated. • **Anterior uveitis** is usually present and is characterized by miosis, aqueous flare, ± fibrin, iris hyperemia, conjunctival hyperemia, and chemosis.	• **Surgery is suggested if the ulcer is greater than halfway through the cornea.** Refer the animal to an ophthalmologist immediately. In the case of deep ulcers, don't apply antibiotics unless you first obtain a specimen for bacterial culture. Don't place a third-eyelid flap because the pressure may cause the globe to rupture, and because it will need to be removed for primary corneal repair anyway. • Pre-op: Atropine 1% TID • Cytologic exam and bacterial culture and sensitivity. Infected or melting ulcers should be treated immediately with either a combination of triple antibiotic and gentamicin or tobramycin, or with a topical ciprofloxacin (Ciloxan®). Antibiotics can be changed based on cytology and culture/sensitivity. • Assess the eye every 24-48 hours.	**Globe perforation** can cause hyphema, signs of pain, retinal detachment, and phthisis bulbi. Penetrating trauma that perforates the lens capsule may lead to phacoclastic uveitis. Treat tears that are ≤ 2 mm with immunosuppressive doses of systemic prednisone plus topical corticosteroids and atropine. Larger tears may require removal of the lens (phacoemulsification). In cats, ruptured lens capsules may lead to post-traumatic sarcoma formation months to years following the trauma.
OCULAR FOREIGN BODY	• How deep is the foreign body? Determine if the anterior chamber is leaking by using fluorescein stain as with the corneal laceration. Try to determine what the foreign body is. • Assess the consensual PLR. Its presence is a good sign. If it's absent, the animal probably has severe intraocular damage. This patient will probably need an enucleation in the future, but the primary lesion should still be corrected immediately.	**Object penetrating the cornea or sclera:** • Apply topical anesthetics first. Sometimes a sterile Q-tip may be used to remove superficial foreign bodies. A sterile 25-gauge needle may sometimes be used for splinters or thorns. • Use topical atropine (cycloplegic) and antibiotics TID. • Oral topical corticosteroids may be used, but don't use topical steroids until the epithelium has healed sufficiently so that fluorescein stain is no longer retained. Recheck the animal in 3-5 days. **Corneal perforation:** Refer the patient to an ophthalmologist for removal of the foreign object. **Globe perforation** (bad prognosis): Refer the patient to an ophthalmologist for assessment/surgery.	

OCULAR EMERGENCIES (continued)

CONDITION	ASSESSMENT/CLINICAL SIGNS	TREATMENT /PROGNOSIS	SEQUELAE if UNTREATED
GLAUCOMA	Refer to section on glaucoma, p. 15.15.		
HYPHEMA (anterior chamber is filled with blood).	Hyphema is caused by anything that results in hemorrhage elsewhere in the body: trauma, tumor, hypertension (especially in old cats with renal disease), uveitis, coagulopathies, retinal detachment secondary to neovascularization (the retina releases agents that cause neovascularization, and these new vessels may be leaky).	Initially, diagnosis is more important than treatment. Treatment is aimed at resolving the underlying cause (clotting disorders, systemic hypertension). Topical therapy includes corticosteroids and atropine. Monitor intraocular pressure closely when using atropine. Systemic corticosteroids will be beneficial to control uveitis. In cases of trauma, intracameral injection of tissue plasminogen activator (tPA) may help resolve blood clots. Prognosis is guarded if hyphema lasts longer then 14 days.	• Phthisis bulbi (small eyeball) • Glaucoma
LENS LUXATION Terriers are predisposed to lens luxation, usually between 3-6 years of age.	**Refer the patient to an ophthalmologist as soon as possible.** Luxations may be traumatic, hereditary, or caused by glaucoma or anterior uveitis. If the consensual PLR is positive, the lens should be removed. If the consensual PLR is absent, the animal is probably blind in the eye. The eye should be enucleated or an intraocular prosthesis inserted if the eye becomes glaucomatous at a later date. Prognosis is good if the lens is removed and there's no glaucoma or retinal detachment. If the animal has a hereditary predisposition, monitor the second eye for signs of luxation.	An ophthalmologist should remove the lens as soon as possible. Vitrectomy may be required.	• Glaucoma • Corneal edema • Retinal detachment • Anterior uveitis • Cataract
PROPTOSIS	• **Pupil size:** Miotic pupils are a good sign because they indicate that parasympathetic innervation is present. Mydriatic pupils are a bad sign and indicate loss of parasympathetic innervation. The sympathetic innervation may be present, though. Mildly dilated pupils carry a poor prognosis because they indicate loss of both parasympathetic and sympathetic innervation. • **Hyphema:** poor prognosis • **Consensual PLR:** Prognosis may be guarded with lack of consensual PLR. Loss of the consensual PLR may be caused by permanent factors such as retinal detachment, or temporary factors like optic neuritis or intravitreal hemorrhage.	• In brachycephalic breeds, you can usually just pull the eyelids apart and the eye will resume its normal position. With other animals, you can use pre-placed horizontal mattress sutures, a scalpel handle, and ophthalmic lubricant ointment to reposition the eye (under anesthesia). • The eye may require a temporary tarsorrhaphy or third eyelid flap. The tarsorrhaphy should be removed in 14 days. • Topical antibiotics (triple antibiotic ointment) • Atropine 1% TID: mydriatic/cycloplegic • Oral antibiotics may be used for prophylaxis. • Oral corticosteroids (prednisolone 1-2 mg/kg SID)	• Blindness if the optic nerve is severely traumatized • Phthisis bulbi if the ciliary body is severely damaged • Lagophthalmos and exposure keratitis • Strabismus if the rectus muscles are severed

CHAPTER 16: Orthopedics

Orthopedics

Orthopedic Foundation for Animals, Inc. (OFA)
2300 E. Nifong Blvd.
Columbia, MO 65201-3806
(573) 442-0418
Fax: (573) 875-5073
www.offa.org

DRUGS for MANAGING OSTEOARTHRITIS in DOGS

DRUG	DOSE in DOGS
Aspirin (Use buffered aspirin) 65, 81, 325 mg (regular strength) 500 mg tablets (extra strength)	10-25 mg/kg PO with food BID-TID. (This is quivalent to one regular strength aspirin per 25 pounds of body weight. Do not exceed 3 tablets per dose.)
Carprofen (Rimadyl®) 25, 75, 100 mg tablets 50 mg/mL injectable	2.2 mg/kg PO BID or 4.4 mg/kg PO SID. Can also be given SC 2 hours prior to surgery. **Cats:** 1-2 mg SC prior to surgery or post-op. Repeat as needed every 12-24 hours for < 48 hours.
Deracoxib (Deramaxx®) is a coxib class NSAID 25, 100 mg chewable tablets	1-2 mg/kg PO SID as needed. Post-op: 3-4 mg/kg PO SID as needed for ≤ 7 days.
Etodolac (EtoGesic®) 150, 300 mg scored tablets	5-15 mg/kg PO SID.
Meloxicam (Metacam®) 1.5 mg/mL suspension 5 mg/mL injectable	0.2 mg/kg PO initially then 0.1 mg/kg PO SID. **Cats:** Start with the same dose, but by day 3 go to 0.025 mg/kg 2-3 times per week.
Prednisone (last ditch only) 5, 20 mg tablets	0.5-1.0 mg/kg BID. Gradually taper to the lowest possible dose. Only use prednisone as a last ditch effort. It can cause chondromalacia.
Tramadol 50 mg tablets Avoid the form with acetaminophen.	For analgesia: 1-4 mg/kg PO q 8-12 hrs. **Cats:** 4 mg/kg PO BID. (Note: The dose is extrapolated from human medicine.) Long-term safety studies in cats are not yet finished.

SUGGESTED READING:

Piermattei DL, Flo GL, DeCamp CE: Handbook of Small Animal Orthopedics and Fracture Repair. 3rd edition. Philadelphia, WB Saunders, 2006.

ORTHOPEDIC EXAMINATION of the DOG
Conformation and Gait
Palpation

I. **EVALUATE CONFORMATION AND GAIT:** Ask about onset, duration, and timing of the lameness (e.g., is the lameness consistent or intermittent?). With degenerative joint disease, the lameness is worse in the morning and when the animal gets up, but the animal can work out of the stiffness.

   A. **EVALUATE GENERAL CONFORMATION.** Look at:
      1. Limb symmetry
      2. Limb angulation
      3. Rotational abnormalities
      4. Limb length
      5. Varus/valgus deformities
      6. Muscle mass/symmetry
      7. Stance

      Remember to compare the affected limb to the contralateral limb.

   B. **GAIT:** Always observe gait from the side, front, and rear, except in cases of fractures or other injuries such as spinal cord damage. With problems high up on the leg (i.e., hip or shoulder), the pet may not lift its leg much because it's painful to do so. With problems in the lower leg, the animal tends to hold its leg up.
      1. **Front limb lameness:** The animal's head goes up when the lame limb hits the ground so that the pet does not have to bear much weight on the lame leg. The head goes down once the good front leg hits the ground.
      2. **Hind limb lameness:** Often the head does not bob up and down with hind limb lameness, but when it does, it bobs down when the painful limb hits the ground. The dog may hold the lame leg up or walk on its toes. With hip dysplasia, the dog may swing the affected leg and hip. If the dog appears ataxic in the hind end, check for CP deficits. Such deficits indicate neurologic problems and not hip dysplasia, although the animal may have both problems concurrently.

II. **PALPATION:** The goal of palpation is to identify and delineate areas of pain, swelling, increased or decreased temperature, crepitation, and abnormal joint motion.

GENERAL RULES of PALPATION
• Examine the suspect limb only after the other limbs have been inspected and palpated.
• Remember that patients may have bilateral involvement or concomitant musculoskeletal problems.
• Move and palpate one joint at a time.
• Use a gentle, slow approach.
• Also perform a neurologic exam.

   A. **THORACIC LIMB**

COMMON CONDITIONS AFFECTING the FORELIMB in DOGS
• **Osteochondritis dissecans (OCD)** - elbow, shoulder
• **Panosteitis** - humerus, proximal radius, ulna
• **Elbow dysplasia** (± fragmented medial coronoid process, ununited anconeal process, OCD)
• **Osteosarcoma** - proximal humerus, distal radius, ulna (away from the elbow)
• **Bicipital tenosynovitis**
• **Carpal hyperextension**
• **Cervical pain** causing root signature

      1. **Paw**
         a. Examine the **nails** for signs of fracture, exposed quick, or abnormal wear (e.g., dorsal wear may indicate neurologic deficit).
         b. Palpate the **pads and interdigital spaces** for evidence of foreign bodies, lacerations, or draining fistulous tracts.
         c. Palpate each **phalanx** separately, and put each joint through its entire range of motion.
         d. Pay special attention to the **palmar surface of the metacarpophalangeal joints.** Small sesamoids (especially II & VII) in this

area are prone to fracture leading to chronic lameness (especially in Rottweilers).

2. Carpus
   a. Assess the **carpal joint surfaces for inflammation.** A depression should be definable in the normal carpus between the radius and radiocarpal bone if no joint effusion is present.
   b. Flex the foot to **check for a decrease in range of motion.** This may indicate osteoarthritis (degenerative joint disease), swelling and joint effusion, or muscular guarding of painful areas.
   c. Observe the dog bearing weight on the limb to look for **hyperextension.** Often, the dog must be sedated and stress radiographs taken. Hyperextension is characteristic of **palmar carpal ligament injury,** which usually requires carpal arthrodesis. In acute cases of hyperextension, the patient may present with flexion as the flexors attempt to stabilize the carpus.
   d. Palpate the **accessory carpal bone** (located laterally) for pain or displacement that may occur with fractures of this bone and injury to ligaments that originate from here.

3. Radius/ulna:
   a. Palpate the length of the radius and ulna for evidence of pain, swelling, or abnormal movement. The distal radial metaphysis is a common site for:
      i. **Bone neoplasia** in large-breed dogs
      ii. **HOD** in large-breed puppies
      iii. **Panosteitis** (proximal radius and ulna)
      iv. **Growth deformities** (premature distal radial/ulnar closure)
      v. **Fractures** in small-breed dogs

4. Elbow
   a. Palpate the lateral and medial epicondyles and determine the contour of the humerus. The head of the radius can be palpated laterally and proximally with most elbow luxations.
   b. Hyperflexion and hyperextension may result in pain if there's an **ununited anconeal process** within this joint.
   c. A **fragmented coronoid** may produce localizable pain medially but will more often produce signs of elbow osteoarthritis. Flex the elbow and put pressure on the lateral aspect with the thumb. Then do the same with pressure on the medial aspect.

5. Humerus
   a. Palpate the lateral surface of the humerus for pain, swelling, crepitation, or abnormal movement. Fractures occur, but **panosteitis** is the most commonly found lesion of this diaphysis in young, large-breed dogs.

6. Glenohumeral joint
   a. Assessing the relative position of the greater tubercle to the glenoid cavity will generally establish the presence or absence of **shoulder luxation.**
   b. The range of motion in this joint is classically limited in animals with **infraspinatus contracture,** though **osteoarthritis** can considerably decrease the motion, too.
   c. OCD: Hypertension and hyperflexion cause pain in animals with OCD of the humeral head. To limit the stress only to the shoulder joint, grasp the limb and flex it slowly.
   d. Palpate the intertubercular groove and proximal biceps brachii for **bicipital tenosynovitis** or **tendon rupture.** Palpate the tendon by rotating the limb externally and then palpating with your thumb.

7. Scapula
   a. Palpate the cranial angle of the scapula for evidence of pain due to a body **fracture** or excessive movement due to **rupture** of the serratus musculature.
   b. Palpate the spine of the scapula and the acromion process for pain and abnormal morphology.

B. PELVIC LIMB

COMMON CONDITIONS AFFECTING the HINDLIMB in DOGS
• Cruciate rupture
• Osteochondritis dissecans - medial and lateral ridges of the talus, medial aspect of the lateral femoral condyle
• Panosteitis - femur
• Hip dysplasia
• Avascular necrosis of the femoral neck (Legg-Calve-Perthes)
• Patellar luxation
• Osteosarcoma - distal femur and proximal tibia (towards the knee)
• Lumbosacral disease (may mimic hip dysplasia)

1. Tarsus
   a. Inspect for signs of pain or inflammation.
   b. Flex and extend the joint. The normal range of motion is about 90°.
      i. Excessive flexion is usually due to **Achilles** mechanism dysfunction. Palpate the Achilles tendon and gastrocnemius muscle for evidence of pain or enlargement indicating the site of rupture.
      ii. Synovial effusion is easiest to detect medially.
   c. OCD of the hock (usually the medial trochlear ridge, but occurs in the lateral trochlear ridge in Rottweilers) usually produces joint effusion leading to pain on palpation. Place thumb pressure on the medial aspect of the hock to check for pain. Also check for reduced flexion. OCD shows up best on a flexed DP view because this view best shows the medial trochlear ridge.
   d. Determine the medial and lateral stability of the tarsus. **Collateral ligament** injury or **malleolus** fracture is common following trauma to this area.

2. Tibia
   a. Palpate the length of the tibia from the medial side.
   b. Palpate the tibial tuberosity, especially in young animals, for signs of **avulsion fracture.**

3. Stifle
   a. The normal stifle range of motion is > 135°.
   b. **Joint effusion or capsular swelling** results in loss of a palpable depression on either side of the straight patellar ligament. The patella itself may ride further from the patellar groove with severe effusion.
   c. **Check for patellar luxation:** Place your finger on the knee and feel for a trochlear groove. Is the patella displaced? It's usually displaced medially in both small and large dogs. Palpate the patella with your thumb and forefinger while the stifle is moved through its whole range of motion. To check for medial instability, extend the animal's knee, internally rotate it, and place thumb pressure on the lateral aspect of the patella. Conversely, for lateral luxations, slightly flex the stifle, externally rotate the toes, and apply pressure to the medial aspect of the patella. Patellar luxation may be graded 1-4.

GRADING PATELLAR LUXATION	
Grade I	Intermittent patellar luxation: The patella is loose in the groove, so it luxates easily, but it doesn't stay in the luxated position. The pet carries its leg (or skips on the affected leg) occasionally.
Grade II	Frequent patellar luxation: The patella luxates easily and stays out when the leg is flexed. It pops back into place on extension. These pets skip more than those with grade I luxation.
Grade III	Permanent patellar luxation: The patella can be replaced with digital pressure, but it reluxates when the pressure is released. Anatomically, the trochlear groove is shallow, and the tibia and tibial crest are deviated laterally or medially. As a result of the tibial deviation, flexion and extension of the joint causes abduction and adduction of the hock. The animal may bear weight with the stifle held in a flexed position.
Grade IV	Permanent patellar luxation: The patella lies just above the medial condyle or medial to the normal position. It can't be reduced.

    d. Determine **cranial cruciate ligament stability:**
- i. **Cranial drawer sign:** You should be able to elicit a cranial drawer sign in cases of acute, complete ruptures; with partial ruptures, however, the joint may be only mildly unstable. In cases of chronic ruptures, secondary changes may stabilize the joint making it difficult to elicit a drawer sign. You may need to sedate or anesthetize the pet to demonstrate the drawer sign. Place the pet in lateral recumbency. Stand caudal to the pet and place the index finger of one hand on the proximal end of the patella while the thumb is over the lateral fabella. Place the index finger of the other hand on the tibial crest while the thumb is caudal to the fibular head. Slightly flex the stifle and gently push the tibia forward and then caudally. Repeat this motion with the stifle in 90% flexion and then in full extension. Excess movement indicates a cruciate rupture. Subluxation of the tibia caudal to the femur is a **caudal drawer sign** (rare). Always compare the affected leg to the contralateral limb.
- ii. **Tibial compression:** With the pet standing or in lateral recumbency, place the palm of one hand on the distal femur with the index finger on the patella. With the stifle straight, dorsiflex the hock as far as it will go. This tenses the gastrocnemius muscle. The motion presses the femur and tibia together; if the cranial cruciate ligament is torn, the tibia will slide forward.

    e. **Meniscal injury** often leads to an audible or palpable click on joint movement.

    f. Palpate the origin of the **long digital extensor** and the origin of the **gastrocnemius** and fabellae to check for **avulsion** or **fracture** injury.

4. **Femur**
- a. Palpate the length of the femur.
- b. Check the greater trochanter for pain or displacement.

5. **Hip joint (coxofemoral joint):** Osteoarthritis is common in this joint. With the animal standing, extend the legs and put the leg through a whole range of motion. Put the limb through circular motion, abduction, adduction, and extension. Check the neurologic status (CPs, anal and tail tone). Check the lumbosacral area for pain and intervertebral areas for disk disease.
- a. **Coxofemoral luxation:** Luxation is usually craniodorsal with the luxated limb being shorter than the opposite limb. In the standing animal, the luxated side may have a more dorsally positioned greater trochanter. Place a thumb between the greater trochanter and the tuber ischii, and then externally rotate the limb. In a normal limb your thumb will be displaced, whereas with coxofemoral luxation, the femoral head will displace instead of your thumb position. Also, you won't be able to extend the leg caudally in a coxofemoral luxation.
- b. **Ortolani sign** of hip laxity: This usually requires heavy sedation or general anesthesia. Place the animal in dorsal recumbency. Push down on the stifles with the femur perpendicular to the table. Gradually abduct the leg while maintaining pressure. If the joint is lax, you'll feel a solid "clunk" as the femoral head is reduced back into the acetabulum. The angle at which this happens is the angle of reduction. After the reduction, continue maintaining pressure while the legs are adducted back to ventral position. A second clunk may be felt as the femoral head rides over the dorsal acetabulum rim. This is the angle of luxation.
- c. **Barden's sign** of hip laxity in puppies: Apply pressure to the femur in a lateral direction from the medial side. (Pressure misapplied may put pressure on the femoral nerve, creating discomfort for the puppy.)

6. **Pelvis**
- a. Determine the **symmetry** of the pelvis: Evaluate the relationships among the iliac crest, greater trochanter, and ischiatic tuberosity. If the femoral head on one side is not aligned with the femoral head on the other side, the femur is luxated or subluxated.
- b. **Palpate the wings of the ilium and the tuber ischii.** The wing of the ilium shouldn't move when pressure is applied.
- c. **Rectal exam:** Determine the anal tone, pelvic diameter, presence of pelvic fracture, and degree of displacement and instability.

III. **VERIFY FINDINGS WITH RADIOGRAPHS:** Don't forget to palpate the axilla and inguinal area for masses (e.g., schwannomas).

OSTEOARTHRITIS
General Information
Multimodal Approach to Treatment

I. **GENERAL INFORMATION:** Osteoarthritis (also called degenerative joint disease or osteoarthrosis) is a syndrome characterized by pathological changes in synovial joints. It involves articular cartilage deterioration, osteophyte formation, bone remodeling, and low-grade non-purulent inflammation. Despite numerous etiologies, a common molecular pathway leads to the continued damage of the articular cartilage and related structures.

A. **NORMAL PHYSIOLOGY:** Cartilage is comprised of chondrocytes embedded in the extracellular matrix that they produce and maintain. This matrix is made up of **proteoglycans,** a **collagen** framework, and water, all of which are organized to allow the cartilage to distribute force over the underlying subchondral bone and to provide a smooth, frictionless surface for joint movement.
1. **Proteoglycans** consist of a core protein attached to one or more **glycosaminoglycan (GAG) chains** of variable lengths. The chains consist of repeating disaccharides. For instance, **chondroitin sulfate** is made up of repeating dimers of N-acetylgalactosamine-glucuronic acid, and keratin sulfate is made up of N-acetylglucosamine-galactose dimers.
2. Proteoglycans can be classified as **aggregating or non-aggregating.** Aggregating proteoglycans are those that aggregate noncovalently with a glycosaminoglycan called hyaluronic acid. The main proteoglycan that binds this way, **aggrecan,** is the most prevalent proteoglycan in cartilage. It contains both chondroitin sulfate and keratin sulfate.

B. **PATHOPHYSIOLOGY of OSTEOARTHRITIS:** With trauma or damage to the joint, inflammatory mediators such as cytokines and prostaglandins are released. They stimulate chondrocytes, synovial cells, and inflammatory cells to release matrix metalloproteases and aggrecanases. These degrade the existing matrix faster than the matrix can be synthesized. They also stimulate nociceptors, causing pain.
1. In the inflammatory process, cell damage leads to the release of phospholipids from the cell membranes. **Phospholipase A$_2$** cleaves the phospholipids to **arachidonic acid,** which can be converted by **lipoxygenase to leukotrienes.** (Leukotrienes promote inflammation by attracting neutrophils that release inflammatory agents.) Also, **cyclooxygenases** (COX) cleave the phospholipids to inflammatory mediators or compounds that maintain normal physiologic functions. Cyclooxygenase 2 converts arachidonic acid to inflammatory mediators called **eicosanoids** (e.g., thromboxane A$_2$ and prostaglandin PGE$_2$) and to toxic oxygen radicals. Cyclooxygenase 1 converts arachidonic acid to prostaglandins that act on normal homeostasis and have a GI protectant effect.
a. **Prostaglandin E$_2$,** an eicosanoid produced by the action of COX-2 on arachidonic acid, causes vasodilation, increased vascular permeability, and edema. It also decreases the threshold at which nociceptors fire, thereby leading to an enhanced pain response. Theoretically, the ability to decrease prostaglandin formation by inhibiting COX-2 enzymes should decrease both the pain and cartilage degradation.
b. NSAIDs such as aspirin inhibit cyclooxygenases. Since COX-1 leads to products that are necessary for normal homeostasis, and COX-2 leads to increased inflammation and pain, treatments that selectively block COX-2 can theoretically block inflammation without adverse effects on GI, renal, and thrombolytic functions.
c. Most NSAIDs (except for tepoxalin, which blocks both lipoxygenase and cyclooxygenase pathways) do not affect lipoxygenase activity. Thus, leukotriene activity remains high and NSAIDs can't completely control the inflammatory response in the joints.
d. Corticosteroids block phospholipase A$_1$, so arachidonic acid is not formed. This means that inflammatory agents and prohomeostatic prostaglandins are not formed. Thus, corticosteroids can also lead to GI ulcers.

C. **ETIOLOGIES of OSTEOARTHRITIS**
1. Abnormal forces on normal joints; e.g., articular fractures and sprains
2. Normal forces on abnormal joints; e.g., hip or elbow dysplasia

II. MULTIMODAL APPROACH to TREATMENT
   A. **WEIGHT MANAGEMENT** is one of the most important factors in preventing and controlling osteoarthritis. (Watch a video on body condition scoring at www.nerdbook.com/extras).
      1. A study on Labrador Retrievers compared free-feeding with feeding a restricted diet. Results indicated that the dogs on a restricted diet were less likely to develop osteoarthritis, and when osteoarthritis did develop it occurred much later. The Labradors in the control group were mildly overweight (body condition score of approximately 6), whereas those in the experimental group had a BCS of 4-5. Similarly, a study in young Labradors found that those fed 25% below their free-feed amount starting at 8 weeks of age showed a significantly lower incidence and severity of hip dysplasia and osteoarthritis than the control group dogs that were free-fed.
      2. Owners should feed their pets a measured amount and should reserve some of the regular food as treats such that the total amount of daily food intake is appropriate for maintaining the dog at a 4-5 body condition score. To make feeding a more interactive and enriching event, the pet can work to get its food out of a food puzzle. Food puzzles include any of the commercial plastic toys that you place kibble in so that the animal must roll the device around causing food to drop out. For dogs, food can also be placed in a Kong toy and then frozen (with or without water added so that it freezes better). For cats, the food can be placed in a shallow cardboard box with holes strategically cut such that the cat must reach into the holes on the top or sides and bat the food out of the box. These toys can provide both mental stimulation as well as much needed exercise. (See www.lowstresshandling.com, Ch. 19)
   B. **PHYSICAL REHABILITATION and EXERCISE:** Weight control along with exercise can be as effective as NSAIDs for mild to moderate osteoarthritis. Physical rehabilitation is important not only following injuries and surgeries but also long-term. Exercise promotes good muscle tone and better ability to support the joints.
      1. Controlled **water-related exercises,** such as swimming or water treadmill walking, following surgery provide good muscle stimulation and mobility with minimal weight-bearing.
      2. Regular walks at a brisk trot, especially walking in high grass or up stairs or hills, is useful for building and maintaining muscle tone in healthy dogs.
      3. Avoid exercise that leads to sudden starts, stops, and changes of direction. Always let the animal warm up before rigorous exercise, and build up the level of endurance. For dogs with osteoarthritis, regular exercise that does not vary significantly in length or intensity seems to be most effective.
   C. **TREATMENTS**
      1. **NSAIDs:** Many NSAIDs such as aspirin inhibit both COX-1 and COX-2. Inhibition of COX-1 is probably what leads to the adverse GI effects (vomiting, ulcers, hematemesis, melena) and adverse renal effects (vasoconstriction leading to tubular necrosis). It is thought that NSAIDs with the highest COX-2:COX-1 activity have the least side-effects; however, all of the current NSAIDs have reported adverse incidents and even the COX-2:COX-1 ratio is dependent on the type of study performed.

DRUG	DOSE in DOGS	COX-1:COX-2 IC_{50} RATIO*
Deracoxib - a coxib class NSAID (Deramaxx®)	1-2 mg/kg PO SID as needed Post-op: 3-4 mg/kg PO SID as needed for ≤ 7 days	1275
Etodolac (Etogesic®)	10-15 mg/kg PO SID	65
Carprofen (Rimadyl®)	2.2 mg/kg PO BID	3.4
Meloxicam - an oxicam (Metacam®)	0.2 mg/kg PO initially then 0.1 mg/kg PO SID (Start with the same dose in cats, but by day 3 go to 0.025 mg/kg 2-3 times per week.)	COX2>COX1
Piroxicam - an oxicam	0.3 mg/kg PO e.o.d.	COX2>COX1
Aspirin	10-25 mg BID-TID	GI ulcers are decreased with the buffered form.

* Comparison of amount of drug needed to inhibit the activity of COX-1 and COX-2 enzymes by 50%. A larger number indicates more selectivity for COX-2, since it indicates that more drug is needed to inhibit COX-1 than COX-2.

    a.   Individual dogs respond differently to different NSAIDs, so if one does not work well, switch to another. The pet should be off NSAIDs for 3-5 days before starting the new one (and 7-10 days when switching from aspirin). Have owners administer the NSAIDs with food to prevent GI upset, even in those NSAIDs with low COX-1 activity.

    b.   Also be aware that NSAIDs are protein bound, and the non-protein bound fraction is the active fraction. If the animal has low plasma proteins, then the NSAID dose should be decreased.

2. **Dietary fatty acids:** Omega-3 fatty acids such as eicosapentaenoic acid (EPA) act as competitive substrates for phospholipase A, thus preventing the enzyme from working on arachidonic acid. Additionally, the products of EPA are anti-inflammatory. Consequently, the overall effect is that EPA leads to decreased inflammation in the joints. EPA in canines turns off gene expression of aggrecanase, the enzyme that degrades the aggrecan proteoglycans in the cartilage. Omega 3 supplements do not contain EPA in high enough amounts to have this beneficial effect; however, the amount in some prescription diets are much higher and have been associated with a positive response in controlled experiments.

3. **Chondroprotectants and nutraceuticals:** Glycosaminoglycans, such as chondroitin sulfate and glucosamine, inhibit the degradation of cartilage by inhibiting the metalloproteases that degrade it and by stimulating production of more glycosaminoglycans. Because they are nutritional supplements, the FDA does not monitor them; thus, quality control may vary dramatically among different products. According to a June 2002 article in *Consumer Reports*, "Makers of some glucosamine and chondroitin products need to do a better job of producing standardized, appropriately labeled products. " *Consumer Reports* tested 19 brands of chondroitin sulfate and/or glucosamine marketed for humans and found 15 of the 19 brands contained at least 90% of the labeled amount of glucosamine or chondroitin, but 4 of them did not. Two brands recommended a dose that was too low based on human clinical trials, and several others listed a range that included suboptimal doses.

    a.   Doses for dogs are extrapolated from human doses; thus, we do not know the appropriate dose in dogs.

    b.   There have been many conflicting studies in both humans and dogs about the effectiveness of these compounds in the management of osteoarthritis.

4. **Adjunct treatment for pain:** Treatment may also include an opioid analgesic such as tramadol (a partial μ receptor agonist).

ELBOW DYSPLASIA

Elbow dysplasia is a polygenetic hereditary developmental disease that is prevalent in many large breeds of dogs, although it is occasionally seen in small-breed dogs. The disease may be secondary to unequal growth in the radius and ulna, or due to developmental disease of the ulnar notch in which the area of curvature is too small to encompass the humeral trochlea.

DEFINITION	The incongruity becomes evident between 4-6 months of age when the bones are incompletely ossified. The incongruity can result in **osteoarthritis alone or in combination with the following:** • **Fragmentation of the medial coronoid process (FCP)** due to the increased weight on it. The medial coronoid process lies higher than the radius (which usually bears most of the weight in a normal elbow). • **Ununited anconeal process (UAP)** due to micromovement of the cartilage bridge between a separate center of ossification and the olecranon. (This movement is caused by too tight of a fit between the anconeal process and humerus.) • **Osteochondritis dissecans (OCD)** of the medial aspect of the humeral condyle opposite the medial coronoid process, which is lying too high.
BREEDS	Elbow dysplasia occurs most commonly in intermediate and heavy-set breeds such as German Shepherd Dogs, Labrador Retrievers, Bernese Mountain Dogs, Rottweilers, St. Bernards, and Newfoundlands. Over 50% of the affected animals have bilateral involvement.
CLINICAL SIGNS	• The dog may be lame in one or both forelegs. • It may hold its elbows out or hold the leg up.
PHYSICAL EXAM	Look for: • Crepitus and pain on flexion and extension of the elbow joint and deep palpation of the olecranon fossa or medial elbow • ± decreased range of motion • ± effusion
RADIOGRAPHIC CHANGES	The normal elbow joint has small, even joint spaces between the ulnar trochlear notch and the humeral trochlea (lateral view), and among the humeral condyle, radius, and medial coronoid process of the ulna (craniocaudal view). Also on the lateral view, the joint space between the ulnar trochlear notch and the humeral trochlea appears to lie on a continuous arc, as does the joint space between the lateral side of the humeral condyle and the radius. With elbow dysplasia, you may see the following: • **Joint incongruity:** A lateral view reveals an increased humeroulnar joint space in the central area of the trochlear notch and a stair-step at the base of the trochlear notch where it articulates with the radius (because the medial coronoid process is higher than the radius). The craniocaudal view shows increased humeroradial and decreased humeroulnar joint spaces; thus, it looks like a stair-step. (continued on next page)

Orthopedics

ELBOW DYSPLASIA (continued)

RADIOGRAPHIC CHANGES (continued)	• A radiolucent line between the anconeal process and ulna in cases of an ununited anconeal process (UAP). UAPs are seen in dogs that have elbow dysplasia and a separate center of ossification for the anconeal process. Both German Shepherds and Greyhounds have separate centers of ossification. Since elbow dysplasia is not seen in Greyhounds, however, they don't get UAPs, while German Shepherds do. In the normal German Shepherd, bony fusion of the anconeal process occurs between 5-6 months of age. In the case of non-fusion, the bridge remains cartilaginous and develops a cleavage line. If a radiolucent line is present before 5 months of age, it may be the normal anconeal physis and is probably insignificant unless accompanied by compatible clinical signs. You may need to take a flexed lateral view of the elbow to visualize the UAP.

• Direct radiographic visualization of a fragmented coronoid process is usually not possible because typically the piece that fragments lies between the main part of the coronoid process and the radius; thus, it is obscured by the overlying shadows of the bone. The (early) diagnosis of FCP, therefore, is usually based on age, breed, clinical findings, and visualization of sclerotic changes in the area of the medial coronoid process. New bone formation on the anconeal process is also a diagnostic sign.
• A radiolucent area on the medial aspect of the humeral condyle in seen in cases of OCD of the medial humeral condyle. The radiolucent area is visible on the craniocaudal view.
• Sequential osteoarthritis includes:
  • Subchondral sclerosis of the distal area of the trochlear notch
  • Osteophytes on the tip of the anconeal process and where the joint above the anconeal process capsule attaches to the humerus
  • Osteophytes on the medial aspect of the medial coronoid process and on the cranial aspect of the head of the radius
  • Signs of osteoarthrosis on the entire joint, in chronic cases
  • Periarticular lipping of the cranial rim of the radial head |
| **TREATMENT** | Treatment is only palliative. It won't correct the underlying problem. Osteoarthritis is inevitable. Thus, treat as you would for osteoarthritis:
• **Weight reduction:** Keep the animal at a body condition of 4-5 out of 9. For puppies, consider changing to adult dog food at about 6 months of age.
• **Controlled exercise:** Provide low-impact, moderate exercise regularly to maintain muscle strength, but build up to this exercise level gradually.
• **Medication:** Administer NSAIDs and other anti-inflammatory and chondroprotective agents.
• For more information, refer to the osteoarthritis section.

Surgically remove any ununited anconeal process or fragmented coronoid Process, and curette any OCD lesions. This can be done by arthrotomy or arthroscopy. Whether there are benefits of surgical management vs. medical management is controversial. Surgery may decrease the amount of degenerative joint disease that develops. Another option in the case of UAP is to reattach the UAP using Kirschner wires or a lag screw. Elbow replacement surgery may become an option in the future. Since surgery will require cage rest and limited exercise post operatively, dogs should be trained to associate their crates with pleasant experiences and to walk in a controlled manner on leash even when highly excited. For more information, refer to the hip dysplasia section (p. 16.13). To watch videos of some techniques or download client handouts on behavioral techniques go to www.behavior4veterinarians.com. |

HIP DYSPLASIA

Hip dysplasia is a polygenetic hereditary disease of the coxofemoral joint. It affects small, medium, and large dogs and can occur in cats. With hip dysplasia, the hips are normal at birth, but they develop abnormally. One possible reason for this is that the animal's skeleton grows at a faster rate than its musculature; thus, the hip muscles aren't strong enough to hold the femur in the joint. As a result, a dorsal displacement of the head of the femur in the joint occurs, which causes the cartilaginous dorsal rim of the acetabulum to become distorted. The acetabulum then ossifies into a distorted shape (shallow acetabulum). Since the course of the disease is influenced by growth rate, weight, and exercise, the development of hip dysplasia can be minimized by restricting the puppy's exercise and dietary intake so that it doesn't grow too quickly or become overweight.

> Some animals with radiographic evidence of hip dysplasia never show clinical signs. Animals in which an Ortolani sign can be elicited may never show clinical signs of hip dysplasia either. The absence of clinical signs makes it difficult for breeders to realize that they must still radiograph nonclinical animals for hip dysplasia before breeding. Regardless, dogs used for breeding should have their hips OFA certified prior to breeding.

I. CLINICAL SIGNS
   A. **GAIT:** The dog protects the hip by decreasing its motion at the hip joint and swaying its pelvis to throw the leg forward. At a pace slightly faster than a walk, the animal has a tendency to go into a hopping gait. In the young dog ($\pm$ 6 months), before the onset of osteoarthritis, luxation or subluxation may be palpable as the animal walks. That is, you may feel the hips moving in and out of the acetabulum. This can be done by holding your palms over the greater trochanters and walking behind the dog. An animal with subluxation or luxation will demonstrate a "clunk" as the femoral head is driven over the dorsal acetabular rim.
   B. **DIFFICULTY GETTING UP or LYING DOWN**
   C. **MUSCLE ATROPHY** in the affected limb
   D. **DECREASED WILLINGNESS to EXERCISE:** This may appear to the owner as lack of energy, decreased stamina, and a sign of normal aging, when in fact the signs are due to osteoarthritis.

> Sudden onset of hindleg lameness in an animal that has had hip dysplasia all its life is often due to reasons other than hip dysplasia. Rule out cruciate rupture, acute infection in one of the hips, polyarthritis, bone neoplasia, and idiopathic myelopathy before attributing the acute lameness to hip dysplasia. In young animals, rule out local cartilage disorders (such as osteochondrosis), panosteitis, hypertrophic osteodystrophy, and cranial cruciate rupture.

II. DIAGNOSIS can be made using clinical signs, physical exam, and radiography.
   A. **ELICITATION of the ORTOLANI SIGN** (Refer to the orthopedic physical exam section, p. 16.5): When the Ortolani sign is elicited in an awake animal, the animal has hip dysplasia. When the sign is elicited in an anesthetized animal, the animal is most likely dysplastic, but not necessarily radiographically dysplastic (i.e., while awake, muscles are able to compensate for joint laxity and make the joint stable).
   B. **RADIOGRAPHS** can reveal the severity of the hip deformity but do not determine the severity of clinical signs. Some animals with severe deformities have only mild signs and some with mild deformities have marked clinical signs.
      1. Radiographic findings
         a. **Shallow acetabulum:** With a normal hip, the acetabulum should cover 50% of the head of the femur.
         b. **Subluxation of the femoral head:** The acetabulum is shallow and surrounding tissues are relaxed, which predisposes the femoral head to subluxation.
         c. **Thinning of the acetabular rim** may be seen due to uneven pressure of the head in the acetabulum.
         d. **Osteoarthritis** starts at the femoral neck where the joint capsule attaches. With time, the neck becomes thick and distorted.
         e. **Periarticular lipping:** Osteophytes may be produced at the acetabulum to stabilize the hip joint.
         f. Occasionally, **coxa valga** is seen, with the angle of inclination > 135°.
         g. Sometimes, you'll see **increased anteversion,** where the head is rotated away from the acetabulum cranially. (Normal angle is $\pm$ 23°.)
      Two radiographic views are necessary to distinguish between anteversion and coxa valga: VD pelvis and an exact lateral view of the entire femur, or VD pelvis

Orthopedics

and an x-ray beam through the long axis of the femur. Increased anteversion mimics valgus since radiographs are only 2-D. On exact lateral positioning, you may see the femoral head angled too far cranially.

2. Severe hip dysplasia can often be diagnosed as early as 5-6 months; however, hip dysplasia cannot be ruled out on radiographs until 2 years of age.

3. Radiographs determine the phenotypically—not genotypically—dysplastic animals. Those that are phenotypically non-dysplastic may have offspring that are dysplastic.

III. DISEASE COURSE

A. **THE ACUTE PHASE** is the phase of joint instability. Clinical signs are present (abnormal gait), but the animal may not show signs of acute pain until it's 5-10 months of age (following a rapid period of growth). The pain may be due to microfractures of the dorsal cartilaginous rim of the acetabulum. Young dogs may spontaneously improve with conservative therapy.

B. **THE CHRONIC PHASE:** Degenerative changes may stabilize the joint.

1. As the animal becomes older, the joint capsule responds to the unstable hip by thickening. Pressure caused by instability at the sites of joint capsule attachment leads to osteophyte formation. New bone formation at the site of muscle tendon attachment is an enthesiophyte. The joint thickening and osteophyte production stabilize the joint, resulting in a less painful dog. Therefore, a once painful dog may become nonpainful after about 1 year of age, although the joint may have a decreased range of motion. The period in which the joint is not painful may last into mid-adulthood (4-7 years).

2. Later in life, the dog may become painful again due to increasing arthritis and loss of articular cartilage. At this time, most hip joint motion becomes painful. These dogs also have a decreased range of motion in their hips.

IV. TREATMENT: Some animals with radiographic evidence of hip dysplasia never show clinical signs until they reach late adulthood and osteoarthritis is severe. Therefore, it's important that animals that will be used for athletic performance be radiographed for hip dysplasia prior to engaging in intensive athletic training that requires jumping, explosive changes in speed and direction, and extremely lengthy exercise sessions. Additionally, animals with hip dysplasia but no clinical signs should be thoroughly palpated, and owners should be questioned about their dog's gait, activity levels, etc., to help assess pain. Some owners miss subtle signs of lameness and should be aware of the indicators of pain (decreased exercise tolerance, etc.). Animals with radiographic evidence of hip dysplasia may or may not need surgical treatment. Surgery is indicated depending on the degree of pain they exhibit, their response to conservative therapy, whether athletic performance is desired, and whether the owner wishes to slow progression of osteoarthritis and enhance the probability of good long-term limb function.

A. **WEIGHT CONTROL** does not prevent hip dysplasia but decreases the severity of the osteoarthritis associated with it. Animals should be kept at a body condition score of 4-5 out of 9. Use of NSAIDs and nutraceuticals without weight control provides a less than ideal response.

B. **EXERCISE MODIFICATION:** Refer to p.16.7.

C. **PAIN CONTROL:** NSAIDs can be used to address pain and inflammation.

1. **Acute injury:** In cases of acute hip pain, the hip can be iced after all bouts of controlled exercise, and the dog should be under strict cage rest with controlled leash walks to urinate and defecate. NSAIDs can be used for inflammation. Exercise can be gradually increased but in a controlled manner over a week to prevent re-injury.

D. **NUTRACEUTICALS:** Chondroprotectant drugs can slow the degeneration.

V. SURGICAL TREATMENTS

A. **JUVENILE PUBIC SYMPHYSIODESIS** can be performed in puppies 15-20 weeks of age. The caudal pubis is either cauterized or resected to allow fusion. This eventually causes gradual ventroflexion of the iliac shafts, which results in better acetabular cover. A preventive procedure, it is best for dogs with excessive laxity as young pups; however, what's considered excessive is not known for all breeds at all ages. The PennHIP scheme, which measures hip laxity in young animals, may more clearly define which animals are the most appropriate candidates for the procedure.

B. **Triple pelvic osteotomy** (TPO) is a surgery that can be performed in young animals with hip dysplasia where the animal will engage in extensive athletic activity or where the owner wishes to slow the progression of osteoarthritis and thus enhance the probability of good long-term limb function. The most important criteria for determining whether an animal should have a TPO vs. another surgery are the condition of the joint surfaces, the "quality" of the Ortolani sign (i.e., the depth of the acetabulum), and the animal's intended use. If the joint has already undergone degenerative changes (the acetabulum is filled with bone, the dorsal acetabular rim is lost due to eburnation, or the cartilage of the femoral head is destroyed), then a TPO should not be performed.

1. With TPO, the pelvis is cut at 3 sites—the ilium, ischium, and pubis—and then rotated so that the head of the femur sits better in the acetabulum.
2. Treat the side or sides that the animal is clinically dysplastic on. After surgery, the animal should have **strict cage or crate rest along with controlled walks and physical therapy for 4-6 weeks.** Overall, dogs do well with TPOs, with most no longer showing clinical signs of dysplasia.

C. **TOTAL HIP REPLACEMENT** (THR) is a salvage procedure that can be performed on animals over about 20 kg. As with TPOs, surgery is performed on the hip that is clinically dysplastic. With a THR, the head of the femur is removed and a metal implant put in its place. Most dogs return to full function by 8 weeks postoperatively. That is, they have normal gait, near normal range of motion, and normal level of activity with no signs of pain in the hip. Luxation of the joint is the most common cause of early failures. Infection and loosening of the prosthesis account for most of the late failures. THR is contraindicated in dogs that have or have had osteomyelitis in the hip joint, any infectious process, underlying neurologic disease, or cranial cruciate rupture. 50-80% of dogs with bilateral hip dysplasia will do well with only one side replaced.

D. **FEMORAL HEAD OSTECTOMY:** The femoral head and neck are excised allowing formation of a pseudarthrosis. By eliminating bony contact between the femur and the pelvis as scar tissue interposes, pain is relieved in the joint. Slight limb shortening and some loss of range of motion results in a persistently abnormal gait, although the abnormality may be minimal. Femoral head ostectomies can be performed bilaterally or staged 4-6 weeks apart. This technique is especially well suited for cats and small dogs with hip dysplasia. In large and giant breeds where the owner has limited funds, FHO is not ideal but is an alternative to euthanasia.

VI. **POST-OPERATIVE CARE:** All surgical patients require cage rest and carefully supervised physical rehabilitation. For the best outcome, owners need to prevent sudden movements or uncontrolled exercise that could lead to injury of the surgical region.

A. **CRATE TRAINING:** In preparation for the surgery, dogs should be trained to associate their crates with pleasant experiences so that they will accept cage rest willingly. To do this, owners can regularly place the dog's daily meals in the crate while leaving the crate door open. Also, owners can place treats for them to find in their crate randomly throughout the day. When animals willingly go into their crates in the owner's presence and also spontaneously rest in their crates, they have been appropriately crate trained. This process usually takes less than one week.

B. **CONTROLLED WALKING:** In preparation for post-operative care, dogs should also be trained to walk in a controlled manner on a loose leash so that they do not injure themselves while trying to run around. They may need to be leashed as the owner takes them out of their crate to keep them from jumping, running, or making sudden movements that could impair healing during this excitable event. Using a Gentle Leader head halter or a harness where the leash attaches to the front (e.g., the Gentle Leader Easy Walk harness or the SENSE-ation harness) can facilitate training dogs to walk in a controlled manner and to remain calm when they are excited.

C. **PHYSICAL REHABILITATION** includes passive range of motion exercises as well as exercises to improve muscle condition while placing minimal stress on the healing sites. Exercise should be gradually increased. Dogs will do best if their owners have a specific post-operative plan to follow.

VII. **PREVENTION**

A. **ELIMINATING DOGS WITH HIP DYSPLASIA FROM the BREEDING POPULATION** via OFA screening is important for the prevention of hip dysplasia. Additionally, spaying and neutering pets will help prevent unplanned breedings in dogs with hips of unknown status. PennHIP radiographs may have a greater ability than OFA screening to detect laxity at an earlier age and may be more effective in detecting and preventing hip dysplasia.

B. **DIETARY MANAGEMENT:** Dogs that are on a limited diet have less hip joint laxity than those that are free-fed. Large- and giant-breed dogs as well as those already diagnosed with or at risk for hip dysplasia should be fed a measured amount of food on a daily basis and their total calories limited to keep them at a 4-5 out of 9 body condition score. Such feeding has been shown to decrease the onset of osteoarthritis. Dietary restriction also helps reduce the incidence of juvenile orthopedic diseases (e.g., OCD, retained cartilage cores, and HOD).

The Small Animal Veterinary Nerdbook ™

CRANIAL CRUCIATE LIGAMENT RUPTURE

The functions of the cranial cruciate ligament are to limit internal rotation and cranial displacement of the tibia relative to the femur and to prevent hyperextension. Cranial cruciate rupture is one of the most common injuries in the dog and is the major cause of degenerative joint disease in the stifle. Ruptures can occur acutely but are more commonly chronic injuries in which a partial tear gradually progresses to a complete tear. The medial meniscus may be torn acutely when the cranial cruciate is ruptured, or it may be damaged due to chronic instability of the joint. Meniscal injury is present in up to 75% of animals with complete cruciate ruptures.

ETIOLOGIES	• Rupture can occur when the flexed stifle is rotated rapidly or when the joint is forcefully hyperextended. These situations occur when the animal suddenly turns toward the limb with the foot firmly planted or when it steps into a hole or depression while running. • The cranial cruciate ligament normally deteriorates with age due to loss of fiber bundle organization. Whether the ligament actually ruptures depends on many factors, including the activity and weight of the animal. Cruciate ligaments in small dogs deteriorate more slowly than those in large dogs. Since cruciates deteriorate with age, many dogs with one ruptured cruciate also have minor joint effusion in the contralateral stifle, indicating deterioration of the contralateral cruciate. Over 50% of dogs with chronic cruciate ruptures will eventually rupture the other cruciate ligament.
PREDILECTION	• Large-breed dogs (especially Rottweilers, Bull Mastiffs, Labrador Retrievers, Golden Retrievers, Pit Bulls, and Chows) are more likely to develop cruciate ruptures than small-breed dogs. In addition, large-breed dogs usually develop cruciate ruptures at a younger age than small-breed dogs. Over $1 billion is spent yearly in the U.S. on the treatment of ACL ruptures. • Acute traumatic ruptures usually occur earlier in life (< 4 years of age) but can happen at any age. • Chronic ruptures due to normal changes in the cruciate ligament usually occur after 3 years of age in large dogs and later in small dogs. • Obese dogs and dogs that are not conditioned well prior to intermittent heavy exercise are at risk for cruciate rupture. They don't have enough musculature around the knee to protect their intra-articular structures from excessive stress. • Abnormal limb conformation (e.g., bow-legged conformation, internal rotation of the tibia, or straight stifles) puts excessive stress on the cruciate ligaments. In cases where abnormal limb conformation is a major factor, acute and chronic ruptures occur at a young age (and may affect more than one animal in a litter).
CLINICAL SIGNS	Clinical signs may be either acute and associated with a specific traumatic event, or more chronic without a history of distinct trauma. • In many cases of acute lameness due to a cruciate rupture, there's a history of earlier episodic lameness related to bouts of vigorous exercise. This indicates that the animal had a partial cruciate rupture that completely ruptured acutely, or that it had a rupture and then tore the meniscus acutely. • In acute injury to the cruciate ligament, animals initially won't bear weight on the affected limb. Most, however, will start to use the limb within 2-3 weeks and may improve for several months until a gradual or sudden decline in the use of the limb is noted, often due to secondary meniscal damage. By this time, significant secondary degenerative changes have occurred.

CRANIAL CRUCIATE RUPTURE (continued)

DIAGNOSIS	• History and clinical signs • **Cranial drawer signs or tibial compression** (may need heavy sedation or general anesthesia): You should be able to elicit a cranial drawer sign in cases of acute, complete ruptures, but in cases of partial ruptures, the joint may be only mildly unstable. With chronic ruptures, secondary changes may stabilize the joint making it difficult to elicit a drawer sign. (Refer to page 16.5 for instructions on testing for the **cranial drawer** sign or for **tibial compression**). • **Thickened joint or joint effusion:** In chronic ruptures, the medial joint capsule is extremely thickened compared to the sound leg. • **A joint tap** reveals a non-inflammatory effusion and is not very helpful in diagnosing cruciate ruptures. • **Radiographs** (flexed lateral and VD): In acute ruptures, the radiographs may only reveal mild joint effusion. In chronic ruptures, the joint has significant secondary degenerative joint disease and effusion. • **MRIs** are rarely used. • **Exploratory surgery:** Examine the cruciate ligament and the meniscus. Also look for secondary degenerative joint disease and joint effusion.
TREATMENT	More than 100 methods exist for treating ruptured cranial cruciates, but the principles of the methods are similar. The goal is to rest the animal and stabilize the joint long enough to allow secondary joint changes to further stabilize it. • **Conservative (nonsurgical) therapy** is recommended for **cats.** Most regain normal function and range of motion within several months. • In **DOGS UNDER 20 KG, strict rest** and confinement (no running, jumping, or quick movement on the injured leg) often allows the stifle to stabilize due to secondary joint changes. Thus, with small dogs you may wait 6-8 weeks before recommending surgery. • In **DOGS OVER 20 KG,** even in cases of partial rupture, the joint should be **surgically stabilized** to help prevent secondary degenerative changes. In one study, about 10% of dogs > 20 kg did well without surgical stabilization. The three most popular techniques for repair are (1) extracapsular suture stabilizations, (2) tibial plateau leveling osteotomy (TPLO), and (3) tibial tuberosity advancement. Be sure to clean the joint first by removing the degenerative cruciate, a torn medial meniscus, and osteophytes before stabilizing the joint. **Surgical failures** are most often associated with undetected medial meniscal injury.
POST-OP CARE	• Since surgery will require cage rest and limited exercise post-operatively, dogs should be trained prior to surgery to associate their crates with pleasant experiences and to walk in a controlled manner on leash even when highly excited. For more information, refer to the hip dysplasia section (p. 16.13). To watch videos of crate training and other behavior modification techniques or for client handouts on these techniques, visit www.behavior4veterinarians.com. • **Physical rehabilitation** exercises include passive range of motion exercises, leash walks of increasing duration, swimming or water walking, hill or stair climbing, and icing.
PROGNOSIS	With physical rehabilitation, dogs are usually recovered enough to run after 3 months. Dogs used for rigorous sports such as field trials should be rehabilitated methodically over 6 months before returning to work. Prognosis for recovery is good with correct management (85-90% improve with surgery), but the dog will still have degenerative changes in the joint that may hinder its performance as a working dog or cause stiffness and pain later in life. Less than 50% of dogs become completely sound on the affected leg. Many show intermittent lameness. Furthermore, many dogs will rupture the cruciate ligament on the other leg within several years.

Orthopedics

FRACTURES
Fracture Classifications
General Fracture Treatment

Suspect a fracture if you see a deformity or change in angulation of a bone/limb, abnormal motility of the bone, pain or localized tenderness, loss of motion in the affected area, crepitus, or local swelling. Local swelling at the site of a fracture may appear almost immediately or may not appear for up to 24 hours following the fracture incident. The swelling usually lasts for 7-10 days due to disturbed blood and lymph flow.

FRACTURE CLASSIFICATIONS

PRESENCE of a COMMUNICAT-ING EXTERNAL WOUND	• **CLOSED fracture:** The fracture doesn't communicate to the outside. • **OPEN fracture:** The fracture ends communicate through a wound to the outside. These fractures are at high risk of becoming contaminated or infected, resulting in complicated or delayed healing. Surgeons often use external fixation or bone plates, and avoid IM pins when repairing open fractures if they are contaminated.
FRACTURE STABILITY	**STABLE fracture:** The fracture fragments interlock, and resist shortening forces (e.g., transverse, greenstick, impacted fractures). The primary purpose of fixation of stable fractures is to prevent angular and/or rotational deformity. **UNSTABLE fracture:** The fragments do not interlock; thus, they slide by each other and out of position (e.g., oblique, spiral, comminuted fractures). Fixation is indicated to maintain length and alignment and to prevent rotation.
EXTENT of the DAMAGE	**COMPLETE fracture:** The fracture involves the complete cross section of the bone (extends from one side of the bone to another) and is usually accompanied by marked displacement. **GREENSTICK fracture:** Only one side of the bone is broken, while the other is bent. This type of fracture is seen most commonly in young, growing animals. **FISSURE fracture:** One or more fine cracks extend from a surface into, but not through, a long bone.

DIRECTION and LOCATION	• **TRANSVERSE fracture:** The fracture occurs at right angles to the axis of the bone.
	• **OBLIQUE fracture:** The fracture line extends diagonally to the long axis of the bone. Spastic contractions of muscles tend to cause the fragments to slip by each other unless the fractured bone is stabilized with fixation.
	• **SPIRAL fracture:** The fracture line curves around the bone diagonally like the threads of a screw. The fragments tend to slip by each other and rotate unless fixation measures are taken.
	• **COMMINUTED fracture:** The bone is splintered or fragmented, and the fracture lines meet at a common point.
	• **MULTIPLE or segmental fracture:** The bone is broken into three or more segments. The fracture lines do not meet at a common point.
	• **AVULSION fracture:** A small bone fragment occurs at the site of attachment of a ligament and tendon.
	• **IMPACTED fracture:** The bone fragments are driven firmly together.
	• **PHYSEAL fracture:** The fracture occurs at the epiphyseal line or growth plate.
	  • **Salter-Harris I:** The epiphysis is displaced from the metaphysis at the growth plate through the zone of cartilage transformation.
	  • **Salter-Harris II:** The fracture involves displacement of the epiphysis from the metaphysis at the growth plate as with the type I fracture, but it also includes a small corner of metaphyseal bone.
	  • **Salter-Harris III:** The fracture goes through the epiphysis and part of the growth plate, but the metaphysis is unaffected.
	  • **Salter-Harris IV:** The fracture goes through the epiphysis, growth plate, and metaphysis.
	  • **Salter-Harris V:** A portion of the area of chondrogenesis and its blood supply are crushed. This occurs most commonly in the distal ulna.
	• **UNICONDYLAR or CONDYLAR fracture:** The fracture line passes through a condyle (e.g., humerus, femur).
	• **BICONDYLAR fracture (also called a "Y" or "T" fracture):** The fracture occurs between two condyles and the diaphysis.

GENERAL FRACTURE TREATMENT

TREATMENT GOALS	The goal of treatment is to allow early ambulation and complete return of function. The fracture should be **reduced and stabilized as soon as the patient's condition permits.** The longer you wait, the more the muscles will contract. In addition, the inflammatory thickening of the soft tissue increases with time. While in some cases, the fracture can be fixated immediately, often it's advisable to wait a day or more until the patient becomes an acceptable anesthetic risk. However, it's best not to wait until swelling has subsided before reducing and fixing because by that time, hematoma organization and callus formation are well underway. Callus formation obscures fracture lines, nerves, and blood vessels. Surgery prior to the fourth day is accompanied by less hemorrhage. Prior to surgically fixing a fractured extremity, you may place a **bandage** or **cast** for **temporary stability** as long as the joint above and below the fracture can be immobilized.
IMMOBILIZATION	The goals of fixation are to **stabilize the fracture and place the ends in as close apposition as possible** so that the animal can regain use of the fractured bone as soon as possible. In addition, it's best if the animal can use as many joints as possible during the healing period. **EXTERNAL FIXATION** of the limb: CASTS and limb SPLINTS Casts and splints are used for immobilizing stable fractures **distal to the elbow or stifle** (except for radius/ulna fractures in small-breed dogs; these dogs need plate fixation). The cast must immobilize the joint above and below the fracture site and should be placed **within the first 6-8 hours** after a fracture occurs. Splints and casts are indicated in the following circumstances: • Cases with **minor puncture wounds** • As temporary stabilization in cases where the **animal is not stable** enough to undergo surgical fixation • With **stable fractures** (where the periosteum is not ruptured— e.g., greenstick fractures or fissure fractures) **INTERNAL FIXATION:** bone splints (e.g., intramedullary pins, external fixation apparatuses, Kirschner wires, cerclage wires, cortical bone screws, plates, interlocking nails, or a combination of techniques) Internal fixation is indicated as described below. • **IM pins** are indicated in stable contaminated fractures treated within 6-8 hours. Secondary fixation (such as a KE apparatus) is often required for stability. • **Bone screws** or **plates** are indicated when the fracture involves an articular surface or when stability cannot be obtained via less invasive means. • A **KE apparatus** is often indicated when the main fracture area is traumatized and implants must be placed away from the major damage.
CANCELLOUS BONE GRAFTS	These grafts are usually **harvested** from the **greater humeral tubercle, the iliac crest,** or the **greater trochanter** of the femur. Cancellous bone grafts are **indicated** in the following situations: • With **comminuted fractures** • With **bone loss** (e.g., loss of a small fragment of bone at the fracture site) • With all **delayed unions** or **nonunions** (especially avascular ones), to increase the rate of healing • In cases of **infection** (usually after resolution of the infection) • Always when performing an **arthrodesis**

Orthopedics

NUTRITIONAL and METABOLIC BONE DISEASES

DISEASE	DESCRIPTION	CLINICAL SIGNS	PATHOGENESIS
OSTEOPOROSIS (atrophy of bone)	Osteoporosis is caused by **inadequate formation of bone**. It can be **congenital** (osteogenesis imperfecta), **dietary** (lack of available calcium in the diet or inability to absorb calcium from ingesta), or **endocrine** in origin. It can also be caused by disuse (stress and weight bearing are important in maintaining bone mass).	Pathologic fractures	The body does not synthesize enough osteoid, but all of the bone present is adequately mineralized.
RICKETS (vitamin D deficiency in growing animals)	Animals with rickets have **inadequate bone formation** because they have low levels of active vitamin D. (For more info refer to endocrine chapter p.9.23). Rickets can be caused by lack of sunlight, dietary deficiency of vitamin D, or malabsorption of vitamin D. Vitamin D is a fat soluble food, so if fat is not absorbed well and the animal develops steatorrhea, vitamin D won't be absorbed well.	Enlarged costochondral junctions (ricketic rosary) and enlarged joints due to a widened metaphysis Softer bones than usual for young animals (i.e., they bend more easily = osteomalacia)	The osteoid that the body produces is poorly mineralized and does not become bone tissue. As a result, the cartilaginous matrix in the growth plate does not become calcified, and osteomalacia of bone tissue occurs.
OSTEOMALACIA (vitamin D deficiency in adults)	Osteomalacia is caused by **inadequate formation of bone** usually due to a diet low in vitamin D.	Softer, more pliable bones than normal. Osteodystrophy fibrosa is sometimes misdiagnosed as osteomalacia on gross examination because of the pliability of the affected bones.	The osteoid produced is poorly mineralized and does not become bone tissue.

OSTEODYSTROPHY FIBROSA	Osteodystrophy fibrosa is caused by an **increased rate of bone resorption** due to 1° or 2° hyperparathyroidism. **Primary hyperparathyroidism:** A tumor of the parathyroid gland results in excess production of parathyroid hormone. **Secondary hyperparathyroidism:** This is due to renal disease or a dietary imbalance of Ca:P. Osteodystrophy fibrosa reflects faulty bone formation.	May have a rubbery jaw and/or swollen face Late stages: teeth can be pulled out with your fingers Some cases: generalized loss of bone density with coarsening of the remaining cancellous bone and cortical thinning It's sometimes misdiagnosed as osteomalacia on gross examination because of the pliability of the affected bones.	Hyperparathyroidism (> 72 hours) turns on osteoclasts that lyse the bone, leading to osteopenia. Osteoprogenitor cells try to respond by proliferating, but the osteoblasts are unable to differentiate fully. As a result, the matrix that's laid down to replace the missing material has lots of collagen with few bone spicules.
JUVENILE OSTEOPOROSIS (in kittens and puppies on **ALL MEAT** DIETS)	Juvenile osteoporosis is characterized by an **increased rate of bone resorption due to secondary hyperparathyroidism.** The hyperparathyroidism is usually caused by diets with large Ca:P ratios(> 1:7), such as some all meat diets. The ratio should be 1:1. Kittens on **all meat diets** without milk may develop this disease.	Folding fractures Deformed vertebral column Chronic constipation due to fractures and collapse of the pelvis, which impinges on the rectum Thin cortex with an enlarged medullary cavity (may show on radiographs) Cats and dogs: usually other skeletal regions involved more than the head	The prognosis for improvement following correction of the diet is better in puppies than in kittens, since many cats are reluctant to accept a change from an all meat diet.
OSTEODYSTROPHY of mature cats (on **HIGH MEAT DIETS** with low calcium)	This disorder is similar to **juvenile osteoporosis** except that it occurs in mature cats. It's caused by high meat diets with no milk (source of calcium).	Loss of bone density and swelling of long bones A **double outline** of the shafts due to a double cortex; cross section shows a neocortex outside the normal cortex	The prognosis depends upon the amount of periarticular enthesophytes present.
HYPERVITAMINOSIS A (in adult cats on **RAW LIVER DIETS**)	Hypervitaminosis A occurs in mature cats on diets of **raw liver.** Liver is high in vitamin A. Note: Vitamin A toxicosis in kittens causes premature closure of the physes.	**Ossified** tendon insertion lines in regions of frequent movement (especially the cervical spine and elbow joints)	High levels of vitamin A cause chondrocytes in the fibrocartilage insertion lines of tendons to die. The dying cartilage then undergoes endochondral ossification, which may result in the formation of crippling enthesophytes.

Orthopedics

LOCAL CARTILAGE DISORDERS

DISORDER	PREDILECTIONS	CLINICAL SIGNS	RADIOGRAPHIC CHANGES	PATHOGENESIS/PROGNOSIS
EPIPHYSEAL DYSPLASIA "swimmers"	Young dogs with open growth plates	Pups are alert, obviously stunted, and exhibit a clumsy, sprawling gait when forced to walk. Some may not be able to walk. They may stay in sternal recumbency and "swim" with their legs ("swimmers").	Radiographs reveal irregular secondary centers of ossification. This feature is especially prominent in the epiphyses of long bones.	This disorder is probably an inherited defect in endochondral ossification affecting epiphyses. Epiphyseal dysplasia predisposes the dog to developing degenerative joint disease. Treatment involves physical therapy and weight control.
RETAINED CARTILAGE CORE of the DISTAL ULNA	Large-breed dogs (GSDs)	This disorder affects the distal epiphysis/metaphysis of the ulna. It may result in retardation of the growth plate of the distal ulna but with continued growth of the ipsilateral radius, resulting in radius curvus/valgus of the carpus.	Radiographs show a radiolucent core of cartilage extending from the epiphysis to the distal ulna to the metaphysis.	Pathogenesis is unknown. If the animal is being overfed, decrease the amount of food. A retained cartilage core may be an incidental finding in many young, large-breed dogs.
CANINE PANOSTEITIS	Young, growing dogs (5-8 months old) German Shepherds have a higher incidence than other breeds. Males are more commonly affected than females.	At a young age (e.g., 8 months) the animal shows lameness that may start in one leg and migrate to another leg. Once a bone recovers, there's no relapse. Recovery may be prolonged, though. Pain is often elicited on palpation of the affected areas.	Radiographs show increased sclerotic, mottled density in the medullary cavity of the affected diaphysis of the affected bone (enostosis).	Pathogenesis is unknown. Bouts usually subside spontaneously by 2 years of age. Treatment is palliative until spontaneous remission occurs. Animals that are being overfed should be fed less. Keep them at a body condition score of 4-5 out of 9.
CRANIOMANDIBULAR OSTEOPATHY	Primarily Scottish Terriers and West Highland White Terriers. Onset usually occurs in animals around 6-8 months of age.	This disorder affects the cranium and mandible. The dog may have a lumpy calvarial surface, swollen maxilla or mandible, or a massive temporal bulla. The dog can't open its jaw very widely to eat. This disease is very painful and may affect one or all of the listed sites.	Radiographs show roughened osseous proliferations of the mandible, tympanic bulla, and/or thickening of bone plates of the calvarium.	Pathogenesis is unknown. Treatment is palliative (anti-inflammatory drugs).

HYPERTROPHIC OSTEODYSTROPHY (HOD)	Giant-breed dogs (usually around 3-4 months old)	The dog limps and is painful on palpation of the metaphysis of affected bones. The metaphysis may be enlarged due to transient soft tissue swelling in the area. If the animal overcomes the disorder, the bone continues to grow normally. A few of these dogs develop angular limb deformities because the cuffs occasionally bridge the growth plate.	Initially, radiographs reveal a thin, radiolucent line in the metaphysis parallel to the epiphyseal plate. Later, an extraperiosteal cuff of new bone develops along the surface of the metaphysis. In rare cases, radiographs show skull involvement resembling craniomandibular osteopathy.	HOD is a proliferative bone disorder that affects the surface of the metaphysis. There are two clinical patterns. The first pattern is associated with overnutrition of large-breed puppies. These dogs are alert but painful and don't want to walk. Treat by decreasing their food intake to 20% of the free-feed amount or low enough to maintain a 4-5 (out of 9) body condition score. Prognosis for recovery is good. In the second pattern, the dog has a fever and becomes lethargic. Prognosis in this case is guarded.
HYPERTROPHIC OSTEOPATHY (HO)	Primarily in mature animals that have a disease process going on in the chest (e.g., a tumor, *Spirocerca lupi*, heartworm, or chronic infection)	The animal exhibits lameness, reluctance to move, and firm swelling on the distal limbs.	Radiographs show periosteal proliferation of the diaphysis of long bones, beginning in the metacarpals, metatarsals, and phalanges. In peracute cases with swollen limbs, the radiographs may not show periosteal changes for several days.	Pathogenesis is unknown. Thorough diagnostics, especially of the thorax, should be performed. The probability of finding a non-lethal underlying factor is low; thus, the prognosis for recovery is guarded.
ASEPTIC NECROSIS of the FEMORAL NECK	Toy dogs (Legg-Calve-Perthes disease) Any dog can develop this disease if it fractures the femoral neck, interfering with the blood supply to the head.	The animal exhibits pain on palpation of the hip, especially on abduction. Aseptic necrosis is primarily a unilateral disease.	Radiographs may reveal an increased joint space; decreased bone density of the femoral neck; a dense, flattened femoral head; and ± osteophytes of the femoral head and neck. Femoral head density is due to infarction and dystrophic calcification of the affected part of the epiphysis.	Blood vessels going underneath the articular cartilage are damaged, and part of the head loses its blood supply. The cartilage turns pale due to lack of blood supply. Osteoclasts try to get rid of the dead bone and replace it with live bone, so there's no bone in areas of the femoral head to support the cartilage. The articular cartilage collapses down and is no longer smooth. The animal may develop crippling degenerative joint disease. Treatment is the surgical removal of the femoral head (femoral head ostectomy).

Orthopedics

COMMON DRUGS

DRUG	DOSE
Albendazole Hookworm, roundworm, whipworm	25 mg/kg PO BID for 3 days in dogs and 5 days in cats.
Clindamycin (Antirobe®) for *Toxoplasma* and *Neospora* Capsule: 25, 75, 150 mg Liquid: 25 mg/mL in 20 mL bottles	For clinically ill animals **Cats and dogs:** For intestinal infection, use 25-50 mg/kg/day PO or IM divided BID to TID. Systemic: 10-40 mg/kg PO BID or 40 mg/kg PO TID for 14 days.
Diethylcarbamazine Heartworm prevention Roundworm infections	• For prevention of heartworm and roundworm infections in dogs: 6.6 mg/kg PO daily. • Treatment of roundworm infections in dogs and cats: 55-110 mg/kg PO.
Fenbendazole (Panacur®) Paste 100 mg/g Roundworm Hookworm Whipworm Lungworm *Giardia*	**Dogs** • Ascarids: 50 mg/kg PO for 3 days. • *Capillaria aerophila:* 25-50 mg/kg PO BID for 14 days. • *Filaroides:* 50 mg/kg PO BID for 14 days. • *Paragonimus:* 25-50 mg/kg PO BID for 14 days. • *Giardia:* 50 mg/kg PO BID for 3-5 days. **Cats** • Ascarids: 50 mg/kg PO for 5 days. • *Aelurostrongylus abstrusus:* 20-50 mg PO BID for 10-14 days. • *Capillaria aerophila:* 50 mg/kg PO SID for 10 days. • *Paragonimus:* 50 mg/kg PO SID for 10 days.
Ivermectin (Heartgard® and Heartgard Plus®) - heartworm, roundworm, whipworm *Capillaria* Tablets: 68, 136, 272 µg 1% solution	• Heartworm prevention in dogs: 6 µg/kg PO q 30 days. • Microfilaricide before HW adulticide treatment: 50-200 µg/kg PO. • Roundworm, hookworm, whipworm, *Capillaria:* 200 µg/kg PO once.
Melarsomine dihydrochloride (Immiticide®) - adult heartworms	Dogs: 2.5 mg/kg q 24 hr for 2 treatments.
Metronidazole (Flagyl®) - *Giardia* Tablets: 250, 500 mg	Cats: 10-25 mg/kg PO SID for 5 days. Dogs: 30-60 mg PO SID for 5-7 days.
Milbemycin oxime (Interceptor®) Heartworm, roundworm, whipworm Tablets: 2.3, 5.75, 11.5, 23 mg	Heartworm prevention and control of hookworm, roundworm, and whipworm infestations (but not for treatment). **Dogs and cats:** 0.5-0.99 mg/kg PO q 30 days.
Moxidectin for heartworm and hookworm	Dogs: 0.17 mg/kg SC twice yearly.
Piperazine (Pipa-Tabs®) - roundworms Tablets: 50, 250 mg (120 mg OTC)	**Dogs and cats:** 20-30 mg/kg PO once and then again in 3 weeks. Can go up to a dose of 110 mg/kg. Can start in puppies at 3 weeks of age.
Pyrantel pamoate (Nemex® or Strongid®) Roundworm, hookworm Tablets: 22.7, 113.5 mg Suspension: 50 mg/mL	**Dogs and cats:** 5 mg/kg PO. Repeat in 3 weeks.
Praziquantel (Droncit®) - tapeworms (*Dipylidium*)	Refer to package insert.
Sulfadimethoxine (Albon®) - *Isospora* Tablets: 125, 250, 500 mg Oral suspension: 50 mg/mL.	**Dogs and cats:** 50 mg/kg PO for one day. Then 25 mg/kg PO SID for 14-20 days.
Sulfadimethoxine/ormethoprim - *Isospora* Tablets: 100, 200, 500, 1000 mg Sulfadimethoxine fraction	Dogs: 55 mg/kg sulfadimethoxine fraction SID for the first dose. Then 27.5 mg/kg PO SID for 14-20 days.

LOCATIONS of MAJOR PARASITES

PARASITES of DOGS

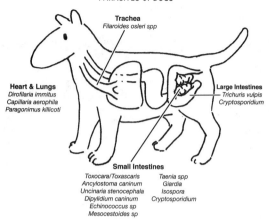

Trachea
Filaroides osleri spp

Heart & Lungs
Dirofilaria immitus
Capillaria aerophila
Paragonimus killicoti

Large Intestines
Trichuris vulpis
Cryptosporidium

Small Intestines

Toxocara/Toxascaris   *Taenia spp*
Ancylostoma caninum   *Giardia*
Uncinaria stenocephala   *Isospora*
Dipylidium caninum   *Cryptosporidium*
Echinococcus sp
Mesocestoides sp

PARASITES of CATS

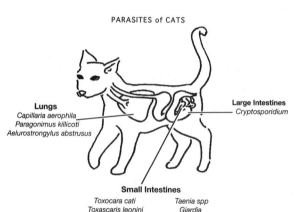

Lungs
Capillaria aerophila
Paragonimus killicoti
Aelurostrongylus abstrusus

Large Intestines
Cryptosporidium

Small Intestines

Toxocara cati   *Taenia spp*
Toxascaris leonini   *Giardia*
Ancylostoma tubaeforme   *Isospora spp*
Echinococcus multilocularis Toxoplasma gondi
Echinococcus sp   *Cryptosporidium*
Mesocestoides sp   *Spirometra*

SUGGESTED READINGS
Companion Animal Parasite Council (CAPC) Guidelines: Controlling Internal and External Parasites in US Dogs and Cats. 2005.

Centers for Disease Control and Prevention (CDC) Guidelines for Veterinarians: Prevention of Zoonotic Transmission of Ascarids and Hookworms of Dogs and Cats. 2006.

Dryden MW, Payne PA, Ridley RK, Smith VE: Gastrointestinal parasites: The practice guide to accurate diagnosis and treatment. Supplement to *Compen Contin Educ Vet* 28:7(A) 3-13. 2006.

PARASITES AFFECTING the LUNGS and HEART in DOGS and CATS

CLASSIFICATION	LOCATION	TRANSMISSION	LIFE CYCLE	CLINICAL SIGNS	DIAGNOSIS
Dirofilaria immitis (heartworm) For more information, refer to p 17.9.	Pulmonary artery	Mosquito bites	Adults in the pulmonary artery release microfilariae into the blood. The microfilariae are taken up by feeding mosquitoes. They mature to L3 and are deposited into another victim where they mature into adults. It takes 70 days for the larvae to appear in the pulmonary artery and 6 months before you see microfilariae in the blood.	Lethargy, exercise intolerance, cough due to pulmonary hypertension or thromboembolism. *D. immitis* vs. *Dipetalonema reconditum*: *D. immitis* (microfilariae) have pointed heads, are larger (308 nm vs. 263 nm), are stationary, and occur in higher numbers than *D. reconditum*.	Knotts test and Difil test for microfilariae Antigen test for adult heartworm antigen (dogs) Antigen and antibody tests for cats
Capillaria aerophila	Lungs	Ingestion of an embryonated egg	Adult worms in the lungs produce eggs that are coughed up and swallowed, then passed in the feces. The eggs embryonate and are ingested by other cats/dogs. Adult worms can inhabit the trachea, bronchi, and, less commonly, nasal cavities and frontal sinuses.	Predisposes the animal to secondary rhinitis, tracheitis, bronchitis. Affected animals may have a deep cough, anemia, and may be emaciated.	Fecal flotation
Paragonimus kellicotti (fluke)	Lungs	Ingestion of an Infected intermediate host	Miracidia penetrate a snail and mature to the metacercaria stage before being released from the snail. They enter the second intermediate host, a crayfish. The infected crayfish is eaten by a cat or dog. Immature flukes migrate extensively and mature in the lungs. Eggs are coughed up and swallowed, then passed in the feces.	Lethargy, intermittent cough	Fecal sedimentation Fecal flotation
Aelurostrongylus abstrusus	Lungs	Ingestion of a Molluscan intermediate host or a transport host (bird)	The larvae are ingested by a snail, which is ingested by a transport intermediate host (e.g., bird). The cat can ingest either the snail or the transport intermediate host. Larvae migrate to the lungs and mature to adults, which produce eggs that hatch and are passed in the feces.	Chronic cough and gradual wasting	Baermann Tracheal wash
Filaroides osleri (canine)	Bifurcation of the trachea	Ingestion of larvae in sputum or feces.	Adults living in the trachea lay eggs that quickly hatch. Larvae are immediately infective upon ingestion. They are coughed up and swallowed, then passed via feces or sputum.	Cough, anorexia, emaciation	Baermann Tracheal wash Endoscopy

Parasitology

PARASITES of the GASTROINTESTINAL TRACT

CLASSIFICATION	LOCATION	TRANSMISSION	LIFE CYCLE	PATHOGENESIS/ CLINICAL SIGNS	DIAGNOSIS
Roundworms (ascarids) *Toxocara cati* *Toxocara canis* *Toxascaris leonina*	Small intestines	Ingestion of eggs or infected paratenic hosts (rodents, rabbits, birds) Transplacental (*canis*) Transmammary (*cati, canis*) Coyotes are a reservoir.	Adult worms lay eggs in the SI, which are then shed in feces. Here, they embryonate in about 2 weeks and are ingested by dogs/cats or rodents. The infected rodent may be eaten by a dog or cat. **Animals < 3 months of age: tracheal migration.** Larvae migrate from the stomach to the liver to the lungs, where they are coughed up, swallowed, and end up in the SI. **Animals > 3 months of age:** Larvae may undergo tracheal migration but are more likely to encyst in muscle. They are activated during pregnancy. **Eggs are very resistant and survive for years in the soil.**	Roundworms affect nearly 100% of pups and kittens, and up to 15% of adult dogs nationwide. Clinical signs include abortion, stillbirth, emaciation, pneumonia, coughing, vomiting, diarrhea, unthriftiness, and death. **Zoonosis: Visceral and ocular larva migrans.** 3-6 million people are affected annually.	Fecal centrifugal flotation 70-75 µm
Hookworms *Ancylostoma caninum* *Uncinaria stenocephala* *Ancylostoma tubaeforme*	Small intestines	Ingestion of infective larvae Skin penetration Transplacental (*Ancylostoma*) Transmammary (*Ancylostoma*)	Adult worms lay eggs in the SI. Eggs hatch in soil and develop to infective larvae, which penetrate skin or are ingested by a dog/cat. **Animals < 3 months old:** tracheal migration. Larvae migrate as with roundworms. **Animals > 3 months old:** Migrating larvae arrest.	In animals < 3 months old: Migrating larvae become adults in the SI and cause tarry diarrhea, weight loss, anemia, unthriftiness. **Zoonosis:** Cutaneous larva migrans	Fecal centrifugal flotation
Whipworm (dogs only) *Trichuris vulpis*	Colon Cecum	Ingestion of embryonated eggs	Adult worms lay eggs in the large intestines. Eggs are passed in feces, embryonate, and are ingested by dogs. Eggs are **very resistant and survive for months to years in the soil.**	Whipworms feed off blood of the large intestines, causing anemia; mucoid, hemorrhagic diarrhea; weight loss; and unthriftiness. Affects about 15% of dogs nationwide. Whipworms affect primarily **mature dogs.** **Zoonosis:** ± intestinal disorders	Daily fecal centrifugal flotation. Few eggs are produced, and shedding is intermittent.
Tapeworms *Dipylidium caninum* *Taenia spp* *Echinococcus spp*	Small intestines	Ingestion of intermediate hosts (fleas, rodents, sheep, pigs)	Posterior segments of adult worms are passed in feces. The eggs are ingested by an intermediate host (flea, rodent, etc.), where they develop into larval tapeworms (metacestodes). The infected intermediate host is ingested by a cat or dog.	No problem. Just aesthetically unpleasant for the owners.	Identify segments in feces or on the anus. Fecal centrifugal flotation (Sheather's sugar solution is best)

Parasitology

Giardia	Small intestines	Ingestion of cysts from feces or contaminated water.	Trophozoites hatch and travel to the SI, where they attach and reproduce. Cysts and feeding stages are passed in the feces 5-10 days after infection. **Cysts are resistant.** Clean the environment with bleach and maintain good sanitation.	Clinical signs range from nothing to acute or chronic explosive, mucoid diarrhea. **Zoonosis:** ± intestinal disorders	Direct fecal smear (trophozoites and cysts). Zinc sulfate fecal flotation (for cysts) ELISA (Alexon) IFA (Meridian)
Coccidia (*Isospora* in dog/cats)	Small intestines	Ingestion of sporulated oocysts Ingestion of infected intermediate hosts	The coccidia invade intestinal cells, and asexual and sexual stages develop in the SI. Unsporulated oocysts are passed in feces, where they sporulate and are ingested by cats or dogs. **Oocysts** are hard to kill and survive up to one year in the environment. Use ammonium hydroxide-containing solutions and maintain good sanitation.	**Young animals** may have watery diarrhea. Treat pets with coccidia when the pet has clinical signs, lives in a kennel or cattery, or when the pet lives with a child or immunocompromised individual (**zoonosis**).	Fecal centrifugal flotation
Toxoplasma (cats only) <u>*Toxoplasma gondii*</u> (protozoa) Disseminated disease in cats, dogs, and people	Small intestines	**Ingestion** of sporulated oocysts **Ingestion** of infected **intermediate hosts** (sheep, pig, rodent; avoid raw meat). **Prenatal infection.** Humans are exposed through cat feces or consumption of uncooked, infected meat.	Sexual stages produce oocysts in the SI, and unsporulated oocysts are passed in the feces, where they sporulate and are ingested by a cat or an intermediate rodent host. Animals only shed for 7-14 **days**, and their **titers remain high** after infection; therefore, high titers indicate present or past infection. Oocysts are very resistant.	Minimal signs in cats (intestinal) **Zoonosis:** Toxoplasma can cause congenital defects in human fetuses. High titers indicate present or past infection.	Toxoplasma titers Fecal centrifugal flotation for oocysts in cats
Cryptosporidia (protozoa)	Small intestines	Ingestion of oocysts	Sporulated oocysts are passed in the feces, where they are ingested. They may also be found in contaminated water.	Organisms invade the microvillous brush borders of the small intestines. We see chronic and severe diarrhea in immunosuppressed dogs/cats and asymptomatic infections in healthy dogs/cats. Diarrhea may occur in **neonatal pups/kittens.** **Zoonosis:** Intestinal disorders.	Fecal float 4-8 µm (sugar) They are tiny and hard to see! ELISA test (Alexon) IFA (Meridian)

ZOONOTIC INFECTIONS

I. **BACKGROUND and PREVENTION of ZOONOTIC INFECTIONS:** Dogs and cats commonly carry intestinal parasites that are a major zoonotic threat to humans. Hookworms and roundworms are among the most concerning. A survey of dogs in animal shelters revealed that nearly 36% of dogs in the U.S. harbor helminthes such as hookworms, roundworms and whipworms. An estimated 10,000 human cases of *Toxocara* infection occur annually in the U.S. and yearly more than 700 of these people experience permanent partial loss of vision. Roundworm eggs can live for 5 years in the environment, and one infected puppy can spread over a million such eggs in the feces per day. Because of the risk GI parasites pose to humans, the CDC (www.CDC.gov) and the Companion Animal Parasite Council (www.CAPCvet.org) have devised guidelines for preventing infection in companion animals and reducing environmental contamination. The guidelines call for regular prophylactic treatment, routine fecal exam, and prompt fecal cleanup.

PARASITE	NOTES
Roundworms • Visceral larva migrans • Ocular larva migrans - leads to unilateral blindness	Nearly 100% of puppies and kittens and up to 15%-36% of adult dogs nationwide harbor roundworms. Pups and kittens require treatment even if they have negative fecal tests because infections can cause serious illness and death even before eggs appear in the feces. Because larvae migrate and mature at different rates, such that parasites are not all in the stage targeted by the medication at one time, treatments should occur every two weeks. This also covers the continued infection from the environment, including the queen's or bitch's milk. Pups should start treatment at two weeks because they can be infected transplacentally. Kittens can be infected when nursing on the queen's milk but are not infected transplacentally; thus, they can start treatment at 3 weeks. Treat the mother and pups/kittens at the same time. The mother can also be treated during pregnancy. • Deworm all **puppies** at 2, 4, 6, and 8 weeks of age. • Deworm **kittens** at 3, 5, 7, and 9 weeks. • For puppies and kittens over 6 weeks of age, deworm for a total of three treatments 3 weeks apart. For prevention, CAPC recommends that dogs and cats receive monthly prophylactic treatment. A convenient way to do so is to treat with monthly heartworm prevention containing pyrantel pamoate or milbemycin (which kills roundworms and controls, but does not kill, hookworms). Adult dogs should receive fecal examinations 1-2 times per year to look for nematodes as well as other parasites. (Pups and kittens 2-4 times per year). If owners cannot afford year-round monthly treatment, they may elect to continue monthly treatment through 6 months of age and then have fecal exams done 2-4 times yearly and treat as needed. • Heartgard Plus®: ivermectin plus pyrantel pamoate (kills both roundworms and hookworms) • Interceptor®: milbemycin oxime (controls hookworms, kills roundworms) • Diethylcarbamazine/oxibendazole (kills roundworms and hookworms) – dogs only
Hookworms • Cutaneous LM	Schedule and treatment is the same as for roundworms.
Tapeworms • ± Diarrhea	Treat when tapeworms are seen either in the fecal sample or on the pet's anus. Inform owners of infectious sources. Treat for fleas. • Treat with praziquantel (Droncit®) • Sulfadimethoxine
Toxoplasma • Fetal abortions • Birth defects	Most cerebral cases in humans are due to reactivation of latent infections or ingestion of infected, undercooked meats. The *Toxoplasma* oocysts are shed by cats and sporulate to their infective form within 1-5 days. Cats shed for only about 14 days, but their antibody titers stay high even after they are no longer shedding. A positive titer means that the cat has been infected earlier in life. Human infection with *Toxoplasma* can be prevented by using gloves when cleaning the litter pan or gardening, and by avoiding undercooked meat. Cats don't leave feces on their body for more than one day, so it's safe to pet the cat.
Giardia • Diarrhea	Treat when the fecal (SNAP giardia test) is positive for *Giardia* regardless of clinical signs. Good sanitation and hygiene are important.
Coccidia • Diarrhea	Treat when the fecal is positive for *Isospora*.

II. DIAGNOSTIC TECHNIQUES
A. **FECAL CENTRIFUGAL FLOTATION** is used to find eggs, cysts, and larvae. The idea is to use a solution with a specific gravity that's higher than that of the eggs so that the eggs will float to the top of the solution. Most eggs float at a specific gravity of 1.2-1.3. If the specific gravity of the solution is too low, then the eggs won't float; however, if the specific gravity is too high, too much fecal debris floats and some cysts collapse. For good results, it's imperative to use a large enough fecal sample and to centrifuge it. Omission of these steps frequently leads to false negatives.
   1. Mix 2-5 grams of feces (5 g = 1 teaspoon) with fecal float solution such as zinc sulfate or a Sheather's sugar solution. Sheather's is better for also recovering *Taenia* due to its higher specific gravity. Avoid passive centrifugation fecal kits such as Ovassay®. They use small fecal volumes and no centrifugation.
   2. To strain out large particles, drain the mixture through a strainer into a centrifuge tube. The sample can then be centrifuged at 1200-1500 rpm for 5-minutes. Centrifugation increases identification of positive samples by 50-100%. The sample can be spun in one of two ways:
      a. **Method 1 (for swinging-head centrifuges):** Overfill the sample such that a meniscus forms. Place a coverslip and then spin the sample for 5 minutes with the coverslip on.
      b. **Method 2 (for fixed-head centrifuges):** Spin the sample without a coverslip for 5 minutes. After spinning, add additional fecal float solution to form a meniscus and place a coverslip on it. Let the sample sit for 10 minutes.
   3. To view the sample under a microscope, place the coverslip, solution side down, onto a microscope slide and view first at 10x and then 40x. To preserve the sample or hold the coverslip still for viewing under oil immersion, nail polish can be placed on the sides of the coverslip.
B. **FECAL SEDIMENTATION** is used to find the same parasite ova as with fecal flotation, but it's also used to find fluke ova (such as *Nanophyetus* and *Paragonimus*). Mix feces with detergent water and pour it through a strainer. Allow the solution to settle for 5-10 minutes and then, using a Pasteur pipette, collect a sample of the sediment and place it on a microscope slide for examination.

C. **A DIRECT FECAL SMEAR** is used for finding protozoal trophozoites (e.g., *Giardia* and *Tritrichomonas foetus*), which are destroyed with salt solution. It is inefficient in looking for other organisms. Use a warm fecal sample (less than one hour old). If you get an older sample (> 6 hours), you can add saline and mix it up well to prevent desiccation of the trophozoite.
   1. **Technique:** Place a drop of saline on a clean glass slide. Add a small amount (size of a peppercorn) of feces to the saline. The prep should be thin enough to just be able to read the fine print of a newspaper through. Add a coverslip and examine at 10x first. Then look at 40x.
   2. *Giardia* moves in a regular fashion whereas *T. foetus* swims in a haphazard, falling leaf motion. *T. foetus* also has 3 flagella and an undulating membrane.

D. **THE INPOUCH™ FECAL CULTURE for *Tritrichomonas foetus*** is a commercial test media (BioMed Diagnostics, Inc., Oregon). Get a fresh specimen of the **diarrheic** stool. Note that the likelihood of getting a positive culture from a normal stool is low. Use a miniscule amount (size of 1/2 a peppercorn). If you take too much stool, bacteria will proliferate and compete for the culture media, and the trophozoites will die quickly. Mix the media by squishing the pouch, and then hang it in the incubator at 37° C for 24 hours. Remove the InPouch3.™ from the incubator, and place it vertically in a cup in a dark space (cupboard or drawer). Once a day look at it under 10x magnification, especially noting the bottom portion and sides of the pouch (trophozoites move to the bottom of the bag). This media does not support the growth of giardia. Sensitivity is 90%, and the pouches are inexpensive. Trophozoites generally appear within 2-3 days. If you haven't seen any by 8 days then the likelihood of culturing *T. foetus* is remote.

E. **THE BAERMANN TECHNIQUE on FECES** is used to find nematode larvae (e.g., *Aelurostrongylus abstrusus* and *Filaroides osleri*). It's based on the idea that larvae will migrate out of feces or soil into warm water (25° C).
   1. **Technique:** Use a 125-225 mL glass or plastic funnel and place a tube over the small end. Clamp the tube shut so that liquid placed into the funnel will not leak. Place 1 mm mesh wire or gauze into the funnel to support the sample, and then

line the wire with Kimwipes®. Add 10 grams of feces onto the wire gauze. Pour warm water into the funnel until the feces is covered. Let the sample sit for at least one hour. Now open the clamp and release 5-6 mL of the solution into a centrifuge tube. Centrifuge the sample for 5 minutes at 1500 rpm. Pipette out the supernatant and place the sediment on a slide for examination under a microscope.

F. DIAGNOSTIC TECHNIQUES PERFORMED on BLOOD
1. **Knotts test for heartworm larvae:** In a 15 mL centrifuge tube, place 1 mL of blood preserved in heparin and add 9 mL of **2% formalin**. Centrifuge the sample for 5 minutes. Pour off the supernatant and add 2 drops of methylene blue to the remaining sediment. Tap the tube to mix the sediment. Place the mixture on a slide and examine the sediment at 100x.
2. **The Difil test (membrane filtration) for heartworm larvae** is similar to the Knotts test but uses a 5 μm millipore filter to concentrate the microfilariae.
3. **The antigen test** is the most widely used screening test because it detects the presence of adult heartworms whether or not microfilariae are present.

III. DRUGS for TREATING GI PARASITES (Refer to page 17.1 for doses.)
In many cases the animal must be dewormed several times. The first deworming kills the adult parasites and the second kills the maturing adult parasites. To know when to give the second treatment and when to recheck for parasites, we must know the prepatent period of the parasite. Recheck for parasites at the end of the prepatent period.

PARASITE	TREATMENT
Coccidia (*Isospora*)	• Sulfadimethoxine (Albon®) • Sulfadimethoxine/ormethoprim
Giardia	• Albendazole • Fenbendazole (Panacur®): Also kills roundworms, hookworms, whipworms. • Metronidazole (Flagyl®)
Heartworm	• Diethylcarbamazine: Higher doses treat hookworms, roundworms. • Ivermectin (Heartgard®) kills heartworms. Higher doses kill hookworms. • Milbemycin oxime (Interceptor®) kills heartworms. • Selamectin (Revolution®) kills heartworms (and roundworms, hookworms in cats).
Hookworm	• Fenbendazole (Panacur®) kills roundworms, hookworms, whipworms. • Diethylcarbamazine: High doses treat hookworms, roundworms. • Ivermectin (24 μg/kg) kills heartworms, hookworms. • Oxibendazole kills roundworms, hookworms, whipworms. • Milbemycin oxime (Interceptor®) prevents but doesn't treat hookworm infections. • Moxidectin (ProHeart®) kills heartworms, hookworms. • Pyrantel pamoate (Nemex®, oral Strongid®) kills roundworms, hookworms.
Roundworm	• Diethylcarbamazine: High doses treat hookworms, roundworms. • Fenbendazole (Panacur®): Also kills roundworms, hookworms, whipworms. • Milbemycin oxime (Interceptor®) kills roundworms, hookworms, whipworms. • Pyrantel pamoate (oral Strongid® or Nemex®) is 98% effective against roundworms and hookworms. Give 2 doses 2 weeks apart. For *T. cati* and *T. leonina*, the prepatent periods are longer; thus, the treatment may need to be repeated for several months and then a fecal performed again at 2-3 months. • Piperazine (Pipa-Tabs®) is for roundworms only.
Tapeworm	• Praziquantel (Droncit®): Give once. To prevent reinfection, control the ingestion of intermediate hosts such as fleas and rodents.
Tritricho-monas foetus	• Ronidazole: 30-50 mg PO BID x 2 weeks (Obtain from a compounding pharmacy)
Whipworm	• Fenbendazole (Panacur®) kills hookworms, roundworms, whipworms. • Milbemycin oxime (Interceptor®) kills heartworms, controls roundworms, whipworms. • Oxibendazole kills roundworms, hookworms, whipworms.

HEARTWORM (*Dirofilaria immitis*) INFECTION in DOGS

About 270,000 dogs and cats nationwide test positive for heartworm each year. Infections are found in most parts of the U.S. Currently, infections are most common in the southern states (Texas: 42,000; Florida: 32,000; Georgia: 17,508), but many hotbeds for infection exist within regions where heartworm is not as common (California: 4,500; New York: 2,100). In areas where heartworm is endemic, nearly 100% of unprotected dogs are infected. The incidence in cats is approximately 10% of that in dogs. Despite good preventative medications, heartworm continues to spread. This is due in part to the relocation of pets from endemic regions, as occurred after Hurricane Katrina, as well as to the presence of wild canids as reservoirs. Estimates state that if 50-80% of the dog and cat population is on preventative medications during the mosquito season, this will provide a blanket of protection for the general population. That is, by decreasing the reservoir population for heartworm, we disproportionately reduce the likelihood of infection and spread, especially in regions of relatively low heartworm prevalence. The guidelines of the American Heartworm Society (www.heartwormsociety.org) are designed with this in mind.

I. **GENERAL INFORMATION**
   A. **LIFE-CYCLE:** Heartworm larvae are transmitted from infected dogs to non-infected animals by mosquitoes. The heartworm microfilariae (L1) accumulate in the mosquito when it feeds on an infected dog. The microfilariae develop to third stage larvae (L3) in the mosquito and then are injected into a non-infected dog, where in 6.5 months (prepatent period) they develop into adults (L5) that produce microfilariae. The adults live in the pulmonary arteries and can cause heart failure, pulmonary hypertension, and pulmonary thromboembolism.

II. **SCREENING TESTS and PROPHYLAXIS:** The animal must be infected with female adult heartworms for the microfilaria or antigen tests to be positive. Since the prepatent period is about 6.5 months for the larvae to mature to adults, testing puppies less than 7 months of age is not justified.
   A. **MICROFILARIA TESTS vs. ANTIGEN TESTS:** Dogs should be placed on monthly heartworm preventative medication within one month of negative screening tests. The medications have a 2-month retroactive effect.
      1. **Antigen tests:** Because many dogs infected with heartworms do not have a detectable microfilaremia, antigen tests (for adult antigen) should be performed as a screening test for heartworm. The tests are virtually 100% specific, and 99% of dogs with mature heartworm infections and microfilaremia are antigen positive. Thus, this test is good for occult infections as well as infections in which microfilariae are present.
         a. **If the test reveals a weak positive,** repeat it, perform a complementary test (such as one for microfilaremia), or take thoracic radiographs (especially in symptomatic animals).
         b. **False positives** are most commonly caused by poor technique (such as inadequate washing); however, in areas with a low incidence of heartworm the number of false positives increases.
         c. **False negatives** occur when mature females are too few or the heartworms are too immature to incite a strong antigen response.
      2. **Microfilaria tests** are run primarily in dogs who have tested positive for heartworms or when dogs will be started or restarted on DEC (see below).
   B. **WHEN to TEST**
      1. **Prior to placing dogs greater than 7 months old on prophylaxis** for the first time, because preventative medications will not treat infection with adult worms. Additionally, any time diethylcarbamazine (DEC) treatments are to be restarted (use the Knotts or Difil test), dogs should be tested first. DEC can lead to a dangerously rapid kill of microfilariae that could result in PTE.
      2. **7 months after possible exposure to heartworm** i.e. the animal is either not on preventative medication or a lapse in monthly prophylactic care (or a 2-day lapse in DEC) has occurred.
      3. **Whenever the type of heartworm preventative** is changed, dogs should be tested immediately prior to changing and again 4 months later for product failure of the first preventative used. The purpose of this testing is to determine product efficacy. A positive test 5 or more months after the switch makes it difficult to determine which product failed.
      4. **Annually** in high incidence regions (including small pocket regions of infection), even if the animal is on year-round therapy. The purpose is to test for lapses in owner compliance as well as breaks in drug efficacy.
   C. **WHEN a TEST is not NEEDED**
      1. Puppies or kittens 8 weeks old need not be tested prior to starting prophylaxis. They can be tested annually starting between 7-12 months of age.

Parasitology

       2. Puppies or kittens born during a season when mosquitoes are not around (i.e., winter in New York) and started on heartworm preventative before mosquito season hits need not be tested, except for annual retesting. If started on prophylaxis after mosquito season starts, test $\geq$ 7 months later.

  C. **HEARTWORM PREVENTATIVE:** Although mosquitoes are seasonal in many parts of the U.S., it is increasingly recommended that dogs and cats be put on year-round therapy because seasons and travel are not precisely predictable, and once infected, pets can serve as a reservoir for other animals. Switching to year-round therapy should increase overall compliance and provide protection without requiring that owners actively keep track of whether they are entering a higher risk region or season. Additionally, many monthly preventatives treat for intestinal helminths. Because an estimated 10,000 human cases of *Toxocara* infection occur annually in the U.S. (http://www.cdc.gov/healthypets/diseases/toxocariasis.htm) and hookworm cutaneous larva migrans is a common condition in endemic areas, roundworms and hookworms are major zoonotic concerns warranting attention from the Centers for Disease Control.

       1. **The macrocyclic lactones**—ivermectin (Heartgard®), milbemycin oxime (Interceptor®), moxidectin (ProHeart®), and selamectin (Revolution®)—are the most commonly used heartworm medications. Given every 30 days, they have retroactive efficacy (or reach-back effect) of at least 2 months. The reach-back effect is not a justification to administer them every 2 months, though. Rather, it is a safeguard in case the medications are inadvertently omitted or delayed. Since these drugs have 8 weeks of retroactive activity, dogs can be started on them at 8 weeks of age without having to be tested for heartworm infection

          a. Some collies and Shetland sheepdogs carry a mutation of the multidrug resistance (mdr1) gene. The gene encodes for p glycoprotein which transports drugs from the brain back into the blood thus preventing levels from accumulating in the brain. Those with the mutated gene synthesize less p glycoprotein. These dogs can develop signs of toxicity if given doses approximately 16x the minimum effective recommended dose. This most frequently occurs with dose miscalculations when administering livestock preparations (an extra-label use). A commercial test is available for detecting the mdr1 mutation (WSU Clinical Pathology Lab).

       2. **Diethylcarbamazine (DEC):** Because DEC has a strong microfilaricidal effect, testing for microfilariae is mandatory before initiating prophylaxis with it. DEC should be given at 6.6 mg/kg daily. Even a 2-3 day lapse voids the protection.

III. DIAGNOSIS

  A. **CLINICAL SIGNS** are due to the reaction of the pulmonary artery endothelium to the heartworms. Signs include exercise intolerance and coughing.

  B. **SCREENING TESTS:** The antigen tests and the microfilaria tests do not rule out heartworm infection. **Dogs showing clinical signs of heartworm infection should be radiographed even if the screening tests are negative.**

  C. **RADIOGRAPHS** may reveal enlarged, tortuous pulmonary arteries (evaluate peripheral branches), pruning of the pulmonary arteries, enlargement of the main pulmonary artery segment, increased right heart size, and associated lung disease.

  D. **CARDIAC ULTRASOUND:** When present in large numbers, heartworms may be visualized within the main pulmonary artery and sometimes in the right heart and vena cava (caval syndrome—very rare).

IV. TREATMENT: The most conventional treatment consists of using a microfilaricide followed by an adulticide. In cases of *caval syndrome,* the adult heartworms should be surgically removed prior to chemotherapy.

  A. ELIMINATION OF MICROFILARIAE:

       1. **Monthly ivermectin, milbemycin, moxidectin, or selamectin** can be instituted immediately to clear microfilariae from infected dogs. Doing so will keep dogs from acting as a reservoir of infection and from being reinfected. Elimination is usually complete after 3-6 months of monthly dosing. With severe infection, some clinicians elect to carry out microfilaricide treatment for up to 6 months prior to treating for adult heartworms.

  B ADULTICIDE TREATMENT: Melarsomine dihydrochloride (Immiticide®)

       1. **Evaluation:** Prior to starting adulticide, the dog should be evaluated for the severity of the infection. The more severe the infection—that is, the more clinical signs and pulmonary changes due to the infection—the more likely the animal is to develop life-threatening pulmonary thromboemboli secondary to treatment.

       2. **Treatment protocol**

a. **One-stage treatment for dogs with mild infection:** Administer 2.5 mg/kg Immiticide® IM 24 hours apart for 2 treatments.

b. **Two-stage treatment for severely affected dogs:** If the dog has severe disease signs and high worm burden, administer a single dose and then one month later administer two doses 24 hours apart.

3. **Pulmonary thromboembolism:** To help prevent the occurrence of PTE, the dog should be under **strict cage or crate rest** and should be taken out only on leash for one month following treatment. Acepromazine can be used for energetic dogs. Owners can also train even energetic dogs to walk calmly on leash prior to treatment (See videos at www.drsophiayin.com).

a. The most severe pulmonary thromboemboli occur within 7-10 days. In mild cases, the dog may show no signs, but in severe cases the dog may show hemoptysis, fever, coughing, syncope, and even heart failure. If clinical signs of pulmonary thromboemboli are seen, the animal should be put on corticosteroids and possibly aspirin. The use of aspirin to treat or prevent heartworm-associated PTE is not recommended.

4. **Retesting:** Dogs should be retested using the antigen test 6 months after treatment because it may take that long for the dying adults to dissolve. Occasionally, despite dramatic improvement in signs, some adult heartworms survive treatment. These residual infections are usually occult; thus, antigen tests are required to detect them. Dogs should be retested for adult antigens in 6 months. If the test is weakly positive, they should be retested again several weeks later. A positive retest does not necessarily mean that the animal must be treated again. Factors such as age of the animal in relation to its lifespan, severity of the remaining infection, the patient's clinical improvement, and the type of performance the owner expects of the animal must be considered.

HEARTWORM INFECTION in CATS

While cats are susceptible to heartworm infection, the prevalence of infection is much lower than in dogs. Infections usually involve 5 or fewer worms, and many involve only 1-2 worms. Even 1 worm, however, can cause clinical signs in a cat.

COMPARISON with infection in dogs	The heartworm life-cycle is similar in cats and dogs; however, in cats, infections may spontaneously clear, and adult heartworms only live 2-3 years. Cats tend to have more aberrant larval migrations than dogs. Cats rarely develop caval syndrome or right-sided cardiac hypertrophy.	
CLINICAL SIGNS	Peracute signs Respiratory distress—may be misdiagnosed as asthma Hemoptysis Seizure or collapse Sudden death	Chronic signs Cough Tachypnea Intermittent vomiting—no relation to eating Signs of right heart failure
DIAGNOSTICS	**Microfilariae tests** are rarely positive because the microfilariae are either destroyed by the cat's immune system or the cats have occult infections. A negative test does not rule out infection. A positive test indicates infection. **Serology** • The **ELISA antigen test** is very specific, but may yield **false negatives** due to low worm burden and because the tests do not detect infection with male heartworms. A negative test does not rule out heartworm infection. A positive test indicates infection. • The **ELISA antibody test** is more sensitive but less specific for heartworm, since the cat can have circulating antibodies from immature heartworms that never fully developed. A negative test lowers the index of suspicion. Using both the antigen and antibody tests together increases the chance of a correct diagnosis. **Thoracic radiographs** show a generalized interstitial lung pattern and/or enlarged, tortuous pulmonary vessels (especially of the caudal right lobar area). The main pulmonary artery segment is often enlarged. **Cardiac ultrasound** may reveal presence of heartworms.	
TREATMENT	Only treat cats that have a positive test and appropriate clinical signs (even if they have radiographic changes). Retest every 6-12 months using antigen and antibody tests to monitor infectious status.	
PROPHYLAXIS	**Ivermectin:** 24 μg/kg PO q 30 days (this is 4x the dog dose). **Milbemycin oxime:** 2 mg/kg PO q 30 days. **Selamectin:** 6-12 mg/kg q 30 days.	

DRUGS COMMONLY USED in PULMONARY DISEASE

DRUG	DOG	CAT
Aminophylline 100 and 200mg tabs, 25 mg/mL liquid	11 mg/kg PO TID	5 mg/kg PO BID (weak effect in cats)
Butorphanol 1, 5, and 10mg tablets	0.05-0.12 mg/kg PO BID-TID	
Dexamethasone SP		Emergency: 0.2-2.2 mg/kg IV, IM, or PO
Dextromethorphan (Pediatric Robitussen®)10 mg tablets, 1.5 mg/mL liquid	1-2 mg/kg PO TID-QID	
Epinephrine (1:1000)		Emergency: 0.1 mL/cat
Hydrocodone (Hycodan® or Tussigon®) 1.5 and 5mg tablets, 0.3 mg/mL syrup	0.22 mg/kg PO BID-QID	
Methylprednisolone acetate (Depo-Medrol®)		10-20 mg/cat IM every 2-8 weeks
Periactin (Cyproheptidine®)		2 mg PO SID-BID as needed
Prednisone 5, 10, and 20mg tablets	1 mg/kg PO BID, then taper to 0.5 mg/kg PO BID, then go to alternate day dosing.	2.2 mg/kg PO BID for 3-5 days, then 1-2 mg/kg PO BID. Continue to taper.
Prednisolone Sodium Succinate	Emergency: 20 mg/kg IV	Emergency: 10-20 mg/kg IV
Terbutaline 2.5mg and 5mg tabs, 1 mg/mL liquid	1.0-5.0 mg/dog PO SID-TID	0.625 mg/cat (up to 1.25 mg/large cat) PO BID. Emergency: 0.01 mg/kg IV,SC, IM
Theophylline (Theocap or Theochron™, Inwood Labs) 100, 200, 300 mg tablets	10 mg/kg PO BID. Start with 1/2 dose for 3-4 days and if well tolerated go to full dose.	20 mg/kg SID in the evening

Pulmonary

NASAL DISCHARGE

Nasal discharge can be unilateral or bilateral, serous, mucopurulent, or hemorrhagic. The characteristics of the discharge are helpful in determining the etiology.

RULE OUTS	DIAGNOSTICS
FOREIGN BODY (e.g. foxtail) Unilateral discharge	• The nasal discharge is often preceded by paroxysmal sneezing (e.g. the dog sneezes frequently for a day, stops sneezing, then develops a nasal discharge). Signs often recur when antibiotics are finished. • **Radiographs** may reveal fluid/mucus on the affected side and sometimes reveal a radiodense foreign body. • **Rhinoscopy:** Look for the foreign body.
TOOTH ROOT ABSCESS or ORONASAL FISTULA Unilateral discharge	• **Exam:** Look for swelling below the eye and one-side chewing. • **Oral exam:** Look for periodontal disease/fistulas. • **Radiographs:** Intraoral radiographs are best for evaluating the teeth. Look for radiolucent areas at the root apex. • **Rhinoscopy:** Look for a fistula.
FUNGAL INFECTION *Cryptococcus* (primarily in cats) *Aspergillus* (primarily in dogs, especially rottweilers) Unilateral or bilateral discharge	• **Clinical signs:** Discharge often starts on one side and progresses to the other side. Pets can develop swelling over facial bones, draining fistulas, submandibular lymphadenopathy, and nasal soft tissue masses. If the CNS is affected, the pet can develop neurologic (e.g. seizures) and/or ocular signs (chorioretinitis). • Make a **smear of the nasal discharge, skin lesion,** or **draining tract** (or CSF of a cat with neurologic signs): Stain the sample with india ink, new methylene blue, or Wright's stain. Positive samples contain 3-30μm large organisms with wide capsules (*Cryptococcus*) or fungal hyphae (sometimes with *Aspergillus*). If cytology is positive, then no further tests are required. • **Fungal titer:** The fungal antigen test detects *Cryptococcal* capsular antigen in the serum or CSF. This test is good for monitoring response to treatment. It can be run at a diagnostic lab or using a test kit. The titer test for *Aspergillus* is an antibody test. False negatives are possible with nasal aspergillosis. • **Radiographs** of the nasal region may reveal turbinate destruction. Thoracic radiographs may reveal an interstitial or multifocal nodular pattern. • **Rhinoscopy** may reveal fungal plaques or granulomatous masses. Take deep biopsies of any mass or plaque and take multiple biopsies (especially with *Aspergillus*).
TUMOR • Squamous cell carcinoma • Fibrosarcoma • Adenocarcinoma • Undifferentiated carcinoma • Lymphosarcoma Unilateral or bilateral discharge	• Often starts as a unilateral discharge and progresses to bilateral. • **Radiographs:** On nasal radiographs, look for turbinate or other bony destruction and mass lesions. CT scan is more sensitive. Also perform a thoracic metastasis check for completeness. • **Rhinoscopy:** Look for the mass. Pets can get **secondary bacterial and fungal infections** as well as **marked inflammation** with nasal tumors; therefore, a biopsy is often not representative. That is, nasal biopsy in a dog with a nasal tumor may reveal inflammation, bacterial infection, or fungal infection rather than revealing the underlying tumor. As a result, the biopsy may need to be repeated when the discharge recurs or does not clear up. Surgical exploration and histopathology are often required.
FELINE UPPER RESPIRATORY INFECTION Refer to p. 11.16	Infectious agents include Herpes, Calici, Chlamydia, Mycoplasma. Diagnosis is based on history and physical exam. The **bilateral** nasal discharge is often associated with conjunctivitis, ocular discharge, sneezing, and oral ulcers.
ALLERGIC Bilateral nasal discharge	Diagnosis is usually based on **history** and the subsiding of signs once the instigating allergen is removed. It can be complicated to diagnose as it can mimic all the other etiologies. Typical history is sneezing and/or mucopurulent or serous nasal discharge that's seasonal or associated with irritants such as smoke, perfume, pollens, kitty litter, cleaning agents, and old or new carpets. Eosinophils may be prominent in the CBC, cytology, or on histopathology.
COAGULOPATHY Bilateral nasal discharge (bloody)	Coagulopathies can cause bloody nasal discharge (epistaxis). Epistaxis can also be caused by nasal foreign bodies, tumors, fungal infections, and hypertension (check blood pressure). • Clotting panels and bleeding times are prolonged • CBC: $\pm$ anemia, thrombocytopenia

18.2

NASAL DISCHARGE: WORK-UP and TREATMENT

HISTORY	• Try to determine whether the animal was **sneezing** prior to the onset of the nasal discharge. Paroxysmal sneezing that precedes nasal discharge suggests a foreign body. • Describe the **character** of the discharge (e.g. mucoid, purulent). Is it **unilateral** (foreign body, tooth root abscess, fungal, neoplasia) or **bilateral** (allergy, upper respiratory infection, coagulopathy, fungal infection, neoplasia)? Has it progressed from one side to both? • Are there systemic signs of illness? • Are the signs seasonal or related to exposure to environmental irritants?
PHYSICAL EXAM	• **Oral exam:** Look for evidence of tooth root abscesses, oronasal fistulas, foreign bodies, or oral ulcers. • **Facial symmetry:** Most tumors are malignant and cause lots of bone destruction which eventually leads to facial deformity. Fungal disease can also cause facial deformity. • **Fundic exam** may reveal **chorioretinitis** (check for *Cryptococcus*). • **Neurologic signs:** seizures, abnormal mentation, etc.
RADIOGRAPHS or OTHER IMAGING	• First look at the nostrils to determine whether one or both are occluded with discharge. If needed, check airflow by holding a mirror or microscope slide to each nostril. • Look for **increased density** (and decreased turbinate pattern) due to fluid, fungal mass, or neoplasia. • Look for **destruction of the turbinates** and/or of the nasal bone. Neoplasia and fungi cause bone destruction. Inflammation, chronic rhinitis, or previous rhinoscopy can cause bony destruction too. • **Dental arcade:** Look for radiolucent areas at the tips of the tooth roots. Radiolucent areas indicate bone loss which is usually caused by endodontic disease (**tooth root abscess**). • **Frontal sinus shot:** The frontal sinuses should be wide open and black. They should be symmetrical. Obstructions appear as soft tissue densities. They may be due to mucus building up secondary to a mass preventing sinus drainage, or they may represent active disease itself. • **Cribriform plate:** Check that it's intact (CT scan or MRI is better for this). Neoplasia and fungal disease often destroy the cribriform plate.
RHINOSCOPY and BIOPSY	You must be aggressive in order to get a good sample. Tumors are often difficult to identify because they are surrounded by a superficial layer of chronic inflammation and may be associated with secondary fungal or bacterial infections. Take multiple deep biopsies. Also look for increased eosinophils indicating allergic etiology.
FUNGAL TITERS	*Cryptococcus:* Stain nasal exudate with New Methylene Blue or india ink for *Cryptococcus*. A positive smear reveals organisms that are 3-30µm big and contain a thick capsule. Alternatively, you can run the capsular antigen test on serum or CSF. This test is good for monitoring response to therapy. *Aspergillus* is a normal nasal inhabitant. A small amount is normal, but the presence of fungal plaques is abnormal. Fungal titers can be performed. Negative titers do not rule out *Aspergillus*. Since *Aspergillus* is an opportunistic infection, look for an underlying etiology (e.g. neoplasia).
TREATMENT	**FUNGAL** • **Clotrimazole in dogs with *Aspergillus* infections (best performed by a specialist):** Bathe the nasal sinus with clotrimazole or econazole by blocking the caudal nasal pharynx with an inflated foley catheter inserted through the oral cavity. Infuse the drug via urinary catheter into the dorsal meatus, and block flow out through the nares by inflating the cuff of a 3rd catheter just inside the nares. Let the drug sit for one hour (the animal is anesthetized and rotated every 15 minutes), then let the drug flow out the nares. Repeat in 2 weeks if needed. Dogs can be treated with oral itraconazole instead of or in addition to the nasal infusion just described. Itraconazole is more convenient but less effective. • **Cats with *Cryptococcus*:** Fluconazole (penetrates best), intraconazole, or amphotericin B can be used. Treat for 1 month past resoluton of signs and one month after the antigen test is negative (often 3-6 months). Prognosis in cats without CNS signs is fair to good. **ALLERGIC:** Remove the inciting agent if possible. Try antihistamines such as chlorpheniramine (2.2 mg/kg PO BID-TID in dogs; 2 mg/cat PO BID-TID), loratadine, or prednisone (0.25 mg/kg BID until signs resolve and then taper the dose).

Pulmonary

UPPER AIRWAY OBSTRUCTION

CLINICAL SIGNS	• **Respiratory distress:** May be exacerbated by exercise or hot weather. Respiratory distress can lead to syncope and can be accompanied by **hyperthermia.** • **Inspiratory stridor** or **snorting/stertor.** • **Change in voice** is specific for **laryngeal disease** (e.g. laryngeal paralysis).
RULE OUTS	• **Laryngeal paralysis** is a common cause of upper airway disease that occurs as a result of damage to the recurrent laryngeal nerve. Etiologies include neoplasia (thyroid carcinoma may invade the nerve), trauma, hypothyroidism (possibly—they may just occur concurrently, without cause and effect), iatrogenic (following surgery to the area), or idiopathic. It's rarely caused by a myopathy or neuropathy. • **Brachycephalic breeds** often have stenotic nares, everted saccules, an elongated soft palate ± a hypoplastic trachea. • **Neoplasia** • **Pharyngeal or laryngeal inflammation** • **Foreign body** • **Collapsing trachea:** Occurs most commonly in middle-aged or older toy and miniature breeds. Usually it just causes coughing, but sometimes it can cause upper airway obstruction. More commonly though, upper airway obstructions exacerbate the collapsing trachea.
DIAGNOSIS	LISTEN FOR STRIDOR: You should be able to hear stridor without using a stethoscope. If you hear stridor, determine which area is affected (larynx or trachea) and whether to perform diagnostics. If the animal is in distress, you may have to stabilize it and administer a sedative so it can calm down and breath more easily. The patient may also need **oxygen** via mask, oxygen cage, intubation, tracheostomy, or a make-shift set-up (e.g. oxygen flowing into a clear plastic bag encompassing the pet). Additionally, the pet may need **corticosteroids** (10 -20 mg/kg prednisolone sodium succinate IV) to decrease upper airway inflammation. (For more information, refer to the emergency section on respiratory distress p. 8.16) PHYSICAL EXAM: • **Palpate the trachea** to check its size (hypoplasia is common in brachycephalic breeds) and try to elicit a cough. If a cough is easily elicited, think collapsing trachea or other causes of inflammation of the trachea. (Also refer to other causes of coughing p. 18.5). • **Evaluate the nares for stenosis:** Brachycephalic breeds often develop upper airway obstruction due to stenotic nares. Check whether air can flow through the nares. ORAL EXAMINATION (laryngoscopy) under anesthesia: • Check for **laryngeal paralysis:** Anesthetize the dog (light plane of anesthesia) with thiopental (2-4 mg/kg boluses) or propofol, and with the animal in sternal recumbency, look down the throat using a laryngoscope. Watch the vocal folds and arytenoids as the animal breathes and wakes up. Assess the motion. Can the arytenoids open up in a coordinated fashion to allow air to pass? With paralysis, they don't open. You must distinguish organized motion from vibrations due to air being forced into the trachea. Dopram® can be used to accentuate this test. • Check for **erythema, swelling, masses, and foreign bodies.** Biopsy any abnormal looking tissue. Look for **eversion of the saccules** and/or an **elongated soft palate.** RADIOGRAPHS: Take a lateral chest radiograph that extends from the nasopharynx to the cranial cervical trachea. Look for foreign bodies, soft tissue masses, and collapsing trachea. BRONCHOSCOPY: If all other tests are negative and the pet has recurrent upper airway obstruction or the obstruction does not resolve with medical treatment, perform bronchoscopy to look for a collapsed trachea, tumor, or foreign body within the upper airway.
TREATMENT	Laryngeal paralysis: Perform a laryngeal tie back. Brachycephalic breeds: Surgically open the nares by removing a triangular wedge of tissue. Shorten the soft palate. Remove inflamed, everted saccules.

18.4

COUGHING
Etiologies
Diagnostics
Specific Diseases

Coughing can be seen with diseases of the trachea, major bronchi, and pulmonary parenchyma, as well as with cardiac disease (due to pulmonary edema or collapse of the mainstem bronchi). Occasionally it indicates disease of the pleural space (more commonly we see dyspnea in this case).

I. **ETIOLOGIES OF COUGHING**

UPPER AIRWAY	LOWER AIRWAY	PULMONARY PARENCHYMA
• **Collapsing trachea** due to chondromalacia or mass lesions outside the trachea.	Chronic **bronchitis** (feline lower airway disease-FLAD)	Cardiogenic edema Noncardiogenic edema (e.g. electrocution and upper airway obstruction leading to wide swing in pleural pressure)
• **Infectious** tracheobronchitis (Bordetella, distemper, etc.)		
• **Parasitic** (Filaroides osleri, Capillaria aerophila)	Foreign body	Neoplasia Infectious (mycotic, bacterial, viral)
• **Intraluminal foreign body** or tumor	Parasitic (lungworms, heartworm)	Inflammation (PIE, allergic pneumonitis)
• **Upper airway obstruction** (e.g. stenotic nares, everted saccules) can contribute to the progression of collapsing trachea.	Cilia dysgenesis	Foreign body Parasitic (lungworms, heartworm)

II. **DIAGNOSTICS**
    A. **PHYSICAL EXAM**
        1. **Observe breathing:** Is inspiratory effort increased? Are inspiratory or expiratory phases prolonged? Is there an increased abdominal component?
        2. **Tracheal palpation:** Cough is usually easy to elicit on tracheal palpation regardless of etiology. Listen to the cough. Is there an end-expiratory snap suggesting intrathoracic collapse?
        3. **Thoracic auscultation** for heart and lung sounds. Does the heart sound muffled or is there a heart murmur? Do you hear crackles or wheezes? Listen to all lung fields and over the trachea. (Sometimes they are difficult to hear in cats and small dogs due to low tidal volume.)
    B. **RADIOGRAPHS of the neck/thorax:** Look in an orderly fashion for an abnormal pulmonary pattern, abnormal cardiac silhouette, or lymphadenopathy (e.g. enlargement of the hilar lymph nodes). Also look for collapsing trachea.
        1. Foxtails often cause pneumonia in the dorsal caudal lung field.
        2. Aspiration pneumonia is usually concentrated in the right middle lung lobe (assuming the animal was sternal or upright when it aspirated).
        3. An enlarged heart or enlarged chamber (commonly the left atrium) can push up on the trachea and collapse the mainstem bronchi. This occurs primarily in dogs.
        4. Enlarged, tortuous pulmonary vessels that end abruptly along with an enlarged main pulmonary artery indicate heartworm disease.
        5. In order to diagnose collapsing trachea, take inspiratory and expiratory films. The intrathoracic trachea is more likely to collapse during expiration and the extrathoracic trachea is more likely to collapse during inspiration.
    C. **FLUOROSCOPY**
    D. **TRANSTRACHEAL WASH or BRONCHOALVEOLAR LAVAGE (BAL) plus culture** may reveal intracellular bacteria (indicating infection), eosinophils (suggesting allergy or parasitic infection), neoplastic cells, etc.
    E. **BRONCHOSCOPY** may reveal foreign bodies, inflammation, infection (BAL), or masses. Bronchoscopy is recommended to rule out chronic bronchitis, infection, other inflammatory diseases, or collapsing trachea.
    F. **LUNG ASPIRATE or BIOPSY** can be performed in animals with intrathoracic mass lesions that contact the thoracic wall. Fluoroscopic or ultrasound guidance is highly recommended.
    G. **BLOOD-GAS ANALYSIS** provides information about pulmonary ventilation and perfusion.

III. **SOME SPECIFIC DISEASES**
    Infectious Tracheobronchitis (Refer to Infectious Disease chapter p. 11.7)
    Collapsing Trachea
    Chronic Bronchitis in Dogs
    Chronic Bronchitis in Cats (Feline Lower Airway Disease-FLAD)

Pulmonary

COLLAPSING TRACHEA in DOGS

Collapsing trachea refers to the flattening of the tracheal rings or presence of a redundant dorsal tracheal membrane. Always consider collapsing trachea as a cause of coughing in middle-aged or old dogs, especially in overweight toy or miniature breed dogs. Collapsing trachea can also develop secondary to left atrial enlargement, which compresses the mainstem bronchi. Some breeds are predisposed to this condition, indicating a hereditary component; however, signs may be initiated or exacerbated by other factors that cause tracheal inflammation or that increase the resistance of airflow through the trachea. Such conditions include chronic bronchitis, infection, and upper airway obstruction (e.g. laryngeal paralysis, elongated soft palate, eversion of laryngeal saccules, stenotic nares).

CLINICAL SIGNS	• Dry, hacking, non-productive cough that's easily elicited on tracheal palpation. With intrathoracic collapse, a snap on end-expiration (due to the dorsal tracheal membrane hitting the ventral wall of the trachea) can sometimes be heard. • No crackles are associated with this cough. • Signs are worse with exercise, excitement, collar pressure on the neck, and overheating. In severe cases dogs may become cyanotic or have syncopal episodes.
SITES of COLLAPSE	Collapse may be intra or extrathoracic and can involve the mainstem bronchi. • **Intrathoracic tracheal collapse** causes expiratory dyspnea ± an audible snap on end-expiration. • **Extrathoracic tracheal collapse** causes inspiratory dyspnea.
DIAGNOSIS	The diagnosis is often made in the exam room but frequently requires bronchoscopy. • Elicit a cough/retch on palpation of the trachea. • Auscultation of the trachea may reveal an end-expiratory snap. • **Radiography:** Take inspiratory films of the neck and thorax (to look for cervical collapse) and expiratory films (to observe for intrathoracic collapse). Don't forget to evaluate the area near the carina. Tracheal collapse can frequently be diagnosed using radiographs, however, negative findings do not rule out tracheal collapse. Fluoroscopy or bronchoscopy may be required. • **Bronchoscopy** is a more sensitive test for tracheal collapse, especially for intrathoracic collapse. Collapse of the mainstem bronchi is fairly common. Bronchoscopy can also be used to identify contributing conditions that can be treated, such as chronic bronchitis, elongated soft palate, etc. • **Transtracheal wash or BAL** help rule out any concurrent respiratory infection (look for intracellular bacteria).
TREATMENT (Continued next page)	Collapsing trachea is not curable. The goal of treatment is to control the problem and remove or alleviate contributing factors such as chronic bronchitis, elongated soft palate, etc. • **Avoid inciting factors** such as excitement. Tranquilize the animal prior to an exciting situation (e.g. guests). • **Avoid collars and choke chains:** Use a head halter (e.g. Halti® or Gentle Leader®) or a harness where the leash attaches in the front (Easy Walk™ or Sensation® harness) rather than one that attaches in the back. Back-attaching harnesses encourage dogs to pull. • **Correct obesity:** A majority of dogs with collapsed trachea are obese. Fat reduces the ability of the thorax to expand. These dogs should lose weight prior to being put on corticosteroids. • **Correct contributing problems** such as everted saccules, laryngeal paralysis, and stenotic nares. Also address chronic bronchitis and infection, since any inflammation contributes to chondromalacia of the cartilage rings and increases mucous and other secretions. Secretions decrease the airway diameter, making it more difficult to move air. Additionally, avoid environmental pollutants such as cigarette smoke.

COLLAPSING TRACHEA, continued

TREATMENT continued	• **Bronchodilators:** Use in cases of chronic bronchitis. Bronchodilators open up the airways by dilating bronchi distal to the mainstem bronchi. Treatment is usually life-long. Terbutaline, a ß2 agonist with little effect on cardiac ß1 receptors has fewer side effects than theophylline, a methylxanthine, which has weak chronotropic and inotropic effects. • **Antibiotics:** Treat secondary infections as identified on culture. Doxycycline, ciprofloxacin and enrofloxacin, TMS, and clavamox penetrate the respiratory epithelium. Doxycycline is often a good first choice. Gentamicin (3-5 mg/kg) can be delivered by nebulizer through a face mask for about 10 minutes/day. Avoid giving theophylline and enrofloxacin together as this elevates plasma levels of theophylline. • **Antitussives:** Address concurrent diseases such as chronic bronchitis before using antitussives. Cough suppressants allow mucus to build up in the bronchi which can contribute to additional problems. Once coughing is controlled, decrease the dose. 　• **Dextromethorphan (Pediatric Robitussen®):** 1-2 mg/kg PO q 6 -8 hours. OTC cough suppressants are not as effective as prescription medications. 　• **Butorphanol:** 0.05-0.12 mg/kg PO q 8-12 hours (controlled) 　• **Hydrocodone Bitartrate (Hycodan®):** 0.22 mg/kg PO q 6-8 hours (controlled substance) • **Corticosteroids** can be used to control inflammation if there is no infection. For tracheal inflammation, 3-5 days is often sufficient. For chronic diseases such as bronchitis or eosinophilic pneumonia, treat long term but taper to the lowest dose. • **Surgery:** Fixing upper airway problems such as stenotic nares, elongated soft palate, and other conditions that increase the resistance within the trachea make a collapsing trachea easier to manage. Surgical splinting of the trachea is occasionally performed in severely affected dogs. This procedure can now be done with bronchoscopy.

CHRONIC BRONCHITIS in DOGS and CATS

Chronic bronchitis is characterized by a persistent cough lasting ≥ 2 months for which other causes of cough (cardiac, neoplastic, parasitic, or infectious diseases) have been ruled out.

CLINICAL SIGNS	**DOGS:** The cough is similar in nature to that seen with collapsing trachea. It's a chronic, **dry, honking cough** easily elicited upon tracheal compression and often induced by drinking, excitement, exercise, etc. The cough is usually non-productive but often occurs in paroxysms that end with a **gag** or **retch** (due to coughing up and then swallowing mucus and exudate). The animal may also wheeze and exhibit exercise intolerance. Dogs can present in respiratory distress characterized by **expiratory hyper-effort ±** wheezing. These episodes occur in association with exposure to inciting allergens. **CATS:** Coughing or respiratory distress are the main complaints but sometimes cats present with an acute onset of respiratory distress (tachypnea, expiratory hyper-effort) that is quickly relieved with oxygen and/or bronchodilators and corticosteroids.
PATHO PHYSIOLOGY	In both cats and dogs, chronic bronchitis is most likely induced by environmental irritants such as cigarette smoke. The resulting inflammation causes a reversible constriction of the small airways, stimulates exudate formation, and causes the airways to become hyperreactive. The decrease in airway diameter leads to an exponential increase in resistance to airflow. If the process continues for about 2 months, irreversible changes start occurring. The epithelium becomes denuded, destroying the ciliary mechanism for transport of material out of the airways. Additionally, goblet cells increase. The net result is that there are increased secretions and less cilia to transport the resulting mucus out.
HISTORY	History is important to help to identify the irritants (e.g. fireplace smoke, forced air heat with filters that aren't changed often, household aerosols, and perfumes). For cats, ask about the litter box. Covered litter boxes, scented litters, and dusty litters (even those that claim to be low in dust) may all act as respiratory irritants. Recent moves to a new household in which items in the house are packed and unpacked can expose pets to low-lying dust, carpet, and other allergens

Pulmonary

DIAGNOSIS	RULE OUT OTHER CAUSES OF COUGHING • **FECAL FLOAT**, fecal sedimentation, Baermann, and heartworm tests rule out pulmonary parasites that can cause a hypersensitivity reaction. • **THORACIC RADIOGRAPHS** can help rule out cardiac disease, collapsing trachea, neoplasia, pneumonia, pulmonary edema, and foreign bodies in the airways. In cases of bronchitis, thoracic radiographs may reveal a **bronchiolar pattern** ("doughnuts" and "tram lines") due to thickened bronchial walls (especially in chronic bronchitis). **Bronchiectesis**— dilatation of the airway walls due to chronic disease— can occur with chronic bronchitis and indicates more serious disease. About 15% of cats with chronic bronchitis have hyperinflated lungs. • **BAL or TRANSTRACHEAL WASH:** A normal sample contains macrophages and neutrophils. Elevated numbers of eosinophils can be seen with chronic bronchitis and other conditions. Intracellular bacteria may be visible with bacterial pneumonia. Note: if your sample contains salmonsiella (2-3x the size of a neutrophil) or squamous cells, it is contaminated with oral contents. Do not culture this sample. • **CBC** may reveal a mild eosinophilia • **CULTURE:** Perform a culture to rule out concurrent pneumonia. Infection is common in dogs but not in cats with chronic bronchitis. • **BRONCHOSCOPY** is invaluable for diagnosing collapsed trachea/bronchi and for inspecting the bronchiolar mucosa. In chronic bronchitis, airways are erythematous, thickened, edematous, and have excess mucus.

TREATMENT	The primary goals are to **CONTROL AIRWAY INFLAMMATION** and **relieve bronchospasm**. Treat promptly and appropriately to avoid permanent, pathologic airway changes.
	• **ELIMINATE THE SOURCE:** If you can determine what the pet is allergic to, remove it from the environment (e.g. cigarette smoke, perfume, etc.)
	• **BRONCHODILATORS** open up the airways. Use when expiratory hyper-effort, air-trapping, or bronchiolar patterns are seen.
	    • **Theophylline** (Theocap ER: Sustained release formulation by Inwood Laboratories): 10 mg/kg PO BID in dogs. Start with 1/2 dose for 3-4 days and if well tolerated, go to the full dose. Use carefully in cats due to the low therapeutic window. When combined with enrofloxacin it can quickly reach toxic levels.
	    • **Aminophylline:** 11 mg/kg PO TID in dogs. Weak effect in cats.
	    • **Terbutaline:** 1-5 mg/dog PO SID-TID in dogs (start at low dose). 0.625-1.25 mg/cat PO BID. **Periactin®** (cyproheptadine): An antihistamine with serotonergic activity, may be an effective substitute in cats. Use it only as needed (2 mg PO SID-BID).
	• **NEBULIZATION** helps break up mucus plugs.
	• **HYDRATION:** Keep the animal hydrated so that the airways remain hydrated. This facilitates mucociliary clearance.
	• **CORTICOSTEROIDS:** Chronic bronchitis usually requires several months of treatment with pred before it can be discontinued. Start with 1 mg/kg PO BID and taper to 0.5 mg/kg PO BID over two weeks. Then decrease to q 48 hours or less frequently over several months. Sometimes it can be discontinued after several months. **Cats** should respond to corticosteroids within 3 days. Start with an immunomodulatory dose: 2.2 mg/kg PO BID for 3-5 days, then decrease to 1-2 mg/kg PO BID and continue tapering for 2-3 months. For owners unable to give oral medications, methylprednisolone acetate (Depo-Medrol®) may be given at 10-20 mg/cat IM every 2-8 weeks. Inhalant corticosteroids can also be used to minimize systemic effects (eg. diabetic cats).
	• **ANTITUSSIVES:** Use with caution and try to reserve use for cases where other treatments have not been successful. (Doses on p.18.7)
	• **ANTIBIOTICS:** Treat concurrent bacterial infections if present.

EMERGENCY THERAPY IN CATS	**Provide oxygen** **Administer terbutaline** or **corticosteroids**. Response should be seen within 30 minutes. **Terbutaline** (0.01 mg/kg IV, SC, or IM) is a ß2 adrenergic agonist that relaxes smooth muscle in the airways. **Prednisolone sodium succinate:** 10-20 mg/kg IV or IM. **Dexamethasone SP:** 0.2-2.2 mg/kg IV, IM, or PO. **Epinephrine** (1:1000) 0.1 mL/cat IV Has both α and ß effects and can induce arrhythmias. Use only in the short-term emergency situation. **Albuterol inhalants**. Use for emergencies and exacerbations of dyspnea.

Canine Eye Registration Foundation (CERF)

VMDB/CERF
P.O. Box 3007
1717 Philo Rd., Suite 15
Urbana, IL 61803-3007
(217) 693-4800 www.vmdb.org/cerf.html

Orthopedic Foundation for Animals, Inc. (OFA)
2300 E. Nifong Blvd.
Columbia, MO 65201
(573) 442-0418
www.offa.org

University of Pennsylvania Hip Improvement Program
www.PennHIP.org

SUGGESTED REFERENCES:
Ackerman, L: The Genetic Connection: A Guide to Health Problems in Purebred Dogs
Lakewood, CO. AAHA Press, 1999.

Feldman EC, Nelson RW: Canine and Feline Endocrinology and Reproduction. 3rd edition.
Philadelphia, PA. WB Saunders, 2004.

Gough A, Thomas A: Breed Predispositions to Disease in Dogs & Cats. Ames, Iowa. Blackwell
Publishing, 2004.

Tsutsui T, Mizutani W, Hori T, et al: Estradiol benzoate for preventing pregnancy in mismated
dogs. *Theriogenology* 66: 1568-1572. 2006.

Reproduction

PHYSICAL EXAMINATION of BREEDING ANIMALS
General Physical Exam and History
Examining the Bitch
Examining the Dog

The breeding animal is most commonly examined for two reasons: (1) to determine if the animal is suitable in a breeding program, or (2) to determine the cause of breeding failure if indicated.

I.   **THE GENERAL PHYSICAL EXAM and HISTORY**
   A.   SOME QUESTIONS to ask when taking a history include:
      1.   **Drugs:** Is the male or female being medicated? Include antiparasiticals, vitamins, supplements, coat conditioners. Bitches should not be bred when on teratogenic compounds. Avoid "fertility" supplements and calcium prenatally.
      2.   **Past cycles:** Has the bitch had ovulation timing performed in the past? Does she cycle regularly with normal interestrus intervals? What's her breeding history?
      3.   **Diet?**
   B.   PHYSICAL EXAM: When performing a general physical exam, be sure to pay special attention to possible hereditary and reproductive problems (Breed Predispositions to Disease in Dogs & Cats by Alex Gough and Alison Thomas; The Genetic Connection: A Guide to Health Problems in Purebred Dogs by Lowell Ackerman). It's best to have an idea of the hereditary problems specific to the breed. The breeder should know of the breed-specific problems, too, but if he/she doesn't, you should direct him/her to resources (AKC Web site, local breed clubs' code of ethics) for such information. Pay special attention in all breeding animals to:
      1.   **Skin** problems such as atopy, generalized demodicosis
      2.   **Heart murmurs** and arrhythmias
      3.   **Malocclusion,** missing teeth, or extra teeth
      4.   Obvious **ocular** disorders such as entropion, cataracts, corneal lesions, and retinal lesions, as well as those requiring a fundic exam by an ophthalmologist.
      5.   **Lamenesses,** especially if you suspect hip dysplasia, elbow dysplasia, osteochondritis dessicans, luxating patellas
      6.   Obvious **behavioral problems** such as aggression or fear
      7.   Poor conformation

   C.   SCREENING TESTS: Prior to breeding, the animal should undergo a series of **screening tests** including an eye exam and certification, and radiographs for hip and elbow dysplasia. Echocardiographic examination is indicated in breeds at risk.
      1.   Breeding animals over 10kg should have their hips certified as normal by the Orthopedic Foundation of America (OFA) or PennHIP (www.PenHip.org) after 2 years of age. Breeds predisposed to developing elbow dysplasia should also have their elbows certified by the OFA.
      2.   Breeding animals should have their eyes certified yearly as clear of hereditary defects by a board-certified ophthalmologist.
      3.   Some breeds are routinely tested for other hereditary defects. For example, Dalmatian puppies are hearing tested as puppies before they are sold to prospective buyers.
      4.   *Brucella* testing: *Brucella* can cause neonatal death, and abortion and infertility in otherwise healthy animals. Plus, it is zoonotic; therefore, breeding animals should be tested for brucellosis using serologic testing. Bitches should be tested before each breeding; stud dogs should be tested annually. This method can yield false positives, so if the test is positive, perform a more specific test such as the AGID test (Cornell University).

II.   **EXAMINING THE BITCH**
   A.   THE MAMMARY CHAIN: Examine the mammary chain for masses or abnormal nipples.
   B.   VULVAR ANATOMY: The vulva should be readily visible. Some are recessed and covered by a skin fold. This anatomical formation can predispose the animal to perivulvar dermatitis, urinary tract infections, or urethritis but may resolve after the first heat cycle. If causing problems, the anatomical defect should be surgically corrected. Also look for abnormal vaginal discharge, and palpate for any vaginal strictures at the vestibulovaginal junction that would interfere with breeding or whelping.

VAGINAL DISCHARGES in the BITCH

TYPE OF DISCHARGE	ETIOLOGY	DIAGNOSIS
Bloody	Proestrus	History and clinical signs Vaginal cytology Estrogen levels (not advised)
	Estrus	History and clinical signs Vaginal cytology Progesterone levels LH testing
	Subinvolution of placental sites	History: recent whelping No treatment required Monitor PCV, TP
	Severe vaginitis or cystitis	Culture and physical exam Abdominal ultrasound Vaginoscopy
Greenish-black or dark bloody	Separation of placental sites	History: pregnant bitch Abortion
	Post-partum lochia	History: whelped within the last 6-8 weeks. A normal finding.
Reddish-brown, yellow, thick, malodorous	Open-cervix pyometra	History: intact bitch in diestrus Complete blood count: neutrophils may be elevated Radiographs/ultrasound: may indicate fluid in the uterus Culture Chemistry panel: azotemia
	Metritis	Bitch is sick 2-7 days after whelping Purulent vaginal discharge Poor mothering
	Severe vaginitis	As above for severe vaginitis
Straw-colored	Estrus	History and clinical signs Vaginal cytology Progesterone levels Normal in late pregnancy Puppy vaginitis (benign)

C.   VAGINAL CYTOLOGY and CULTURE

1.   **Culture:** You don't need to culture the female unless the bitch has an abnormal vaginal discharge. The normal bacterial flora in the distal vagina/urethra consists of gram-positive and gram-negative bacteria plus mycoplasma. This flora is the same as the mixed fecal flora. Bacteria in low numbers are normal, but if the discharge grows a pure culture (i.e., of *E. coli*) the dog most likely has an infection. A vaginal culture is only appropriate when open pyometra or severe localized septic vaginitis is present. Normal bitches do not have sterile vaginas. An intrauterine culture can be obtained with a transcervical sample using a cystourethroscope, such as is used for transcervical inseminations, and a guarded micro swab used for bronchoscopy.

2.   **Cytology:** For ovulation timing, it's best to perform vaginal cytology every other day if possible, starting at proestrus and continuing into early diestrus so that the owner has a good record of the bitch's estrous cycle. This also permits prediction of whelping dates. You can teach the owner to make and date the vaginal smears for you to evaluate.

3.   **Digital examination** for strictures. Strictures may be circumferential or septate. When you find a stricture, you must decide whether the bitch can get pregnant and whether she can whelp. Sometimes the circumferential strictures break down on their own or relax under the influence of estrogen and relaxin when whelping. You can use artificial insemination to impregnate these bitches, but a cesarean section might be necessary. Septate strictures should be transected. It is not known if strictures are heritable.

4.   **Vaginoscopy:** Use a pediatric proctoscope as a vaginoscope/cystourethroscope. Insert the endoscope with or without insufflation and look at the vaginal mucosa. The normal vaginal mucosa is pink and has folds. During proestrus, the vaginal folds become puffy and pink. After

Reproduction

ovulation, the folds become wrinkled. Vaginoscopy can be more reliable than cytology in determining when to breed.

You can also use vaginoscopy to locate the origin of a vaginal discharge and to evaluate for cranial strictures. The discharge may be coming from
   a. The cervix (uterus)
   b. A mass
   c. The urethral area (bladder)
   d. A foreign body
5. **Hormone levels:** Serial progesterone levels or LH tests can be used to evaluate ovulation and time breeding.

D. **VACCINATION AND PARASITE CONTROL**
   1. Vaccinations in the breeding bitch should be current (within 3 years) prior to proestrus. The bitch can be vaccinated in early proestrus but should not be vaccinated once pregnant unless necessary due to inadequate vaccination schedules.
   2. Parasites: Fenbendazole can be given in late gestation (after day 40) if needed for roundworms and hookworms.

III. **EXAMINING the MALE DOG:** Check the scrotum, prostate, prepuce, penis, and testicles. The testes should be symmetrical and nonpainful. Cryptorchid dogs should not be bred.
   A. **TESTICULAR TUMORS: Estrogen-secreting tumors** are a concern because estrogen in both the male and female may affect the bone marrow, causing irreversible pancytopenia or aplastic anemia. Testicular tumors rarely metastasize. They usually don't cause problems unless they secrete estrogen or alter the sperm-blood barrier. You can't always tell by clinical signs however, whether the tumors are secreting estrogen (i.e., gynecomastia or bilateral endocrine alopecia, atrophy of the contralateral testis).

ESTROUS CYCLES and BREEDING
Onset of Maturity
Estrous Cycle in the Dog
Clinical Breeding Protocol
Artificial Insemination
Estrous Cycle in the Cat

I.   **THE ONSET of MATURITY:** Bitches attain sexual maturity about one to two months after achieving their adult height and weight. Thus, small breed dogs reach sexual maturity at a younger age than large breed dogs.

CYCLES/ INTERESTROUS INTERVALS in DOGS	
Sexual maturity	4-18 months
Most dogs cycle by	18-24 months
Interestrous interval	4.5-8 months
Interestrous interval in African breed dogs	12 months

II. **THE ESTROUS CYCLE in the DOG:** Before reading the following section, read the chart on the estrous cycle. (pp.19.6 & 19.7)

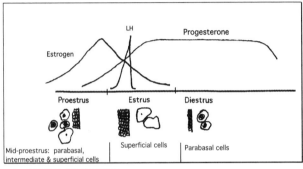

A. **GENERAL INFORMATION**
1. The cervix is open during proestrus and estrus, thus **red blood cells** can get from the uterus into the vagina. In addition, if the cervix were not open, sperm would not be able to get into the uterus.
2. Parabasal cells are also called noncornified cells. Superficial cells are also called cornified or keratinized cells.
3. There are two definitions for the end of estrus. The first definition is that estrus ends when the female stops standing. The other definition is based on vaginal cytology. When vaginal cytology is comprised primarily of parabasal cells (less than 50% superficial cells), estrus has ended. The distinction between these two definitions is important in predicting whelping dates and in assessing breeding dates. Some bitches breed several days into diestrus (as determined by vaginal cytology).
4. The bitch's most fertile period occurs during the last four days of estrus (4-6 days after the LH surge). You can always count back from the first day of diestrus to determine when the bitch was most fertile. You can also count back 7-9 days to determine the day of the LH surge.
5. **Preventing cycling:** Currently, no safe drug is available in the U.S. to stop cycling in the bitch.
6. **Progesterone assay kits** are not advised. Quantitative testing via a commercial lab is superior, and 12-24 hour turnaround is available. A progesterone level of < 1 ng/mL is a baseline reading. If you monitor a dog that is in proestrus every other day, ovulation should occur within 24-48 hours from when you first see the progesterone level increase to 2-3 ng/mL. The eggs will mature in another 24-36 hours, and the bitch will be fertile in 3 days, continuing through the 7th day. If the bitch is examined for the first time and her progesterone levels are > 5 ng/mL, you won't be able to determine when she ovulated.

Reproduction

THE ESTROUS CYCLE

	PROESTRUS	ESTRUS	DIESTRUS	ANESTRUS
DEFINITION	Begins when vaginal bleeding is first seen and ends when the bitch allows a male dog to mount and breed her.	The time during which the bitch allows a male to mount and breed her.	Begins with the cessation of standing heat and continues throughout the time during which progesterone is secreted by the corpora lutea.	The phase following diestrus during which the uterus involutes. Begins with whelping and ends with proestrus.
DURATION	Usually: 6-11 days Average: 9 days Normal variation: 1-25 days	Usually: 5-9 days Normal variation: 1-20 days	Pregnant bitch: 56-58 days Non-pregnant: 60-80 days	4-10 months
CLINICAL SIGNS	Behavior: The female attracts males but discourages mounting. Bloody vaginal discharge (from intrauterine hemorrhage). Swelling (turgidity) of the vulva.	Behavior: When you press on the bitch's perineum, she lifts her tail. Female allows the male to mount. Vaginal discharge may become straw-colored. The swollen vulva becomes flaccid.	The bitch no longer attracts males. Vulva returns to normal anestrual size. Mammary glands: Increasing prolactin initiates glandular development in mammary tissue. Prolactin concentration rises as progesterone concentration decreases during the final 1-3 weeks of gestation, causing overt lactation. Behaviorally there is no difference between anestrus bitch and a non-pregnant diestrus bitch. No difference between a pregnant and non-pregnant bitch in early diestrus except an increase in relaxin in the pregnant bitch.	Not readily discernible from diestrus in the non-pregnant bitch. It's difficult to tell if a bitch has been spayed or is intact and in anestrus without assaying pituitary hormones, FSH and LH. These hormones would be dramatically elevated in the spayed bitch.

HORMONE CHANGES	**Rising estrogen:** The bitch in proestrus is under the influence of estrogen secreted by ovarian follicles. The estrogen brings about the behavior changes, attraction of males, vaginal discharge, and uterine preparation for pregnancy. Just prior to proestrus, estrogen increases above 15 pg/mL. In early proestrus, levels rise above 25 pg/mL. In **late proestrus** they may rise to > 60-70 pg/mL.	**Estrogen:** The peaked estrogen levels start to decline. **Progesterone** levels rise above baseline. The two events together result in standing heat and also feedback to the hypothalamus and pituitary, resulting in a surge in FSH and LH. LH surge results in ovulation.	**Progesterone** concentrations rise and then plateau (15-60 ng/mL 2-3 weeks into diestrus). In the pregnant bitch the luteal phase ends abruptly at the onset of parturition, while in the non-pregnant bitch it declines more gradually.	Fluctuations in LH.
UTERINE ANATOMY		The follicles mature as signaled by decline in estrogen. Ovulation occurs 24-72 hours after the LH surge.	Progesterone supports **hypertrophy** of uterine glandular tissue. Maximum non-pregnant uterine size occurs at 20-30 days diestrus and coincides with the higher progesterone levels. Implantation: about 14 days after fertilization. Fetuses are palpable at 30 days.	The uterus is undergoing self-repair. Externally the vet will detect little change in the palpable uterus once involution reduces uterine size to one that's comparable to bowel loops.
VAGINAL CYTOLOGY	Estrogen increase causes rapid increase in the number of cell layers lining the vaginal vault. **Early:** Parabasal cells and RBCs **Mid:** Increasing intermediate and superficial cells and fewer RBCs **Late:** > 80% superficial cells, no WBCs, ± RBCs	Superficial cells > 80% **No neutrophils** unless there's inflammation. RBCs may be seen.	Superficial cells < 20% You may see neutrophils and sheets of cells. **The diestrus cytology is clearly demarcated from that of a bitch nearing the end of estrus.** Ovulation occurs about 5-6 days prior to day 1 of diestrus.	Primarily **parabasal** cells. Few neutrophils. RBCs usually absent. Normal bacterial flora.

Reproduction

7. An **LH assay** is used primarily in cases of infertility, or artificial insemination with frozen semen (and less commonly with chilled semen), where timing is especially crucial. It is always used in conjunction with the progesterone assay. Based on serial vaginal cytology, vaginoscopy, and LH and progesterone tests, determine when the bitch is fertile. The bitch is most fertile 4-6 days after the LH surge.

III.   CLINICAL BREEDING PROTOCOL

CLINICAL BREEDING PROTOCOL

Breeder clients should notify the clinic when they first notice their bitch is in season. They should watch for vaginal discharge or vulvar swelling and attraction to males; however, even the most astute owner can fail to notice the true onset of proestrus for a few days.

- Early proestrus should be documented by vaginal cytology (less than 50% cornification/superficial cells).
- A baseline progesterone level (usually 0-1 ng/mL) might be informative if the true onset of the cycle is unknown.
- Vaginal cytology should be performed every 2-4 days until a significant progression in cornification is seen, usually above 70% superficial cells.

At that point, serial hormonal assaying should begin. For routine breedings, progesterone testing may be done every other day, until a rise in progesterone above 2 ng/mL is identified. The day of the initial rise in progesterone above 2 ng/mL is identified as day "zero." Breedings are advised on days 2, 4 and 6.

When increased accuracy of ovulation timing is necessary (e.g., frozen or chilled semen breedings, infertility cases, breedings with subfertile stud dogs), daily LH testing is recommended. Once the LH surge is identified, breeding days may be planned. The day of the LH surge is also day "zero."

- It is useful to perform vaginal cytology every 2-3 days until full cornification (>90% superficial cells) occurs. This maximal cornification usually occurs before the fertile period is reached and continues until the onset of diestrus, which is usually a few days after the end of the fertile period. Vaginal cytology may be continued until the diestral shift is identified; this provides a retrospective evaluation of the breeding just completed.
- In addition, at least one progesterone assay should be performed after the LH surge/initial rise in progesterone is identified to document that levels continue to rise. This illustrates sustained corpus luteum function and strongly suggests that an ovulatory cycle has occurred.
- Extended chilled breedings should occur on days 4 and 6, or 3 and 5, after day "zero." Which two days are chosen can depend upon overnight shipping possibilities and the involved clients' schedules. Frozen semen breedings should occur on day 5 or 6 after day "zero."

If client economics dictate minimal testing, serum can be batched on a daily basis and quantitative progesterone tests performed as advised above. When the initial rise in progesterone is identified, the batched serum can be specifically evaluated for the day of the LH surge, confirming identification of day "zero."

Vaginoscopy may be performed throughout the cycle as an adjunct to vaginal cytology and hormonal assays, especially when evaluating an unusual cycle.

Behavioral and other observations should also be made at each examination, but less weight should be put on these parameters. The clinician should keep in mind that the most accurate ovulation timing occurs when information from several tests is pooled (vaginal cytologies, vaginoscopy, and progesterone or LH tests).

IV. **ARTIFICIAL INSEMINATION** is an easy procedure. The difficulty is in collecting semen from the male.
   A. **PHASES**
       1. After the dog mounts the bitch, ejaculation of a **sperm-free prostatic fluid** takes place during the initial 15-60 seconds. Following pelvic thrusting, the male typically dismounts by placing both front legs to one side of the bitch, lifting one hind leg over her back, and standing tail to tail with her. Full engorgement of the bulbus glandis makes withdrawal of the penis from the relatively small vaginal opening impossible. The dogs are locked together for **5-60 minutes** and may drag each other around during this period.

2. **Semen collection and evaluation:**
   a. Collect the sperm-rich fraction for 1-2 minutes, usually just after the male stops thrusting and turns.

SEMEN COLLECTION

	CONTENTS	TIME	AMOUNT
Fraction 1	Prostatic fluid Seminiferous fluid	20-60 seconds	1-2 mLs
Fraction 2	Sperm-rich fluid	1-2 minutes	0.5-1.5 mLs (cloudy)
Fraction 3	Prostatic fluid	About 20 minutes	Copious clear fluid, up to 30 mLs.

   b. Examine the semen. Sperm quality decreases with concurrent disease. The semen must be warm to evaluate motility.

SEMEN ANALYSIS

Normal progressive motility	> 70%
Normal morphology (some 2° changes are caused by collection techniques)	> 80%
Normal numbers	200-400 million sperm per ejaculate

(Number of sperm/mL ejaculate) x (mL collected) = sperm/ejaculate

   c. Keep the semen out of UV light.
   d. Note: For shipping, don't store the sperm in prostatic fluid because prostatic fluid *in vitro* is toxic to sperm. Use a commercially prepared buffer according to manufacturer directions.

3. **Inseminating the female:** Attempt to inseminate the bitch within 10-15 minutes of collection if possible. Semen can be extended and stored chilled for 48 hours and shipped within that time. To inseminate the bitch, draw the semen into a sterile 12-20 mL latex-free syringe. Attach the syringe to a clean insemination pipette. Gently place your non-lubricated index finger (lubricants may be spermicidal) into the vaginal vault, palm up. Slide the insemination catheter into the cranial vagina. Flush semen into the vaginal vault (use air to empty the catheter) and remove the catheter. Now use your index finger to stroke the perineal region (feathering technique). This sometimes causes obvious vaginal contractions. Elevating the hindquarters is not necessary.

4. **Insemination protocol:** To optimize the chances of success, perform AI 2-6 days post-LH surge or 2-6 days after the initial rise in progesterone.

5. **Success rate:** Generally, AI is associated with good conception rates (70-90% of normal). AI is best when the stud dog has good quality semen and the bitch is relatively young (2-4 years of age) and healthy.
   a. The conception rate is lower with frozen semen (40-50%) than with chilled semen. Insemination with fresh, chilled semen is usually 70-80% successful.

V.. **ESTROUS CYCLE in CATS:** Cats are induced ovulators and are seasonally polyestrus, cycling from around January to September. Estrus lasts about one week .
   A. **INDUCTION of OVULATION:** Ovulation can be induced by inserting a cotton swab (as for a vaginal smear) into the vagina (or by breeding the queen). This will stop her signs of heat. It won't decrease the length of estrus, though. Instead of the female coming out of estrus and going into a 7-10 day interestrous, she will go into pseudopregnancy for 30-45 days.
      1. In the cat, the placenta produces progesterone late in gestation.

   B. **OTHER FACTS about FELINE PREGNANCY**
      1. Cats can breed and become pregnant while they are lactating.
      2. Queens can become impregnated by multiple males and can breed more than 20 times in a 24-hour period.

Reproduction

PREGNANCY and PARTURITION
Diestrus in the Pregnant vs. Non-pregnant Bitch
Pregnancy Diagnosis
Nutrition
Stages of Labor
Dystocia
Whelping Monitoring Equipment
Abortion, Resorption, Stillbirth
Post-partum Concerns
Pseudopregnancy
Mastitis
Pregnancy Termination
Pyometra

I. **DIESTRUS in the PREGNANT vs. NONPREGNANT BITCH:** Diestrus lasts 57 days in a pregnant bitch (longer for smaller litters and shorter for larger litters) and 60-80 days in a non-pregnant bitch. Diestrus is shorter in the pregnant bitch because the stressed fetus makes ACTH, which causes $PGF_{2\alpha}$ release, which in turn lyses the corpus luteum. This leads to a decline in progesterone and induction of parturition.

II. **PREGNANCY DIAGNOSIS in the BITCH**

METHOD	DAYS OF GESTATION*	FINDINGS
Ultrasound	• 21-25 days • > 23-38 days	• Fetus • Fetal heart beats
Palpation	• 20-30 days • > 30-35 days	• Individual fetuses palpable • Diffuse uterine enlargement
Relaxin Assay (Synbiotics)	• 30-35 days	• A positive result is reliable. • False negatives can occur with small litters.
Radiographs	• > 42-45 days	• Fetal skeletons

* Gestational age is based on the day of the LH surge.

A. Ultrasound is the best method for determining whether the puppies are alive and healthy (fetal heartbeats). Wait until about day 28 after breeding to ultrasound the bitch.

B. Radiographs may be better than ultrasound for counting the number of fetuses later in gestation. They are less helpful than ultrasound in determining fetal death unless profound changes have taken place. Mummified fetuses have osteopenic skeletons since they are being reabsorbed. They may have folding fractures and contain gas.

III. **NUTRITION in the PREGNANT BITCH:** The current recommendation is to feed a diet adequate for all life stages starting at the time of breeding. You may need to feed the bitch in multiple small meals since her enlarged uterus will make it difficult to eat large amounts at one time. In addition, during lactation, you may want to feed the bitch in an area away from the puppies so that she is undisturbed while eating. Many bitches won't leave their puppies.

NUTRITION DURING PREGNANCY and LACTATION

TIME	AMOUNT of GOOD COMMERCIAL DOG FOOD
4th week of diestrus	Normal
5th-6th week of diestrus	Normal + 25%
8th-9th week of pregnancy	Normal + 50%
2nd-3rd week of lactation	Normal + 100% to 200%
4th week of lactation	Gradually taper the amount down once the pups are weaned, after the bitch has regained her condition.

IV. **STAGES of LABOR:** 10-14 hours after the decline in progesterone, the bitch's rectal temperature falls to < 100°F. This drop in temperature precedes Stage I labor by 10-24 hours.

A. **Stage I** is comparable to the longest phase of human labor. It begins with the onset of **uterine contractions** and ends when the cervix is fully dilated. These contractions of the uterine musculature are not visible externally.
  1. **Characteristic:** Cervical dilatation
  2. **Duration:** 6-24 hours
  3. **Clinical signs:** Nesting behavior, restlessness, nervousness
  4. **Whelp watch:** Uterine activity can be monitored (tocodynamometry) using intrauterine monitor (WhelpWise, Veterinary Perinatal Services, www.whelpwise.com).

B. **Stage** II begins with full dilatation of the cervix and ends with complete expulsion of the fetus. The owner typically calls with problems during this stage.
  1. **Characteristic:** Expulsion of the fetus with visible abdominal contractions.
  2. **Duration:** The first puppy should come out within one hour.
C. **Stage** III begins after expulsion of the fetus and ends with expulsion of the placenta. The placenta is usually passed within 5-15 minutes, but the bitch may eat it before the client sees it.

Bitches move between Stages II and III until all fetuses and placentas are delivered. The placentas may lag in delivery.

V. **DYSTOCIA**
  A. **DIAGNOSING DYSTOCIA:** When should the bitch be treated?

CRITERIA FOR DIAGNOSING DYSTOCIA	
Prolonged gestation	• > 70-72 days after the first day of breeding • > 58 days of diestrus • > 66 days of gestation measured from the LH surge date
Pelvic obstruction	• Breed likelihood (pug, bulldog, etc.) • Presence of a mass lesion or previous fracture
Strong contractions without expulsion of a puppy	• > 45-60 minutes without expulsion of a puppy
Weak contractions unresponsive to medications	• ≥ 1 hour without expulsion of a puppy
Failure to enter Stage I labor	• 24-36 hours after the rectal temperature initially falls below 100°F
Bitch is in obvious pain. Excessive hemorrhage	• Due to failure to expel a puppy
Obvious radiographic abnormalities	• Stressed fetuses (HR < 200) by ultrasound or Doppler • Malposition • Fetal oversize (usually a single puppy) • Fetal death (overlapping of skull bones, intrauterine gas, collapse of spinal column)
Previous history of dystocia	• C-section isn't always required after a previous C-section
Stillbirths, sluggish puppies or clearly sick bitch	

  B. **CAUSES OF DYSTOCIA IN THE BITCH**

CLASS OF DYSTOCIA	TREATMENT
1° uterine inertia Failure of sufficient uterine contractions to expel the fetus. This is more common in large breed dogs with large litters.	**Calcium gluconate 10%:** Give 1 mL/5 kg SC q 4-6 hours to improve contraction strength. (Safe even in eucalemic bitches and queens.) If obstructive dystocia is ruled out, next give **oxytocin** 0.25-2.0 units SC or IM q 30-90 minutes to increase the frequency of contractions. Use caution if the cause of dystocia is not known and a uterine monitor (**tocodynamometry**) is not available. Monitor fetal heart rates (Doppler or ultrasound). If they drop in response to oxytocin, discontinue oxytocin and perform a cesarean section. Excessive oxytocin can compromise placental circulation and fetal oxygenation, and can rupture the uterus. IV oxytocin is not advised in the bitch or queen.
2° uterine inertia Uterine fatigue as a result of fetal obstruction (too large a fetus, small birth canal due to pelvic fracture or congenital formation, malpositioning, or vaginal stricture). Brachiocephalic breeds are more likely to have 2° uterine inertia.	C-section (medical management is not indicated).
Nervousness Occurs more in toy breeds.	Provide a quiet area for whelping.

C. **TREATMENT:** Perform a thorough physical exam to determine whether the bitch is truly in dystocia and whether the dystocia is obstructive (surgical case) or non-obstructive.

1. Evaluate her physically and biochemically: PCV TP ionized calcium and blood glucose minimally. Stabilize the bitch (fluids, etc.) if she is unstable.
2. **Digital examination** and **abdominal radiograph or ultrasound** for puppies: number, position, viability.
3. **Ultrasound or Doppler** to assess the fetal viability and stress (heart rate should be > 170 – 200 bpm).
4. Radiographs will tell you the following:
   a. If the bitch has fetuses to deliver and if dystocia is obstructive.
   b. The spines of the puppies should be dorsal. Make sure puppies aren't stuck. Bitches in dystocia should remain in the clinic, even in a quiet room with their owner, until the delivery is complete.
   c. **Fetal death:** Overlap of cranial bones and presence of gas in the uterus with time. Acute death is not evident radiographically but can be determined immediately with ultrasound or Doppler.
5. Medical management of uterine inertia: Refer to the above chart.
6. **Surgical management: C-section.** The indications for a C-section include:
   a. Obstructive dystocia where you can't reposition the puppy so that the puppy can be delivered, or where the puppy is too large to be delivered.
   b. Failure of medical management.
   c. Systemic illness—the bitch is in shock or septic.
   d. Excessively prolonged Stage II labor where fetal distress is evident.
   e. Improved chance of delivering live, vigorous puppies
   f. If the puppies are dead and are not passing.

VI. **WHELPING MONITORING EQUIPMENT:** The WhelpWise monitoring system can be used to help monitor labor. It consists of a Doppler monitor for fetal heart beats plus a sensor that monitors intrauterine and intra-amniotic pressures to detect contractions. It's especially useful for inexperienced breeders, bitches with a history of whelping problems, those with excessively large or small litters, and bitches six years of age or older (although it's best not to breed bitches at this age).

A. The system is strapped onto the shaved portion of the caudal abdomen of the pregnant bitch starting one week prior to the calculated whelping date. Measurements should be taken 1-2 times a day with the dog lying down calmly.
B. Normal fetal heart rate should be 180-200 bpm. Heart rates at or below 170 indicate problems with a fetus.

VII. **ABORTION, RESORPTION, STILLBIRTH**

A. **THE TIME SCALE**

ABORTION, RESORPTION, STILLBIRTH	
Resorption	< 35 days
Abortion	>35 days
Stillbirth	> 60 days

B. **CAUSES OF ABORTION**

ETIOLOGIES	DIAGNOSIS
Poor bitch health	• Physical exam of the bitch
Trauma	• History
Toxin, drugs	• History
Fetal defects	• Necropsy
Chromosomal abnormalities	• Karyotype the fetus
Infectious	• Culture the uterus, placenta and fetal tissues • PCR fetus/placenta for herpes • Histopathology of fetus
Toxoplasmosis	• Paired titers (3 weeks apart)
Premature labor	• Virus isolation from the fetal tissues • Detect with uterine monitor on the next pregnancy when all other causes of abortion are ruled out (normal bitch, unremarkable pathology of aborted fetuses) • Rule out use of raspberry leaves in bitch's diet
Brucella Any brucella present is significant.	• Slide/tube agglutination, confirm negatives (uses *B. ovis* antigen), positives suggest brucella infection • AGID or culture confirms positives • Repeat testing if tests are neg. but suspicion is high

VIII. PERI- and POST-PARTUM CONCERNS in the BITCH

PROBLEM	SIGNS	TREATMENT
Acute metritis (retained placenta/fetus, trauma, infection)	Lethargic + discharge 1-7 days post-whelping.	Antibiotics Spay Prostaglandins
Eclampsia	Post-partum restlessness, painfulness, convulsions. Occurs most commonly 1-3 weeks post-partum, during peak lactation.	3-20 mLs 10% calcium gluconate IV
Septic mastitis	Off-colored milk, ± sick	Antibiotics Drain the glands
Non-septic mastitis (Galactostasis)	Swollen, painful mammary glands	Improve nursing
Hypoglycemia	Weakness, seizures, sepsis	IV glucose, frequent feedings, parturition or C-section
Hyperglycemia/ketosis	PU/PD	Parturition or C-section
Diabetes mellitus	Hyperglycemia, abortion, hypoglycemic puppy	Spay Hard to regulate with insulin

A. **SEPARATION of PLACENTAL SITES:** A vaginal discharge of any color during pregnancy is a concern. Near the end of pregnancy, a hemorrhagic dark, red, or black vaginal discharge may indicate tearing of the placenta away from the uterus. This causes intrauterine bleeding and reduced placental blood supply to the fetus. Since separation of placental sites often occurs too early in gestation for a C-section to produce live puppies, our only treatment option may be to rest the dog and to check for infection.

B. **SUBINVOLUTION of PLACENTAL SITES** is when the placental sites have not healed post-weaning, and bright red discharge persists. The normal bitch has a brick red, vaginal discharge due to subinvolution of placental sites for up to 16 weeks post-whelping. This subinvolution is not associated with any long-term problems unless blood loss is significant. Check for other coagulopathies.

C. **ECLAMPSIA** is severe hypocalcemia that occurs most commonly in small breed dogs within the first 3 weeks of lactation. It does also occur in other dogs, as well as in cats. Eclampsia is due to loss of calcium during lactation and decreased food intake that may occur due to stress, leading to lower calcium intake. Supplementation with excess calcium pre-partum predisposes bitches to eclampsia.

> Any time you see a **lactating bitch** with **CNS signs** (nervousness, muscle twitching, seizures), think **eclampsia**. Also check for hypoglycemia, since hypoglycemia often accompanies hypocalcemia.

1. **Clinical signs:** Early signs of eclampsia include restlessness, pruritus, nervousness, pacing, lack of attentiveness to the puppies. These can progress to more severe signs of muscle twitching and seizures within minutes or hours.

2. **Calcium levels:** Total serum calcium is usually < 7mg/dL, and ionized serum calcium is also low, but presumptive diagnosis can be made based on history, signalment, and signs prior to obtaining chemistry results; thus, therapy can be initiated upon presentation.

3. **Treatment:** Administer 0.5-1.0 mL/kg (or 5-15 mg/kg) of **10% calcium gluconate** IV at a rate of 1 mL/minute over at least 10-30 minutes. The animal should start improving early in treatment, but if not, continue infusing to the high-end dose and beyond over the 30 minutes, if indicated by serum calcium levels. Monitor with EKG and cease administration if **bradycardia**, S-T elevation, or QT shortening are seen. Effects of calcium gluconate last 1-12 hours. Always re-dose with SC calcium gluconate diluted in an equal amount of saline every 6-8 hours until the bitch is eating vigorously and on oral supplement. Weaning the puppies (or kittens) may be necessary, if eucalcemia is not obtained with supplementation. Send the bitch home on 100-150 mg/kg of calcium carbonate (Tums®; 750 mg/tab) divided BID while the bitch is still lactating. In some cases, you can just hand feed the puppies (or kittens) for 12-24 hours so that they nurse less on the bitch during this period. Do not give oral calcium supplements during gestation as a prophylactic measure to prevent eclampsia because doing so may worsen post-partum hypocalcemia.

Reproduction

IX. **PSEUDOPREGNANCY** is the external and behavioral manifestation of pregnancy in a non-pregnant bitch. Bitches that undergo false pregnancy can exhibit all the same signs as a pregnant bitch. They can even lactate. Bitches are predisposed to pseudopregnancy because they are spontaneous ovulators, and their progesterone stays high for 2-3 months. The drop in progesterone induces false pregnancy, a normal response. What's variable is the bitch's reaction (sensitivity) to increased prolactin. Some show no change, but others begin to lactate. The steepness of the decline in progesterone affects the onset of pseudopregnancy. **The steeper the drop, the higher the prolactin levels and the more likely the chance of pseudopregnancy.**

    A. **TWO SCENARIOS in WHICH PSEUDOPREGNANCY OCCURS:**
        1. At the end of normal diestral phase.
        2. When the veterinarian spays the animal during late estrus or diestrus: The loss of the ovaries results in a steep decline in progesterone.

    B. **TREATMENT**
        1. **No medical treatment** is recommended in clinical pseudopregnancy, primarily because most dogs remain in this condition for only 1-3 weeks. The endocrine changes associated with the end of diestrus will progress, and the signs of pseudopregnancy will cease. If the bitch is lactating, though, the owner can do several things to dry her up:
            a. Stop stimulation of milk letdown by preventing the bitch from licking her mammary glands.
            b. Avoid hotpacking mammary glands, as this stimulates lactation.
        2. **Progesterone therapy** (not recommended) will return the bitch to diestrus and will alleviate signs of clinical pseudopregnancy. Once discontinued, however, you may see pseudopregnancy again, or you may predispose the animal to developing pyometra. Any other steroid (i.e., testosterone) will work, too, but is not recommended. Some females become aggressive with steroid treatment. The steroids feed back to the pituitary and turn the pituitary off so that less prolactin is secreted.
        3. **Cabergoline** is a prolactin inhibitor that will diminish lactation.

X. **MASTITIS:** Bacterial mastitis occasionally occurs in lactating bitches. It's characterized by warm, painful, firm mammary glands. The bitch is usually not systemically ill but can become lethargic and develop a fever. She may not allow the puppies to nurse. The glands can be aspirated and cultured or milk can be expelled and cultured. The most common bacteria isolated include *E. Coli*, streptococci and staphylococci. Treat with appropriate antibiotics (Clavamox and Cephalexin are good first choices). Continue letting the puppies nurse to drain the other mammary glands. Alternatively, if she will not let them nurse, then hotpack the glands and drain them manually. If the glands become necrotic, then they should be debrided surgically and any abscesses flushed and drained. Cabergoline can be used to diminish lactation.

XI. **MISMATING and PREGNANCY TERMINATION:** Spaying is 100% effective. $PGF_{2\alpha}$ is one effective medical treatment. Oral dexamethasone is effective, with monitoring. Follow-up ultrasound must be performed. Other drugs are less reliable or have been studied less, but alternatives are being developed (synthetic prostaglandins, antiprogestationals). Medical treatment with prostaglandins can be expensive, because dogs should be kept in the hospital for at least 24 hours to watch for side effects and to confirm that abortion is complete. Prostaglandins should not be dispensed to owners. They should be administered in the hospital.

	MISMATING	PREGNANCY TERMINATION
$PGF_{2\alpha}$ Not 100% effective	0.10-0.20 mg/kg BID for at least 5 days starting at 30+ days gestation. A progesterone level can also be performed while the dog is receiving $PGF_{2\alpha}$ to test whether progesterone levels have fallen. Concurrent use of misoprostol (PGE) hastens abortion; 1-2 µg/kg once daily into the vagina.	Refer to the section below on $PGF_{2\alpha}$
Dexamethasone		0.1-0.2 mg/kg BID for 10+ days. If started around day 30, resorption occurs. After 45 days, abortion occurs. Ultrasound at 10th day to determine endpoint.

A.   **PGF$_{2\alpha}$** (Lutalyse) is the most reliable drug for terminating pregnancy (with the
   longest therapeutic window) in dogs and cats. Giving PGF$_{2\alpha}$ to pregnant bitches
   after 30 days of gestation and to queens after 40 days of gestation results in
   100% abortion.
   1.   PGF$_{2\alpha}$ causes a decline in progesterone levels and myometrial contraction in
      the bitch. The bitch goes into Stage II labor and delivers the fetuses; she may
      also lactate.
   2.   PGF$_{2\alpha}$ **-induced** abortion should be delayed until the second half of gestation,
      when the presence of viable fetuses can be identified via ultrasound to confirm
      pregnancy. Ultrasound is important in determining when all of the fetuses have
      been delivered. Premature discontinuation of treatment can result in the
      eventual whelping or queening of remaining fetuses.
   3.   **Dose for bitches:** 0.10 mg/kg given subcutaneously every 8 hours for the
      first 48 hours and then 0.2 mg/kg SC every 8 hours until all of the fetuses are
      expelled. Hospitalize the bitch so that it does not expel the fetuses at home.
   4.   The bitch treated with PGF$_{2\alpha}$ usually returns to proestrus within four months
      following treatment and then cycles normally and can have a successful
      pregnancy.
   5.   **Side effects:** Lochia, panting, nesting, defecation/urination, emesis, trembling,
      and straining.
   6.   Giving 1-3 μg/kg misoprostol intravaginally once daily may hasten the abortion
      (softens the cervix).
B.   **ESTROGEN** (not recommended) predisposes the bitch to future development of
   pyometra and can cause bone marrow dyscrasias.

XII. **PYOMETRA:** Pyometra is an infection of the uterus. Any intact bitch that is ill should
   have pyometra on her list of differential diagnoses.

GENERAL INFO	Pyometra occurs under the influence of **progesterone**. It occurs only during **diestrus** and most commonly occurs 2-10 weeks after the end of estrus. In both cats and dogs, the most common organism found is *E. coli.* Pyometra occurs under the influence of progesterone because progesterone: • Suppresses leukocyte response to infectious stimuli • Decreases myometrial contractility • Stimulates endometrial glands to develop and produce more fluid (making the uterus a good culture plate for bacteria)
SIGNALMENT	The **older bitch/queen:** Older cats and dogs are more prone to pyometra. **Young females who have been treated with estrogens** for early pregnancy termination: Estrogen treatments make animals more susceptible to developing pyometra.
CLINICAL SIGNS	• Anorexia, lethargy, vomiting/diarrhea • 85% of queens and bitches have a **purulent vaginal discharge.** The other 15% have **closed-cervix pyometra** and are much sicker. • Increased white blood cell count • Palpable uterus • Radiographs and ultrasound show a severely enlarged uterus.
TREATMENT	**Ovariohysterectomy** is the best treatment. In cases of open-cervix pyometra where the animal is young, **prostaglandins** can be used. Administer 0.1-0.25 mg/kg SC SID for 3-5 days. They have side effects, though (vomiting, diarrhea, salivating, etc.). Treat concurrently with antibiotics and with fluids if indicated. Recheck the pet in 2 weeks. Examine for vaginal discharge, palpable uterine enlargement, and fever. Repeat ultrasound or radiographs may be required on follow-up.

Reproduction

SUGGESTED READING
Peterson ME, Talcott PA: Small Animal Toxicology. Second ed. St. Louis: Elsevier Saunders, 2006.

Poppenga RH, Volmer PA: Toxicology. Veterinary Clinics of North America: Small Animal Practice. Philadelphia: WB Saunders, Vol. 32, No. 2, March 2002.

ASPCA National Animal Poison Control Center (NAPCC)
NAPCC is manned by licensed veterinarians and board-certified veterinary toxicologists.
It receives calls 24 hours per day.
www.aspca.org/apcc
(888) 426-4435
$55.00 consultation fee
Veterinary hospitals can join the Veterinary Lifeline Partner Program.

Toxicology

A PARTIAL LIST of TOXICANT RULE-OUTS by CLINICAL SIGNS

CLINICAL SIGNS	RULE-OUT
Anemia (hemolysis, Heinz bodies)	Onion toxicity Metals • Iron • Lead • Zinc (pennies) NSAIDS and acetaminophen
(coagulopathy)	Rodenticides (anticoagulant rodenticides)
Arrhythmias	• Any stimulant (e.g., methylxanthines, pseudoephedrine) • Oleander plants/digitalis glycosides
GI signs (vomiting, diarrhea, hematemesis, etc.)	Metals • Lead • Zinc • Arsenic • Zinc phosphide (rodenticide) plus all other rodenticides Insecticides: Organophosphates and pyrethrins Plants NSAIDS Tricyclic antidepressants
Hyperexcitability	• Methylxanthines • Pseudoephedrine • Tricyclic antidepressants and other drugs of abuse such as amphetamines and cocaine
Liver disease signs	Acetaminophen, zinc, iron, cycad palm, xylitol, mushrooms
Renal disease signs	Ethylene glycol, cholecalciferol, NSAIDS, Lilium, Hemerocallis, grapes, raisins, aminoglycoside antibiotics.
Seizures	Insecticides • Carbamates • Chlorinated hydrocarbons • Organophosphates • Pyrethrins Metals • Lead Ethylene glycol Rodenticides • Strychnine • Metaldehyde • Bromethalin • Zinc phosphide Fungal: Any moldy food (penitrem, roquefortine) Tricyclic antidepressants Xylitol, Calycanthus, Brunfelsia, isoniazid, methylxanthines (caffeine, theobromine)

EXCRETION of DRUGS FROM the BODY

When an animal is exposed to a drug or foreign product, it can eliminate the drug in several ways. It may excrete the drug intact in the urine (depending on the drug's size and acid-base characteristics), or it may first modify the drug via oxidation and conjugation to make the drug more soluble for excretion into the urine. The rate at which the animal can rid itself of the drug (represented by the half-life) depends on many factors including the rate at which the body metabolizes the compound, the pH of the urine, and the animal's age, species, diet, and other health conditions.

I.   **PHASE I and II REACTIONS:** Drugs are often metabolized to more water-soluble compounds that can be excreted into the urine. Sometimes these metabolites are more toxic than their precursors.

    A.   **PHASE I, OXIDATION:** The compound is oxidized to make it more water soluble. This can make the substance more or less toxic. Oxidation is performed by the cytochrome P_{450} system in liver microsomes, in the gut, and in the lungs.

    B.   **PHASE II, CONJUGATION:** A handle is synthesized onto the molecule to make it more water soluble. Most major species differences in metabolism arise as a result of phase II differences.

        1.   The three most common handles are: **glutathione**, **glucuronide**, and **sulfate**. **Acetylation** and the addition of **amino acids** to the molecule also make the molecule more water soluble.

        2.   The glutathione and sulfate pools are very shallow, while the glucuronide pool is large. The problem in the cat is that the glucuronyl transferase can conjugate endogenous compounds well, but it doesn't work well with foreign substances. This is why substances such as Tylenol® (acetaminophen) that require glucuronide conjugation are so toxic in cats.

II. **HALF-LIFE** is the time needed to reduce the amount of substance in the body by one-half. It takes 5-7 half-lives before a compound is essentially gone. For example, if an animal ingests a toxicant that inhibits synthesis of coagulation factor VII (e.g., anticoagulant rodenticides), the total concentration of factor VII gradually diminishes. Since the half-life of factor VII is 5-6 hours, it takes 25-40 hours for factor VII concentrations to fall close to zero. Consequently, hemostatic signs of the toxicant don't appear for 1-2 days. On the other hand, if the toxicant inhibits factor IX synthesis (half-life = 13 hours) hemostatic signs don't appear for 3-5 days.

    A.   **THE HALF-LIFE of a GIVEN COMPOUND** can be altered by the presence of other compounds.

        1.   Some compounds, such as acetylcysteine, act as **building blocks for glutathione**, a molecule used in phase II conjugation. As a result, they accelerate the metabolism of some compounds. Acetylcysteine (Mucomyst®) is given to patients with acetaminophen toxicosis to speed up elimination of the acetaminophen.

        2.   Some substances (i.e., barbiturates) induce their own metabolism by up-regulating the liver microsomes. Chloramphenicol and cimetidine inhibit the microsomal cytochrome P_{450} system.

    B.   **HALF-LIFE can be ALTERED by ACID/BASE CHARACTERISTICS and ION TRAPPING:** At neutral pH, weak organic acids such as aspirin are ionized. At acidic urine pH, they are unionized, so they can cross membranes down their concentration gradient from the nephron into the blood stream. If you make the urine basic by adding bicarbonate, the acid stays ionized. As a result, it isn't resorbed into the blood stream. Instead, it's excreted with the urine. Many drugs are weak acids.

        1.   The ion trapping principle can be used to treat aspirin toxicosis by alkalinizing the urine (administering bicarbonate) and keeping the animal on fluids for at least 24 hours after vomiting and diarrhea have stopped.

Toxicology

PRINCIPLES of TREATING TOXICOSIS
(Also refer to p. 20.3 on excretion of drugs from the body)

When an owner calls you because his/her dog has come into contact with something toxic but is not showing any signs, you can advise as follows:

- **Toxic ingestion:** Bring the animal in so that you can evaluate it and induce vomiting if indicated. You may not want to advise the owner to induce emesis because he/she may do so incorrectly or ineffectively, thus wasting time, or the pet may not be in an appropriate condition for emesis. Emesis is contraindicated for some toxicants such as acids and alkalines (e.g., toilet bowl cleaners, batteries); rather, dilution with milk or water is recommended in these cases. Also avoid emesis in rodents or rabbits (They are unable to vomit.), animals at risk for aspiration, and animals that have vomited already. If the animal is healthy and the amount ingested is known and can be quantified upon recovery, consider inducing emesis.

- **Toxin in contact with the skin:** Have the owner wash the animal with mild liquid hand dishwashing detergent and lukewarm water (while wearing gloves). Be sure to rinse the pet well. Do not use solvents on the pet because solvents disperse the substance. In addition, some solvents may enhance the permeability of the skin to a toxin. After bathing the animal, the owner should bring the animal in for medical evaluation. If the pet is unstable, it should be taken to the veterinary hospital prior to bathing.

- **Toxin in the eye:** Have the owner attempt to rinse the eye out immediately with tepid water (or saline eyewash solution) for at least 20-30 minutes. If the eyes are too painful for the animal to allow the owner to flush them, the owner will need to take the animal to a hospital where it can be sedated prior to flushing the eyes. The eye should also be evaluated for corneal ulcers.

If the animal is showing signs of toxicosis, forego the above steps and have the owners bring it in for evaluation and stabilization.

I. **STABILIZE the VITAL SYSTEMS.** Control of life-threatening signs (treating the patient) takes precedence over obtaining a detailed history. If intoxication is suspected, try to get a history to determine the type of toxin and route of entry. If possible, have the owner bring in the toxin and its original packaging.

II. **REMOVE the TOXIN.** Also have the owner remove the source of poison if it is still present to prevent additional exposure to the patient or to other animals.
   A. **INDUCE EMESIS** (only in asymptomatic animals) and examine the vomitus. More toxin is removed if the stomach contains food. A small amount of food may be fed to some animals requiring emesis to increase the amount of toxin recovered. Emesis usually must be induced within an hour of ingestion and often even sooner.
   1. **Apomorphine** is the most consistent emetic in both dogs and cats (1/2 tablet subconjunctivally is preferred route, as excess can be flushed from the eye after the animal has finished vomiting). It usually takes effect within 5-10 minutes, and vomiting lasts for several minutes. If a pet develops respiratory depression, administer naloxone 0.01 mg/kg IV or 0.04 mg/kg IM. Generally, if the initial dose of apomorphine is not successful, a repeat dose is not likely to work.
   2. **Syrup of ipecac:** Syrup of ipecac is less than ideal. Results are variable, and when vomiting does occur, it may not happen for 30 minutes. If a pet does not vomit, some pets could be at risk for cardiotoxic effects from the ipecac. If this is the only emetic available, make sure you have syrup of ipecac and not ipecac extract.
   3. **3% hydrogen peroxide** (1 mL/kg to a maximum dose of 45 mL): If the animal does not vomit within 15 minutes, it can be dosed one more time. Hydrogen peroxide is extremely irritating to the GI epithelium. The peroxide must be fresh (look for bubbling when placed with organic material), and it is more effective when food is in the stomach. Some cats develop hemorrhagic gastroenteritis after treatment with hydrogen peroxide, so use with caution in cats.
   4. **Xylazine** can be used in healthy cats at a dose of 1.1 mg/kg IM or SC. It can profoundly decrease cardiac output as well as cause cardiac arrhythmias, so cats should have an intravenous catheter placed prior to administration. Cats with cardiac disease should not receive xylazine as an emetic. Xylazine is reversible with 0.1 mg/kg yohimbine IV (cats and dogs), and it should not be used unless an IV catheter is placed and the reversal agent is available.

5. **Do not induce emesis in:**
   a. **Rodents or rabbits**
   b. Animals at risk for **aspiration** (e.g., animals that are **comatose**, lack a pharyngeal reflex, or are **seizuring**)
   c. Animals that have already **vomited repeatedly**
   d. Animals that have **ingested strong acids** (undiluted toilet bowl cleaner, car batteries, pool sanitizers), **alkalis/corrosives** (automatic dishwasher detergents, radiator flushes, some batteries), or **petroleum products** (heating oil, turpentine): These substances can further damage the esophagus if vomited, or they may be aspirated, causing pneumonia. These animals can be given milk/egg whites to help dilute ingested products, decrease risk of burns, and coat the GI lining.
   e. Animals that have ingested wood glue, such as Gorilla glue®, containing isocyanates or diisocyanates, since this may lead to esophageal obstruction

B. **GASTRIC LAVAGE** may be performed in animals where emesis is not recommended. Animals must be anesthetized, and a cuffed endotracheal tube used to protect the airway. Use the largest bore stomach tube appropriate to the size of the pet. Instill 5-10 mL/kg of normal saline or water at body temperature, then allow gravity to drain it into a container. Repeat until the lavage fluid returns as a clear liquid. In cases where you must remove the entire ingested toxin, then after the gastric lavage give a high enema until clear fluid appears in the stomach tube (**enterogastric lavage**). Follow the lavage with instillation of activated charcoal suspension via the stomach tube. **Do not perform gastric lavage** in animals that have **ingested strong acids, strong alkaline/caustic products, or petroleum distillates,** or in animals that have ingested **wood glues with isothiocyanates,** as these glues expand with the addition of water.

C. **ADMINISTER an ADSORBENT:** Adsorbents are used to bind with toxins not removed by emesis or lavage. Activated charcoal is the most common adsorbent. Administer 1-4 g/kg body weight mixed with 50-200 mL of water orally within 1-2 hours of toxic ingestion. Some dogs will eat it if the slurry is mixed with canned dog food. It can also be given via gastric tube with the animal under sedation and an endotracheal tube in place. If the animal has ingested a compound that undergoes extensive enterohepatic circulation, such as acetaminophen, digoxin or ivermectin, then additional doses of charcoal should be administered at 6-8 hour intervals. Remember to tell the owner that the pet may have black diarrhea for several days following charcoal administration.

D. **CATHARTICS** draw water into the GI tract allowing the toxin to be moved through the GI tract faster. Prepared activated charcoal products usually contain a cathartic such as sorbitol. Avoid cathartics if the animal already has diarrhea or is dehydrated. If multiple doses of activated charcoal are needed, only use cathartics with the first dose. A common cathartic is 70% sorbitol, which can be purchased through drugstores. Give 1-2 mL/kg.

E. **ENEMA:** Warm water enema. Do not use a phosphate enema.

F. **FLUID ADMINISTRATION:** To prevent renal shutdown, consider keeping the animal on fluids and possibly on mannitol, dopamine, or lasix. Monitor fluid in/out rate, heart rate, and blood pressure.

G. **ION TRAPPING:** Acidify the urine to facilitate the excretion of basic toxins, or alkalinize the urine to facilitate excretion of acidic compounds. Determine the animal's acid-base status first. To avoid causing imbalances, do not give either acidifying or alkalinizing substances unless you are able to monitor the acid-base status.

H. **ALSO REMEMBER** to have the owner **remove the toxin from the environment** so that the animal is not re-exposed when it goes home.

III. **ADMINISTER the ANTIDOTE:** A few poisons have specific antidotes, but most toxins do not. The key to successful treatment is effective decontamination, close monitoring for potential signs, and effective symptomatic and supportive care.

IV. **SUPPORTIVE TREATMENT:** Control seizures, prevent dehydration, regulate temperature, etc.

V. **OBSERVE the ANIMAL UNTIL it is STABLE.**

Toxicology

TOXIC FOODS
Chocolate, onions, grapes, moldy foods, macadamia nuts, xylitol

I. **CHOCOLATE** is the most common toxic ingestion in pets. The primary toxin is theobromine, a methylxanthine found in cocoa, baker's chocolate, dark chocolate, and milk chocolate. Some chocolates contain a second methylxanthine, caffeine (which can also be found in tea, coffee, and diet pills).

 A. **MECHANISM of ACTION:** Methylxanthines inhibit phosphodiesterase (PDE), an enzyme involved in the cyclic AMP cascade that's triggered in the fight or flight response. Phosphodiesterase down-regulates this cascade by degrading cyclic AMP, the first step of the cascade.

 B. **CLINICAL SIGNS** occur within 1-4 hours.
   1. **Gastrointestinal signs** occur first and include vomiting and diarrhea.
   2. **Neurologic signs:** Once the methylxanthines are absorbed into the blood, the animal may show neurologic signs including hyperexcitability, weakness, ataxia, seizure, and coma.
   3. **Cardiac signs:** Animals may also exhibit PVCs or other arrhythmias, which may result in death.

 C. **AMOUNT CAUSING TOXICITY:** When calculating toxicity, add the ingested theobromine and caffeine together to get the total methylxanthine ingested. The lethal dose (LD_{50}) is 110-200 mg/kg, but animals start showing signs at much lower doses. Animals vomit and appear restless after ingesting about 20 mg/kg of methylxanthine, have arrhythmias at 40-50 mg/kg, and seizure at 50-60 mg/kg.

TOXIC AMOUNTS* of THEOBROMINE and CAFFEINE

SOURCE	AMOUNT of METHYLXANTHINE	TOXIC DOSE (10 kg dog)	TOXIC DOSE (20 kg dog)
Cocoa bean mulch	56-900 mg/oz**	0.5-1.0 oz	1.0-2.0 oz
Unsweetened cocoa	700 mg/oz	0.75-1.5 oz	1.5-3.0 oz
Baking chocolate	400 mg/oz	1.25-2.5 oz	2.5-5.0 oz
Semisweet chocolate or instant cocoa	140 mg/oz	3.5-7 oz	7.0-14 oz
Milk chocolate	64 mg/oz	10-20 oz	20-40 oz
Coffee (caffeine)	40 mg/oz	12.5-25 oz	25-50 oz
Espresso (caffeine)	100 mg/oz	5-10 oz	10-20 oz

*Based on 50-100 mg/kg—the amount that causes seizure to the low end of the lethal dose range) **Calculations use 900 mg/oz.

 D. **TREATMENT** includes the standard emesis (within 2 hours) and activated charcoal administration. Since methylxanthine undergoes extensive enterohepatic circulation, repeat charcoal administration every 3-6 hours.
   1. **Control seizures and hyperexcitability** with diazepam (2.5-20 mg IV to effect).
   2. **Fluid therapy** aids in renal excretion of the compounds.
   3. **Treat arrhythmias.**

 E. **PROGNOSIS** is good if treatment is instituted within several hours of ingestion.

II. **ONION TOXICITY:** Both cooked and raw onions pose a threat. They may be ingested in large amounts acutely or in moderate amounts chronically. The most common source is dehydrated onions or onion powder such as in onion soup.

 A. **MECHANISM of ACTION:** Onion ingestion results in irreversible oxidative denaturation of hemoglobin (resulting in formation of Heinz bodies), oxidation of membrane lipid sulfhydryl groups, and methemoglobin formation. The damaged red blood cells are less deformable than normal cells and lyse easily, resulting in intravascular hemolysis in severe cases. Extravascular hemolysis occurs when Heinz bodies are cleared from the red blood cells by the spleen, Heinz body formation and red blood cell destruction peak several days following onion ingestion.

 B. **CLINICAL SIGNS** are initially due to GI upset (diarrhea, vomiting), but anemia is the cause of the primary signs (exercise intolerance; lethargy; pale, cyanotic, or icteric mucous membranes). Animals can also become hemoglobinuric.

 C. **DIAGNOSIS**
   1. **History** of being fed onions (onion soup, dehydrated onions, etc.).
   2. **Regenerative anemia:** It takes several days for the animal to mount a regenerative response, but when it does, the response is usually very dramatic

and often includes **nucleated red blood cells.** The anemia is associated with the following:

  a. **Heinz bodies:** Heinz body formation is the highest within the first week after ingestion. Dogs get multiple small Heinz bodies, whereas cats develop single large Heinz bodies in their red blood cells.
  b. **Intravascular hemolysis** occurs in severely affected animals.
  c. **Icterus** (or increased icterus index) can occur due to extra- and intravascular hemolysis.
  d. **Urinalysis** may reveal mild hemoglobinuria and the presence of urobilinogen.

  D. **TREATMENT**
    1. **Emesis** within 2 hours of ingestion
    2. Activated **charcoal administration**
    3. **Fluid therapy** to encourage renal excretion
    4. **Blood transfusions** are sometimes required
  E. **PROGNOSIS** is good.

III. **GRAPES and RAISINS:** Grapes and raisins involved in toxic ingestions have been commercially purchased, home grown, organic, non-organic, and of many different varieties. The lowest documented ingestion leading to renal failure was 0.7 oz raisins per kg of dog. Four to five grapes were toxic to an 8.2 kg dog. Thus, one to two grapes in a small dog is a potentially significant exposure, even if the dog has eaten grapes in the past with no adverse effects.
  A. **MECHANISM of ACTION:** Neither the toxic agent nor the mechanism of action is known, but some grapes and raisins can cause **renal failure** within 72 hours of ingestion.
  B. **TREATMENT**
    1. **Emesis** within 6-12 hours post-exposure.
    2. Follow with fluid diuresis for 48 hours minimum even if raisins or grapes were vomited on emesis, unless you know that all of the raisins and grapes were vomited, and emesis was induced early. Diuresis can be SC if there's no evidence (on urinalysis or chemistry) of renal failure.

IV. **MOLDY FOODS:** Mold can grow on fruits, walnuts, cheese, compost, and road kill. A wide range of fungi can produce tremorgenic mycotoxins. The overall effect is the same, although the specific mechanism of action may vary.
  A. **CLINICAL SIGNS:** Tremors that progress to seizures, plus GI signs such as vomiting. The neurologic signs can also start out as hyperactivity and progress to coma.
  B. **TREATMENT:** Early decontamination is essential. Animals that die do so usually within the first 2-4 hours.
    1. **Methocarbamol** should be used for the tremors. **Diazepam** can be used for hyperesthesia. The animal may need to be anesthetized with propofol and barbiturates.
  C. **DIAGNOSIS:** If the owners want to try to identify the cause, stomach contents and vomitus can be sent to Michigan State University's Diagnostic Center for Population and Animal Health (www.animalhealth.msu.edu, 517-353-1683) and a gas chromatography run for common toxins (GCMS Toxin Screen) for approximately $80.00. Turn-around time is 5-7 days. Gas chromatography can be used to identify strychnine, insecticides, metaldehyde, zinc phosphide, methylxanthines, drugs of abuse, bromethalin, and tremorgenic myoctoxins (roquefortine, penetrim), among other substances.

V. **MACADAMIA NUT** ingestion (about 1 nut per kg dog) causes weakness, depression, vomiting, ataxia, and tremors within 24 hours of ingestion, with a peak at around 12 hours. Most dogs can be managed with supportive care at home, but those with pre-existing conditions or older dogs should be managed at the veterinary hospital.

VI. **XYLITOL** is a sugar substitute found in sugar-free gums, candies and baked goods. Upon absorption it stimulates insulin release for several hours leading to **hypoglycemia**. Signs of hypoglycemia can be seen in 15-30 minutes. Treatment involves emesis (charcoal may not absorb xylitol well) and CRI of dextrose for symptomatic dogs. Asymptomatic animals can be fed frequent small meals with added sugar. Some dogs have subsequently developed liver failure after ingesting xylitol-containing products, so liver values should be monitored.

Toxicology

DRUG TOXICITIES
NSAIDs
Acetaminophen
Pseudoephedrine
Phenylpropanolamine and Amphetamines

I. **NSAID TOXICITY**

A. **MECHANISM of ACTION:** NSAIDs work by reversibly inhibiting the **cyclooxygenase enzyme** step in **prostaglandin synthesis.** Prostaglandins are important mediators of local inflammation. In addition, renal prostaglandins regulate renal blood flow (vasodilation) and glomerular filtration rate, while gastric prostaglandins are important in gastric protection (inducing bicarbonate secretion and mucus production). Prostaglandins also act on the hypothalamus to increase temperature. Consequently, administration of NSAIDs reduces fever and inflammation, and NSAID toxicity causes gastric ulcers and renal damage.

B. **COMMON NSAIDS INVOLVED in TOXIC INGESTION:** Repeat doses are more often responsible for severe disease than single acute doses.
   1. **Aspirin:** 80 mg (baby), 325 mg (regular strength), 500 mg (extra strength)

SPECIES	TOXIC DOSE
Dogs	50 mg/kg TID (3 regular strength tablets in a 20 kg dog)
Cats	25-100 mg/kg SID (0.5-1.5 regular strength tablets per 5 kg cat).

   2. **Ibuprofen, naproxen, and ketoprofen are chemically similar NSAIDs.** The most common generic drug toxicity is due to ibuprofen (Advil®, 200 mg tablets). Little has been documented about toxicity and pharmacokinetics of naproxen (Aleve®, 25 mg tablets) and ketoprofen (Orudis®, 12.5 mg tablets).

SIGNS	ONE DOSE
GI (in 12 hrs-5 days)	• 50 mg/kg in dogs (2.5 tablets in a 10 kg dog) • 25 mg/kg in cats
Renal failure (in 24 hrs-5 days)	• 150 mg/kg (7.5 tablets in 10 kg dog)
CNS (in 2-12 hrs)	• >400-600 mg/kg (20 tablets in a 10 kg dog)
Acute death	• >600 mg/kg (30 tablets in a 10 kg dog)

C. **CLINICAL SIGNS:** GI signs related to ulceration include vomiting and hematemesis and may occur within 5 days post-exposure. Within 1-5 days, signs of renal dysfunction such as polyuria, oliguria, depression, seizure, and coma may occur.

D. **BLOODWORK** may show evidence of anemia due to GI bleeding.
   1. **Heinz bodies:** Cats may have Heinz bodies.
   2. Plasma, urine, and serum can be tested for common NSAIDs. Results may not be available for 5-7 days, though.

E. **TREATMENT:** Treat by decontamination (emesis, charcoal, cathartics).
   1. Also treat gastric ulcers as per the GI section on gastric ulcers (p. 20.4).
   2. Diurese and treat for renal disease as per the section on renal disease (p. 21.20).

II. **ACETAMINOPHEN**

A. **MECHANISM of ACTION:** The cytochrome P_{450} system converts acetaminophen to a very hepatotoxic compound that also oxidizes hemoglobin to methemoglobin. Under normal circumstances, methemoglobin is reduced back to hemoglobin by glutathione. But with acetaminophen toxicity, the glutathione pool is decreased due to conjugation to acetaminophen, and it is not large enough to keep up with formation of methemoglobin or toxic metabolites. The toxic metabolite also causes oxidative damage to hepatocyte membranes, resulting in hepatic necrosis.

B. **TOXIC DOSE** (325 mg and 500 mg tablets)

SPECIES	TOXIC DOSE
Dogs	>100 mg/kg can cause liver injury >200 mg/kg can cause methemoglobinemia
Cats	50-100 mg/kg (1-2 pills can be fatal)

C. CLINICAL SIGNS
1. **GI Signs:** Vomiting, anorexia, abdominal pain
2. **Liver Signs:** Icterus, bilirubinuria
3. **Additional signs in cats (and dogs at doses >200 mg/kg):** Cats may show the following signs within one hour of ingestion:
   a. Cyanosis and dyspnea due to Heinz body anemia
   b. Swollen face and paws
   c. Death

   Keratoconjunctivitis sicca has been reported in some dogs 72 hours after exposure to acetaminophen.
D. **BLOODWORK** reveals Heinz body anemia, methemoglobinemia, hemoglobinuria, and increased liver enzymes.
E. **TREATMENT** is the same as for aspirin, plus the following:
1. **Oxygen** therapy for cyanosis.
2. **Acetylcysteine** (Mucomyst®): Acetylcysteine provides building blocks for glutathione. Thus, more glutathione becomes available for conjugation to acetaminophen. In cats and dogs, give 140 mg/kg IV or PO initially, 70 mg/kg 6 hours later PO or IV, and then continue with this dose q 6 hours for seven treatments. You can also use a 10-20% solution (100 mg/mL and 200 mg/mL solutions available in 4, 10, and 30 mL vials) for IV use. Oral administration may be more effective since acetylcysteine is almost 100% absorbed, and all that is absorbed goes straight to the liver where it is needed.
3. **Ascorbic acid:** 30 mg/kg PO q 6 hours to treat for the methemoglobinemia.
4. **Methylene blue** is no longer recommended.
5. **Hepatoprotectants** such as SAM-E can be used.

III. **PSEUDOEPHEDRINE** is a decongestant found in many sinus, allergy, and cough preparations. It's rapidly absorbed. Cough medications also include products such as caffeine, alcohol, antihistamines, and dextromethorphan. Extended release products may have delayed onset of signs and prolonged duration of signs. Toxic doses in dogs: 5-6 mg/kg (clinical signs include agitation, hyperactivity, hyperthermia); 10-12 mg/kg deaths have been reported.
A. **CLINICAL SIGNS** are due to sympathetic overstimulation and include agitation, hyperactivity, hyperthermia, disorientation, seizures, mydriasis, tachycardia and vomiting. Because it's rapidly absorbed, signs can occur within an hour of ingestion.
B. **TREATMENT** is the same as for PPA and amphetamines (See below).

IV. **PHENYLPROPANOLAMINE and AMPHETAMINES:** Phenylpropanolamine is a sympathomimetic used for urinary incontinence in dogs. It's available in a chewable form. Signs are caused by increased sympathetic tone. Amphetamines are CNS stimulants that work by increasing both catecholamine and serotonin release and inhibiting catecholamine reuptake.
A. **TOXIC DOSES** of PPA in dogs:
1. 1-5 mg/kg—tachycardia, vomiting, hyperactivity
2. 5-10 mg/kg—hypertension, vomiting, hyperthermia, tachycardia
3. > 20 mg/kg—potentially life-threatening CV and CNS signs, including seizures
B. **CLINICAL SIGNS:** Tachycardia, panting, hypertension, tremors. Dogs can be **bradycardic** secondary to the **hypertension.** Dogs tend to present as either depressed, bradycardic, and hypertensive or as agitated, tachycardic, and hypertensive. The hypertension can cause retinal detachment.
C. **TREATMENT:** Standard decontamination. Promote **emesis** within 1 hour of ingestion if no serious signs present. Use activated charcoal and administer fluids to help prevent renal failure and speed excretion.
1. **Acepromazine** can be used for agitation. Use the premedication dose, and titrate dose up as needed (May require large dose depending on amount ingested).
2. **Cyproheptadine** is a serotonin antagonist. It can be used if signs of serotonin syndrome develop (disorientation, aggression, hyperthermia). Try up to 4 doses (1.1 mg/kg) in a 24-hour period.
3. Once agitation is under control, treat residual **tachycardia** with **propranolol** 20-60 μg/kg IV over 10 minutes in dogs and 40 μg/kg IV in cats.
4. Treat **seizures** and hyperactivity with acepromazine Diazepam is contraindicated. **Do not treat for the bradycardia.** It's a reflex bradycardia. Rather, treat the hypertension. **Nitroprusside** can be used to decrease blood pressure.
5. Tachycardia can be treated with **propranolol.**

Toxicology

MISCELLANEOUS HOUSEHOLD TOXINS
Paintballs, wood glue, shampoos, glow-in-the-dark jewelry, potpourri

I. **PAINTBALL** formulations vary between manufacturers, but in general, they contain products such as glycerol and polyethylene glycol (PEG), which are osmotic cathartics. Ingestion of large amounts leads to GI loss of water and, consequently, hypernatremia.
    A. **CLINICAL SIGNS:** Ataxia, disorientation, etc., are due to **hypernatremia.** Signs usually start within 3 hours.
    B. **TREATMENT:** Treat any dog that has eaten ≥ 5 paintballs per 10 kg dog. Treat even if the dog is asymptomatic, because the paintballs melt quickly in the stomach.
        1. **Induce emesis but avoid activated charcoal.** The cathartics included with charcoals may make the condition worse. If treated before signs occur, then monitor for 4-5 hours before sending home.
        2. **Treat seizures** with diazepam. Use **methocarbamol** for tremors if needed. You can give gas or propofol.
        3. **Manage hypernatremia:** Warm water enemas often normalize the hypernatremia quickly.
            a. IV administration of sodium free or low sodium fluids.
            b. It's okay to correct acute hypernatremia quickly (vs. chronic hypernatremia, which should be corrected slowly). If we correct the hypernatremia slowly the dog may develop chronic hypernatremia, which makes it much more difficult to manage quickly.
        4. Manage acidosis by first controlling the clinical signs (emesis, seizures) . If the animal is still acidotic, redo blood gases to see if these need to be addressed.
        5. Continue with fluids to prevent secondary renal disease.
    C. **PROGNOSIS:** Signs normally subside over 12-24 hours with aggressive treatment. Refractory cases lasting 24 hours are more guarded because of the chronic hypernatremia.

II. **WOOD GLUES such** as Gorilla Glue®, Elmer's ProBond®, and other brands contain **isocyanates** or **diisocyanate**. These chemicals draw in water from the environment and then expand and fill up the joints. The stomach has lots of moisture, so the glue expands and forms a foreign body in the stomach. If the dog has eaten a paper towel with the glue on it, then the foreign body is probably small. If the owner has found a chewed bottle of glue, then the foreign body is likely to be large.
    A. **TREATMENT:** The foreign body usually forms within 40 minutes to 2 hours.
        1. Avoid inducing emesis, as it may cause an expanding foreign body in the esophagus. Additionally, do not dilute with fluid; it will make the foreign body larger.
        2. The foreign body should be removed surgically. Most are huge and form a cast of the gastric mucosa and cause angry mucosal irritation.

III: **NON-IONIC and ANIONIC DETERGENTS** such as sodium laurel sulfate shampoos, body, and hand soaps, some household cleaners, etc. If cats walk through these products or the products are applied to their skin but not washed off, and the cats inhale and ingest the products upon grooming, then they develop vomiting, diarrhea, hypersalivation, and dyspnea. Radiographs often reveal pulmonary edema.
    A. **TREATMENT:** Treat supportively for the dyspnea (e.g., oxygen cage and Lasix if indicated). Also wash the products off the fur.

IV **GLOW-IN-THE-DARK JEWELRY** contains dibutyl phthalate, a low toxicity compound with a bitter taste. When cats bite into it, they are shocked by the bitter taste. They often try to run away from the taste and drool profusely. They may hide and also become aggressive. Owners can feed tuna or tuna water to help wash out the bitter taste. Then take the cat into a dark room and wipe off anything that's glowing.

V. **LIQUID SIMMERING POTPOURRI:** Cats may lick this household fragrance from the container or off of their fur if it spills on them. These products contain cationic detergents, which cause ulceration of the oral and GI mucosa, as well as CNS depression and dermal irritation. They should be treated as a corrosive/alkaline toxicosis. Dilute with milk or water, avoid emesis and activated charcoal, and place on pain medications, sucralfate and other GI protectants. Provide supportive care.

ETHYLENE GLYCOL TOXICITY

SOURCE	Antifreeze, some photographic solutions, brake fluids
ACUTE LETHAL DOSE*	Dogs ≥ 4.2-6.6 mL/kg • 5 kg dog = 25 mL • 15 kg dog = 75 mL • 30 kg dog = 150 mL	Cats ≥ 1.5 mL/kg • 5 kg cat = 8 mL
MECHANISM of ACTION	Ethylene glycol is no more toxic than ethanol; however, it's metabolized in the liver by **alcohol dehydrogenase** to a number of products that are much more toxic than ethanol. They cause acidosis and destroy the renal tubular epithelium. Furthermore, oxalic acid, the final product, combines with calcium to form calcium oxalate, which precipitates in the renal tubules causing further destruction. Fifty percent of ethylene glycol is excreted unchanged in the urine, and the other 50% is rapidly metabolized to toxic compounds.
CLINICAL SIGNS	Any animal with a history of acute renal failure or with CNS signs plus polydipsia is a possible ethylene glycol toxicosis suspect. **Early signs** (0-12 hours following exposure) are due primarily to unmetabolized ethylene glycol and are **similar to signs of ethanol intoxication** (e.g., animals act "drunk"). Peak absorption occurs at 1 hour in cats and 3-6 hours in dogs. Signs can start within an hour of ingestion. Absorption is slower if the stomach has food in it. • Vomiting • Ataxia, knuckling • Depression within 1-3 hours • Polydipsia due to increased osmolality • Muscle fasciculations **Transition** (12-24 hours): The initial signs may progress to seizures or coma, or the animal may temporarily get better and then go into acute renal failure. This temporary improvement only occurs in dogs. **Late signs** (24-72 hours following exposure in dogs and 12-24 hours following exposure in cats) are caused by ethylene glycol metabolites. In this stage, the animal develops signs of **acute renal failure**. • Severe depression, coma • Seizures • Anorexia • Oral ulcers/salivation • Oliguria, which progresses to anuria

*Dose reported to cause acute death from acidosis, inebriation. Dose needed to cause potentially fatal renal injury is likely lower.

ETHYLENE GLYCOL TOXICITY (continued)

BLOOD ANALYSIS	**Early stage:**
	• **Commercial test kit:** EGT kit for ethylene glycol levels in the blood. This test detects levels above 50 mg/dL, a toxic level in dogs. It is not sensitive enough to detect the lowest lethal levels in cats. That is, negative results in cats do not rule out ethylene glycol intoxication. For cats, consider testing at a human hospital or diagnostic laboratory. Treat at whatever levels the lab indicates would warrant treatment in humans. False positives can occur with exposure to formaldehyde, metaldehyde, glycerin/glycerol, and propylene glycol. Some formulations of activated charcoal may contain glycerin or glycerol.
	• **Increased osmolar gap:** Serum osmolality increases within 1 hour of ingestion and remains elevated for up to 18 hours. The normal osmolar gap is about 10 mOsm/kg. An **osmolar gap of > 50 mOsm/kg suggests ethylene glycol toxicity.** Multiplying osmolar gap x 6.2 gives the ethylene glycol concentration in the blood in mg/dL.
	OSMOLAR GAP = Measured serum - Calculated serum osmolality osmolality
	• **Acidosis** within 3 hours. • **Hyperphosphatemia** without elevated BUN is due to phosphate in antifreeze, not due to renal failure.
	Late stage: • Chemistry changes associated with **renal failure** such as elevation in BUN, creatinine, phosphorus, potassium. • Decreased calcium due to chelation with oxalate.
URINALYSIS	• **Isosthenuric** by 3 hours due to **hyperosmolarity,** which results in polyuria and osmotic diuresis. Later, the isosthenuria is due to renal failure. • **Acidic pH** due to the weak acids formed by metabolism of ethylene glycol. • **Calcium oxalate crystals** may occur as soon as 3-6 hours post-ingestion but often are not seen and are a late finding. These crystals come in a wide variety of shapes. Calcium oxalate crystals can also be seen in animals with calcium oxalate calculi in the bladder or kidney and in some normal animals that haven't been exposed to ethylene glycol. To diagnose ethylene glycol toxicity, you must correlate the history, clinical signs, and other diagnostic findings with the finding of calcium oxalate crystals in the urine. • **Casts** (all types) indicate renal damage (white blood cell casts, red blood cell casts, granular casts, etc.). • **Wood's lamp:** Ethylene glycol may contain fluorescein dye. So, if you shine a Wood's lamp on urine collected from an animal with ethylene glycol toxicity, the urine will fluoresce for up to 6 hours post-exposure. Vomitus early in the toxicity will fluoresce, too. A negative result does not definitively rule out exposure.
OTHER TESTS	**Radiographs/ultrasound:** The kidneys may appear radiodense on radiographs or hyperechoic on ultrasound due to the precipitation of calcium oxalate in the kidneys. **Renal biopsy:** Finding masses of calcium oxalate crystals in the renal tubules is diagnostic for ethylene glycol toxicity.

ETHYLENE GLYCOL TOXICITY (continued)

THERAPY	Remove ethylene glycol from the system: Induce vomiting or perform gastric lavage within 1 hour of ingestion. Inhibit conversion of ethylene glycol to toxic metabolites. • In dogs, administer 4-methylpyrrazole (fomepizol: Antizol-Vet™): 4-MP is a noncompetitive inhibitor of alcohol dehydrogenase that effectively decreases the metabolism of ethylene glycol when given up to 36 hours after ingestion. If given within 3 hours of ingestion, 90% of the ethylene glycol is excreted unchanged in the urine. One vial is enough to treat a 25 kg dog. • Dose 1: (time 0) = 20 mg/kg IV • Dose 2: (12 hours) = 15 mg/kg IV • Dose 3: (24 hours) = 15 mg/kg IV • Dose 4: (36 hours) = 5 mg/kg IV • In cats, administration of 4-methylpyrrazole must be started within 3 hours of exposure to ethylene glycol. • Dose 1: (time 0) = 125 mg/kg IV • Dose 2: (12 hours) = 31.25 mg/kg IV • Dose 3: (24 hours) = 31.25 mg/kg IV • Dose 4: (36 hours) = 31.25 mg/kg IV • Administer ethanol IV: Ethanol is a competitive inhibitor of alcohol dehydrogenase. The disadvantages of using ethanol are that it can cause severe depression and coma at the doses needed, and it increases osmolality so that we can no longer use osmolar gap to determine the amount of ethylene glycol in the blood. The ethanol must be given in doses high enough to keep the animal "drunk." Use a 20% solution of ethanol. This can be obtained by diluting vodka (80 proof, 40%) with an equal amount of saline or by mixing Everclear (180 proof, 90%) with 3.5x the amount of saline (e.g., 1 mL of Everclear to 3.5 mL of saline). Protocol: • Dogs: 5.5 mL/kg IV every 4 hours (5x), then every 6 hours (4x) • Cats: 5.0 mL/kg IV every 6 hours (5x), then every 8 hours (4x) • Alternatively, administer ethanol at a constant rate infusion of about 1.3 mL/kg of 30% ethanol as a slow bolus, then 0.42 mL/kg/hr slow IV for 48 hours. To do this, mix the 30% solution in an IV bag, mixing enough for at least 24 hours. For example, dilute 750 mL of vodka with 250 mL of saline, or dilute 330 mL of Everclear with 670 mL of saline. • Sometimes alcohol can be given orally (if it's sweet tasting, dogs may drink it, or you can tube the dog). This is only appropriate if the animal is conscious and has good control of its swallow reflex. Supportive care: • Fluids: Fluid administration is very important because it aids excretion of unmetabolized ethylene glycol. The ethanol can be piggy-backed into the fluid line. • Administer bicarbonate to correct the acid-base balance.

SAMPLE TREATMENT REGIMENS USING ETHANOL

20% ETHANOL	5 kg DOG	10 kg DOG	30 kg DOG
*Boluses	25 mL bolus	75 mL bolus	150 mL bolus

*Boluses should be administered over 10-15 minutes.

Toxicology

INSECTICIDES
Cholinesterase Inhibitors—Organophosphates (OPs) and Carbamates
Pyrethrins and Pyrethroids

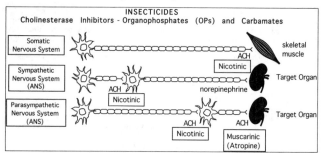

I. CHOLINESTERASE INHIBITORS—ORGANOPHOSPHATES (OPS) and CARBAMATES

RECOGNIZE the NAMES	Organophosphates (OP) usually have **phosph-** in their names (e.g., phosphate, phosphorothioate, phosphoramide, etc.). For example, Dursban® (chlorpyrifos) is a phosphorothioate. Other common OPs include malathion, fenthion, diazinon. **Carbamate** insecticides usually, but not always, have **carbam-** in their names (e.g., methylcarbamoyl, methylcarbamate).
COMMON SOURCES of EXPOSURE	**Organophosphate and carbamate insecticides** are used to control ectoparasites in dogs and cats as well as in livestock. They are also used in agricultural pest control and termite control. • **Dogs** are often exposed by ingesting OPs and carbamates. • **Cats** are more sensitive to OPs and carbamates. They are more likely to develop toxicity from prolonged exposure to a contaminated environment or by ingesting toxic amounts of insecticides through grooming.
CLINICAL SIGNS	**Onset:** Signs can occur within minutes to hours of exposure but can also be delayed for up to 5 days (delayed onset occurs primarily in cats and most commonly with chlorpyrifos, aka Dursban®). Oral exposure may lead to a more rapid onset of signs. Clinical signs can last from several days up to a month (the longer duration is due to the lipophilic nature of some OPs). **Signs** of OP and carbamate toxicosis are due to overstimulation of the parasympathetic nervous system. Signs can be divided into three groups: **muscarinic** (GI, respiratory, and urinary = SLUD), **nicotinic** (muscle), and CNS. This distinction is important in the treatment plan. **Early signs** are usually due to the muscarinic effects. • **Gastrointestinal effects:** vomiting, diarrhea, salivation, GI pain • **Respiratory effects:** bronchial constriction and secretions causing tachypnea and dyspnea. • **Urinary effects:** incontinence, frequent urination • **Cardiac effects:** bradycardia (sometimes see tachycardia instead - sympathetic) • **Ocular effects:** Either miosis or mydriasis can occur. **Nicotinic signs** may soon follow: muscle twitching, muscle stiffness, weakness, paresis, paralysis. **CNS signs:** anxiety, disorientation, hyperactivity, seizure, mental depression, coma, depression of vital centers. Cats with chlorpyrifos toxicosis may suffer from anorexia and behavior changes following an acute exposure. **Death is usually due to respiratory failure** attributed to the muscarinic effects (increased secretions and bronchiolar constriction), nicotinic effects (paralysis of the diaphragm and intercostal muscles), or CNS effects (inhibition of the medullary respiratory drive), or to a combination of the three. **Delayed neuropathy** (axonal degeneration) is rare but occurs with some OP exposure (e.g., triorthocresyl, triorthotoyl, tricresyl phosphate). Onset occurs 7-21 days post-exposure. It's characterized by hindlimb weakness, ataxia, CP deficits, and hindlimb paralysis, which may progress to the forelimbs.

ORGANOPHOSPHATES and CARBAMATES (continued)

MECHANISM of ACTION	Organophosphates and carbamates are **anticholinesterase** insecticides; they work by **inhibiting acetylcholinesterase (AChE)**, an enzyme responsible for breaking down **acetylcholine (ACh)** at cholinergic nerve endings. By breaking down ACh, **acetylcholinesterase** prevents overstimulation of the post-synaptic membrane or effector organ. Consequently, AChE inhibitors cause overstimulation of the post-synaptic membrane or effector organ. OPs and carbamates inhibit ChE by **reversibly** phosphorylating or carbamylating the active site of the enzyme. OPs have a higher binding affinity for the ChE enzyme than do carbamates. Thus, animals are more likely to show clinical toxicity with OPs than with carbamates, and the clinical effects of OP toxicity last much longer than those seen with carbamates. Some OPs undergo an aging change that causes them to become **irreversible** enzyme inhibitors. This makes early treatment (within a few hours) especially crucial.
DIAGNOSIS	History and clinical signs are important. **Measuring cholinesterase activity** in the brain and blood (whole blood or serum): The activity is reduced in affected animals (50-75% reduction suggests ChE toxicity). With dogs, use whole blood if possible because the RBC AChE is more likely to be depressed after a clinically significant exposure, whereas any exposure can depress the serum AChE regardless of the clinical significance. RBC AChE is not a significant factor for cats, so either sample is acceptable. Cats are very sensitive to ChE inhibitors, and clinically normal cats may have low ChE activity. Low ChE activity in cats indicates exposure to ChE inhibitors but must correlate with the clinical signs for diagnosis of OP or carbamate toxicity. Brain (cerebrum) ChE activity is more diagnostic but can only be performed post-mortem. ChE activity should not be used as a prognosticator since cats with very low ChE activity can still recover from the toxicity. **Chemical analysis** for poisons in the ingesta or from the suspected source. **Response to low dose atropine administration:** Administer 0.02 mg/kg atropine IV. If the muscarinic effects (watch for tachycardia, mydriasis) aren't controlled, the signs may be due to toxicity. **Response to treatment** **Rule out** other causes of the signs.
TREATMENT	**Support vital functions:** temperature, respiration, electrolytes. **Control seizures** with valium (2.5-5 mg/kg IV as needed) or phenobarbital (6 mg/kg IV as needed). **Remove the poison:** Activated charcoal may even benefit clinically affected cats several days post-exposure to chlorpyrifos. Bathe in mild detergent. **Administer atropine and 2-PAM:** • **Atropine** (0.2 - 0.4 mg/kg, give 1/4 IV and 3/4 SQ or IM): Atropine is a parasympatholytic agent, so it counteracts the muscarinic (SLUD) effects of OP toxicity. It doesn't alleviate the nicotinic effects, though (e.g., muscle weakness). To avoid over-atropinization, redose only as needed to control the respiratory and cardiac effects of toxicity (e.g., dyspnea due to bronchiolar constriction and secretions, bradycardia). Use the lowest dose that will control clinical signs. Signs of over-atropinization include intestinal stasis, tachycardia, and hyperthermia. Do not substitute glycopyrrolate for atropine since glycopyrrolate does not get into the CNS; thus, it cannot block the central effects of excessive ACh. • **2-PAM chloride** (Protopam Chloride, pralidoxime chloride: Wyeth-Ayerst Lab, Philadelphia) acts competitively to break down the phosphorylated enzyme complex, freeing AChE and at the same time tying up the OP, making it available for hydrolysis and excretion. 2-PAM alleviates the **nicotinic** as well as **muscarinic** signs of ChE toxicity. Use it for 24-36 hours (20 mg/kg every 12 hours IM or IV initially and then IM or SC). If there's no improvement, discontinue use. If there's improvement, continue use until the patient becomes asymptomatic. 2-PAM is used primarily for OP poisoning. • **Use 2-PAM and atropine together** with OP toxicity, particularly early in therapy. • **Diphenhydramine** (2-4 mg/kg PO or IM every 8-12 hours) may help control muscle weakness (nicotinic signs).
PROGNOSIS	The prognosis is good in cases of early, aggressive therapy. Even with delayed therapy, many recover. Full recovery may take 2-4 weeks.

Toxicology

II. **PYRETHRINS and PYRETHROIDS:** Pyrethrins are found in flowers of plants belonging to the *Chrysanthemum* genus. Pyrethroids are synthetic pyrethrins. They are more stable and more potent than naturally occurring pyrethrins.

RECOGNIZING the INSECTICIDE NAMES	Names usually contain -thrin, –chrysanthemate, or -cyclopropaneate (e.g., **phenothrin**) or end in **-benzeacetate** (as with fenvalerate). Several compounds for use in cats have been marketed as non-pyrethrins when they are pyrethrins. Two such compounds are **phenothrin** (which the EPA has linked to toxicities in young cats) and **etofenprox** (a non-ester pyrethrin).
COMMON SOURCES of EXPOSURE	Pyrethrins and pyrethroids are found in many house and garden insecticides as well as in agricultural insecticides. Toxicity occurs primarily in **cats.** In general, pyrethrin-containing dips and sprays that are labeled for use in cats are safe to use at the labeled recommendations. Problems occur when products are used improperly (e.g., sprays for dogs are used on cats, products are not diluted correctly, products are used too copiously). Some products for dogs contain 45-65% permethrin. When pyrethrin products (including spot-ons) are placed on dogs, the dog must be kept separated from the cat for several days. Some individual cats may be more sensitive to pyrethrins, including phenothrin and etofenprox. Many pyrethrin-containing insecticides contain **synergists** that increase the toxicity and effectiveness of the product by inhibiting liver cytochrome P_{450}. Examples of such synergists include piperonyl butoxide (PBO), N-octyl-bicycloheptene dicarboximide (MGK 264), and 5KF525A.
MECHANISM of ACTION	Pyrethrins affect the voltage-dependent sodium channels in nerves, leading to either repetitive discharge or membrane depolarization. Some pyrethrins also work by blocking the GABA receptor. GABA receptors operate chloride ion channels and are the major inhibitory receptor in the nervous system. By blocking this receptor, pyrethrins cause hyperexcitability of nervous tissue.
CLINICAL SIGNS	Onset: usually within several hours of exposure Duration: 24-72 hours Clinical signs are similar to those seen with OP and carbamate toxicity. • **CNS:** hyperexcitability, ataxia, tremors, seizure • **Muscle:** muscle fasciculation, muscle weakness • **Hyperthermia:** especially in young animals • **Respiratory:** respiratory distress, possibly due to weakness of the respiratory musculature • **Other:** vomiting, diarrhea, anorexia, salivation, cardiovascular distress
DIAGNOSIS	History and clinical signs There are no specific tests for diagnosing pyrethrin toxicity and no specific findings on necropsy. Some diagnostic toxicology labs can confirm exposure. Determining cholinesterase activity is helpful in differentiating between OP/carbamate toxicity and pyrethrin toxicity.
TREATMENT	Treatment is primarily **symptomatic** and **supportive** since no specific antidotes exist. Control **seizures** and muscle **fasciculations** with one of the following: • Methocarbamol (Robaxin®): (50-150 mg/kg IV slowly to effect; no more than 330 mg/kg/24 hours). Start with 50-75 mg/kg or, if actively seizuring, use 150-200 mg/kg. If seizures are not controlled, use barbiturates (pentobarbital: 4-20 mg/kg IV; they do slow metabolism of pyrethrins). Diazepam doesn't control the tremors well, but once treated with methocarbamol, it can help alleviate signs of hyperesthesia (diazepam: 0.2-2 mg/kg IV). Remove the toxic compound by inducing emesis early on and administering activated charcoal. Remove product from skin by bathing. Monitor temperature and electrolytes. Keep the animal warm. Atropine can be used to control salivation and pulmonary secretions, but it hasn't been shown to increase survival rates.

RODENTICIDES and MOLLUSCICIDES
Rodenticides That Cause Coagulopathies (Coumarin Rodenticides)
Vitamin D Rodenticides (Cholecalciferol)
Zinc Phosphide
Rodenticides/Molluscicides That Cause CNS Signs (Strychnine, Bromethalin, Metaldehyde)

I. COUMARIN RODENTICIDES CAUSE COAGULOPATHIES

RECOGNIZING the RODENTICIDE NAMES	First generation • Coumarin compounds (short-acting): warfarin • Indandione compounds (long-acting): diphacinone **Second generation** coumarin rodenticides were developed because some rodents developed a tolerance to warfarin. They include: bromadiolone, brodifacoum, chlorphacinone, diphacinone, difelthialone.
MECHANISM of ACTION	These compounds inhibit the vitamin K-dependent coagulation factors by blocking conversion of vitamin K to its active form. The vitamin K-dependent factors are II, VII, IX, and X. Signs of coagulopathy don't occur until the level of coagulation factors has significantly dropped. The rate at which this occurs depends partly on the half-life of the coagulation factors. It takes 5-7 half-lives before a compound is essentially gone. The coagulant factor VII has the shortest half-life (5-6 hours) of the affected coagulation factors. So you generally don't see signs of anticoagulant poisoning for 3-7 days. Factor IX has a half-life of 13 hours, so you don't see signs due to factor IX synthesis inhibition for 3-5 days.
CLINICAL SIGNS	GI signs: Vomiting and lethargy can occur on the day of ingestion. Signs of coagulopathy occur 3-7 days following exposure to a toxic dose. The clinical effects last 4-7 days with warfarin and 2-4 weeks with diphacinone. Signs are caused by hemorrhage and vary depending upon the location of the hemorrhage. • Lethargy, painful abdomen, and fever may be present. Animals may be found dead or depressed and cold to the touch. • Physical evidence of anemia and bleeding include bruises, pale mucous membranes, etc.
DIAGNOSIS	• History of toxic ingestion and clinical signs • PIVKA (Thrombotest®) is prolonged. This is the most sensitive test for determining deficiency of the vitamin K-dependent coagulation factors. • Prothrombin time (PT): factor II, VII (shortest half-life), X • Activated partial thromboplastin time (APTT): II, IX, X • Activated coagulation time (ACT) • Response to therapy • Some diagnostic labs can evaluate blood and liver samples for anticoagulants (3-5 mL of blood or serum needed).
TREATMENT	Treat with vitamin K_1 (expensive). Avoid vitamin K_3 as it can cause severe methemoglobinemia and Heinz body anemia. Always retest the clotting parameters 48-72 hours after discontinuing therapy. Give a 5 mg/kg loading dose of vitamin K_1 (phytonadione; Aquamephyton®) in multiple sites SC. If the animal is hypotensive, then SC absorption will be slow. In this case IV administration is an option, although there's a risk of anaphylaxis. Diluting the drug in fluids and pre-treating with antihistamines are good precautions. After the first 24 hours, give 2.5 mg/kg vitamin K_1 orally (Maphytone®, 5 mg tablets) BID with canned food (e.g., a high fat meal). • For warfarin, the vitamin K_1 maintenance dose range is 1.25-2.5 mg/kg. One week of treatment is sufficient, but retest the clotting parameters 48-72 hours after last treatment. • For diphacinone and 2nd generation anticoagulants, the vitamin K_1 dose range is 2.5-5.0 mg/kg. Continue treatment for 2-4 weeks and then retest 48-72 hours after the last dose. • Unknown anticoagulant: You can either treat conservatively as for warfarin and then check to see if this was long enough, or you can treat as for longer-acting anticoagulants and retest upon discontinuing the therapy.

Toxicology

COUMARIN RODENTICIDES (continued)

OTHER TREATMENT CONSIDER-ATIONS	• Dogs presenting as severely depressed and anemic with declining PCV should receive **fresh** or **frozen plasma** IV (50-100 mL) immediately upon presentation (and possibly again in 4 hours) plus vitamin K₁. This will provide needed **clotting factors** to stop localized areas of bleeding. By the time these factors are utilized, the coagulation proteins induced by vitamin K are being produced. • For dogs that present with severe depression, anemia, and marked respiratory distress, distinguish whether **pulmonary, pleural,** or **pericardial hemorrhage** is present and then treat appropriately (surgical intervention to drain the pericardium, thoracocentesis, etc.). If the respiratory dyspnea is due to severe anemia, then whole blood transfusion is necessary (20 mL/kg). • If a poor clinical response to vitamin K₁ is observed (evident within 12-24 hours), perform a platelet count to evaluate the possibility of **secondary platelet involvement** such as DIC, **immune-mediated phenomenon,** or a misdiagnosis with a primary platelet problem or DIC as the root cause.

II. CHOLECALCIFEROL (A vitamin D rodenticide)

MECHANISM of ACTION	Cholecalciferol, vitamin D3, enhances calcium absorption from the bone and kidney leading to thinning of the bones, pathologic calcification, and consequential death in rodents in 4-6 days.
SOURCE	**Brand names:** Quintox®, Rampage®, and Mouse-Be-Gone® (although some of the products are now bromethalin—so check the label)
CLINICAL SIGNS	One or more days following ingestion you'll see depression, anorexia, PU/PD. If the client does not detect these signs, the dog may be found dead with no apparent cause. Signs are those associated with uremia or heart failure. The course of poisoning lasts 2-3 weeks.
DIAGNOSIS	**Hypercalcemia** (13-16 mg/dL or greater): If the animal is treated for initial ingestion of bait, take a pre-serum sample for comparison. Then recheck the calcium every 24 hours for 3-5 days. If the calcium is elevated, then initiate therapy. Serum calcium can be elevated within 24 hours following exposure. **Serum phosphorus** is generally elevated and often rises slightly before serum calcium. **Bradycardia** and shortening of the Q-T interval can occur with hypercalcemia. • **BUN** and **creatinine** may be elevated if renal damage is present due to the hypercalcemia. • Some laboratories can measure cholecalciferol.
TREATMENT	• **Fluids and diuresis** will help decrease serum calcium levels. • **Prednisolone:** High doses (2-3 mg/kg) can decrease Ca²⁺ levels. • If **calcitonin** can be obtained from a human pharmacy, administer it at 10 units/kg. It has an **antidotal** benefit in reducing the serum Ca²⁺ concentrations. Use salmon calcitonin since it has been shown to be effective in various animal species. Some animals will become refractory to calcitonin. • **Pamidronate** (Aredia®) can be used **instead** of salmon calcitonin. (1.3-2.0 mg/kg slow IV over 2 hrs). It inhibits osteoclastic bone resorption and generally lowers calcium levels to normal within 48 hours. Repeat in 5-7 days if needed. • If the animal shows cardiac effects (bradycardia with heart block) due to extremely high serum calcium levels (e.g., 20 mg/dL), use **sodium EDTA** (25-75 mg/hr IV infusion) and monitor cardiac rhythm with ECG. Once the animal is stabilized, it can be sent home on prednisone and furosemide, and it should be rechecked in 2 weeks.

III. ZINC PHOSPHIDE

CLINICAL SIGNS	Acute respiratory distress, hemorrhage, seizures. Onset is from < 1 to several hours. Death can occur in as little as 3 hours post-ingestion. 1 tbsp is toxic to a 10 kg dog. Damage is due to oxidative damage to cells.
DIAGNOSIS	Send frozen stomach contents, liver, and kidney samples to diagnostic labs that test for phosphine.
TREATMENT	**Treatment:** aggressive decontamination and support. Phosphine gas produced is toxic to veterinary personnel. Insure adequate ventilation and minimize exposure to fumes from vomitus.

IV. RODENTICIDES and MOLLUSCICIDES CAUSING CNS SIGNS

	CLINICAL SIGNS	MECHANISM of ACTION	DIAGNOSIS	THERAPY
Strychnine	Initial uneasiness and stiffness (sawhorse stance) Cyclic repetitive tetanic spasms and seizures that are induced by noise Death results from exhaustion and asphyxiation. Death can occur within 15 minutes to 2 hours or longer after ingestion.	Interferes with neurotransmitters of Renshaw cells, resulting in obliteration of inhibitory reflexes on incoming impulses (glycine)	History of using rodenticide baits in the area (Often baits contain dye.) **Clinical signs:** stimulus-induced tetanic spasms Look at **stomach contents:** These animals usually don't vomit; thus, we find a full stomach with strychnine in it. The contents are often green or other colors due to dye in the bait. Some labs can test for strychnine in stomach contents or liver tissue.	There's no specific antidote. Remove the poison with gastric lavage. Give activated charcoal before signs appear. Acidify the urine if the patient is not already acidotic, and support renal function. Control seizures and acid-base abnormalities. Metaldehyde may be helpful in managing tremors, convulsions. **Keep the animal in a quiet location.** **Prognosis:** If caught early, the animal is likely to respond well to therapy. The animal should respond in 12-24 hours.
Metaldehyde Some molluscicides contain carbamates, too, which may make clinical signs more complicated.	Signs occur within 0.5-1 hour. Incoordination, anxiety. Muscle fasciculations contribute to severe hyperthermia (up to 110°F). Continuous muscle tremors lead to convulsions. The dog may become comatose. Profuse salivation, the eyes are unresponsive or dilated (whereas organophosphates = miosis). Death may occur as soon as 2-12 hours (respiratory collapse).	Metaldehyde blocks the inhibitory GABA neurotransmitters (1/3 of the neurotransmitters in the brain are GABA receptors).	History of eating snail bait **Clinical signs: shake and bake syndrome.** These seizures are not induced by sound as are strychnine seizures. Some **diagnostic labs** can analyze stomach contents, serum, urine, and liver for metaldehyde.	Treatment is similar to treatment for strychnine poisoning (Refer to strychnine treatment). Decontaminate with gastric lavage and activated charcoal before clinical signs appear. Then provide supportive care. Prognosis is good for those that survive the first 24 hours and that are treated early. Those that have not received a lethal dose may fully recover in several days to several weeks.
Bromethalin Assault®, Trounce®, Vengeance®	**Peracute** with high doses. Animals exhibit neurologic signs that resemble those seen with compound 1080. **Subacute:** Associated with low ingestion. Vomiting, depression, paralysis, terminal seizures. These signs may have a delayed onset (several days).	Causes uncoupling of oxidative phosphorylation (affects the Na/K pump in nervous tissue), results in increased CSF pressure and intramyelinic edema.	History, clinical signs **CSF pressure** is increased. EEG abnormalities persist if the animal recovers clinically. Diffuse vacuolization of myelin sheaths are seen on histology.	Supportive Often doesn't respond to steroids or mannitol, but it's acceptable to try steroids anyway. Administer activated charcoal (0.5 g/kg) every 4 hours for 3-5 days. Prognosis is poor if severe CNS signs have developed.

Toxicology

METAL TOXICOSIS

METAL	SOURCE	CLINICAL SIGNS	DIAGNOSIS	TREATMENT
Lead toxicity	Auto parts, paint, fishing sinkers, linoleum, some pottery glazes, weights (e.g., curtain weights), stained glass	**CNS:** seizures (petit or grand mal), personality changes **GI:** vomiting, diarrhea, anorexia	**Clinical signs/history** Anemia (microcytic, hypochromic) due to inhibition of hemoglobin production **Basophilic stippling:** Lead blocks an enzyme that metabolizes pyrimidines, thus pyrimidines accumulate causing the stippling. **Whole blood lead levels:** This is the best test for indicating exposure. Radiographs may reveal evidence of a metal foreign object or visualization of lead lines (at the metaphysis of the metacarpals, etc.).	Remove the source prior to chelation. **Chelation with one of the following:** **Calcium EDTA** binds lead so that the lead is excreted in the urine. Use it 5 days in a row then 2 days off. If still needed, use it 5 days again; otherwise you risk renal damage. **Penicillamine** (12.5 mg/kg QID orally) and **British anti-lewisite** are almost obsolete. **Succimer** has fewer side effects than EDTA; however, it is more expensive and may be more difficult to obtain. Give 10 mg/kg PO TID for 10-17 days. **Magnesium sulfate and sodium sulfate** PO (e.g., milk of magnesia) bind lead in the gut.
Iron toxicity	Iron tablets (Geritol®) and iron-coated pills taste sweet.	GI signs (vomiting, diarrhea) can occur within 30 minutes of ingestion. Hepatic necrosis CNS depression Cardiovascular collapse Hypotension/shock	Serum iron levels or total iron binding capacity (TIBC) Normal serum iron: 0-100 µg/dL Iron toxicity: > 350 µg/dL or when TIBC is > 80% of serum iron	Remove the source prior to chelation. **Chelation:** **Deferoxamine** (Desferal®) IM at 40 mg/kg every 4-8 hours or IV as a CRI at 15 mg/kg/hour Fluids and supportive treatment
Zinc toxicity	Pennies made after 1983, galvanized metal (e.g., some cage nuts and bolts), diaper rash ointments containing zinc oxide	Icterus AIHA signs Lethargy Pancreatitis signs	History of exposure Clinical signs Submit serum or RBCs for zinc analysis. Don't use a rubber-stoppered tube because the stopper contains zinc. Use a trace mineral tube.	Remove the zinc source once the animal is stabilized. Zinc levels rapidly decline following removal of source. Calcium EDTA is the suggested chelating agent, but it does not work particularly well. Intravenous fluids to minimize risk of renal injury secondary to hemoglobinuria

CHAPTER 21: Urinary

Urinary

URINARY TRACT INFECTIONS (UTI)
Consequences
Simple vs. Uncomplicated
Diagnosis
Principles of Treatment
Treatment of Uncomplicated UTIs
Treatment Failure
Treatment of Complicated UTIs
Treatment of Mixed Infections

Up to 17% of all dogs admitted to veterinary hospitals for any reason have urinary tract infections. UTIs are much more common in female dogs than male dogs. While some animals present with clinical signs such as pollakiuria, fever, lethargy, hematuria, or visibly abnormal urine, many patients with UTIs exhibit no signs. This makes it especially important to rely on laboratory tests for diagnosing UTIs rather than relying on clinical signs alone. UTIs are usually caused by intestinal bacteria that ascend the urethra into the bladder. Most infections involve only one bacterial species, but 20% of UTIs are mixed bacterial infections. Urinary tract infections are **not common in cats** (< 1 % of cats presenting to veterinary hospitals). They are more common in older cats, especially those with chronic renal failure.

A. **POSSIBLE SEQUELAE OF UTIs**: Whether or not an animal with a UTI has clinical signs, the UTI should be treated. Lack of treatment can result in serious consequences which include:
1. Pyelonephritis
2. Prostatitis
3. Urinary calculi
4. **Septicemia**: Animals with UTIs can develop septicemia, especially if they are treated with high doses of immunosuppressive agents (corticosteroids, antineoplastic drugs). As a result, it is important to rule out UTIs before putting an animal on these drugs, and to monitor for UTIs during therapy.
5. **Discospondylitis** occasionally develops secondary to a UTI.
6 UTIs can cause infection of the spermatic cords and testicles and can cause infertility in both sexes.

B. **UNCOMPLICATED UTIs vs. COMPLICATED UTIs**:
1. **UNCOMPLICATED UTIs** have no underlying cause for infection (i.e. no structural or functional abnormalities of the urinary tract, no immunosuppression, etc). These cases are easy to treat.
2. **COMPLICATED UTIs** involve an underlying etiology. Such cases are more difficult to treat. The infection is often persistent or recurring. Examples of underlying etiologies include:
   a. Urolithiasis or another nidus of infection (e.g. prostate, renal)
   b. Neurogenic disorders of micturition (e.g. leading to increased residual urine volume in the bladder, decreased voiding, etc.)
   c. Decreased immunity
   d. Neoplasia
   e. Increased urine pH
   f. Anatomical defects (e.g. patent urachus, vestibulovaginal stricture, etc.)

C. **DIAGNOSIS**: Urinary tract infections are definitively diagnosed by **urinalysis and/or culture** performed on samples collected and processed using sterile technique. Cystocentesis provides the best sterility. A **culture** should be performed in order to identify the pathogenic organism(s) and pick the appropriate antibiotic.

1. **Sterile collection and handling of the sample**: Collect the urine via cystocentesis because other methods of collection are not sterile. (With catheterization, the catheter travels through the distal urethra, picking up bacteria which contaminate the sample and can produce an iatrogenic UTI. Voided urine samples flow past the distal urethra and become contaminated with bacteria from the distal urethra). Once you collect the sample, evaluate it within fifteen minutes or refrigerate it (bacteria can double in number every 30 minutes). Samples to be cultured should not be refrigerated for more than 12-24 hours because extensive refrigeration can kill the bacteria, resulting in false negative culture results.

2. **Components of the urinalysis**: Evaluate the sediment for crystals, cells, and bacteria (gram stain). Also measure protein, glucose, ketones, bilirubin, and specific gravity.

21.2

3. **When to culture:** Culture the urine if the urine fits any **one** of the three boxed criteria below, or if the animal is known to be immunosuppressed, has concurrent disease (e.g. hyperadrenocorticism, diabetes, pyelonephritis, etc.), or if it has chronically dilute urine (e.g. renal failure).

CULTURE the URINE IF:

• Bacteria are seen
• > 3 WBC/hpf
• Specific Gravity < 1.015

Evaluate the WBC count and urine specific gravity to help determine whether the urine should be cultured or not. Bacteria are not always visible on microscopic evaluation of infected urine. Urine must contain $\geq$ 10,000 rod-shaped bacteria/mL or $\geq$ 100,000 cocci/mL in order for the bacteria to be visualized.

4. **If the urine was collected via free catch or catheterization,** the presence of a single bacterial population (rather than a mixed population) indicates infection. Additionally, if quantification is performed, > 10,000 bacteria/mL from a catheterized sample and > 100,000 bacteria/mL from voided sample indicate a bacterial infection rather than sample contamination.

MICROBIOLOGY RESULTS from COMMON UTI BACTERIA			
ORGANISM	**GRAM STAIN**	**BLOOD AGAR**	**MacCONKEY**
Staphylococcus	Positive cocci	Bright white, opaque, small colonies; often hemolytic $\pm$ double zone of hemolysis on cow blood (green zone)	No growth
Streptococcus	Positive cocci	Tiny pinpoint colonies; partial hemolysis (green zone)	No growth
Proteus mirabilis	Negative rod	Usually swarms (i.e. doesn't form discrete colonies)	Colorless (Lac negative)
Pseudomonas	Negative rod	Gray or greenish colonies; fruity or ammonia odor; often hemolytic	Colorless (Lac negative)
E. coli	Negative rod	Smooth, gray, opaque, colonies; may be hemolytic	Pink colonies (Lac positive)
Klebsiella	Negative rod	Mucoid, grayish, white colonies	Pink, often slimy colonies (Lac positive)
Enterobacter	Negative rod	Smooth, gray colonies	Pink colonies (Lac positive)

E. coli is the most common cause of UTIs in dogs followed by *Proteus, Staphylococcus, Streptococcus,* and *Klebsiella. Enterobacter* and *Pseudomonas* infections are less common.

D. **PRINCIPLES OF TREATMENT**
   1. Bacterial UTIs are most commonly caused by one of seven bacteria. Ideally, a culture and sensitivity should be performed on all urine samples to determine the most effective antibiotic therapy. If you are unable to perform a sensitivity, you can still make an educated guess as to which antibiotic to use.

BACTERIA	ANTIMICROBIAL AGENTS
Escherichia coli	**Trimethoprim/sulfa** (TMS), Cephalosporins, Gentamicin, Enrofloxacin, Clavamox
Proteus mirabilis	**Penicillin** (ampicillin or amoxicillin), TMS, Cephalosporins, Gentamicin, Enrofloxacin, Clavamox
Staphylococcus	**Penicillin** (ampicillin or amoxicillin), Cephalosporins, TMS, Chloramphenicol, Gentamicin, Clavamox
Streptococcus	**Penicillin** (ampicillin or amoxicillin), TMS, Gentamicin, Clavamox
Pseudomonas	**Tetracycline**, Gentamicin
Klebsiella	**Cephalosporin** (cephalexin or cefadroxil), Gentamicin, Clavamox
Enterobacter	**Trimethoprim/sulfa** (TMS), Clavamox

* Trimethoprim/sulfa (TMS) + Cephalosporin = cephalexin or cefadroxil

Urinary

    a. **Ampicillin** is about 100% effective. Clavamox, trimethoprim/sulfa, or enrofloxacin will treat about 80% of UTIs.

    b. **Amoxicillin/Clavulanic acid** is effective against all of these bacteria except *Pseudomonas*.

    c. **Enrofloxacin** (and possibly ciprofloxacin and other fluoroquinolones) is bactericidal and has a wide margin of safety. Considered a "big gun" antibiotic, it is generally effective against bacteria that are resistant to other drugs. As a result, try to reserve it for the difficult cases rather than using it as a first choice.

    d. **Gentamicin** (an aminoglycoside) can only be given parenterally. Because aminoglycosides can be nephrotoxic, use them with caution.

If you are unable to perform a culture, you can base your treatment on gram staining characteristics.

GRAM-STAIN CHARACTERISTICS	ANTIMICROBIAL AGENTS
Gram positive cocci	Penicillin (ampicillin or amoxicillin)
Gram negative rods	Trimethoprim/sulfa*, Clavamox, or enrofloxacin**

*Avoid Trimethoprim/sulfa in Dobermans (and possibly Rottweilers) due to suspected breed hypersensitivity.

**Enrofloxacin is expensive but often effective against bacteria that are resistant to other drugs. Try to reserve enrofloxacin (Baytril®) for difficult cases.

2. **MIC:** Most antibiotics used in treating UTIs are rapidly excreted into the urine resulting in high urinary concentration of the antibiotic compared to blood concentration of the antibiotic. Due to the high urinary concentration, you can use antibiotics that would normally be ineffective against the pathogenic bacteria. An antibiotic is likely to be effective in combating a UTI if it reaches a concentration in the urine that is $\geq$ 4x the MIC for that specific pathogen. Note that some labs report MICs based on anticipated serum antibiotic concentrations rather than urine antibiotic concentrations, thus many antibiotics that would be effective are reported as ineffective. Also, with pyelonephritis and thickened bladder walls, the antibiotics may not reach expected urine concentrations within the affected tissues.

COMMON ANTIMICROBIAL DOSAGES

Antimicrobial	Daily Dose	Mean urine concentration + SD
Penicillin G	40,000 U/kg TID	294 ± 211 U/mL
Ampicillin	25 mg/kg TID	309 ± 55 µg/mL
Amoxicillin	11 mg/kg TID	202 ± 93 µg/mL
Amoxicillin/clavulanic acid*	11 mg/kg TID	202 ± 93 µg/mL
Tetracycline	20 mg/kg TID	138 ± 65 µg/mL
Chloramphenicol	33 mg/kg TID	124 ± 40 µg/mL
Cephalexin	5 mg/kg TID	805 ± 421 µg/mL
Cefadroxil	5 mg/kg TID	800 ± --- µg/mL
Trimethoprim/sulfa**	2.2 mg/kg BID	55 ± 19 µg/mL
Enrofloxacin	2.5 mg/kg BID	43 ± 12 µg/mL
Gentamicin***	2.2 mg/kg TID	107 ± 33 µg/mL
Amikacin***	2.2 mg/kg TID	100 ± --- µg/mL

* Based on the amoxicillin fraction. ** Based on the trimethoprim fraction. ***All of the dosages in this table are for oral administration except for gentamicin and amikacin which are given parenterally (subcutaneously).

3. In order to get the best effect, the owner should try to prevent the animal from urinating until just before it's about to receive its next antibiotic dose. Many owners elect to give the antibiotic at bedtime after the animal has gone outside to urinate.

4. **Duration of treatment:** Treat long enough to eradicate the bacteria from the urine and to prevent re-infection until the normal urinary tract defenses have recovered enough to protect the urinary tract.

    a. With uncomplicated UTIs, 14 days is usually adequate.

    b. With chronic infections where tissue damage may be severe, you may need to treat for extended periods.

    c. Male dogs with urinary tract infections should be treated as complicated cases (treat for at least 3 weeks).

    d. Intact male dogs should be treated for prolonged periods (at least 4 weeks) in order to prevent the high probability of prostatic colonization. It is advisable to use antibiotics that penetrate the prostate.

    e. Animals with suspected pyelonephritis should be treated for at least 4-8 weeks. Chronic or complicated cases of pyelonephritis must be treated for longer periods than acute pyelonephritis.

E. MANAGING UTIs

STEPS for MANAGING UTIs

1. **Diagnose UTI via urinalysis** (gram stain of the urine sediment and ideally a culture and sensitivity). Cystocentesis is the most sterile collection method.

2. **Select an appropriate antibiotic** (based on culture results) and place the animal on medication for 14 days. If the UTI is chronic or is in a male dog, especially an intact male dog, you will have to treat for more than 14 days.
   a. Neutered male dogs should be treated for a minimum of 3 weeks.
   b. Intact males dogs should be treated for a minimum of one month (possibly using antibiotics that penetrate the prostate).
   c. Animals in which pylonephritis is suspected should be treated for at least 4-8 weeks (chronic pyeloephritis and complicted cases of pyelonoephritis must be treated for longer periods than acute pyelonephritis).

3. Because some animals with UTIs have no clinical signs, do not rely on clinical signs alone to determine whether the antibiotic is working effectively. **Reculture the urine in 3-7** days to see if the antibiotic is working well. If it is, continue therapy as planned. If it isn't, repeat the urinalysis, culture, and sensitivity and change to the appropriate antibiotic. Keep the patient on the new antibiotic for 14 days (more in chronic cases, etc.) and repeat the urinalysis again in 3-7 days.

4. **Recheck/reculture the urine 5-7 days** after treatment is finished to see if the infection is recurrent or persistent.

F. TREATMENT FAILURE:

1. In cases of treatment failure, consider the following:
   a. **If the recurrent infection is caused by the same bacteria (a relapse)**, consider the following:
      i. **Antibiotic-related reasons:** Inappropriate antibiotic choice, inappropriate duration of treatment, the bacteria have developed resistance, the owner is not administering the medication, the animal has GI disease preventing adequate absorption.
      ii. **Nidus of infection** (e.g. kidney, prostate, uroliths)
      iii. Underlying **immune** problem
      iv. **Iatrogenic** (catheterization)

   b. **If the recurrent infection is due to a different bacteria**, consider:
      i. Underlying immune problems or predisposing conditions such as hyperadrenocorticism, a neurologic deficit of the urinary tract, anatomic abnormality, neoplasia, etc.
      ii. Iatrogenic (catheterization)

2. **Work-up recurrent infections** in which the etiology is not related to antibiotic choice, duration, etc.
   a. **Drug history:** Has the pet been on chronic steroids of any kind (e.g. shampoo, creams, ear or eye meds, etc.)?
   b. **Hemogram/Chemistry panel:** Rule out systemic diseases such as Cushing's disease or pyelonephritis.
   c. **Radiographs:** Check for uroliths, neoplasia, etc.
   d. **Ultrasound, excretory urogram, double contrast cystogram:** These tests can reveal anatomic abnormalities, neoplasia, uroliths, prostatic cysts or

Urinary

hyperplasia, and possibly pyelonephritis. Pyelonephritis is usually difficult to diagnose and is often diagnosed by ruling out other causes of UTI. Indicators of pyelonephritis include fever and leukocytosis. Positive culture from a renal aspirate provides a diagnosis of pyelonephritis.

3. Once the underlying problem is found, try to correct it.

G. **MANAGING COMPLICATED UTIs (PERSISTENT OR RECURRENT UTIs):**

1. Treat with appropriate antibiotics for 4-6 weeks and provide careful follow-up. Remember to use antibiotics that are safe for long-term use (e.g. Trimethoprim/sulfa can cause KCS when used over prolonged periods).

2. If the animal gets **frequent infections that can't be cured** (they recur after the animal is taken off antibiotics and you can't find or correct the underlying cause), you may need to keep the animal on antibiotics for extended periods of time (possibly for the rest of its life). Some owners elect just to treat the frequent, individual UTIs rather than keeping the animal on antibiotics long-term.

LONG-TERM TREATMENT of PERSISTENT/RECURRENT UTIs

- First control the infection.
- Keep the animal on 1/3 the dosage of the effective antibiotic once a day for 6 months (at night after the pet voids). Perform a monthly urine culture.
- If the animal gets a UTI while on the low-dose antibiotics, perform a culture and sensitivity and treat appropriately. Once this infection is controlled, decrease the antibiotic to 1/3 the dose and proceed as previously described.
- If the animal is bacteria-free for 6 months, you may discontinue antibiotic therapy, but continue to perform urine cultures once a month for three months to rule out recurrence.

H. **TREATING MIXED INFECTIONS:** Up to 20% of UTIs in dogs involve mixed bacterial infections.

PRINCIPLES of TREATING MIXED INFECTIONS

- Try to use just one antibiotic unless you are sure that two different antibiotics are needed. Check for drug interactions (i.e. they may inactivate each other).

- Ideally, use an antibiotic that will work against both/all of the infectious agents. For example, if the infection involves *Proteus* and *Staphylococcus,* you can treat with amoxicillin.

- If you can't effectively treat both bacteria with one drug, treat one bacteria and then treat for the other bacteria. For example, if you have an infection with *E. coli* and *Pseudomonas,* treat the *E. coli* first with trimethoprim/sulfa. Once you have eradicated *E. coli,* treat the *Pseudomonas* infection with tetracycline. UTIs with *Pseudomonas* are usually fairly easy to treat.

PROSTATIC DISEASES

A number of diseases can affect the prostate. The most common include benign hyperplasia, acute bacterial prostatitis, chronic bacterial prostatitis ± prostatic abscess, and neoplasia.

PROSTATIC DISEASES	• **Benign prostatic hyperplasia:** Normally, the prostate of an intact male dog undergoes continuous hyperplasia as the dog ages. This predisposes the dog to developing bacterial prostatitis. • **Acute bacterial prostatitis** is typically painful and is characterized by a urethral discharge and an enlarged prostate. • **Chronic bacterial prostatitis** is usually not painful and involves few systemic signs of illness. It is often characterized by recurrent urinary tract infections (UTIs). • **Prostatic adenocarcinoma** and **transitional cell carcinoma (TCC)** are the most common neoplasms (affecting the canine prostate. The tumors are locally invasive and may metastasize to sublumbar lymph nodes, lumbar vertebrae, and the pelvis. Prostatic neoplasia occurs with approximately the same frequency in castrated and intact male dogs. • **Intraprostatic or periprostatic cysts**
HISTORY	Recurrent urinary tract infections (UTIs) may indicate chronic bacterial prostatitis. All male dogs with recurrent UTIs should be evaluated for prostatic disease.
CLINICAL SIGNS	• **Tenesmus**— due to an enlarged prostate blocking passage of feces from the colon. **Stranguria** and **pollakiuria**—due to blockage of urine. • Hemorrhagic or purulent **urethral discharge** • Fever, lethargy • **Painful** gait or pain on palpation of the caudal abdomen or prostate (via rectal exam) • The dog may show **no signs**, especially with chronic prostatitis or benign prostatic hyperplasia
DIAGNOSTIC FINDINGS	Clinical Signs and history should suggest prostatic disease. **Physical Examination:** On rectal examination, the prostate may be enlarged, asymmetric, or irregular (suggests neoplasia) — but it can also be normal in size (common with chronic bacterial prostatitis). Prostatic enlargement is usually due to hyperplasia rather than inflammatory changes. In cases of acute bacterial prostatitis, the prostate is usually painful. **Prostatic neoplasia** should be high on the differential list for castrated dogs that have a normal to enlarged prostate that is fixed in place. **Radiographs** often provide information about the size and position of the prostate gland. A positive contrast cystogram helps differentiate bladder from prostate. It's important to remember to look for sublumbar lymphadenopathy or evidence of metastasis to the lumbar vertebrae/sublumbar tissues. Also, calcification of the prostate is highly suggestive of neoplasia. **Ultrasound** is better than radiography for evaluating the prostate. It can reveal size as well as homogeneity of the prostate (cysts, abscesses, and other hypoechoic areas can be identified). Invasion of the urethra with cells indicates a prostatic tumor. **Cytology and culture of the prostatic fluid:** There are a number of methods for collecting prostatic fluid. The most definitive method is the ultrasound-guided aspirate. This method is invasive, but other less-invasive methods may contain bacterial contamination from sources other than the prostate, making results difficult to evaluate. • **Ultrasound-guided prostatic aspirate:** Aspirate and culture prostatic cysts. A positive culture indicates bacterial infection. Negative results can mean that the prostate is not infected, or that the infected area within the prostate was not obtained. One disadvantage to a prostatic aspirate is that if you aspirate an abscess, you may seed the peritoneal cavity with bacteria. • **Examination and culture of urethral discharge** and semen evaluation. • **Prostatic massage:** Prostatic fluid collected via this method will always be contaminated with urine, but the procedure is minimally invasive.

Urinary

MANAGEMENT of PROSTATIC DISEASES

MANAGEMENT OF PROSTATIC HYPERPLASIA	Normally, the prostate of intact male dogs undergoes hyperplasia continuously as the dog ages. This makes them more susceptible to bacterial prostatitis. If the hyperplasia is asymptomatic, the animal does not need to be treated. If it is causing problems, the best treatment is a castration. Once the dog is castrated, the prostate gradually involutes over a three month period.
MANAGEMENT OF PROSTATIC NEOPLASIA	There is no effective treatment. Prognosis is grave.
MANAGEMENT OF BACTERIAL PROSTATITIS	ANTIBIOTICS: The bacteria causing prostatitis are the same as those that cause urinary tract infections. Choose an antibiotic based on culture and sensitivity results. When selecting an antibiotic, choose one that attains high concentrations in the prostatic tissue and fluid. • For **acute prostatitis**, keep the dog on the antibiotics for > 21 days. Reculture the prostatic fluid prior to discontinuing therapy and 3-5 days after discontinuing therapy. • For **chronic prostatitis**, choose an appropriate antibiotic. Reculture the prostatic fluid about every 2-3 weeks while the dog is on antibiotics; continue until prostatic fluid is culture-negative two times in a row. **This may take several months.** Finally, retest the dog in 30-60 days. In some cases, the animal must be on permanent low dose antibiotics to control secondary UTIs. CASTRATION is recommended for both acute and chronic prostatitis to decrease prostatic hyperplasia TOTAL PROSTECTOMY is an option but is not ideal. Note: Acute bacterial prostatitis and prostatic abscesses may be life-threatening. Ruptured abscesses may lead to peritonitis and septicemia. Take care to avoid rupturing abscesses during sample collection. If you aspirate a hypoechoic area that turns out to be an abscess or your rupture an abscess, you may need to support the animal with fluids and electrolytes in addition to putting it on the appropriate antibiotics. Abscesses should be drained or surgically removed.

BACTERIA and ANTIBIOTICS in PROSTATIC DISEASE

BACTERIA COMMONLY INVOLVED in PROSTATITIS	ANTIBIOTICS that REACH the PROSTATE
• *Escherichia coli* • *Staphylococcus* • *Streptococcus* • *Klebsiella* spp. • *Enterobacter* • *Proteus mirabilis* • *Pseudomonas*	• Chloramphenicol • Clindamycin • Erythromycin Fluoroquinolones (e.g. enrofloxacin - Baytril®) • Trimethoprim/sulfa • Tetracyclines

URINARY CALCULI
General Information and Diagnosis
Management of Selected Canine Urinary Calculi
Feline Urinary Calculi

I. **GENERAL INFORMATION and DIAGNOSIS:** Most canine urinary calculi are composed of a **series of concentric rings** that represent sequential deposition of mineral substances from the center outward. Each layer can be made up of one compound or a mixture of compounds (e.g., one layer may be struvite and the next layer may be struvite and calcium oxalate).

COMMON CALCULI	Struvite (magnesium ammonium phosphate) Calcium oxalate Urate salts Calcium phosphate (apatite and brushite) Silica Cystine (in dogs)
DIAGNOSTIC APPROACH	**Clinical signs:** The animal may have signs of concurrent UTI or may have a history of recurrent UTI. Hematuria may also be present. **Physical exam:** Occasionally, stones are palpable within the bladder. **Radiographs:** • Calcium oxalate, calcium carbonate, and struvite calculi are radiopaque. • Uric acid and xanthine calculi are often radiolucent, so they must be identified using a contrast study or ultrasound. • Cystine calculi are variable. • A **double contrast cystogram** can be used to identify calculi if ultrasound is not available or if ultrasound does not give a definitive diagnosis. A double contrast urethrogram may be needed to identify urethral stones. **Ultrasound** is a more efficient method for diagnosing bladder and renal calculi than plane film radiography if no gas is in the GI tract; however, it does not show the pelvic urethra. **Urinalysis:** The presence of a high number of crystals in the urine may indicate stone formation. If you palpate a stone, the urinalysis may help determine the kind of stone present. It will also tell you if the animal has a concurrent UTI. • **Struvite** (triple phosphate crystals): On urinalysis, triple phosphate crystals look like little coffins. Struvite is more likely to precipitate in basic urine. • **Calcium oxalate** precipitates in acidic urine.
MANAGEMENT (GENERAL PRINCIPLES)	**Surgical removal:** In dogs, urinary calculi should be removed surgically and sent to a urinary stone analysis lab for analysis of the different layers. The analysis is important in determining the proper management for preventing recurrence. Often the animal must be maintained on a special calculolytic diet to prevent urolith recurrence. **Control of UTIs:** A urinalysis should be performed and a culture run if indicated. If the animal has a concurrent UTI (the urolith acts as a nidus of infection), place the animal on appropriate antibiotics and follow the UTI management protocol. Animals may have to be on antibiotics for extended periods of time, since uroliths can cause extensive urinary tract inflammation and the tissue may take awhile to recover. **Dietary management:** In cases of feline struvite urolithiasis and in some cases of urolithiasis in canines (e.g., struvite and urate), dietary and/or medical **dissolution** of the stones can be attempted. This method puts male dogs at risk of developing urethral obstructions, and owners must be instructed to watch for signs of obstruction. In addition, canine uroliths have multiple layers and often have more than one type of compound involved in the different layers; thus, the dietary considerations used to treat one layer may not be effective for treating the next layer, or the diet may be useful for one component of a given layer but not the other component of the same layer. Dietary dissolution is a viable option, though. Diet is often important in preventing urolith recurrence. Animals with uroliths should be encouraged to **drink more water** to form dilute urine. Adding water or a small amount of salt to their food can help (calculolytic diets may contain increased sodium chloride to promote polydipsia).

Urinary

II. MANAGEMENT of SELECTED CANINE URINARY CALCULI

A. STRUVITE or STRUVITE/APATITE STONES in DOGS: Virtually all struvite-containing calculi in dogs are induced by staphylococcal UTI. Both *proteus* and *staphylococcus* contain the enzyme urease, which degrades urea to CO_2 and ammonia. The net result is an increase in pH and an increase in ammonium and phosphate formation (two of the components of struvite).

1. **Dietary dissolution (to acidify the urine):** Dietary dissolution of struvite stones in dogs can be attempted, but it's not as successful as in cats because it only works when the stones are greater than 80% struvite. In dogs, the stones are rarely > 80% struvite in all layers. In addition, in male dogs, the resulting small stones and crystals may become lodged in the os penis or another portion of the urethra, resulting in **obstruction** (a medical emergency). Struvite dissolution through diet is best reserved for cats and female dogs.

2. **Dietary management may be used to decrease the incidence of new stone formation.**
   a. The goal of dietary therapy is to keep the pH between 6 and 6.5 and to encourage the animal to drink water so that the urine is dilute. The diet should contain moderate levels of protein. Animal-based protein is better at acidifying the urine than is vegetable-based protein. Some diets also contain a urinary acidifier such as dl-methionine or ammonium chloride. (These acidifiers must be listed in the ingredients before sodium chloride to be present in significant enough amounts to acidify the urine.) To determine the efficacy of the diet, the urine pH should be measured about 4 hours after a meal (alkaline tide peaks at about this time).
   b. Struvite calculolytic diets are also usually low in ash.
   c. Calculolytic diets are not good maintenance diets and should not be used in lactating bitches, growing dogs, or working dogs. They also shouldn't be fed to dogs with congestive heart failure, hypertension, or nephrotic syndrome.
   d. To increase water uptake, add water to the food.

3. **Control the associated urinary tract infection.** If the urinary tract infection is not controlled, struvite uroliths will reform. You may need to keep the dog on low dose antibiotics (1/3 the regular dose) for several months and follow the culture protocol.

B. CALCIUM OXALATE STONES form in acidic urine. The prevalence of such stones has increased in the last 10 years, possibly due to the increased use of acidifying diets. Treatment consists of removing the stone surgically, radiographing to check that all have been removed, and then putting the dog on a diet that makes the urine alkaline (use a diet with vegetables as the primary source of protein). The diet can be supplemented with a small amount of salt to increase the animal's water intake so that its urine is more dilute, or water can be added to the food. A diet that moderately restricts protein, calcium, and oxalate, and has a normal amount of phosphorus and magnesium may be helpful in preventing recurrence of calcium oxalate uroliths after surgical removal.

C. URIC ACID CALCULI in DALMATIANS: This is primarily a disease of male Dalmatians. Dalmatians are uniquely predisposed to developing uric acid calculi because they have a heritable defect in uric acid metabolism. Although uricase is present in sufficient amounts in the liver, it's unable to convert enough uric acid to allantion. In addition, Dalmatians don't reabsorb as much of the filtered uric acid in the proximal tubules of the kidney as other breeds do. As a result, they have a higher concentration of uric acid in their urine.

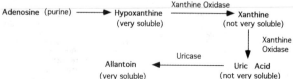

1. Dalmatians have a much higher urate concentration in their blood and urine.

MEDIUM-SIZED DOG	24-HR URINE URATE EXCRETION	URINE URATE/CREATININE RATIO
Normal Dalmatian	400-600 mg	0.5:0.5 (values as high as 1.5 have been seen in Dalmatians)
Normal non-Dalmatian	10-60 mg	

2. **Treatment of uric acid stones in Dalmatians:** As with the other canine uroliths previously discussed, treatment for uric acid stones must include medical and dietary therapy because 30-50% of all urate stones surgically removed recur. Surgery, however, is the ideal method in most Dalmatians for removing uric acid stones, but medical and dietary dissolution may be attempted. Again, this method places the male dog at risk of obstruction (emergency).
   a. **Surgically remove the stones.**
   b. **Dietary management: Change to a high quality, low purine, low protein diet.** The amount of dietary purine and protein greatly influences the concentration of uric acid in the urine of Dalmatians. The dog will be on this diet for life.

   c. **Allopurinol** is a **xanthine oxidase inhibitor** that partially blocks the purine degradation pathway to uric acid, thus decreasing the amount of uric acid in the urine. It must be given for the rest of the dog's life. Before starting the dog on allopurinol, the animal should already be on the low purine diet that it will be maintained on for the rest of its life. Start with a daily oral dose of 10 mg/kg TID for about 3 weeks following surgery. Then do a 24-hour uric acid excretion to determine the patient's specific allopurinol needs on the diet being consumed. A one-time urine urate:creatinine ratio is not an accurate approximation of the 24-hour uric acid excretion amount since the urate:creatinine levels fluctuate throughout the day.

   The goal is to keep the amount of urine uric acid produced per day to about 300 mg (0.3 urine urate/creatinine ratio). If it's much higher, increase the dose of allopurinol. If it's lower, decrease the dose. When too much allopurinol is given, the dog is at risk of forming xanthine calculi.

   > The amount of allopurinol the dog needs is dependent on the dog's diet. Consequently, you should make it absolutely clear to the owners that the dog must be on a strict low purine diet for the rest of its life.

   d. Urate stones are seen primarily in male Dalmatians and are more common in the liver-spotted Dalmatians.
D. **URIC ACID STONES in NON-DALMATIANS** are most commonly (80% of the time) caused by a **liver shunt**. Clinical signs of a liver shunt include PU/PD, stunted growth, and neurologic signs. Diagnosis is made via ultrasound and/or nuclear scintigraphy. (Refer to the GI subchapter on liver disease p. 10.19, for specific information on liver disease and liver function tests.) The vascular shunt should be corrected and the urolith surgically removed. Urine pH should be kept around 7.5 and protein intake should be regulated.

III. FELINE URINARY CALCULI

A. **URINARY CALCULI in CATS** are usually composed of a single mineral substance, with struvite and calcium oxalate being the most common minerals. Unlike with dogs, the struvite calculi in cats are usually not associated with urinary tract infections.

B. **MANAGEMENT of STRUVITE CALCULI in CATS**
1. Because the struvite calculi in cats are usually 100% struvite, dietary dissolution of the calculi using an acidifying diet low in calcium, magnesium, and phosphorus is often successful. Stones should dissolve in 2-4 weeks. Radiograph the abdomen 6 weeks after the diet is initiated to monitor the progress of stone dissolution. If stones are not visible, no further therapeutic effort is necessary. If stones are still present, they should be surgically removed at this time.
2. The urine should be cultured at the time of the urolith diagnosis to rule out concurrent UTI. UTI should be treated with appropriate antibiotics while the cat is on the calculolytic diet.
3. Cats should be maintained on a maintenance **calculolytic** diet indefinitely following stone dissolution or surgical removal. The most important component of the calculolytic diet is the urine acidification. High protein, low carbohydrate diets in cats are acidifying, and cats on such diets tend to drink more water. The pH should be maintained between 6.0 and 6.5. Ammonium chloride (not dl-methionine, which can be toxic in cats) can be used to acidify the urine. Do not use an acidifying diet in conjunction with ammonium chloride.

C. **MANAGEMENT of CALCIUM OXALATE CALCULI** in cats: **Calcium oxalate uroliths can't be dissolved** with dietary management, but they may be prevented with the right diet. Use a moderately protein restricted, calcium and oxalate restricted diet. Increase water intake by either feeding canned food or adding water to the dry food. Feed in meals to promote alkaline tide. The goal is to maintain a pH of about 7.0. Do not add sodium to the diet because it may lead to increased calcium in the urine. Calcium oxalate uroliths should be removed surgically. Blood work should be performed to look for underlying calcium regulation problems.

URINARY INCONTINENCE
Nervous Control of Micturition
Micturition Problems
Diagnosis
Treatment

Micturition is the process in which urine is passively stored and actively voided. Animals can experience problems in both the storage phase as well as the voiding phase (i.e., unable to void). Urinary incontinence is the involuntary leakage of urine during the storage phase of micturition.

I.   **NERVOUS CONTROL of MICTURITION:** Micturition is controlled by a combination of autonomic (parasympathetic and sympathetic) as well as somatic innervation.

   A.   **THE SYMPATHETIC NERVOUS SYSTEM predominates during the urine storage phase.**

      1.   Sympathetic neurons emerge from spinal segments L1-L4 via the hypogastric nerve. The preganglionic hypogastric nerve fibers synapse in the caudal mesenteric ganglion. The postganglionic fibers terminate in the detrusor muscle of the bladder.

      2.   The postganglionic fibers consist of both α– and ß-adrenergic fibers.

         a.   **α–adrenergic fibers** terminate on the smooth muscle fibers of the trigone and urethra, which form the internal urethral sphincter when they contract. Contraction of this sphincter holds urine in the bladder.

         b.   **ß-adrenergic fibers** terminate on the detrusor muscle and cause it to relax, which allows the bladder to fill.

      3.   When the sympathetic autonomic system dominates, the detrusor muscles are relaxed (ß-adrenergic stimulation) and the internal urethral sphincter is closed (α–adrenergic stimulation), allowing urine to be stored in the bladder. Additionally, sympathetic stimulation inhibits urination by blocking the parasympathetic system.

   B.   **THE PARASYMPATHETIC NERVOUS SYSTEM predominates during the voiding stage of micturition.**

      1.   Parasympathetic neurons emerge from spinal segments S1-S3 via the pelvic nerve. Stimulation of this nerve results in depolarization of the pacemaker fibers within the detrusor muscle, leading to contraction of the detrusor muscle.

      2.   Motor nerves to the external urethral sphincter also emerge from S1-S3. They travel through the pudendal nerve to the external urethral sphincter. When the parasympathetic system is activated, it inhibits the pudendal nerve, thereby causing the external urethral sphincter to open.

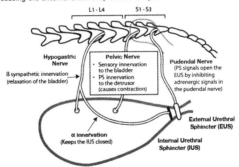

   C.   **GENERAL SCHEME**

      1.   As the bladder fills, bladder pressure increases and the smooth muscle of the bladder wall elongates. When the bladder reaches a certain pressure limit, sensory fibers in the bladder wall discharge. The signal travels up the **pelvic nerve** into the spinal cord, then up the spinal cord to the brain.

      2.   When it's appropriate to urinate, signals travel from the cortex down the spine to the parasympathetic system such that the pelvic nerve causes detrusor

Urinary

contraction. At the same time, the sympathetic signals that close the internal urethral sphincter and the somatic system signals (pudendal nerve) that close the external urethral sphincter are inhibited. Thus, the urine is voided.

3. Once the bladder is empty, the sympathetic system once again predominates. The internal urethral sphincter contracts and the detrusor muscle relaxes allowing filling.

II. **MICTURITION PROBLEMS** can be divided into two categories based on bladder size: (1) disorders leading to a large, distended bladder and (2) those leading to a small or normal-sized bladder. Incontinence can occur in both categories.

   A. **DISORDERS LEADING to a LARGE, DISTENDED BLADDER** can result in incontinence if pressure within the bladder builds up to a point where it exceeds outflow resistance. Etiologies for such disorders include the following:

      1. Both **upper and lower motor neuron disorders**

         a. LMN disease results in a large, flaccid bladder that's easy to express. Overdistention of the bladder for prolonged time periods for any reason can cause loss of detrusor muscle tone, leading to incontinence. The perineal reflex should be tested as a sign of LMN disorder.

         b. UMN disease results in a large bladder that's difficult to express because the external urethral sphincter is hyperreflexic.

      2. **Outflow obstructions** (urethral stones, struvite/mucous plugs, neoplasia): If the bladder is distended and difficult to express, ease of catheterization aids in determining whether the problem is neurologic or due to a physical obstruction.

      3. **Reflex dyssynergia** results when the detrusor actively contracts during attempts to void, but the internal urethral sphincter fails to relax because α-adrenergic input is not inhibited during voiding. These animals start to urinate a normal stream, but then the stream quickly becomes narrow and may be reduced to short spurts. A catheter can be easily passed.

   B. **DISORDERS LEADING to a SMALL (OR NORMAL-SIZED) BLADDER**

      1. **Inflammation (e.g., UTI, FLUTD)** leads to increased urgency to urinate and consequently pollakiuria.

      2. **Urethral sphincter incompetence** is more common in older, spayed female dogs, and the incontinence is most prominent when the animal is lying down or asleep. It often responds to hormone therapy (to diethylstilbestrol in spayed females or to testosterone in neutered males). α-adrenergics (such as phenylpropanolamine) are commonly effective. If either class of drug alone is ineffective, then try both together (hormones and α-adrenergics).

      3. **Congenital abnormalities** of the urinary tract, such as ectopic ureters (where the ureters drain directly into the urethra or vagina), a pelvic bladder (often associated with poor urethral sphincter tone), or vaginal strictures can lead to incontinence. Suspect congenital abnormality if the signs emerge when the animal is very young or in certain breeds such as English Bulldogs.

III. **DIAGNOSIS**

   A. **HISTORY:** Ask about the amount of urine voided to help determine whether the pet is pollakiuric or voiding normal amounts. A sudden change in housebreaking can indicate UTI or other inflammatory disorders, hormone responsive problems, cognitive dysfunction (in older dogs), or disorders causing PU/PD. Incontinence following recent trauma is most commonly related to neurologic problems.

   B. **PHYSICAL EXAM**

      1. Palpate the bladder to see whether it's large or small, and if large, whether it's easy or difficult to express.

      2. Digital palpation: Check for an enlarged prostate, which could predispose the animal to UTI or, if severe, could be associated with obstruction. Also palpate for urethral obstructions.

      3. Vaginal exam: Check for strictures.

   C. **A NEUROLOGIC EXAM** may reveal a lesion causing UMN or LMN signs relating to the bladder. Be sure to check the perineal reflex.

   D. **URINALYSIS:** All patients with urinary incontinence should have a urinalysis to check for primary or secondary bacterial infections and other factors associated with inflammation.

   E. **IMAGING**

      1. Survey radiographs can reveal a pelvic bladder, enlarged prostate, or radiodense uroliths or ureteroliths.

2. **Intravenous urography** and retrograde vaginourethrography can help reveal congenital ectopic ureters as well as **obstructions** (stones, neoplasia).

F. **URETHRAL PRESSURE PROFILES** (UPP) are used to determine urethral sphincter function during the storage phase of urination. They can identify areas of increased urethral tone or resistance (e.g., due to stricture).

1. A UPP is required for a definitive diagnosis of urethral sphincter incompetence. Decreased urethral tone can be treated with DES or phenylpropanolamine since α-adrenergic tone contributes the most to smooth muscle contraction in the urethra. (DES most likely works by sensitizing the sphincter to α-adrenergic signals). Trial drug therapy is often used to try to determine whether urethral sphincter incompetence exists.

2. UPPs are useful tests in patients with ectopic ureters because the results may tell whether the patient will need to be on medical therapy after surgical correction of the ureters.

3. Increased or normal UPPs in animals that are unable to urinate suggest functional urethral obstruction or an inability to coordinate relaxation with detrusor contraction.

G. **CYSTOMETROGRAM**: A CMG records change in intravesical pressure during filling and contraction of the bladder. It can be used to evaluate the detrusor reflex, bladder compliance and capacity, and maximum contraction pressure. Abnormal CMGs can be seen with disorders of either the storage or emptying phases of urination.

1. **Decreased compliance** during the storage phase can be due to fibrosis, inflammation, or neoplasia.

2. **Detrusor hyporeflexia** is caused by neurologic impairment.

3. **Detrusor hyperreflexia** can be caused by inflammation, tumor, calculi, or neuropathies.

IV. TREATMENT
A. MEDICAL TREATMENT of NON-NEUROGENIC CAUSES

DRUG and INDICATION	DOSE	SIDE EFFECTS
Diethylstilbesterol (for spayed females)	Dogs: 0.1-1.0 mg per dog SID for 3-7 days. If a response is seen, taper the dose interval to the lowest possible interval such as 1-2 times a week. Cats: 0.05-0.1 mg per cat PO SID for 3-5 days, and then taper to the lowest interval such as every 3-7 days.	Estrus, bone marrow toxicity, endocrine alopecia, hypertension, restlessness
Testosterone (for neutered male dogs)	Dogs only: 1-2.2 mg/kg q 30 days	Aggression, prostatomegaly
Phenylpropanolamine (α-adrenergic agonist)	1.0-4.0 mg/kg PO BID to TID This should take effect within 2-3 weeks. After the 2nd week, the dose may be increased or DES added if needed.	Hypertension, restlessness, anxiety, possible aggression
Bethanechol (a parasympathomimetic agent for detrusor atony) Rule out obstruction first.	Dogs: 5-15 mg PO TID Cats: 1.25-5.0 mg PO TID SC injections may be more effective. Start at the lowest possible dose. The maximal amount with either form is realized when the patient starts to salivate.	Salivation, lacrimation, vomiting, diarrhea, arrhythmias (Signs usually occur within 1 hour of administration)

1. Some neutered animals respond to hormone administration (estrogen in females and testosterone in males). These hormones may increase the sensitivity of the bladder to α-adrenergic stimulation.

2. α-adrenergic agonists such as phenylpropanolamine cause detrusor relaxation and contraction of the internal urethral sphincter.

3. **Parasympathomimetics** such as bethanechol are used to increase detrusor contractility in cases of detrusor atony (such as with LMN disease). Rule out urethral obstruction prior to administering this class of drugs.

B. **ECTOPIC URETERS** can be treated surgically.

1. Urinary tract infections must be cleared prior to surgery.

2. A UPP should be performed to help predict clinical outcome and the likelihood of needing medications following surgery.

Urinary

FELINE LOWER URINARY TRACT INFLAMMATION (FLUTI)

Feline lower urinary tract disease (FLUTI) is a syndrome that can be caused by a number of diseases. It's characterized by signs of lower urinary tract inflammation, which include hematuria, stranguria, and pain on urination. It may be obstructive or non-obstructive.

SIGNALMENT	Overweight cats (possibly due to increased total magnesium intake since they eat more food overall) Primarily indoor cats (may just be noticed more in these cats) Cats on dry food diets (may be due to increased fecal water loss resulting in decreased urine volume) Male cats (They obstruct more commonly then females because mucus and struvite often lodge in the narrow penile urethra)
CLINICAL SIGNS	• **Urinating outside the litter box** • **Stranguria**: The cat spends a long time in the litter box and may yowl due to pain while urinating. The owner may think the cat is constipated. • **Hematuria** • **Pollakiuria** • **Depression/lethargy** and signs of uremia if a partial or complete obstruction is present
ETIOLOGIES	FLUTI can be categorized into cases with crystalluria and inflammation and those without crystalluria or uroliths. • **Crystalluria or uroliths:** Struvite or calcium oxalate crystals are the most common crystals. Struvite crystals can be found in normal cats with alkaline urine, too (or calcium oxalate crystals if in acidic urine). • **Urinary tract infection** (< 10% of cases) • **Neoplasia** • Urethral stricture and other **structural abnormalities** • **Idiopathic sterile inflammation:** This is the most common etiology. • **Behavioral problems** can cause inappropriate elimination. Rule out the medical problems before diagnosing a behavioral problem.
DIAGNOSTIC FINDINGS	• History and clinical signs • A large, painful bladder that does not express well with gentle pressure indicates partial or complete obstruction. • **Urinalysis and culture:** Rule out urinary tract infection and crystalluria. • **Radiographs and contrast cystograms** help rule out uroliths and neoplasia. They can also identify thickened bladder walls and bladder rupture. • **Ultrasound** gives similar information as contrast cystograms. • A **contrast urethrogram** can identify urethral neoplasia or uroliths. • **Catheterization** can reveal urethral obstruction. • **Cystoscopy is used to** visualize and evaluate the mucosal wall. • **Chemistry/CBC:** Look for complications caused by obstruction. These include acidosis, hyperkalemia, azotemia, dehydration (elevated total protein and hematocrit), and other evidence of renal failure.
MANAGEMENT of NON-OBSTRUCTIVE DISEASE	**UTI:** If signs are caused by a **urinary tract infection**, treat with appropriate antibiotics. **Sterile cystitis:** If there's no infection, antibiotics are not required. In cases of idiopathic sterile cystitis, cats usually improve spontaneously within 5-7 days. If they don't improve, try an anticholinergic (e.g., propantheline) to reduce bladder spasms caused by detrusor hyperreflexia. Corticosteroids have not been proven to help, but in cases where a UTI has been ruled out, it's okay to try corticosteroids. Subcutaneous fluid therapy for 1-3 days may help flush out the bladder. **Struvite or calcium oxalate crystals:** Refer to the same topics under managing obstructive disease on the following page. **Pain management:** Consider opioids for pain management.

FLUTD (continued)

MANAGING OBSTRUCTIVE DISEASE	**Unblock the cat.** If the cat is extremely depressed, you may be able to place a catheter without anesthesia, but if it's bright and alert, you will need general anesthesia. There are many methods for unblocking the cat. Tomcat catheters are often used (round-ended or open-ended). Place the catheter in the urethra and flush saline to distend the urethra and dislodge the sediment. If you are unable to dislodge the sediment using a catheter, you may need to perform a cystocentesis prior to further attempts. If the bladder is already friable, doing a cystocentesis may cause the bladder to rupture, so use a very small needle. Once you unblock the cat, you may want to replace the rigid tomcat catheter with a softer one because the rigid catheter may cause more mechanical damage. Try to keep the catheter in overnight to be sure that the cat doesn't immediately reblock. If you're unable to leave a urinary catheter in, you may need to express the cat's bladder 4-6 times a day because some cats develop temporary detrusor atony, especially if they've been blocked for over 24 hours. **Set up a closed urine collection system** to keep track of urine production. These patients may develop infections from the urinary catheter, so periodically check the urine sediment and treat with antibiotics if indicated. **Administer IV fluids** to correct dehydration and electrolyte imbalances. Often cats develop post-obstructive diuresis. **ECG:** Evaluate for hyperkalemia using an ECG if potassium levels can't be obtained immediately (look for bradycardia, prolonged P-R interval, wide QRS, spiked T wave, flat or absent P wave, or ventricular arrhythmias). If the ECG or potassium levels indicate hyperkalemia, treat by first correcting the acidosis with fluid and bicarbonate therapy (0.3 x base deficit x weight in kg or 1-2 meq bicarbonate/kg slowly IV). If this is not adequate, administer insulin (0.25-0.5 U/kg IV) and dextrose (2g/U insulin given slowly IV). **Blood work:** Check the kidney status (BUN, creatinine, phosphorus, etc.). **Parasympatholytics** such as propantheline can be used to prevent detrusor spasms (7.5-30 mg PO TID). If the cat blocks repeatedly, a **perineal urethrostomy** may be indicated. This surgery prevents future blockage, but the animal may still develop signs of cystitis. **Struvite crystals:** If the obstruction is due to struvite crystals, maintain the urine pH at 6.0-6.5 with diet (a prescription acidifying diet that doesn't contain excess magnesium or calcium) or with urinary acidifier drugs such as ammonium chloride. Encourage water drinking (keep fresh water readily available) and encourage voiding (clean, abundant litter). **Calcium oxalate crystals** may be prevented with appropriate dietary management. Use a diet that's moderately protein restricted, and calcium and oxalate restricted. Increase water intake by either feeding canned food or adding water to the dry food. Feed in meals to promote alkaline tide. The goal is to maintain a pH of about 7.0. Do not add sodium to the diet because it may lead to increased calcium in the urine. **Do not use bethanechol.** It's a parasympathomimetic. It causes contraction of the smooth muscle of the urinary bladder.

Urinary

POLYURIA and POLYDIPSIA

Polyuria (PU), excessive urination, and **polydipsia (PD)**, excessive water intake, can be caused by a number of diseases. Either the polyuria or the polydipsia can be the primary problem; the other feature usually follows out of necessity.

SIGNS	• Nocturia or urination accidents in the house • Increased need for the litter box to be changed • Drinking from the toilet, puddles, etc., and increased need to refill the water bowl
NORMAL	Normal water consumption in dogs and cats is 50-100 mL/kg per day Normal urine production is 30-50 mL/kg per day or less. Polyuria = > 100 mL/kg per day (often can be > 200 mL/kg per day) These values can change with environmental conditions such as: <u>Increased water consumption</u> <u>Increased urine volume</u> Heavy exercise (panting) High water content of diet High environmental temperature Low environmental temperature Salty or dry dog food Vomiting/diarrhea
REGULATION of WATER INTAKE	Water intake is regulated by the hypothalamus. Decreased blood volume or increased blood osmolality triggers the hypothalamic thirst center to make ADH. ADH is stored in the posterior pituitary and released into the blood. It travels to the distal tubules and collecting ducts of the kidneys and causes increased permeability to water. This allows more water to be reabsorbed back into the body (more concentrated urine). Prolonged absence of ADH results in **medullary washout,** which in turn decreases the normal kidney's ability to concentrate the urine until a high osmolality is re-established in the medulla.
ETIOLOGY of PD	Primary polydipsia is psychogenic, due to abnormal function of the hypothalamic thirst center. Primary polydipsia is rare.

ETIOLOGIES of POLYURIA (DIABETES INSIPIDUS)	Diabetes insipidus (DI) is polyuria caused by a decrease in ADH synthesis or secretion, or a decrease in the kidney's ability to respond to ADH. It can be divided into central or peripheral causes.
	
	Central diabetes insipidus (CDI) is a decrease in synthesis or secretion of ADH. Partial insufficiency is called partial CDI. CDI can be congenital (primary) or acquired (secondary).
	• Primary (congenital) CDI occurs in young animals and is rare.
	• Secondary (acquired) CDI is idiopathic or secondary to a brain tumor. It can occur in an animal of any age.
	
	Nephrogenic diabetes insipidus (NDI) results when renal tubules can't respond to ADH. This occurs because ADH either can't bind to receptors or because the kidney doesn't respond sufficiently. Possible reasons for the latter include: (1) the renal medullary gradient is insufficient due to low BUN or washout, (2) Na transport out of the urine at the loops of Henle is inhibited due to administration of loop diuretic or a similar compound, or (3) other reasons. As with CDI, NDI can be partial or complete. ADH levels are normal or increased with NDI.
	• Primary (congenital) NDI occurs in young animals and is rare.
	• Secondary (acquired) NDI is the most common form of diabetes insipidus. It involves several renal and metabolic disorders, and is potentially reversible when the underlying disorders are corrected.
	    • Hypoadrenocorticism and hyperadrenocorticism
	    • Hyperthyroidism
	    • Diabetes mellitus
	    • Renal insufficiency
	    • Post-obstructive diuresis
	    • Hypercalcemia (usually due to renal disease or lymphosarcoma)
	    • Hypokalemia
	    • Drug-induced (Lasix, steroids, estrogen)
	    • Pyometra
	    • Hepatic insufficiency (The NDI is due to decreased BUN leading to a decrease in the renal medullary concentration gradient)
	    • Renal medullary solute washout (due to excessive water intake or temporary decrease in ADH production or secretion)

PU/PD (continued)

DIAGNOSIS
 	
First,
rule out
secondary
nephrogenic
diabetes
insipidus.
	First rule out causes of **secondary nephrogenic DI.** Most dogs and cats with PU/PD have secondary NDI.
	History: Any history of trauma or medications?
	Urinalysis and culture: The urine will probably be too dilute to reveal bacteria on microscopic exam. Establish the degree of isosthenuria or hyposthenuria. Hyposthenuria indicates that the kidney is able to dilute the urine, and the animal is not in renal failure. Proteinuria may indicate glomerulonephritis or early renal disease. Glucosuria may suggest diabetes mellitus.
	Complete blood count and blood chemistry including T$_4$: This helps rule out the following:
	  • Hyperthyroidism (elevated T$_4$)
	  • Diabetes mellitus (hyperglycemia)
	  • Hepatic insufficiency (elevated liver enzymes, low albumin, etc.)
	  • Renal insufficiency (increased BUN, CRT, ± phosphorus, Ca^{2+})
	  • Hypercalcemia
	  • Hypokalemia
	  • Infection (e.g., neutrophilia, leukocytosis, left shift)
	Lymph node aspirate: If hypercalcemia is found or if the animal has lymphadenopathy, aspirate the lymph nodes to look for lymphosarcoma.
	Abdominal radiographs or ultrasound: Rule out pyometra or pyelonephritis (ultrasound).
	ACTH stimulation test: Rule out hyper- and hypoadrenocorticism.

DIAGNOSIS Second, rule out all other etiologies.	Once you've ruled out secondary nephrogenic diabetes insipidus, perform tests to **rule out central diabetes insipidus, primary nephrogenic diabetes insipidus, and psychogenic water drinking.** This can be done by trial therapy with ADH. Primary nephrogenic DI and psychogenic water drinking are very rare. **Trial therapy with ADH** tests for central diabetes insipidus. Administer DDAVP (synthetic ADH; 0.1 mg and 0.2mg tablets). The recommended starting dose is 0.1 mg PO TID for 20 kg dogs and 0.2 mg PO TID for 40 kg dogs. Administer for about 7 days. Dogs and cats with CDI should improve markedly. With NDI, improvement is minimal. DDAVP nasal drops (1-4 drops BID) can be used in place of the oral medication but are much more expensive, and results are more variable. **The modified water deprivation test** is no longer used due to safety issues. If trial with ADH indicates CDI, perform a neurologic exam, CT scan or MRI in older pets, and CSF tap to look for the underlying cause. For animals with primary NDI, consider a renal biopsy in the older pet.
TREATMENT	• Treat the underlying disease. • If the animal has **CDI or primary NDI,** treatment is not completely necessary as long as the animal has unlimited access to water and urination areas. Keep in mind that even short-term water deprivation (for several hours) in these patients may be devastating. • **CDI** can be treated with synthetic **vasopressin** (DDAVP-desmopressin). As stated in the diagnostics section, a common starting dose is 0.1 mg PO TID in small dogs (20 kg) and 0.2 mg PO TID in larger dogs (40 kg). Adjust doses for cats and larger dogs. If a clinical response is seen within 7 days, then the dose can be adjusted such that the lowest dose possible is used at the lowest dosing interval (SID or BID). Do not overdose. Rather, wait until the dog has mild PU/PD before giving the next dose. • **Other drugs for CDI** include chlorpropamide and chlorothiazide diuretics. They are usually minimally helpful.
PROGNOSIS	**Primary CDI:** Prognosis is good if there's no underlying brain tumor. **Secondary CDI** due to trauma can be controlled with DDAVP. Signs often resolve on their own within several weeks. **Primary NDI:** Prognosis is poor. The disease is not very responsive to medications. **Secondary NDI:** Prognosis depends on the underlying disease. Treat the underlying etiology.

Urinary

RENAL FAILURE
Acute Renal Failure vs. Chronic Renal Failure
Acute Renal Failure
Chronic Renal Failure

Sixty-five to 75% of the kidney must be destroyed for it to lose most of its compensatory ability, resulting in uremia and clinical signs of renal disease. Detection of disease prior to this time allows us to significantly delay the progression of disease.

I. **ACUTE RENAL FAILURE (ARF) vs. CHRONIC RENAL FAILURE (CRF):** The kidneys may be damaged acutely or more slowly. In both cases, clinical signs include anorexia, dehydration, vomiting, diarrhea, lethargy, and oral ulcers/uremic breath. Additionally, with acute renal failure, animals become oliguric (or anuric), whereas with chronic renal failure they become polyuric.

	ACUTE RENAL FAILURE	CHRONIC RENAL FAILURE
CLINICAL SIGNS (that differ)	Anuria (rare) or oliguria	Polyuria/polydipsia Weight loss Edema or ascites (low albumin)
DIAGNOSIS	Isosthenuria in the presence of dehydration (elevated total protein and BUN) indicates renal failure. Urinalysis: isosthenuria ± proteinuria and casts (active sediment) CBC: may be normal Chemistry changes tend to be much more pronounced in acute renal failure than in CRF. • **BUN:** moderate to marked elevation • **Creatinine:** moderate to marked elevation • **Phosphate:** moderate to marked elevation • **Calcium:** normal, high, or low • **Potassium:** moderate to marked elevation • Total **protein** and **hematocrit:** elevated due to dehydration Radiographs/ultrasound: large or normal-sized kidneys	Isosthenuria in the presence of dehydration (elevated total protein and BUN) indicates renal failure. Urinalysis: Isosthenuria ± proteinuria CBC: normocytic, normochromic, non-responsive anemia Chemistry: • **BUN:** mild to moderate elevation • **Creatinine:** mild to moderate elevation • **Phosphate:** mild to moderate elevation • **Calcium:** normal or hypercalcemic (renal 2° hyperPTH); hypocalcemic (due to PU/PD and low Vit D conversion)in endstage disease. (See Ca/P chapter, p. 9.23). • **Potassium:** mild to moderate elevation; may also be decreased Radiographs/ultrasound: small kidneys that are often irregularly shaped

II. ACUTE RENAL FAILURE
   A. TREATING the CRISIS
      1. **Remove any inciting factors** such as nephrotoxic drugs and toxins that have been ingested. (Refer to the toxicology section, p. 20.2 and 20.4.)
      2. **Rehydrate** the animal with appropriate fluids, and treat the acidosis by administering bicarbonate if indicated.
         a. Administer bicarbonate if the blood bicarbonate is < 14 meq/L, the base deficit is < 10 meq/L, or the pH is < 7.2.

> Amount of bicarbonate = 0.3 (animal's weight in kg) (base deficit)

   Give 1/4 to 1/2 of the calculated dose over 30 minutes, then recheck the acid-base status.

      b. **Treat the hyperkalemia:** Hyperkalemia can lead to life-threatening cardiac conduction abnormalities including bradycardia, atrial standstill, ventricular tachycardia, and ventricular fibrillation. Treating for the acidosis helps alleviate the hyperkalemia. If potassium is < 6.5 meq, just treat the acidosis. If it's > 6.5 meq (cardiotoxic range), treat with regular insulin (0.25-0.5 U/kg IV) and dextrose (2 g/U of insulin given). This treatment drives potassium from the extracellular fluid into the cells.

3. **Re-establish urine output:** Place a urinary catheter in the animal and monitor urine output. Kidneys in acute failure may produce little or no urine. As a result, the animal may become overhydrated. The animal must be adequately hydrated before diuretics are used.

   a. **Lasix** is a loop diuretic. It does not affect the glomerular filtration rate, but the diuresis alone helps the animal by getting rid of toxic substances (azotemia). Start with 2-4 mg/kg IV and keep track of urine output.

   b. **Mannitol** (0.25-0.5 g/kg IV of a 20-25% solution) is an osmotic diuretic. It pulls fluid into the renal tubules. This action also helps remove casts and other material that's plugging the damaged nephrons. Do not use mannitol if the animal is in heart failure. If there's no diuresis in one hour, than discontinue this treatment. If the kidneys respond well, decrease to a maintenance dose of 1 mg/kg/minute mannitol as a constant rate infusion. DO NOT USE MANNITOL IF THE PATIENT IS DEHYDRATED.

   c. **Dopamine** (2.5 µg/kg/minute) increases glomerular filtration rate. It's used in dogs since cats may not have dopamine receptors in their kidneys.

B. **PROBLEMS ASSOCIATED WITH RENAL FAILURE:** Once the above problems are addressed, the acute crisis can then be treated the same as with chronic cases.

III. **CHRONIC RENAL FAILURE:** In the past, clinicians usually diagnosed CRF only after 2/3 of kidney function was lost and the animal was showing significant signs of uremia. Now, clinicians are encouraged to monitor for earlier signs of renal failure to allow for earlier intervention.

A. **THE PROCESS of RENAL FAILURE**

   1. **Inciting factor:** Many factors—such as exposure to toxins (e.g., certain antibiotics, NSAIDS), hypotension, and infection—can damage the kidney either gradually or in one major episode.

   2. **Functional progression:** Once the kidney is damaged, a number of processes may lead to further damage. For instance, hypertension leads to renal tissue hypoxia as well as increased renal capillary pressure, which can contribute to proteinuria. Loss of urine concentrating ability leads to calcium loss and consequently hypocalcemia. This triggers secondary hyperparathyroidism, which leads to hypercalcemia and hyperphosphatemia. When the calcium x phosphorus product rises above 60-70, it results in dystrophic calcification. These processes occur independent of the primary cause of renal damage.

   3. **Uremia:** Once enough renal function is lost, azotemia occurs, leading to many of the clinical signs associated with renal disease.

B. **FOUR STAGES of CHRONIC RENAL FAILURE devised by the International Renal Interest Society (www.iris-kidney.com):** This staging is based on clinical suggestion of renal failure plus creatinine levels in the hydrated patient.

STAGE	AZOTEMIA	CREATININE (mg/dL) in DOGS	CREATININE (mg/dL) in CATS
I	None	< 1.4	< 1.6
II	Mild	1.4-2.0	1.6-2.8
III	Moderate	2.1-5.0	2.9-5.0
IV	Severe	> 5.0	> 5.0

   1. **Stage I:** The animal has proteinuria or some other indication of possible renal disease, such as hypertension, but is not azotemic.

   2. **Stage II:** Same as stage I, but the animal is mildly azotemic. By catching animals in stages I and II, we can intervene before the irreversible processes have been set in motion. Animals in stage I or II may have had a transient non-progressive renal insult and do not automatically require intervention at this point, though.

   3. **Stages III and IV:** The animal has more prominent clinical signs such as PU/PD and vomiting and is now moderately to severely azotemic. These are the stages where owners often notice the clinical signs and where over 65-75% of the nephrons have already been destroyed.

C. **DIAGNOSIS:** Suggestions of early renal disease may be found during routine physical exam, or pre-anesthetic work-up, or due to owner recognition of abnormalities. Such indicators include:

   1. **Non-specific clinical signs:** The animal may have vague signs, such as unexplained dehydration, weight loss, or poor hair coat, that alert the veterinarian and suggest that diagnostics be performed.

   2. **Urinalysis** may reveal abnormalities:

   a. The urine may be **less concentrated** (specific gravity of < 1.025 in cats or repeated isosthenuria in dogs).

      b. **Proteinuria** may be present. 1+ protein in dilute urine (< 1.025 in the cat) may be significant and suggests that a urine protein:creatinine should be performed. Upc > 0.4 in cats and > 0.5 in dogs indicates significant proteinuria.

3. **Signs of hypertension** such as tortuous retinal vessels or retinal detachment may be found on fundic exam.

4. **Creatinine** may reveal stage I or II CRF, or may be high enough to be associated with uremia.

5. **Renal imaging:** If any of the above changes are seen, radiographs or ultrasound can be performed to look for abnormalities in size, shape, and to look for calculi.

D. **THERAPEUTIC APPROACH to CRF:** Therapy consists of (1) finding the primary disease (e.g., pyelonephritis) and treating it, (2) checking for functional or biochemical abnormalities that should be treated (e.g., proteinuria, hypertension), and (3) controlling the clinical signs (such as vomiting and GI ulceration).

    1. **Minimize azotemia:** Azotemia occurs when the damaged nephrons are unable to filter waste products out of the blood. As a result, nitrogenous wastes accumulate. Keep the BUN below the level where clinical signs occur. Many cats can tolerate 60 mg/dL. Treat based on signs rather than the absolute number.

      a. **Hydration:** Dogs on dry food drink more to accommodate their lower water intake. Cats on dry food, however, do not.

        i. Cats that are polyuric should be on **canned food** or should have water added to their dry food. Additionally, they should have easy access to water from multiple sources and even from a fountain water bowl if it helps.

        ii. Some owners can also give **subcutaneous fluids;** however, many cats dislike the process and thus, it can cause anxiety in both cat and owner. To condition the cats to tolerate or enjoy the treatment, the fluids can be paired with meals or treats. This must be done in a manner that teaches the cat a pleasant association with the process rather than accidentally teaching it to dislike its food because the food is associated with the treatment. For instance, the owner can start the desensitization/counter-conditioning process by just pinching the cat's skin while giving treats and discontinuing the pinch action as soon as the cat finishes the treat. If the cat ignores the pinching, then owners can try inserting the needle as the cat is eating but removing it before the cat shows signs of discomfort and just before the cat finishes the treat or stops eating. Owners should start with short fluid administrations (short enough so that the cat shows no signs of aversion) and increase the length over several tries. In such a manner, they avoid going over the cat's tolerance threshold and instead desensitize the cat to the fluid administration, teaching it to associate administration with pleasant experiences. (See video of the technique at www.behavior4veterinarians.com)

      b. **Diet:** Provide adequate calories and high quality protein or the body will use its own protein for energy, which will result in elevated BUN. Cats with azotemia feel nauseous and may learn to associate foods with this nausea. Consequently, finding a diet these cats will eat can be difficult. Placing an esophageal or gastrostomy tube for long-term feeding and fluid and drug administration can be useful; these tubes are well tolerated.

    2. **Treat hypokalemia (cats):** Polyuria in cats can lead to hypokalemia, which in turn results in muscle weakness (e.g., inability to climb or jump and decreased energy). Owners may perceive this weakness as a significant decline in well-being and may euthanize when actually these clinical signs can be controlled with supplementation. Because most potassium is intracellular, once we start to see decreased serum potassium levels, the cell levels are dangerously low. Therefore, start supplementing when potassium levels reach the lower half of the normal range.

      a. **Supplement with potassium citrate** or feed a renal diet. They are high in potassium.

    3. **Prevent or treat hyperphosphatemia:** Non-functional nephrons are unable to excrete phosphate into the urine. A calcium:phosphorus ratio > 60-70 predisposes the animal to calcification in tissues.

      a. Place the animal on a low phosphorus diet.

      b. If diet alone does not control the phosphorus, add phosphate binders. Aluminum hydroxide (100 mg/kg/day) is the safest but is not as easy to find as calcium carbonate. Be careful with calcium carbonate as the presence of the calcium can contribute to hypercalcemia or an elevated Ca:P ratio. Phosphate binders should be given with a meal since they work by binding the phosphorus in the GI tract.

4. **Manage hypercalcemia:** In renal failure, the calcium is initially low because vitamin D is not being converted to its active form in the kidney. Phosphate is high due to decreased renal function (decreased excretion). The low calcium triggers an increase in parathyroid hormone secretion leading to **secondary hyperparathyroidism.**

   a. Diuresis with saline can bring the calcium down quickly.
   b. **Administer calcitriol (vitamin D)** to increase calcium levels in the normocalcemic or hypocalcemic animal. Only use it when the phosphate levels are controlled (Ca x P of < 50), because it works to increase both Ca and P. If levels increase above 60 or 70 mg/dL, the animal will develop dystrophic calcification. Start with 1.5-2.5 mg/kg/day in cats and dogs, and evaluate ionized calcium as well as phosphorus levels weekly for a month. Then measure the levels every 2 weeks for up to 6 months. If the medication has no effect within 2 months, then discontinue. It's also good to monitor PTH. Calcitriol administration can markedly delay progression of the renal failure. Calcitriol should be prepared by a compounding pharmacy.

5. **Correct significant metabolic acidosis:** Bicarbonate is usually secreted by the kidneys. With PU/PD, excess bicarbonate is lost. Occasionally check the total bicarbonate, and if it's below 18-22 meq/L, then supplement with potassium citrate.

6. **Treat clinical anemia:** Anemia in chronic renal failure occurs due to bleeding from GI ulcers induced by azotemia, and also because the damaged kidney secretes less erythropoietin. If the cat has clinical signs of anemia, human recombinant erythropoietin (epogen or darbepoetin, which has a longer half-life) can be administered. Because these are human products, many cats will develop antibodies; however, in most cases the product can just be discontinued if this happens.

7. **Control hypertension:** Renal disease can lead to hypertension through several mechanisms, including decreased sodium excretion or reduced renal blood flow leading to activation of the RAAS. Hypertension and the associated high perfusion in turn can damage renal capillary beds, cause renal vasoconstriction, and lead to capillary hypoxia. **Systolic blood pressure should be kept below 160 mmHg.** If it's above this, treat with ACE inhibitors such as enalapril or benazepril. If ineffective, add a calcium channel blocker such as amlodipine (0.25 mg/kg) PO SID. Amlodipine has an immediate effect on blood pressure, whereas ACE inhibitors take longer since they affect the RAAS. If the urine protein:creatinine ratio is high and the animal is normotensive, then give ACE inhibitors to reduce proteinuria and delay disease progression.

DRUG	CLASS	DOSE	INDICATIONS
Benazepril	ACE I	0.5 mg/kg PO SID-BID	Hypertension, proteinuria
Enalapril	ACE I	0.4 mg/kg PO SID-BID	Hypertension, proteinuria
Amlodipine	CCB	0.25 mg/kg PO SID	Hypertension

8. **Diet:** If the animal is azotemic, then put it on a diet that is protein restricted, has low phosphorus, and that is high in omega-3 fatty acids. Restricted protein diets can double the lifespan of the CRF animal. When going to a restricted protein diet in cats, do not drop the level suddenly to the lowest protein possible as this may result in muscle catabolism. Rather, you may need to decrease in a stepwise manner as the disease progresses. Start with a medium protein diet such as one of the senior diets (which are also lower in phosphorus), and if needed switch to a prescription renal diet later.

9. **Recheck** every 4-6 months and perform a urinalysis and culture. Animals with dilute urine lack the protective elements present in more concentrated urine and consequently are more prone to infection. They, especially cats, may show no outward signs of urinary tract infection and so the urine should automatically be cultured in dogs with isosthenuria and renal disease cats with SG < 1.030.

Urinary

RENAL PROTEINURIA
Renal Proteinuria
Glomerulonephropathy

I. **RENAL PROTEINURIA** is often the first sign of early renal disease and indicates damage primarily of the glomeruli (glomerulonephropathy).
   A. **PATHOPHYSIOLOGY of RENAL PROTEINURIA**
      1. In the **Bowman's capsule,** the small molecules (smaller than albumin) pass through the glomerular basement membranes into the urine, but larger molecules remain in the capillaries. Some smaller proteins do get through, but they are reabsorbed by receptor-mediated endocytosis so that the urine contains very little protein. Damage to the walls of the capillaries in Bowman's capsules (such as with formation of immune complexes) cause smaller proteins like albumin to leak into the ultrafiltrate. The amount of proteins exceeds the ability of receptors to resorb them, leading to a **selective proteinuria** consisting primarily of **albumin.** Leakage of proteins through the glomerular capsule is termed **glomerulonephropathy.** Glomerulonephropathy is characterized by the selective loss of albumin in the urine. In the early stages the nephrons are not affected; thus, the urine is concentrated and creatinine is normal.
      2. As renal disease progresses the interstitium becomes diseased, and tubular damage occurs. Now, larger molecular weight proteins appear in the urine, too. Once 2/3 to 3/4 of the nephrons are damaged, renal failure ensues and we see the clinical signs related to the inability to concentrate the urine (PU/PD) and azotemia (anorexia, vomiting, nausea).
   B. **PROTEINURIA can be PRE-RENAL, RENAL or POST-RENAL.** In terms of renal health, we are concerned primarily with renal proteinuria.
      1. **Pre-renal** proteinuria is when the glomerular capillary walls have normal permaselectivity (small molecules pass through, but larger ones like albumin remain in the blood), but the content of the plasma proteins is abnormal (e.g., presence of immunoglobulin light chains; a.k.a. Bence-Jones proteins). This results in more proteins being filtered than can be reabsorbed.
      2. **Renal** proteinuria occurs due to a structural or functional lesion within the kidney that allows more protein to diffuse into the ultrafiltrate than can be reabsorbed.
      3. **Post-renal** proteinuria is caused by the entry of protein into the urine after the urine enters the renal pelvis. This may be due to hemorrhage or inflammation of the ureter, bladder, or urethra.
   C. **IMPLICATIONS of RENAL PROTEINURIA**
      1. Regardless of the cause, persistent renal proteinuria—even low grade—is associated with bad outcomes. Dogs and cats with bad proteinuria develop renal disease more quickly and die sooner than others.
   D. **CONTROLLING RENAL PROTEINURIA:** In cases where the asymptomatic animal is proteinuric on serial UPCs performed every two weeks for three or more tests, treatment to control the protein is likely to be beneficial. Urine protein levels vary from day to day, but they must change by 30-50% to be sure the underlying magnitude has changed.

ACTION in NONAZOTEMIC DOGS & CATS	UPC RATIO
Monitor only	≥ 0.5
Look for underlying causes	≥ 1.0
Intervene	≥ 2.0

   1. **Start with ACE inhibitors** and then monitor the UPC one month later. If on enalapril and the UPC is not decreased by 50%, then increase the dose. The higher the UPC to start with, the better the effect of ace inhibitors.
      a. Benazepril 0.5 mg/kg PO SID-BID
      b. Enalapril 0.4 mg/kg PO SID-BID (starting dose)
   2. **Restricted protein diet:** Place animals on a diet of high quality, low quantity protein, such as a renal diet (in dogs). Remember that with cats, we may need to avoid changing quickly to an ultra-low protein diet because cats cannot adapt that quickly and will catabolize their muscles. Thus, we might switch initially to a senior diet.
   3. **Higher omega-3 diets** lead to lower proteinuria.

II. **GLOMERULONEPHROPATHY** is frequently classified as either glomerulonephritis (inflammation of the glomerulus) or amyloidosis (deposition of amyloid in the glomeruli). Glomerulonephritis can be caused by any chronic antigenic stimulation. Amyloidosis can be caused by neoplastic (e.g., multiple myelomas) or inflammatory processes, or it can be familial (Abyssinian cats and Chinese Shar-Pei dogs).

```
                SOME  CAUSES  of  GLOMERULONEPHRITIS
Infectious
  • Chronic bacterial infection (pyometra, endocarditis, foxtail
    granuloma, brucellosis, diskospondylitis, etc.)
  • Viral (canine adenovirus I, FeLV, FIP, FIV)
  • Ehrlichia/tick-borne disease
  • Parasitic (Dirofilaria immitis-especially occult infections)
Neoplastic
Immune-mediated
  • SLE
  • Pancreatic necrosis
  • Anti-glomerular basement membrane
```

A. CLINICAL SIGNS may be due to protein loss, renal failure, loss specifically of antithrombin III, and/or hypertension.
   1. Signs due to **albumin** loss include **ascites or edema** (when albumin is < 1-1.5 g/dL), weight loss (decreased muscle mass), and lethargy. These signs often occur in the absence of other signs of renal disease.
   2. If the nephrons are also damaged significantly, then we see signs of **renal failure** including PU/PD, vomiting, anorexia, weight loss, and lethargy.
   3. **Loss of antithrombin III** in the urine can lead to pulmonary thromboembolism (rare) and other hypercoagulation signs.
   4. **Hypertension** occurs in response to the decreased glomerular filtration rate and contributes to further glomerular membrane damage. It can lead to blindness or vision deficits due to retinal detachment and optic nerve degeneration.

B. DIAGNOSTIC FINDINGS: The combination of proteinuria, hypoalbuminemia, ascites or edema, and hypercholesterolemia is called **NEPHROTIC SYNDROME.** It strongly suggests glomerulonephropathy.
   1. **Urine protein:creatinine** (UPC) > 2.0 is high (< 1.0 is normal and 1-2 is in the grey zone). We usually see signs with a ratio > 4.0. UPC can be affected by diet, exercise, increased temperature, and UTI (increased protein). UTI can easily cause a ratio of > 6.0 and up to 14. Rule out UTI via examination of the urine sediment of bacteria, crystals, WBCs, casts, and a urine culture.
   2. **Chemistry panel**
       a. **Decreased albumin** (Total protein may be low, too.)
       b. **BUN, phosphorus, and creatinine** may be normal in early glomerulonephropathy until about 75% of the nephrons are nonfunctional.
       c. Total serum **calcium** is influenced by **albumin** levels.
       d. **Hypercholesterolemia:** The liver reacts to loss of proteins by making more of everything.
   3. A **CBC** helps rule out causes of glomerulonephropathy. For example, eosinophilia may indicate parasites.
   4. **FIV, FeLV, and heartworm test:** Animals with positive tests may have high globulin levels, and the globulin-antigen complexes may be deposited at the glomerular membranes.
   5. **Blood pressure:** Animals may become hypertensive in response to the decreased glomerular filtration rate.
   6. A **renal biopsy** helps determine whether the glomerulonephropathy is due to amyloid or immune complexes. Signs are usually more severe with amyloidosis.
   7. **Check for Bence-Jones proteins in the urine** to help rule out multiple myelomas.
   8. **Radiographs/bone scan:** Multiple myelomas may appear as multiple lytic lesions in the bone.

C. TREATMENT
   1. Eliminate the source of antigen (rare).
   2. Administer **immunosuppressive drugs** such as Leukeran® and Imuran®. Don't use prednisone unless the animal has SLE. Prednisone causes protein catabolism, which may exacerbate the proteinuria. It may also cause hypertension.
       a. **Cyclophosphamide** (Cytoxan®): 50 mg/m2 q 48 hours or in a cycle of SID PO for 3-4 days and then off for 3-4 days
       b. **Azathioprine** (Imuran®; use in dogs only): 50 mg/m2 PO SID or every other day
       c. **Cyclosporine** (dogs only): 15 mg/kg PO SID
   3. **Aspirin therapy** may be used to help prevent thrombosis due to decreased AT-III (3-10 mg/kg PO SID-BID in dogs and 25 mg/kg PO q 48 hours in cats).
   4. **Treat as for** proteinuria, hypertension, and renal failure where appropriate.

Urinary